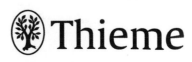

Audiology Treatment

Third Edition

Jason A. Galster, PhD, CCC-A, FAAA
Director of Clinical Research
Advanced Bionics LLC
Valencia, California

304 illustrations

Thieme
New York • Stuttgart • Delhi • Rio de Janeiro

Acquisitions Editor: Delia K. DeTurris
Managing Editor: Prakash Naorem
Director, Editorial Services: Mary Jo Casey
Production Editor: Shivika
International Production Director: Andreas Schabert
Editorial Director: Sue Hodgson
International Marketing Director: Fiona Henderson
International Sales Director: Louisa Turrell
Senior Vice President and Chief Operating
    Officer: Sarah Vanderbilt
President: Brian D. Scanlan

Library of Congress Cataloging-in-Publication Data
Names: Galster, Jason A., editor.
Title: Audiology treatment / [edited by] Jason A. Galster.
Description: Third edition. | New York : Thieme, [2018] | Preceded by
    Audiology / [edited by] Michael Valente, Holly Hosford-Dunn, Ross J.
    Roeser. 2nd ed. 2008. | Includes bibliographical references and index. |
    Identifiers: LCCN 2018018090 (print) | LCCN 2018018992 (ebook) |
    ISBN 9781626233294 | ISBN 9781626233287 (hbk.) |
    ISBN 9781626233294 (e-book)
Subjects: | MESH: Hearing Loss--therapy | Hearing Aids
Classification: LCC RF290 (ebook) | LCC RF290 (print) | NLM WV 270 | DDC
    617.8--dc23
LC record available at https://lccn.loc.gov/2018018090

© 2019 Thieme Medical Publishers, Inc.
Thieme Publishers New York
333 Seventh Avenue, New York, NY 10001 USA
+1 800 782 3488, customerservice@thieme.com

Thieme Publishers Stuttgart
Rüdigerstrasse 14, 70469 Stuttgart, Germany
+49 [0]711 8931 421, customerservice@thieme.de

Thieme Publishers Delhi
A-12, Second Floor, Sector-2, Noida-201301
Uttar Pradesh, India
+91 120 45 566 00, customerservice@thieme.in

Thieme Publishers Rio de Janeiro,
Thieme Publicações Ltda.
Edifício Rodolpho de Paoli, 25ª andar
Av. Nilo Peçanha, 50 – Sala 2508
Rio de Janeiro 20020-906, Brasil
+55 21 3172 2297

Cover design: Thieme Publishing Group
Cover image: Courtesy of Starkey Hearing Technologies

Typesetting by DiTech Process Solutions, India

Printed in India by Replika Press Pvt. Ltd.   5 4 3 2 1

ISBN 978-1-62623-328-7

Also available as an e-book:
eISBN 978-1-62623-329-4

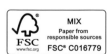

Contents

Preface

In recent years, the impacts of untreated hearing loss have become an increasingly larger part of public conversation around health and wellness. Evidence to suggest that untreated hearing loss may be a predictor of accelerated cognitive decline has emerged. We have also learned that untreated hearing loss may precipitate poorer academic performance, reduced quality of life, decreased social engagement, and increased fatigue. Although we cannot draw direct ties between the treatment of hearing loss and mitigation of these conditions, proactive management of hearing loss is associated with clear benefits to the individual with very few contraindications.

With this book, it is our goal to provide an introduction to fundamental practices and considerations associated with the audiologic treatment of hearing loss. The most common treatment for hearing loss is the provision of hearing aids. For this reason, the majority of this textbook focuses on modern concepts related to the treatment of hearing loss with hearing aids in populations that range from childhood to adulthood. Physical properties of hearing aids and verification (i.e., measurement) of acoustic performance are reviewed. Methods of audio signal processing to shape and filter sound in a manner that addresses the reduced audibility of speech are reviewed, followed by a detailed introduction to the prescription hearing aids.

Also included are chapters on the treatment of hearing loss through bone conduction devices, which have seen improvements through advancements in direct-drive technologies. Cochlear implants provide a surgical option for treatment that bypasses acoustic hearing by electrically stimulating the auditory system. In recent years, candidacy for cochlear implants has expanded to new patient populations as the quality and consistency of outcomes has improved.

These technologically oriented treatments for hearing loss are often complemented by the provision of assistive listening devices that make audible speech more accessible through direct transmission to a hearing device, whether it is a hearing aid, cochlear implant, or headset. The remaining chapters in this text address the assessment of patient needs and measurement of posttreatment outcomes, hearing protection devices, and management of tinnitus and hyperacusis.

I would like to acknowledge the authors who contributed their valuable time to this text and the staff at Thieme Medical Publishers for their support during the coordination and preparation of this material. Finally, I would like to thank the readers for their interest and invite suggestions for future editions of this text.

Jason A. Galster, PhD, CCC-A, FAAA

Contributors

Harvey B. Abrams, PhD
Courtesy Professor
Department of Communication Sciences and Disorders
University of South Florida
Tampa, Florida

Samuel R. Atcherson, PhD
Professor and Director of Audiology
Department of Audiology and Speech Pathology
University of Arkansas at Little Rock;
Adjunct Clinical Associate Professor
Department of Otolaryngology, Head and Neck Surgery
University of Arkansas for Medical Sciences
Little Rock, Arkansas

James R. Curran, MS
Consultant
Audiology Research
Starkey Hearing Technologies
Eden Prairie, Minnesota

Brian J. Fligor, ScD, PASC
Chief Development Officer
Lantos Technologies Inc.
Woburn, Massachusetts;
Adjunct Professor
GSO College of Audiology
Salus University
Elkins Park, Pennsylvania

Jason A. Galster, PhD, CCC-A, FAAA
Director of Clinical Research
Advanced Bionics LLC
Valencia, California

William Hodgetts, PhD
Associate Professor
Corbett Hall, University of Alberta;
Department of Communication Sciences and Disorders
University of Alberta;
Program Director, Bone Conduction Amplification
Institute for Reconstructive Sciences in Medicine (iRSM)
Edmonton, Alberta, Canada

Andrew J. Johnson, MSEE
Senior Electroacoustic Engineer
Starkey Hearing Technologies
Eden Prairie, Minnesota

Ryan W. McCreery, PhD
Director of Research
Central Research Administration
Boys Town National Research Hospital
Omaha, Nebraska

Erin M. Picou, AuD, PhD
Research Assistant Professor
Department of Hearing and Speech Sciences
Vanderbilt University Medical Center
Nashville, Tennessee

David A. Preves, PhD
Former Chair of ANSI-ASA
Working Group S3-48, Hearing Aids;
Former US TAG Chair of IEC TC29 Electroacoustics;
Former Technical Patent Manager
Starkey Hearing Technologies
Eden Prairie, Minnesota

John Pumford, AuD
Director of Audiology and Education
Audioscan
Dorchester, Ontario, Canada

Ayasakanta Rout, PhD
Associate Professor and Program Director of Audiology
Director, Hearing Aid Research Laboratory
Department of Communication Sciences and Disorders
James Madison University
Harrisonburg, Virginia

David Smriga, MA
Senior Audiology Consultant
Audioscan
Dorchester, Ontario, Canada

Christopher Spankovich, AuD, PhD, MPH
Associate Professor and Vice Chair of Research
Department of Otolaryngology and Communicative Sciences
University of Mississippi Medical Center
Jackson, Mississippi

Sarah A. Sydlowski, AuD, PhD
Audiology Director, Hearing Implant Program
Cleveland Clinic
Cleveland, Ohio

Dennis Van Vliet, AuD
Senior Clinical Educator
Bloom Hearing Specialist Network
Miami, Florida

1 Introduction: On the Treatment of Hearing Loss

Jason A. Galster

The World Health Organization (WHO) estimates that more than 5% of the global population, 360 million people, suffer from disabling hearing loss, making hearing loss one of our greatest societal disease burdens.[1] In the United States alone, nearly 75% of people aged 70 and older have high-frequency hearing loss of at least moderate severity.[2,3] Over the next three decades, it is expected that the number of individuals in the United States between the ages of 65 and 84 years will double, while those over the age of 85 years will triple.[4] Given the fact that the handicapping nature of hearing loss increases with severity, and severity of hearing loss increases with age, the demand for hearing care services is expected to increase precipitously. Estimates for this demand on hearing care are not available, however, the demand for physician services has been cited as increasing by 60% over the same period of time.[5]

The societal effects of hearing loss have caught the attention of government and professional organizations. In 2017, three reports, one from the WHO and two from the United States' National Academies of Sciences Engineering and Medicine (NAS) summarized *the costs of unaddressed hearing loss and cost-effectiveness of interventions*[6] and *hearing health care for adults, priorities for improving access and affordability*[7] and *the promise of assistive technology to enhance activity and work participation*.[8] The WHO's findings indicate that annually, the global cost of untreated hearing loss falls between $750 and $790 billion USD. This extreme financial burden attempts to capture three dimensions of cost: (1) direct cost: those incurred by health care and educational systems; (2) indirect cost: those incurred as a result of lost productivity or inability to contribute; and (3) intangible/societal costs: those motivated by stigma-induced behavior, withdrawal from social activity or grief.

Pearl

In a 2017 report, the WHO presented a compelling case for the treatment of hearing loss in their financial-minded analysis of the cost of unaddressed hearing loss.

1. The cost of unaddressed hearing loss is estimated at $750 to $790 billion USD, annually.
2. Unemployment and premature retirement, resulting from untreated hearing loss, cost $105 billion USD annually.
3. The annual cost of childhood hearing loss is estimated between 24 and 47 billion USD, with a dependency on a country's GDP and the inclusion of cochlear implantation.

These staggering statistics have motivated action on the part of the WHO. During the 17th World Health Assembly, a resolution was issued that will urge governments to do the following:

- Integrate strategies for hearing care within primary health care systems.
- Establish training programs for ear and hearing health.
- Improve access to affordable, cost-effective, high-quality, assistive hearing products.
- Ensure universal access to hearing loss prevention and hearing care.

The 2017 NAS consensus report *The Promise of Assistive Technology to Enhance Activity and Work Participation* was prepared with a scope that included and extended to treatment of disabilities beyond hearing loss. The committee preparing this report noted that assistive products and technologies may reduce handicapping effects and increase an individual's contribution to society. Nine barriers to treatment and benefit were identified in the report; five of which are included below, in the original language. Each of these conclusions present considerations that are addressed in this text book. For the reader new to hearing care and the treatment of hearing loss, these will read as insights that should be the prime interest in reading the chapters of this text book. The reader experienced in the treatment of hearing loss may be surprised that these statements, written in the context of treatment of many different disabilities, resonate strongly as value statements for the rehabilitative services provided by the audiologist.

1. Assistive products and technologies hold promise for partially or completely mitigating the impacts of impairments and enhancing work participation when appropriate products and technologies are available, when they are properly prescribed and fitted, when the user receives proper training in their use and appropriate follow-up, and when societal and environmental barriers are limited.

2. When matching individuals with appropriate assistive products and technologies, it is important to understand the complexity of factors that must be optimized to enhance function. Selecting, designing, or modifying the correct device for an individual and providing training in its use, as well as appropriate follow-up, are complex but necessary elements for maximizing function among users of assistive products and technologies.

3. Education regarding the availability of assistive products and technologies and knowledge and training that empower users to self-advocate or have a significant other (e.g., family member, friend, or professional) advocate for them are important elements in achieving successful access to appropriate assistive products and technologies and related services.

4. Professionals involved in disability determinations cannot assume that because an individual uses an assistive product or technology, this device is always effective for that person, that it mitigates the impact of the person's impairment, or that it enables the person to work. Environmental, societal, and individual factors must also be considered.

5. Additional research is needed to understand how the specifications for and use of assistive technologies and products and related services impact inclusion in society and work

participation for individuals with disabilities. Such research may not only enhance knowledge in these areas, but also inform the development of rational resource utilization, including informing cost/benefit analyses and coverage for devices and related services.

Narrowing the focus to treatment of hearing loss, two organizations work to aggregate data on the treatment of hearing loss with hearing aids. The first of these is the United States' Hearing Industries Association (HIA); membership of the HIA consists of corporations that provide products and services for the treatment of hearing loss. The HIA, in partnership with the Better Hearing Institute, developed a periodic MarkeTrak report that documents consumers' (i.e., patients') experience with hearing aids in the United States. The second and similar group, the European Hearing Instruments Manufacturers Association (EHIMA), sponsors ongoing market research to understand the impact of treating hearing loss throughout the European Union and other parts of the world, not including the United States. Both the HIA and EHIMA hold interest in increasing public awareness of hearing loss and ensuring high standards of hearing care. Similar to the MarkeTrak report, EHIMA sponsors a periodic EuroTrak report.

▶ **Fig. 1.1**[9] combines data from MarkeTrak and EuroTrak. Shown as yellow bars are estimates for the prevalence of self-reported hearing loss across EHIMA-tracked countries. Red bars show the proportion of a country's total population that suffer from hearing difficulty and the yellow bars show the proportion of people, with hearing difficulty who have pursued hearing aids (also described as hearing aid uptake). At 14.1%, Japan reports the lowest uptake of hearing aids with Norway, at 42.5%, reporting the highest. Of the countries assessed, the United States ranks third with uptake of 30.2%. The factors that contribute to hearing aid uptake are complex, including social and societal contributors, as well as the nature of a country's distribution channel, service providers, and health care policies.

When considering the uptake of hearing aids, it would be natural to assume that countries with state organized health care, providing free hearing aids, would have greater rates of hearing aid uptake. While countries with free market health care, in which patients pay for hearing aids, may have comparatively lower rates of hearing aid uptake. Based on data provided in 2016, it's clear that the United Kingdom (state organized health care) ranks higher at 41.1%, when compared to the United States at 30.2%.

Conclusions can be drawn across health care systems and countries. Firstly, patient outcomes and satisfaction are improving over time. This trend

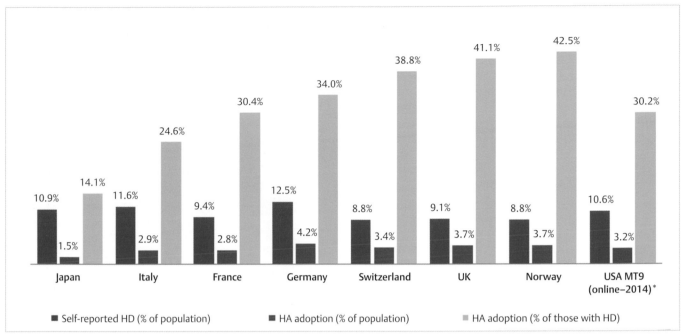

Fig. 1.1 Data from EuroTrak and MarkeTrak 9 reports are shown for countries around the world. Blue bars show estimated proportion of the population that self-reports hearing difficulty (HD). Red bars show estimated proportion of the population that reports hearing aid ownership. Yellow bars show estimated proportion of the population with hearing difficulty who have pursued hearing aids.

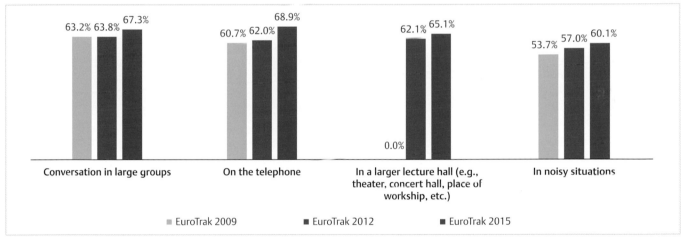

Fig. 1.2 Data from EuroTrak 2009, 2012, and 2015 are shown for four challenging listening conditions. Hearing aid wearers report a small but consistent improvement in satisfaction over time for all assessed conditions: large groups, telephone, lecture hall, and noisy situations.

is observed in both the MarkeTrak and EuroTrak, across a variety of questions intended to probe different domains of interest. ▶ **Fig. 1.2** shows data from EuroTrak 2009, 2012, and 2015, in which 4,133 hearing aid users rated their satisfaction when listening with hearing aids in large groups, telephone, lecture hall, and generally noisy situations. Small but consistent improvements are observed in each category over time. Because many hearing aid technologies are designed to positively affect listening in these and similar listening conditions, these findings stand as testimony for the forward advancement of technological solutions for treating hearing loss.

1.1 Best Practice in the Treatment of Hearing Loss

No single treatment plan will accommodate the needs of every patient, for this reason, the information presented here should be viewed as guidance and not a literal recipe to be explicitly followed. This is reflected in most best practice documentation that are presented as guidelines and written in a manner that arms the clinician with the information necessary to support evidence-based decision making. Two examples of guidance documents, provided by the American Academy of Audiology are named below. Both of these documents can be freely accessed at http://www.audiology.org

1. Guidelines for the Audiologic Management of Adult Hearing Impairment
2. American Academy of Audiology Clinical Practice Guidelines: Pediatric Amplification

This text book introduces the reader to fundamentals in the treatment of hearing loss, while describing the best practices that should be considered when structuring a rehabilitative treatment plan. A series of general components are common to most treatment plans. By minimally accommodating these components, a logical progression of care is assembled that can be applied to most of the treatment, whether it is hearing aids, cochlear implants, or a bone conduction solution. ▶ **Fig. 1.3** shows a series of thematic components that are common to most plans for the treatment of hearing loss.

Every treatment plan begins with the assessment of patient needs, which includes but is not limited to diagnosis of hearing loss and characterization of hearing ability, measurement of speech understanding ability, and collection of pretreatment subjective reports that describe a patient's perception of their own function or expectations from the treatment.

Next, in the case of technological treatment, verification and validation of that treatment is included. Verification describes a type of measurement that objectively documents the manner in which a treatment compensates for the diagnosed hearing loss; Chapters 7 and 8 provide a detailed information on the verification of hearing aids. Following verification, behavioral validation of effectiveness provides evidence that the treatment is beneficial and addresses activity limitations that may be of concern.

Post-treatment patient reports are the most common method of outcomes assessment. A clinician's choice of outcome measure is often discretionary and may be motivated by a multitude of factors that are discussed in Chapter 10.

Finally, the treatment plan should include elements of auditory rehabilitative care and/or therapy. Rehabilitative care often involves one-to-one or group counseling sessions, in which participants focus on the pragmatics of managing their hearing loss. It is also common practice to prescribe regimented auditory training, which often takes the

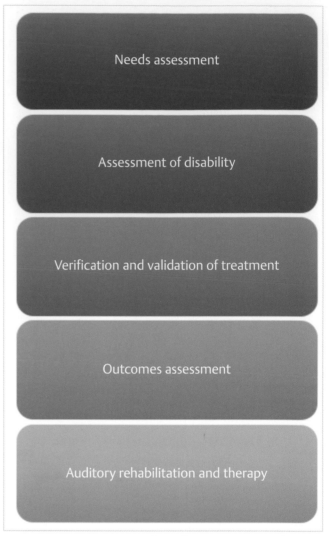

Fig. 1.3 Five steps, central to a best practice workflow in the treatment of hearing loss are shown. These provide a high-level framework, within which more detailed protocols and treatment strategies may be developed.

form of a game-like task of speech understanding in noise that patients complete in an effort to improve their listening ability.

These fundamental steps offer a clear framework around which an individualized treatment plan can be constructed. Options for that treatment are presented throughout this textbook, ranging from technological solutions (i.e., hearing aids or cochlear implants) to rehabilitative tools and strategies that facilitate the success of a technology-based treatment.

References

[1] World Health Organization. Prevention of blindness and deafness. http://www.who.int/pbd/deafness/en/. Accessed 25th June, 2017
[2] Lin FR, Thorpe R, Gordon-Salant S, Ferrucci L. Hearing loss prevalence and risk factors among older adults in

the United States. J Gerontol A Biol Sci Med Sci. 2011; 66(5):582–590

[3] Lin FR, Niparko JK, Ferrucci L. Hearing loss prevalence in the United States. Arch Intern Med. 2011; 171(20):1851–1852

[4] U.S. Department of Health and Human Services. Physician supply and demand: projections to 2020. https://bhw.hrsa.gov/sites/default/files/bhw/nchwa/projections/physician2020projections.pdf Accessed 25th June, 2017

[5] U.S. Department of Health and Human Services. The physician workforce: projections and research into current issues affecting supply and demand, 2008. https://bhw.hrsa.gov/sites/default/files/bhw/nchwa/projections/physiciansupplyissues.pdf Accessed 21st March, 2018

[6] World Health Organization. The costs of unaddressed hearing loss and cost-effectiveness of interventions. http://apps.who.int/iris/bitstream/10665/254659/1/9789241512046-eng.pdf?ua=1. Accessed 25th June, 2017

[7] National Academies of Sciences, Engineering, and Medicine. Hearing Health Care for Adults: Priorities for Improving Access and Affordability. Washington, DC: The National Academies Press; 2016

[8] National Academies of Sciences, Engineering, and Medicine. The Promise of Assistive Technology to Enhance Activity and Work Participation. Washington, DC: The National Academies Press; 2017

[9] Hougaard S. Hearing aids improve hearing and a lot more. Hearing Review 2016

2 Fundamentals of Hearing Aid Acoustics and Hardware

Andrew Johnson

2.1 The Advancement of Hearing Aid Technology

In the early days of hearing aid development, manufacturers were vertically integrated (i.e., they manufactured their own components used in building their instruments). In time, manufacturers became dependent on specialized suppliers to the industry to furnish these parts; Knowles Electronics and Sonion are examples of modern transducer suppliers. Competition between manufacturers and between suppliers eventually became the natural engine for significant improvement in function and form. Now, even the smallest hearing aid types incorporate many of the latest technological advances. Recent trends (in the last 10 years or so) reflect a market dominance of behind-the-ear (BTE) styles.[1] The BTE hearing aid can be subdivided into two categories: receiver in canal (RIC) and receiver in the hearing aid (RITA). Both will be discussed later in this chapter. The most popular hearing aid style has, in a way, come full circle, because BTE hearing aids were the predominate style in the 1960s and 1970s, giving way to a strong presence of the custom hearing aid market in the 1980s, 1990s, and for a few years after 2000. The custom hearing aid market comprises mainly of the following styles: in the ear (ITE), in the canal (ITC), and completely in the canal (CIC).

Hearing aid designers must somehow devise small, high-performance devices that are powered by low-voltage batteries having limited capacity (expressed as a milliamp-hour rating). Manufacturers continually strive to reduce the battery current used by hearing device components, while at the same time, increasing performance and available features. The conflicting requirements of packaging superior performance into a small size have encouraged manufacturers to design their own custom integrated circuits for wireless transceivers (radios) and signal-processing chipsets. Most leading hearing device manufacturers work closely with their suppliers to mutually develop novel transducers, radios for wireless communication, signal processors, and rechargeable battery solutions that are uniquely suited for hearing device applications.

2.2 Hearing Aid Styles

As new hearing aid styles are introduced to the marketplace, electroacoustic quality is usually not an issue because advances in transducers, circuitry, and assembly techniques have made electroacoustic performance much less of an issue than it was in previous decades.

Popularity trends in hearing aid styles have changed and continue to change with time, often being motivated by technological advancement. For example, body-style and eyeglass hearing aids were popular in the 1940s and 1950s, but are extremely rare today. A motivating contributor to the development and use of eyeglass hearing aids was the need to control whistling feedback that was common among analog hearing aids that did not offer feedback suppression—which requires digital signal processing (DSP) capability. A second example is modern high-power BTE hearing aids that have replaced the most powerful body aids. Current BTE hearing aids produce 2cc coupler gain as high as 80 dB and OSPL90 (output sound pressure level [SPL] with a 90 dB SPL input signal) values up to 145 dB SPL peak. These numbers together, known as the "matrix" of a hearing aid, are just two of several figures of merit that will be described in the following chapters.

Terminology: Hearing Aid Matrix

The amplification characteristics of a hearing aid are expressed as a "matrix." The matrix is a series of numeric values, separated by slashes, that signify the maximum output sound pressure, maximum amplification capabilities, and frequency response "slope." For example, 124/61/5 means that hearing aid can reach a 2cc coupler output sound pressure level of 124 dB SPL, a peak 2cc coupler gain of 61 dB, and the gain frequency response "slope" (difference in gain between low and high frequencies) of 5 dB. Today, the slope value is not included, as digital hearing aids allow for adjustment of the hearing aid response slope through the programming software.

The coupler section of chapter 10 explains how different couplers affect acoustic responses. This means the matrix numbers will change depending on the acoustic coupling (e.g., ANSI 2cc or on a real ear).

2.2.1 Behind the Ear

The BTE style of hearing aid is one of the oldest styles and remains the most popular form factor today. This is largely due to a combination of flexibility in use and durability. ▶ **Fig. 2.1** shows a typical BTE with several points of interest that are often explained to patients. Most BTE hearing aids will offer an electronic switch or push button that allows for manual control of the hearing aid settings. Actuation of the switch may increase or decrease the hearing aid amplification or change among predetermined settings call programs, each of which is tailored for listening in a different situation. The BTE battery compartment is almost universally located at the base of the hearing aid with a small indentation or protrusion that allows patients to easily open the battery door for

battery replacement. At the time of this publication, rechargeable hearing aids are becoming commonplace, some of which include a sealed battery compartment that is not accessible by the patient.

The BTE microphones are mounted at the top of the hearing aid, this aligns the microphones in a manner that provides unobstructed access to ambient sounds and aligns multiple microphones on a horizontal plane—a consideration that allows for beneficial acoustic signal processing that is discussed in Chapter 6. The BTE earmold is attached at the hearing aid ear hook, a piece of curved rigid plastic that passes over the top of a patient's ear. The ear hook connects the physical BTE housing to the replaceable tubing that couples to a patient's ear via a custom earmold or standard ear bud, see Chapter 4 for information on ear coupling methods.

The BTE hearing aid shown in ▶ **Fig. 2.1** is of the RITA configuration. This means that the hearing aid receiver (loudspeaker) is encased inside hearing aid. In contrast, a second BTE style referred to as RIC moves the receiver from the hearing aid case to the patient's ear canal. In professional conversation, audiologists seldom use the terms RITA and RIC; rather the RITA style is simply referred to as a BTE, while the counterpart style is referred to as a RIC. From this point forward, we will follow this vernacular, referring to the RITA style as BTE and RIC as such.

Terminology: BTEs Both RIC and RITA

BTE hearing aids sit behind the ear. However, there are two categories of BTEs: the traditional form factor may be referred to as RITA; a second, and more modern form factor, is designed with the hearing aid receiver (speaker) placed ITE canal. This second style is commonly referred to as RIC. This alternative naming works well for "standard" hearing aids (i.e., off the shelf with no customization), but custom hearing aids have receivers that are both in the aid and ITE.

The RITA style of BTE tends to be larger than their RIC counterparts because the receiver is in the case. BTEs may have multiple ear-level user controls such as volume wheels or up-down switches and multifunction buttons. BTEs are more likely to have external pins for direct audio input (DAI) or FM receiver attachments. Directional microphones and telecoils are standard on most BTE sizes, and the acoustic tubing is easily swappable between many choices. Advanced sensors are most often included in the BTE style. The BTE style is also most likely to include pediatric features, such as an LED indicator, because this style is considered to be the most kid-friendly. BTEs are available in the widest range of batteries, from the large 675 to the smallest 10 A.

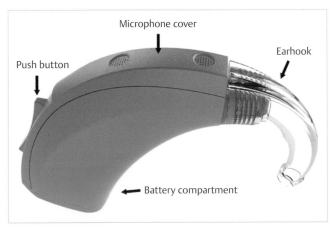

Microphone cover

Push button

Earhook

Battery compartment

Fig. 2.1 A behind-the-ear (BTE) hearing aid is shown. This is a receiver-in-the-ear (RITA) style of BTE.

2.2.2 Receiver in Canal

The RIC style of hearing aid rose to prominence quickly. Introduced in 2003, it accounted for two-thirds of all hearing aids sold in 2016.[1,2] Shown in ▶ **Fig. 2.2**, this style is a modification of the BTE, with the receiver moved out of the case and into the ear canal. Other than the receiver location, the RIC shares most of the same standard features and theory of operation with the BTE style. There are several advantages of the RIC over the traditional BTE style. First, the hearing aid case can be significantly smaller without the receiver inside. Secondly, the cable from the case into the ear canal can be extremely thin and discrete, as it needs to contain only two small-gauge electrical wires instead of a wider acoustic tube for sound.

The RIC receiver and cable are typically ordered as a combined single unit that is sized by the audiologist to fit a patient's ear. The RIC cable combination is detachable making them easily replaceable. A damaged receiver is easily replaced in the audiologist's office, because receivers are a common point of failure for many hearing aids; this reduces the number of hearing aids that are sent to the manufacturer for repair. Lastly, the RIC is well liked because it is considered an "instant fit." Patients can be fit at their first appointment and begin their field trial without waiting for custom earmolds to be ordered. The modularity of the RIC receiver also allows a single BTE unit to accommodate both high- and low-power receivers, accommodating a broad range of hearing losses.

Receiver cables are available in different lengths for various ear sizes. Flexible earbuds also come in various sizes and attach to the end of the receiver spout. The buds may be occluded or well vented to allow for an open fit. The RIC cable may also have a flexible strip of plastic that follows the curvature of the concha bowl, providing retention—this is casually referred to as a sport lock (▶ **Fig. 2.3**).

The RIC receiver may also be fit with a custom shell that is molded to the patient's ear geometry. The occluding nature of the custom earmold makes this application well suited for severe to profound hearing losses.[3]

2.2.3 Custom Hearing Aids

Introduced in the 1970s, the custom hearing aid places all components inside the patient's ear. The manner in which the custom hearing aid fills the ear dictates the naming convention. While there are countless variations on these naming conventions, three categories can be identified and are shown in ▶ **Fig. 2.4**. The first of these is the ITE hearing aid.

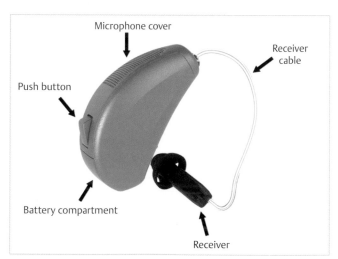

Fig. 2.2   A receiver-in-the canal (RIC) hearing aid is shown. This style of behind-the-ear hearing aid moves the receiver out from the case of the hearing aid into the ear canal of the patient.

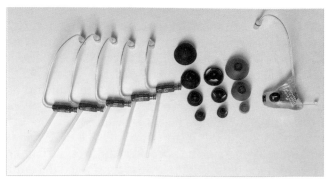

Fig. 2.3   Receiver-in-canal (RIC) stock and custom receiver cables with stock earbuds.

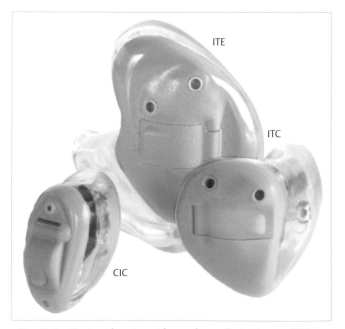

Fig. 2.4   Custom hearing aids are shown for in the ear (ITE) in the canal (ITC), and completely in the canal (CIC) form factors.

The ITE style fills the ear canal, concha bowl, and extends into the helix. This is the largest of the custom styles, offering the best retention and most room for placement of electrical components; it is also the most outwardly visible of the custom styles. The next smallest size is ITC. The ITC style fills the ear canal with a small portion that extends beyond the aperture of the ear canal without completely filling the concha bowl. The smallest size is CIC. The CIC custom hearing aid will fill the ear canal and extend only to the ear canal aperture. The CIC hearing aid is the smallest and least outwardly visible of the custom hearing aid styles. The small size of the CIC hearing aid makes them difficult to manufacture, as all components must be packaged in a small space. This size also limits the severity of hearing loss that can be treated with a CIC hearing aid as the proximity of the microphone, receiver, and internal components increases the likelihood of whistling feedback.

Early studies demonstrated that the custom ITE family of instruments provide some acoustic advantages over the other types of hearing instruments. Specifically, the position of the microphone in custom ITE hearing aids produces about 4 to 6 dB enhancement of the high frequencies compared with BTE aids with identical performance and components.[4,5]

When a hearing aid receiver is used in a custom ITE hearing aid instead of a BTE model, the tubing-related resonance normally found in the BTE hearing aid at approximately 1,000 Hz disappears because the receiver is now contained within the ear shell, close to its tip, and only a very short length of tubing is used.[6] The absence of the 1,000-Hz frequency response peak may allow the hearing aid volume control to be turned up higher without exceeding loudness discomfort levels for hearing aid wearers that have greater hearing loss in the higher frequencies than at the lower and middle frequencies.[7] Also, by moving the receiver closer to the tympanic membrane, as is the case for deep-fitting CIC hearing aids, there is a smaller residual volume, indicating less gain is required in the hearing aid itself to provide an appropriate frequency response for a given hearing loss, when compared with an equivalent BTE hearing aid fitting. This same advantage may exist for RIC hearing aids having deeply fitted custom earpieces.

Recall that the earmold tubing in a RITA BTE hearing aid acts as a long extension of the hearing aid's internal receiver, routing sound into the ear. It has long been a practice to smooth the BTE frequency response by inserting a damper in the BTE ear hook. If the damper has the appropriate acoustic impedance, it suppresses the 1,000-Hz peak in the BTE hearing aid frequency response, leaving only the higher-frequency peaks that are typical of custom hearing aids.[8] The disadvantage of using a damper to flatten frequency response peaks is that it frequently may become clogged with ear wax and other debris that is present in the ear canal.[9,10] In modern hearing aids, the necessity for physical dampening is lessened, as much of this fine tuning of the frequency response can be managed via DSP.[11]

2.2.4 Other Hearing Aid Styles

Today, the majority of hearing aids fall into the categories outlined above. There have been other styles in the past, such as eyeglass aids and body-worn hearing aids, but those have fallen out of use due to the smaller options available. However, new styles could emerge at any time. Hearing aid manufacturers have attempted some style modifications, such as in-the-helix and invisible-in-the-canal (IIC). If the styles of wireless earbuds for normal hearing consumers carry over, there may soon be more focus on standard (i.e., noncustom) in-the-ear hearing aid styles, which have been considered too large and ill-fitting today.

2.3 Hearing Aid Components

Hearing aids are made up of many components. A simplified block diagram lists them in ▶ Fig. 2.5. Sound enters the microphone and is converted to an electrical signal, this signal is amplified and enhanced before being converted back into sound in the ear by the receiver (speaker). The first hearing aids did this signal amplification and enhancement using analog microelectronics.

Every generation of hearing aid sees technological advances that introduce even more components, such as wireless radios and antennas, external audio inputs, sensors, or newly updated transducers. There are also several components that have been used for decades but continue to have usefulness, such as physical volume controls and buttons.[12]

Terminology: Transducer

A "transducer" is any device that converts a signal from one form of energy into another (e.g., acoustic pressure into electricity). In a hearing aid, the microphone, telecoil, and receiver are collectively referred to as transducers.

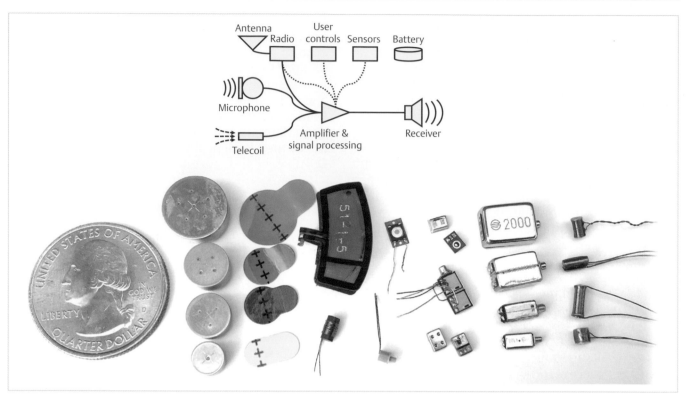

Fig. 2.5 Simplified block diagram of the components found in a hearing aid and various sizes and models of those hearing aid components with a U.S. quarter, for scale. From left to right: Zinc-air batteries with color-coded stickers, radio antennas, buttons, microphones, balanced-armature receivers, and telecoils.

2.3.1 A Note on Logarithms, Decibels, and Frequency Response Plots

In order to understand the performance of hearing aids and their component parts, we must understand how this information is perceived and displayed or plotted visually. Humans perceive sound logarithmically in frequency and amplitude. For example, we hear notes on a piano to be equal steps in frequency, but, in fact, the step size increases substantially with each note. When we determine one sound is twice as loud as another, it is closer to three times the SPL.

Frequency responses of hearing aids and hearing aid components are plotting logarithmically to match human perception. While a normal plot has linearly spaced points (e.g., 1, 2, 3), "log" plots have linearly spaced orders of magnitude (e.g., 1, 10, 100). For humans, the range of audible frequencies covers roughly three orders of magnitude (each called a decade), but the range of pressures is closer to eight. For this reason, the linear unit of pascal (audible from 0.00002 Pa to > 200 Pa) is converted to the logarithmic unit of dB SPL (with a more manageable range of 0–140 dB SPL) (▶Fig. 2.6).

Any graph can be skewed and zoomed to expose or hide important details, but there are standards and conventions for plotting the acoustic frequency response of a hearing aid:

- The frequencies should span at least 100 to 10,000 Hz and at most 10 to 100,000 Hz.
- Every decade (factor of 10) on the frequency axis should be the same length as 50 dB on the vertical axis. This allows for intuition of slopes of lines and severity of bumps and dips.

How do logarithms and decibels actually work? In early telephony, engineers needed an easier way to compare these very large and very small numbers. They invented the Bel (named after Alexander Graham Bell, inventor of the telephone), so that every 1 Bel represented a 10-fold increase in power. Now the decibel (one-tenth of a Bel) is more popular; every 10 decibels represents 10x power. This concept is now used in many disciplines beyond audio, such as radio frequency power levels for wireless transmission.

2.3.2 Microphones

A microphone is a transducer that converts sound (i.e., an acoustic signal) into some other usable signal type (e.g., electrical, digital, etc.). There are many ways to construct a microphone, but the most common type of microphone is called a condenser microphone. Most hearing aids use one or two miniature microphones of the condenser type or a condenser subcategory

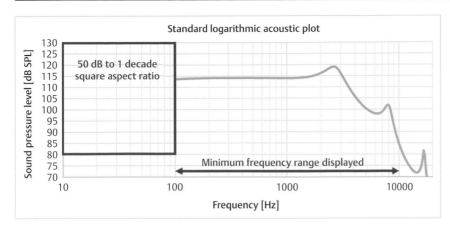

Fig. 2.6 A standard acoustic plot with logarithmic frequency axis and vertical axis with units of decibel. The ANSI-recommended aspect ratio is shown (50 dB per decade).

called "electret." All condenser microphones (also called "capacitor" or "electrostatic" microphones) use the same principle to convert sound to electricity. They have a thin foil diaphragm stretched tightly over a charged backplate. As sound pushes and pulls the diaphragm closer and farther from the backplate, electrons move on and off the diaphragm. This movement of electrons is an electric signal that matches the acoustic sound signal (▶ Fig. 2.7).

The introduction of microelectronic mechanical system (MEMS) technology hearing aids provided opportunities for reliability improvements. The manufacturing methods allow hundreds of MEMS microphones to be fabricated at one time, resulting in tightly matched performance. They are built using a chemical process that involves high temperatures that inherently require the microphones to be robust. Rather than the taut diaphragm found in electret microphones, MEMS microphones use rigid silicon diaphragms that improve

resilience against moisture, temperature, and foreign material such as dust and cerumen.[13]

Microphone Sensitivity Response

Different microphones can produce more or less output signal amplitude for the same input SPL. The term for how much output results from a particular input sound pressure is "sensitivity."

▶ Fig. 2.8 shows a typical free-field omnidirectional microphone frequency response. Note that the sensitivity of a microphone is not the same at all frequencies. There will always be a resonance frequency where the sensitivity gets a boost, and the sensitivity drops off at very high and very low frequencies. Hearing aid developers will made subtle modifications to the microphone hardware in order to place the peak of the frequency response at a desirable frequency.

Terminology: Electret

The backplate of a condenser microphone gets its charge from a power supply (e.g., a battery). Electret microphones simplify the design by using a permanently charged backplate. The name "electret" means "permanently charged" just like "magnet" means "permanently magnetic."

Terminology: Free-field

When discussing microphone responses, the environment near the microphone matters. The term "free-field" means the microphone is in a large empty space with no echoes or objects nearby to affect the sound. This is usually contrasted with "on-head" responses. This microphone location effect is discussed later.

Terminology: MEMS

"MEMS" is an acronym for microelectronic mechanical system. This usually refers to devices that are "grown" out of semiconductor materials instead of assembled by hand or machine. A MEMS microphone, therefore, can use any microphone operating principle. Most MEMS microphones are condenser type rather than electret, because the high heat MEMS microphones can be exposed to would discharge the electret backplate.

Terminology: Linear

When a system is "linear," a change to the input causes a corresponding change to output that can be predicted using a simple multiplier (e.g., "100x" or "+20 dB"). For nonlinear systems, the output to input relationship (i.e., the "gain") is more complicated than this single number. For example, systems with compression are nonlinear, and the output depends on the base gain, the input level, the compression knee point, and the compression level.

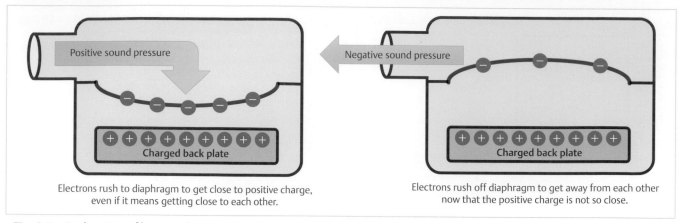

Electrons rush to diaphragm to get close to positive charge, even if it means getting close to each other.

Electrons rush off diaphragm to get away from each other now that the positive charge is not so close.

Fig. 2.7 Explanation of how an electret microphone converts alternating pressure (sound) into alternating current (electricity).

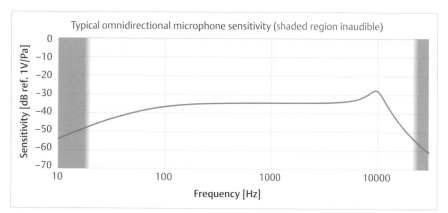

Fig. 2.8 Omnidirectional microphone sensitivity is shown as a function of frequency.

Microphone Limitations

Real microphones have limitations. They can be damaged by intensely loud sounds; the nature of the microphone's diaphragm results in constant miniscule movement that creates random low-level noise referred to as "self-noise."[14] The range between the loudest and quietest acoustic inputs that a microphone can convert to a usable signal is called its "dynamic range."

Every microphone produces self-noise. This can come from the diaphragm or from the built-in electrical amplifier. Either way, it is a constant low-level hissing noise that is always present and usually audible.[15,16] In most listening environments, the sound of interest is louder that the microphone self-noise. This noise, when displayed as a SPL, is referred to as equivalent input noise (EIN). Just like the microphone sensitivity, EIN is different across the frequency range. Unlike sensitivity, which is usually measured with a pure tone sweep, EIN is typically displayed in one-tenth-decade bins. The EIN may also be summarized as a single A-weighted number; in this case, typical microphone EIN will approximate 30 dBA (▶**Fig. 2.9**).

At very high levels, the microphone ceases to be linear near its acoustic overload level (AOL). Not all microphone manufacturers agree on the method of measurement; a common reference will be the

Pearl: EIN is Not Affected by Gain ✔

EIN, as mentioned already, is like an imaginary noise source outside of the hearing aid. The hearing aid output noise is the EIN amplified by the gain at each frequency. EIN is not affected by gain, but output noise is affected by gain. The only way to reduce both is with low-level expansion, noise suppression algorithms, or improving the design of the microphone for lower noise.

level at which a 1-kHz sinusoidal stimulus produces microphone output with 3 to 10% or higher total harmonic distortion (THD). A typical microphone AOL is 120 dB SPL for the referenced tonal input. Speech and music, with comparatively high peak-to-average ratios (a.k.a. "crest factors," may start distorting the system at lower levels, between 100 and 110 dB SPL.[17]

Microphone Directionality

Most microphones are meant to be omnidirectional. This means they pick up sound equally well from all directions and need not be aimed at a sound source. There are times, however, when it is beneficial to have some directionality. Directional microphones will

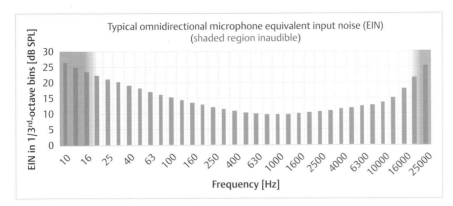

Terminology: Pink and White Noise

The spectral (frequency) shape of some noise can be referred to by different colors. White noise has equal energy at all frequencies and sounds like a light rainfall. Pink noise has a low-frequency emphasis and sounds like heavy rain. Red noise has even less high frequency and sounds like a roaring waterfall. Human speech most closely resembles the spectral shape of pink noise, and pink noise is more perceptually "flat" to human ears. Other random noise types are referred to as "colored noise."

This terminology comes from visible light. Humans can see colors corresponding to frequencies of electromagnetic waves. Frequencies below red (400,000,000,000,000 Hz) are called infrared, while frequencies above violet (789,000,000,000,000 Hz) are called ultraviolet. For sound, this corresponds to infrasonic and ultrasonic frequencies. Between these frequencies, we have all the colors of the rainbow. Combining equal energy at each color frequency creates white light, while a low-frequency emphasis tinges the light pink to red.

amplify sound arriving from a specific direction while attenuating sound from other directions; to state this differently, a patient wearing hearing aids with directional microphones will have better audibility for sound arriving from the front, when compared to sound arriving from the side or behind the same listener.

Polar Patterns and Directivity Index

The amount of attenuation at different angles can be viewed as a polar pattern. A polar pattern shows the relative sensitivity of a microphone viewed from above. Straight ahead is pointing up at 0 degrees; to the left and right are +/− 90 degrees; 180 degrees is directly behind the microphone array or listener. An omnidirectional microphone has a circular polar pattern; no particular angle is less sensitive than any other angle. Directional microphones, however, can have many different polar patterns that show

attenuation at one or more angles. The deepest angles of attenuation are called the null angles.

Pitfall: Free-Field Polar Patterns are Not Realistic

The polar patterns shown in this section are free-field polar patterns, meaning they are measured in a sound field that is free of obstructions (e.g., a human head and torso). That is good for understanding, but the end-wearer will have a degraded polar pattern (▶Fig. 2.10). Additionally, the free-field polar pattern cannot be measured without a large anechoic chamber.[18] With a small sound box, the best approximation is to imagine a straight line through the microphone ports of the hearing aid into the sound box speaker and leave the sound box open to avoid reflections.[19]

The amount of noise field attenuation provided by different polar patterns is reported as directivity index (DI).[20,21] A microphone's or microphone array's DI is a measure of how directional a microphone. Behaviorally, the DI can be interpreted as an effective improvement in signal to noise ratio. The more the directional microphone attenuates sound at angles other than 0 degrees, the higher the DI is. Microphone DI is measured in decibels as the ratio of microphone output for a given input that arrives from directly in front of the microphone to an acoustic input that arrives equally from all directions around the microphone—referred to as a diffuse sound source. By definition, omnidirectional microphone has a DI of 0 dB; it has the same output whether the input is concentrated at one angle or spreads to all angles. Directional microphones with just two sound inlets can have a DI of up to 6 dB.[22] Higher DI can be achieved with more complex directional designs (e.g., more sound inlets or microphones). This is uncommon in single hearing aids but can be achieved with a pair of hearing aids that are wirelessly connected (see binaural beamforming in Chapter 6).

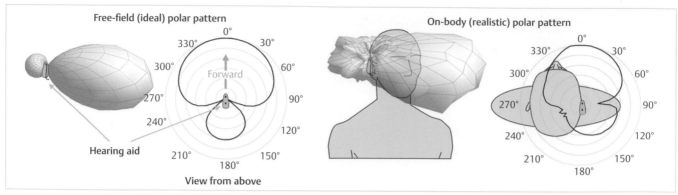

Fig. 2.10 The ideal hearing aid directional polar pattern (shown to the left in both isomorphic and overhead views) is degraded when the hearing aid is placed on a head (shown to the right in both isomorphic and overhead views).

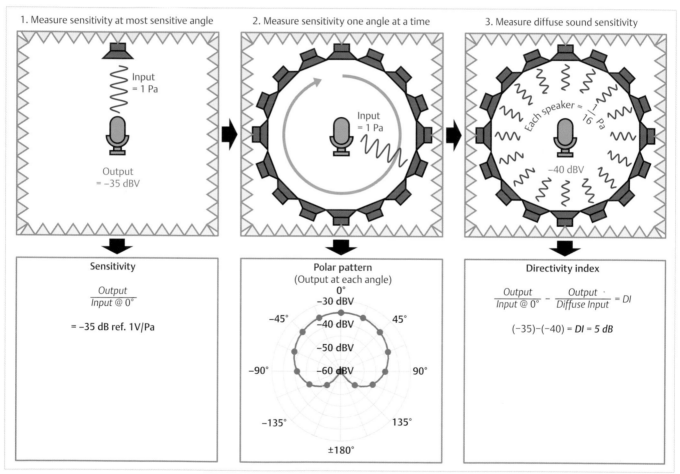

Fig. 2.11 Explanation of microphone sensitivity, polar pattern, and directivity index. The sensitivity is measured from a direct sound from the "front" of the microphone. The polar pattern compares the microphone sensitivity at all other angles to the "front" sensitivity one angle at a time. The directivity index measures the reduction in microphone sensitivity when the sound comes from all directions at once versus just from the front.

In the example shown in ▶ **Fig. 2.11** a directional microphone with a cardioid polar pattern is placed in an anechoic chamber. The sensitivity of the microphone is the ratio of output to input when the input comes from straight ahead. The polar pattern is measured by moving the input to different angles around the microphone, one at a time, and measuring the output at each angle. The DI is measured by spreading the input to all angles simultaneously to see how much the microphone's polar pattern reduces the output (▶ **Fig. 2.11**).

▶ **Fig. 2.12** shows common polar patterns and their corresponding directivity indices. Most single hearing aids are capable of forming polar patterns

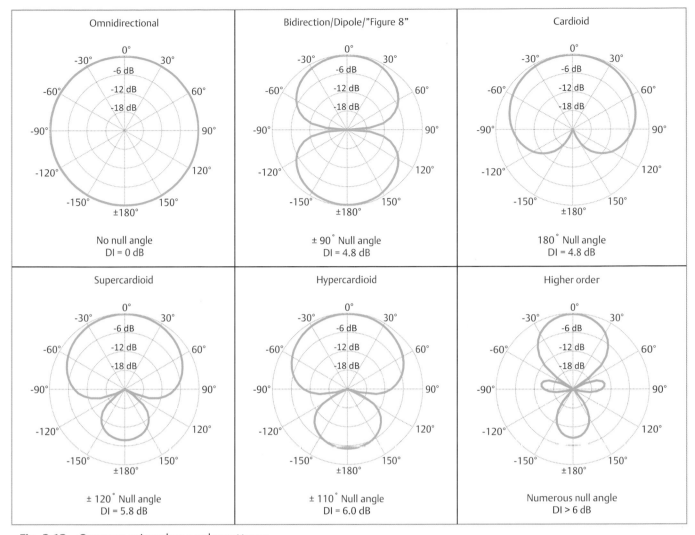

Fig. 2.12 Common microphone polar patterns.

with just one or two lobes. The polar pattern may be fixed with the null angle set by the hardware design, or the null angle may adjust using adaptive digital algorithms in an attempt to best reduce unwanted noise behind the wearer.

An important note is polar patterns and DIs are not the same at all frequencies. For hearing aids, speech frequencies are the most important for maximizing DI. Because of this, there are several conventions for weighting DI over frequency in a manner that is biased toward speech frequencies.

- SII-DI: The speech intelligibility index DI.[23] This weighted average is a current means for accurately representing how increasing directivity may improve speech understanding ability.[24]
- AI-DI: The articulation index DI.[25,26] This weighted average precedes the SII-DI, weighting speech importance across frequency. This deprecated weighting method

is a simple but less accurate form of predicting speech understanding changes.[24]

- Unweighted: The DI average over frequency may be unweighted, meaning every frequency has equal importance.[21,27] In this case, the microphone performance is well represented, but the contribution of increased DI may not clearly translate to improved speech recognition.

Dual Omnidirectional Microphone Arrays

A directional response can be achieved by combining the signals of two omnidirectional microphones in a certain way. When a small delay (several microseconds) is applied to the near microphone, sounds arriving from behind first arrive at the rear microphone and, several microseconds later, the front microphone. This delay aligns the two microphone signals, which when added together will reduce the level of sounds arriving from behind the listener. In the case of adaptive directional microphones, adjusting this delay will result in

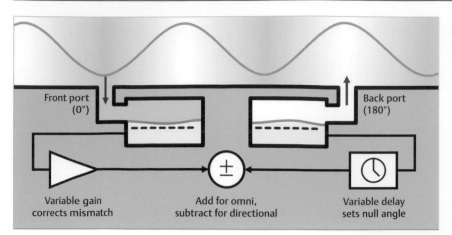

Fig. 2.13   In dual omnidirectional systems, the two signals are combined with variable digital delay and gain to dynamically adjust the directional characteristics.

null steering or a shift in the position of the level reducing directional null (▶**Fig. 2.13**).

One disadvantage of the dual omnidirectional microphone array is the requirement for well-matched omnidirectional microphones. If the microphones differ in sensitivity by more than 1 dB, the resulting directivity will greatly decrease. Even if the microphones are matched to begin with, they can experience shifts in sensitivity over time. This process is called "drift," and can be caused by temperature, moisture, and cerumen.[28] Audiologists should ensure that hearing aid microphone covers are free of debris by cleaning or replacing the microphone covers and verifying directional microphone performance in a test box or through a real-ear measurement.

2.3.3 Induction Coils

An induction coil, also called a "telecoil," is a coil of very fine copper wire wrapped thousands of times around a metal rod. Telecoils use electromagnetic induction to convert magnetic audio signals into electrical signals to be processed as if it were a microphone signal. Magnetic audio signals are generated as a side effect by telephone handsets and induction loops installed in public spaces for the purpose of assistive listening. Amplifying the magnetic audio signal through a telecoil instead of the acoustic audio signal through the microphone provides the advantage of a direct audio signal without contribution from ambient noise.[29]

Telecoils were introduced half a century ago, and their use cases have expanded in that time to include "loop systems."[30] A loop system is a large loop of wire used to transmit magnetic audio signals to telecoils. This loop can be worn around a person's neck or even installed around the perimeter of theaters, taxis, churches, and classrooms. The inductive loop fills a venue with a magnetic signal available that is

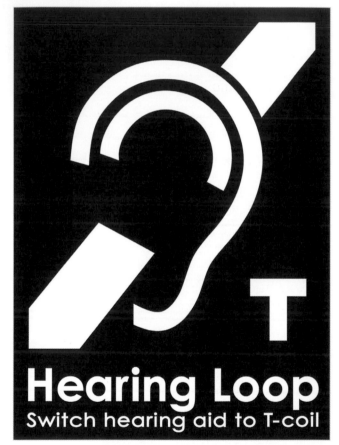

Fig. 2.14   The international standard sign to signify compatibility with hearing aids equipped with an induction coil.

accessible to everyone with a telecoil. Facilities with loops installed often post this international symbol for awareness (▶**Fig. 2.14**).

Induction Coil Operating Principles

An electric current flowing through a loop of wire creates a magnetic field pointing through the center of the loop. Induction coils take advantage of the fact that this principle is symmetric, meaning it works both ways. A magnetic field through a loop of wire induces an electric current through the wire. This means an electric signal can be transmitted wirelessly from one coil of wire to another by converting to a magnetic signal and back again (▶Fig. 2.15).

In a traditional speaker, the coil's alternating magnetic field pushes and pulls the magnet, causing the coil and the cone to move and produce sound. A side effect of this is the speaker coil is radiating a magnetic signal that matches the electrical audio signal intended to produce sound. For decades, every telephone handset had a speaker (receiver) that generated this strong magnetic audio signal. Telecoils take advantage of this fact in order to transmit a clean and isolated signal through magnetic induction instead of relying on the acoustic signal from the phone.

The loop system takes this operating principle one step further. By placing a loop of wire around your neck, around your couch, or even around a

large auditorium and applying an electrical audio signal as if you would to a loudspeaker is enough to provide the magnetic signal needed for induction coil use. Induction coils use many windings to amplify the electrical current for a given magnetic field strength, while loop systems usually just have one "winding." The loop systems having more power available can apply higher electrical currents than the telephone handset, resulting in stronger magnetic fields.

Telecoil Angle

Telecoils are highly directional and will only interact with magnetic fields when the orientation of the coil and the magnetic field is aligned. As an example, ▶Fig. 2.16 and ▶Fig. 2.17 show how the magnetic field of a telephone handset propagates differently from the loop installed in a room. The best

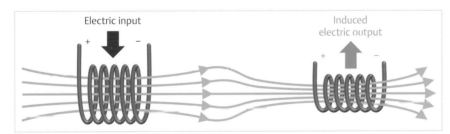

Fig. 2.15 Electromagnetic coupling between induction coils is shown. Note that the signal propagation (shown in blue) travels through the center of the loop.

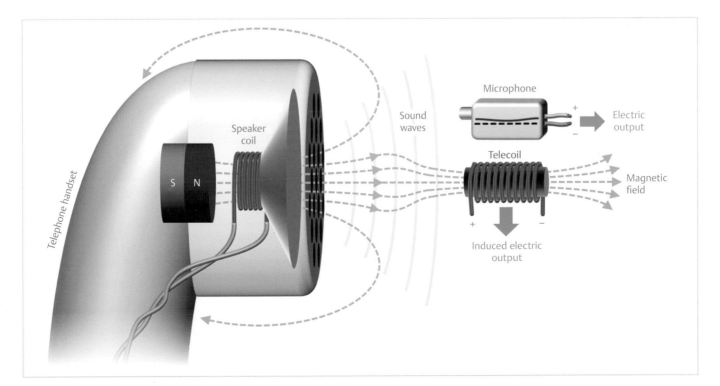

Fig. 2.16 A traditional telephone handset outputs both an acoustic and magnetic audio signal. Both transmit audio from these input sources.

orientation of the telecoil for telephone performance is horizontal in the hearing aid, and the best orientation for loop compatibility is a telecoil pointing up and down in the device. However, the vertical orientation is the preferred compromise, as shown in ▶ Fig. 2.18.[31]

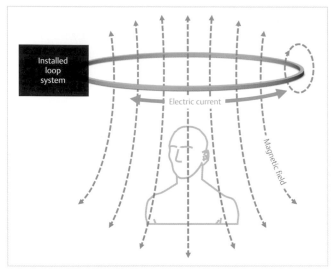

Fig. 2.17 Magnetic loop systems may be large or small. Loops installed into a structure tend to be large, while personal neck-worn loops work only for the wearer.

Telecoil Metrics

▶ **Table 2.1** describes performance metrics defined by ANSI S3.22, which breaks down in the following way.

The absolute measurements (HFA-SPLIV and HFA-SPLITS) are simple measurements that do not require testing in microphone mode. However, that also reduces their usefulness. Every hearing aid can have a different gain that affects these measurements and makes them hard to compare model to model. The tests relative to microphone mode, RTLS and RSETS, are comparable, because the telecoil and microphone gain increase and decrease together to maintain matching. Perfect matching between microphone and telecoil modes is "0 dB." A positive or negative RTLS indicates a telecoil that is too strong or too weak within a loop system, respectively. A positive or negative RSETS means the telecoil is too strong or too weak with a telephone, respectively.[32]

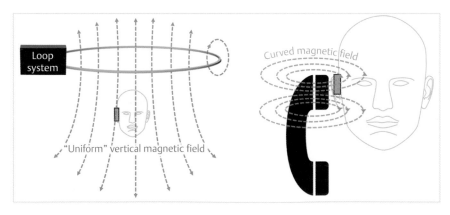

Fig. 2.18 A vertical telecoil takes advantage of the tighter curve of the telephone magnetic field to support loop system and telephone magnetic signals.

Table 2.1 Telecoil performance metrics

Spec/measurement	Hearing aid vertical in uniform vertical field (e.g., large loop)	Hearing aid horizontal in locally curving field (e.g., phone simulator/small loop)
Absolute output in coupler	HFA-SPLIV (high-frequency average sound pressure level in vertical field)	HFA-SPLITS (high-frequency average sound pressure level for an inductive telephone simulator)
Output relative to microphone mode (Want these to be 0 dB)	RTLS (Relative test loop sensitivity)	RSETS (Relative simulated equivalent telephone sensitivity)

Previous versions of the ANSI standard had other names for these metrics. RSETS used to be called simulated telephone sensitivity (STS), and RTLS used to be called test loop sensitivity (TLS).

Pearl: Calculate RSETS and RTLS From Spec Sheet ✔

Not all hearing aid specifications include RSETS and RTLS. However, these metrics of matching can be calculated from the HFA-SPLITS and HFA-SPLIV, if provided.

RSETS = HFA-SPLITS − (RTG + 60)
RTLS = HFA-SPLIV − (RTG + 60)

2.3.4 Hearing Aid Receivers

For decades, hearing aids have used balanced armature receivers. They are called receivers, instead of speakers, to match telephone terminology; the microphone was a transmitter, and the part you put to your ear was a receiver. There are many ways to make a speaker, but the balanced armature design has historically been the smallest and most efficient type of speaker.[33,34]

Balanced armature receivers work similarly to traditional speakers, contrasted in ▶Fig. 2.19. There is a coil of wire, magnet, and a diaphragm, but they are rearranged to fix best in a small box. Instead of moving the entire coil of wire, which can be inefficient, a flexible strip of metal (called an armature) is balanced between two magnets like a diving board. As sound, in the form of electrical current, flows through the coil, the armature is magnetized and pulled toward one magnet or the other. The armature is connected to the diaphragm that drives sound out of the receiver like bellows.

Receiver Sensitivity Response

The receiver has a sensitivity response just like the microphone. Instead of converting sound into electricity, receivers convert electricity back into sound. An example sensitivity is 20 dB relative to Pa/V at 1 kHz. This example means that a 1 V 1 kHz input produces 20 dB higher than 1 pascal (e.g., 1 V in produces 114 dB SPL out). However, the receiver sensitivity response is dependent on the acoustic load. This acoustic load includes tubing and cavities through which the receiver must move air.

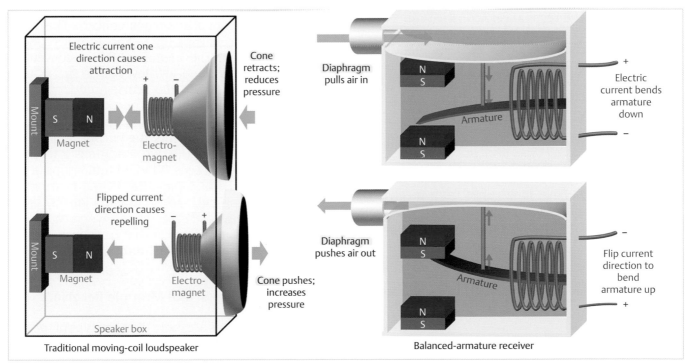

Fig. 2.19 Comparison of the operating principles of a traditional moving-coil loudspeaker (used in the vast majority of speakers, phones, headphones, and earphones) and balanced-armature receivers (used in the vast majority of hearing aids and professional earbuds).

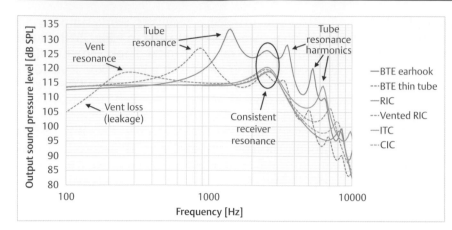

Fig. 2.20 Examples of acoustic output for various tube sizes. All responses shown have the same receiver and coupler; the only difference is the tubing length and diameter. In general, long/skinny tubes move the primary peak to a lower frequency and reduce high-frequency output. Vents introduce a low-frequency resonance and reduce low-frequency output.

Tubing and Resonance Effects

In hearing aids, the receiver moves air in and out of the ear canal through a tube. This system closely matches a classic Helmholtz resonator; you've heard such a resonator when blowing over the top of an empty bottle. For the bottle, the resonant frequency (i.e., the note you hear when blowing over the opening) is mostly determined by three factors[35]:

The longer the neck, bigger the bottle, or skinnier the neck, the lower the resonant note. The same is true for hearing aids. The longer and skinnier the tube, the lower the resonance. Acoustic tubing resonances bring along additional resonances at every harmonic frequency (2x, 3x, 4x, etc.). For many hearing aids, the second harmonic is so high in frequency that it can be ignored. However, if the primary tubing resonance is low in frequency, there may be half a dozen audible tubing resonances, as shown in ▶ **Fig. 2.20**.

RIC and custom hearing aids have the shortest tubes between the receiver and ear canal, so the receiver's natural resonance is not much affected. BTE hearing aids have long tubes from receiver to ear canal that affect the resonance frequency the most. The use of a thin tube further exacerbates this effect.

$$Resonant\ Frequency \propto \frac{Bottle\ Neck\ Diameter}{\sqrt{Bottle\ Volume \times Bottle\ Neck\ Length}}$$

Pearl: Resonance Efficiency Provides "Free" Output ✔

The boost in acoustic output due to a resonance is a passive increase in efficiency, meaning it takes no extra power. BTEs can take advantage of this to achieve higher output with the same receiver and same battery life by having a longer tube.

Pitfall: Tube Length Variability Affects Response ✖

As this section points out, changes to tube length greatly affect the acoustic output at each frequency. BTE hearing aids, therefore, may not have the response that the manufacturer intended once the tube is trimmed for each unique wearer.

Receiver Limitations

Receivers do produce some random noise, but it is low in level and not of audiologic concern. The dominant noise sources in hearing aids are the microphone and preamplifier. The digital to analog conversion stage contributes some low-level noise that is usually only audible when the hearing aid is muted.[36] At the upper limits of their acoustic output, receivers are measured by their maximum possible output (MPO). MPO represents the output limit of the receiver before one of the two conditions is reached. Either distortion exceeds standard limitations or the maximum electrical capabilities of the hearing aid signal processing and battery combination have been reached. In the second case, the receiver is capable of producing louder outputs at that frequency, but the rest of the hearing aid is the limiting factor.

Woofers, Tweeters, and Multiple Receivers

Most audio systems use more than one type of speaker to reproduce sound. The speaker system in a car, for example, might have woofers for low-frequency sound and tweeters for the highest frequencies. The reason for this frequency isolation is to avoid the distortion that can happen when one speaker tries to reproduce all frequencies. The woofer, for instance, has to move so much air that the subtle vibrations needed for high frequencies might be lost.[37]

Most hearing aids have single receiver to reproduce sound, a selection that is largely dictated by the size of the transducers. Dual receivers are used in hearing aids. A dual receiver uses two of the same type of receiver, doubling the acoustic output pressure (+6 dB), but it is also doubling the size. This could also be achieved by increasing the size of a single receiver. However, a key benefit of dual receiver applications is reduced vibration when operating at high output levels. The two oscillating armatures work to cancel vibration inside the hearing aid that may lead to mechanical sources of feedback.[38]

2.3.5 Batteries

Hearing aids are powered by small batteries the size of an aspirin. There are several different types of batteries that are used in modern hearing aids. Each has a unique set of advantages and disadvantages, balancing battery life, size, and rechargeability. For each type, there may also be many sizes available. The next few sections discuss a couple of common battery types.

Zinc-air

The most common type of hearing aid battery for many decades is the zinc-air cell. This battery "chemistry" (i.e., battery type) is the most energy dense battery available.[39] It means that for its size, no other battery chemistry will last as long. Zinc-air batteries have one to five small air holes on the cathode side (positive terminal) to let air in slowly. This exchange of air is necessary in order for a chemical reaction to generate a voltage. If these holes are plugged by water or the stickers they are shipped with, the zinc will not oxidize and no voltage is generated. Conversely, while the holes are open, the battery is discharging whether it is being used or not (▶ Fig. 2.21).

This chemistry produces a voltage around 1.3 V, but the voltage may start at 1.5 V when fresh and droop to below 0.8 V when nearly depleted. This battery type can also appear to die very quickly when exposed to large power surges (e.g., wireless activity or high

acoustic outputs), high heat, or plugged air holes. A typical size 13 zinc-air battery has about 380 mWh. Zinc-air batteries are not rechargeable and come in five standard sizes for hearing aids; each is referred to by model number and color, as shown in ▶ Table 2.2.

Terminology: Milliwatt Hours

The milliwatt hour (mWh) is a measure of how much energy a battery has stored (i.e., it can produce this many milliwatts of power for 1 hour, or 1 mW for these many hours). Some batteries have a specified capacity in milliamp hours (mAh), but not all batteries have the same voltage, so mAh values may not be comparable between battery chemistries.

Silver-oxide

Silver-oxide batteries appear similar to zinc-air batteries (same size and shape), but they lack the holes for gas exchange. This chemistry produces a voltage closer to 1.4 V and can handle large current surges more effectively than a zinc-air battery. However, the silver-oxide battery will not last as long as a zinc-air battery under continuous use (a size 13 silver-oxide battery has ~ 300 mWh capacity). Silver-oxide batteries are not rechargeable and not commonly recommended for use in modern hearing aids due to higher cost and lower capacity.[40]

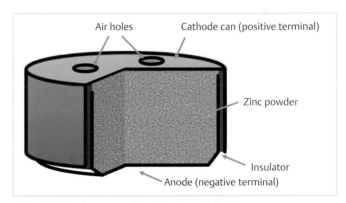

Fig. 2.21 Cross-section of a zinc-air battery.

Table 2.2 Standard hearing aid battery sizes with color codes and typical usage

Battery name	Conventional sticker/ package color	Size (mm)	Common uses
675	Blue	11.6 × 5.4	Power BTEs for profound hearing loss.
13	Orange	7.9 × 5.4	Most common size. All types of hearing aid.
312	Brown	7.9 × 3.6	Second most common size. All types of hearing aids.
10	Yellow	5.8 × 3.6	Smallest custom aids and some small standard aids.
5	Red	5.8 × 2.1	Seldom used.

Silver-zinc

The name "silver-zinc" makes this sound like a combination of zinc-air and silver-oxide battery chemistries, but it is different from both. This battery type is rechargeable and produces an operating voltage around 1.9 V. The silver-zinc battery type comes in the same standard sizes as the zinc-air but has significantly lower capacity, offering a shorter lifespan. Many recent hearing aids are capable of using either zinc-air or silver-zinc with a special battery door.[41]

Lithium-ion

Lithium-ion batteries are common in all manner of rechargeable electronic devices. This chemistry is less energy dense than zinc-air, meaning that the cell must be larger for an equivalent lifespan. Nonremovable versions of lithium-ion batteries are beginning to be included in hearing aids.[42] These applications result in a battery that is not replaceable by the patient. Lithium-ion cells produce an operating voltage of about 3.7 V, but this can vary from 3.0 to 4.2 V over the life of the battery. A size 13 lithium-ion battery would have about 90 mWh of charge.

Battery Life

Independent of battery type, there are many factors that go into the calculation of battery life.[43] Hearing aid specifications often include "idle drain" and "ANSI/IEC drain." The idle drain includes no receiver power or signal processing related to dynamic features such as feedback suppression algorithms. The ANSI/IEC drain measurement has "advanced features" disabled, but includes a standard acoustic input to include some proportion of "typical" receiver battery drain.

As wireless functionality expands in hearing aids, more of the battery's energy must be devoted to maintaining connections and streaming audio and other information. The power devoted to wireless functionality can vary greatly from technology to technology and even manufacturer to manufacturer. For instance, near-field magnetic induction (NFMI) wireless applications have lower power requirements than 2.4 GHz wireless connectivity.

Like any battery-powered electronic device, the battery life depends mostly on how the device is used. Patients with high gain and output who frequently use wireless accessories will have the shortest battery life.

2.3.6 Radios and Antennas

Hearing aids with wireless capabilities need very small radios and antennas. Wireless capabilities can include wireless programming from a professional's computer, button presses from a remote control, and streaming audio between hearing aids and audio accessories, such as a mobile phone.

The term "radio" is used most often to refer to the AM/FM radio systems for broadcasting audio over great distances. This was the first popular radio technology, but the term more generally applies to any device meant to radiate signals wirelessly from one place to another. In a hearing aid, the radio is a small integrated circuit with special programming to convert digital information (audio, programming information, etc.) to and from the format and frequency needed for the antenna to transmit or receive.

Antennas for hearing aids look quite different depending on the wireless technology being used. Antennas meant to radiate at 2.4 GHz or 900 MHz can be as simple as a bent piece of copper wire or look more complicated, like a precisely routed flexible printed circuit board. These antennas can look like whips or loops or have some other topology. They take careful planning, simulation, and testing to make sure they work on and off the human head, which can greatly change the performance.

Antennas for NFMI look almost indistinguishable from telecoils. In fact, they are extremely similar. Both rely on the principle of magnetic induction, but while telecoils are tuned for audio frequencies, NFMI coils are tuned via material and dimensional changes for NFMI transmission and reception (~ 3–10 MHz). NFMI coils are often used for wireless ear-to-ear transmission, since the head has a negligible effect on magnetic fields in this frequency range.[44] For this reason, the NFMI coils are almost universally oriented horizontally in the hearing aid (i.e., they "point" to one another through the head).

References

[1] Strom KE. The RIC as a disruptive technology. Hearing Review. 2014;21(6):6

[2] Strom KE. US hearing aid unit sales increased by 8.7% in 2016. Hearing Review. 2017;24(2):6

[3] Pisa JFD. Power to the people: A RIC for severe-to-profound hearing loss. Hearing Review 2009;16(10):28–34

[4] Griffing T, Preves D. In-the-ear aids Part I. Hearing Instruments 1976;27(3):22–24

[5] Cornelisse LE, Seewald RC. Field-to-microphone transfer functions for completely-in-the-canal (CIC) instruments. Ear Hear 1997;18(4):342–345

[6] Madafarri P, Stanley W. Microphone, receiver and telecoil options: past, present and future. In: Valente M, ed. Hearing Aids: Standards, Options and Limitations. New York, NY: Thieme Medical Publishers; 1996:126–156

[7] Byrne D, Christen R, Dillon H. Effects of peaks in hearing aid frequency response curveson comfortable listening levels of normal-hearing subjects. Aust J Audiol 1981;3(2):42–46

[8] Chasin M. The acoustics of hearing aids: standing waves, damping, and flared tubes. Hearing Review 2013

[9] Staab WJ, Lybarger SF. Characteristics and use of hearing aids. In: Katz J, ed. Handbook of Clinical Audiology. 4th ed. Baltimore, MD: Williams & Wilkins; 1994:694

[10] Pirzanski C. Earmolds and hearing aid shells: a tutorial part 4: BTE styles, materials, and acoustic modifications. Hearing Review 2006

[11] Killion MC. Earmold acoustics. Semin Hear 2003;24(4):299–312

[12] Agnew J. Hearing aid adjustments through potentiometer and switch options. In: Valente M, ed. Hearing Aids: Standards, Options, and Limitations. New York, NY: Thieme Medical Publishers; 1996b:210–251

[13] Lewis J, Moss B. MEMS microphones, the future for hearing aids. Analog Dialogue 2013;47(11):1–3

[14] Davis M. Audio and electroacoustics. In: Rossing T, ed. New York, NY: Springer Handbook of Acoustics. 2014:779–817

[15] Macrae JH, Dillon H. An equivalent input noise level criterion for hearing aids. J Rehabil Res Dev 1996;33(4):355–362

[16] Agnew J. Perception of internally generated noise in hearing amplification. J Am Acad Audiol 1996a;7(4):296–303

[17] Oeding K, Valente M. The effect of a high upper input limiting level on word recognition in noise, sound quality preferences, and subjective ratings of real-world performance. J Am Acad Audiol 2015;26(6):547–562

[18] Preves D. Obtaining accurate measurements of directional hearing aid parameters. Hearing Aid 1975;28(4):13–34

[19] Roberts M, Schulein R. Measurement and intelligibility optimization of directional microphones for use in hearing aid devices. Paper presented at the meeting of the Audiological Engineering Society, New York; 1997

[20] Beranek LL. Acoustics. New York, NY: McGraw-Hill Electrical and Electronic Engineering Series, McGraw Hill; 1954

[21] American National Standards Institute. ANSI S3.35–2010 Method of Measurement of Performance Characteristics of Hearing Aids under Simulated Real-Ear Working Conditions." American National Standard S3.35 2010;17–38

[22] Elko GW. Superdirectional microphone arrays. In: Gay SL, Benesty J, eds. Acoustic Signal Processing for Telecommunication. Boston, MA: Springer; 2000:181–237

[23] American National Standards Institute. ANSI S3.5–1997 Methods for Calculation of the Speech Intelligibility Index. American National Standard S3.51998;1–22

[24] Hornsby BWY. The speech intelligibility index: what is it and what's it good for? Hear J 2004;57(10):10–, 12, 14, 16–17

[25] French NR, Steinberg JC. Factors governing the intelligibility of speech sounds J Acoust Soc Am 1947;19:90–119

[26] American National Standards Institute. ANSI S3.5–1969 Methods for the Calculation of the Articulation Index. American National Standard S3.51969;1–22

[27] Ricketts TA, Henry PP, Hornsby BW. Application of frequency importance functions to directivity for prediction of benefit in uniform fields. Ear Hear 2005;26(5):473–486

[28] Ellison J. Silicon microphone technology. Innovations 2015;5(1):22–27

[29] Preves D. Standardizing hearing aid measurement parameter and electroacoustic performance tests. In: Valente M, ed. Hearing Aids: Standards, Options, and Limitation. New York, NY: Thieme Medical Publishers; 1996:1–71

[30] Lybarger S. Development of a new hearing aid with magnetic microphone. Electrical Manufacturing; 1947

[31] Compton C. Providing effective telecoil performance with in-the-ear hearing instruments. Hear J 1994;47(4):23–33

[32] Teder H. Quantifying telecoil performance: understanding historical and current ANSI standards. Semin Hear 2003;24(1):63–70

[33] Miller T, Bellavia A. WP03—The Science of Premium Sound Using Miniature Transducers. Itasca, IL: Knowles Corporation; 2015

[34] Sonion. What is Balanced Armature Receiver Technology? Roskilde, Denmark: Sonion Academy; 2016

[35] Kinsler L, Frey A, Coppens A, Sanders J. Fundamentals of Acoustics. New York, NY: Wiley; 2000:285

[36] Lewis JD, Goodman SS, Bentler RA. Measurement of hearing aid internal noise. J Acoust Soc Am 2010;127(4):2521–2528

[37] Hoefler D. Basic Audio Course. New York, NY: Gernsback Library, Inc; 1955:154

[38] Killion M. Hearing aid transducers. In: Crocker M, ed. Encyclopedia of Acoustics. New York, NY: Wiley & Sons; 1997:1979–1990

[39] Dopp R. Zinc air technical introduction. Rayovac Battery Symposium, Madison, WI; 1996

[40] Bloom S. Today's hearing aid batteries pack more power into tinier packages. Hear J 2003;56(7):17–18, 20, 22, 24

[41] Freeman B, Ortega J, Dueber R. What's the state of rechargeable batteries for hearing aids? Hearing Review. 2016;22(9):28

[42] Heuermann H, Herbig R. Hearing aid batteries: the past, present and future. Audiology Online, 2016;18176

[43] Staab W. Hearing Aid battery life can vary widely. Hearing Health Matters; 2016

[44] Galster J. A new method for wireless connectivity in hearing aids. Hear J 2010;63(10):36–39

3 Standards for Assessing Hearing Aid Performance

David A. Preves

3.1 The Need for Standards and the Standards Development Process

When hearing aid performance began to be reported many years ago, hearing aid engineers made measurements and reported hearing aid performance on specification sheets using different methods. Such measurements are needed so that electroacoustic data can be provided to hearing aid dispensing professionals and to government agencies that relate to both quality control and actual performance during use. For those attempting to use these specification sheets, it was impossible to assess and compare performance of hearing aid devices from different manufacturers since the measurement methods they used to assess performance differed. Stakeholders and others affected soon realized that there was a need for standardizing hearing device performance measurement methods to provide consistent procedures that were widely understood and replicable for those needing to generate and use this performance data.

Standardized measurement procedures are achieved by consensus and are typically the result of widely used practices by those in the field. In the standardization process, after the need for standardization has been established, the next step is to identify members of a committee or working group (WG) to draft a new standard or to update an existing standard. A WG consists of experts in the technology area involved, and those who have financial support and can volunteer their time to participate in drafting and reviewing the draft standards and attending WG meetings.

Early on, a consensus is needed within the WG about the scope for a new standard or the scope for changes to an existing standard. Determining how, when, and where the committee will meet is also an early task. In-person meetings usually occur once or twice a year. In between in-person meetings, WG members communicate via email, telephone, and web meetings.

In the case of hearing aid–related standards, the American National Standards Institute (ANSI) publishes standards drafted by WGs and standards committees of the Acoustic Society of America (ASA). Every five years, ANSI standards must reaffirmed, revised, or withdrawn.[1] The purpose of these standards is to ensure that the same measurements made on a hearing aid at different facilities give substantially the same results using different test equipment, as long as that equipment complies with the requirements and follows the procedures described in the standards.

Existing standards cannot be instantly modified to bring them up to date with current practice. Instead, they must go through the same consensus and approval process that a new standard undergoes. Once a new or revised ASA standard has consensus within the standards WG, it is ready to go to the parent ASA committee for balloting the members and individual experts. (For hearing aid standards, the parent committee is Accredited Standards Committee S3 on Bioacoustics, which is sponsored by the Acoustical Society of America.) At about the same time, a call for public comments is published in ANSI's *Standards Action*. Negative votes and comments resulting from the ballot or public comment need to be resolved by the WG and, after the WG makes corrections in the draft standard, it is circulated again by ASA S3 for final approval. Again, a call for public comments is published. This process continues until there are no negative votes, and the new or revised ASA standard is sent to ANSI for final approval and published as an American National Standard.

3.2 Regulatory Applications of Standards

Procedures described in ANSI standards are voluntary unless they are adopted and required by a regulatory agency. One example of a standard whose procedures are required is ANSI S3.22, Specification of Hearing Aid Characteristics, which was first created in 1976 at the request of the Food and Drug Administration (FDA), and last revised in 2014. Federal law requires that hearing aid manufacturers must report the parameters specified in S3.22 using the measurement methods of S3.22 for published data in their hearing aid specification sheets.[2]

Hearing aid performance data of interest includes, but is not limited to, measurements of amount of amplification (acoustic gain), maximum output sound pressure level, frequency response, frequency range, distortion, internal circuit noise, battery current drain, induction coil (telecoil) sensitivity, directionality, and automatic gain control (AGC).

Normative annexes that are included in an ANSI standard are considered to be part of the body of the standard.[3] However, informative annexes in ANSI standards provide additional information and are not treated as part of the body of a standard. Any tests defined in informative annexes are therefore optional.

3.3 ANSI and IEC Standards

The International Electrotechnical Commission (IEC) has developed hearing aid–related standards of its own which fill the need for specifying consistent methods to measure and verify the performance of hearing devices in most of the world, including European, Asian, and Latin countries. Hearing aid manufacturers selling their devices in these countries must use the measurement tests and report the parameters specified in IEC standards. Some ANSI standards are also used by countries other than the United States, for example, Canada and Australia, to measure and verify hearing aid performance. If different test parameters and/or test conditions are specified in corresponding ANSI and IEC standards, hearing aid manufacturers must provide two sets of data, resulting in potential hardship from the need to test and conform to both ANSI and IEC standards to sell their products in the countries that use ANSI and IEC standards. This potential hardship has led standards committees drafting corresponding ANSI and IEC hearing aid–related standards to try to harmonize them as much as possible so that the same tests and test conditions are specified.

ASA-ANSI and IEC hearing aid standards working groups have not always worked well together to achieve harmonized standards.[4] Consequently, in past years, there have been several ANSI and IEC standards that use somewhat different measurement procedures and parameters to cover the same topics. Recently, for some standards, there has been good progress within ANSI WGs and their counterpart IEC WGs to achieve a large degree of harmonization. In many cases, ASA-ANSI hearing aid WG members are also members of IEC hearing aid–related WGs, so each has input into what is contained in the other's standards. Perhaps the epitome of harmonization between corresponding ASA-ANSI and IEC standards is the adoption by ANSI of an IEC standard, as is, without any changes. Recent examples of this are ANSI S3.42-Part 2, which is a nationally adopted international standard, IEC 60118–15 Methods for characterizing signal processing in hearing aids with a speech-like signal, and ANSI S3.55-Part 5, which is adopted as is from IEC 60318–5 Simulators of human head and ear—Measurement of hearing aids and earphones coupled to the ear by means of ear inserts.

There are many ASA-ANSI and IEC standards that cover similar tests for the same hearing aid–related parameters, but they are too numerous to include in this chapter, so only a few are discussed. Examples of ASA-ANSI standards and their IEC standard counterparts that cover the same topics are as follows:

3.3.1 Hearing Aid Electroacoustic Testing and Tolerancing for Quality Control Purposes: ANSI S3.22 Specification of Hearing Aid Characteristics and IEC 60118–7 Measurement of Hearing Aids for Quality Inspection for Delivery Purposes

These two standards are closely aligned except for a few tests, for example, differences in telecoil tests in the body of the two standards: ANSI S3.22 uses the Telephone Magnetic Field Simulator (TMFS) fixture to simulate the 31.6 mA/m magnetic field produced by a typical telephone handset. The most recent revision of S3.22 (2014) has tests for induction loop sensitivity in a vertical magnetic field in the body of the standard as well. IEC 60118–7 has an induction loop test in a vertical magnetic field only and does not use the TMFS because most applications for telecoils in countries other than the United States involve picking up inductive room loop signals. Also, IEC 60118–7 defines the Maximum High Frequency

Average magneto-acoustical sensitivity level (HFA MASL) of the induction pickup coil.

Recently added in ANSI S3.22 is the option of obtaining frequency response curves using a complex signal for the test signal, such as the speech-spectrum noise specified in ANSI S3.42-Part 1 Testing hearing aids with a broadband noise signal. This provision is designed to speed up testing as compared to using swept sinusoidal signals. IEC 600118–7 does not specify the use of a complex test signal. Another difference between the two standards is in the use of annexes for specifying additional tests. There are no annexes in IEC 60118–7. Instead, additional measurements for further characterizing hearing aids are simply specified as such at the end of the IEC standard, whereas there are several informative annexes in the ANSI S3.22 standard that describe additional optional tests. Among the many additional optional tests included in informative annexes of S3.22 are AGC tests (which used to be in the main body of the standard, but were recently made optional by moving them to an annex), tests for harmonic distortion as a function of frequency, hearing aid output noise spectrum, maximum induction coil sensitivity, and harmonic distortion for induction coil, difference frequency distortion, and the effect of gain control, tone control, and output limiting control on frequency response.

In an extraordinary example of harmonization between ANSI and IEC standards, the latest revision of IEC 60118–0 Measurement of the performance characteristics of hearing aids is even more aligned with ANSI S3.22 than is IEC 60118–7 and IEC 60118–0 will likely eventually replace IEC 60118–7 for quality control purposes. For example, IEC 60118–0, which for many years in the past used only the IEC 711 Occluded ear simulator (now IEC 60318–4), now specifies default use of the 2-cm³

coupler, with optional use of the occluded ear simulator, and incorporates additional measurements with the TMFS fixture for predicting telecoil performance with a telephone.

3.3.2 Testing Hearing Aids with a Broadband Noise Signal ANSI S3.42-Part 1 and IEC 60118–2 Amendment 2 (Now Abandoned)

The need for this standard arose from the recognition that measuring hearing aid performance with discrete pure tones is not indicative of how they will perform with complex input stimuli in actual listening situations. The result was the development of ANSI standard S3.42-Part 1, which specifies techniques for assessing the performance of hearing aids with a broadband, steady-state, speech-shaped noise input signal, rather than utilizing a sinusoidal (pure tone) input, as specified in the ASA-ANSI S3.22 standard. This need was identified particularly for hearing aids that utilize nonlinear signal processing algorithms, for example, automatic gain control AGC and noise reduction because of a low-frequency "blooming" artifact that occurs when determining the hearing aid frequency response at different input levels with a swept sinusoidal input signal.[5] The family of frequency response curves obtained for a hearing aid with AGC in accordance with ANSI standard S3.42-Part 1 does not have the blooming artifact, as shown in ▶ Fig. 3.1. Among the tests described, ANSI standard S3.42-Part 1 are saturation sound pressure level, gain, frequency response, family of frequency response curves, and output versus input characteristic, all obtained with the specified speech-shaped broadband noise input.

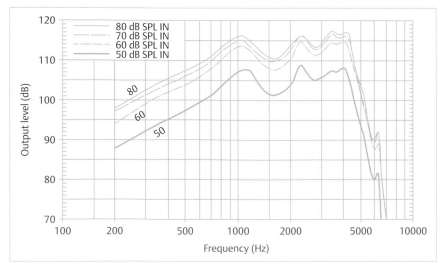

Fig. 3.1 Example of a family of frequency response curves obtained for an AGC hearing aid in accordance with ANSI S3.42-Part 1 with four broadband noise input levels.

3.3.3 Characterizing Signal Processing in Hearing Aids with a Speech-like Signal IEC 60118–15 and ANSI S3.42-Part 2

Performance of hearing aids in actual use may differ significantly from that determined with test procedures in ANSI S3.42-Part 1, which uses a steady-state noise input signal. Realizing this, the ASA S3/WG48 committee for standardizing hearing aid measurements attempted for many years to develop an extension of the original ASA-ANSI S3.42 (now Part 1) standard that would utilize a temporally varying signal for an input rather than the steady-state broadband noise input specified in S3.42-Part 1. Because consensus could not be achieved within the ASA WG, this endeavor did not result in an ASA-ANSI standard. Meanwhile, however, the European hearing aid manufacturers[6] had been working in parallel toward the same goal and had reached consensus on a temporally varying test signal. Ultimately, the European Hearing Instrument Manufacturers Association (EHIMA) effort resulted in the IEC 60118–15 standard, which uses a nonsteady state, speech-like test signal with the hearing aid set to specific settings. This standard describes a recommended speech-like test signal,[7] the International Speech Test Signal (ISTS), and a method for the characterization of hearing aids using this signal with the hearing aid set to actual user settings or to the manufacturers recommended settings for one of several "typical" audiograms in a reference set of audiograms. The ISTS is formulated by taking excerpts from six languages and concatenating them, resulting in an unintelligible test signal that simulates normal speech. Thus, this standard takes into consideration the combination of the hearing aid, the fitting software which programs it, and tests with a signal-like actual speech. The IEC 60118–15 standard filled the need for the desired extension of ASA-ANSI S3.42–1 to use a temporally varying signal and was adopted by ASA-ANSI, in total, as ANSI S3.42-Part 2 and the original ANSI S3.42 discussed above then became S3.42-Part 1.

3.3.4 Using a Manikin Such as KEMAR to Test the Simulated Effect of the Human Head and Torso on the Performance of Hearing Aids, Including Directionality: ANSI S3.35 and IEC 60118–8

These documents provide guidance on how to use KEMAR to estimate hearing aid performance *in situ*, that is, taking into account the head and torso diffraction caused by an average hearing aid wearer. As shown in ▶ Fig. 3.2, ANSI S3.35 contains tests for measuring directivity index (DI) in three dimensions,[8] whereas IEC 60118–8 calculates the DI in only two dimensions (in a horizontal plane). However, IEC 60118–8 has correction factor tables for converting free field to

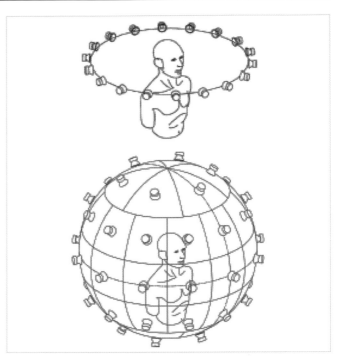

Fig. 3.2 Illustration of recommended loudspeaker locations for 2D (top) and 3D (bottom) directional measurements. With permission from Preves and Burns.[8]

hearing aid microphone inlet SPL for different types of hearing aids, to account for the microphone location effect (MLE), whereas ANSI S3.35 does not.

3.3.5 Ear Simulators for Testing Hearing Devices—ANSI S3.25 and IEC 60711 and IEC 60318–4

Whereas couplers, for example, the 2-cm^3 coupler, provide a stable fixture for measuring the electroacoustic performance of hearing aids, they do not mimic the average acoustic impedance across frequency of ear canals. To better represent the acoustic termination provided by human ear canals, ear simulators were developed many years ago, and have been widely used for hearing aid characterization. The original values for transfer impedance in ANSI S3.25 (which originally described only the modified Zwislocki ear simulator) and in IEC 60711 were very close, S3.25 differing from the values in IEC 60711 by 1 dB or less at a few frequencies between 100 and 8,000 Hz. However, these small differences resulted in the modified Zwislocki ear simulator not meeting the IEC 60711 transfer impedance tolerances, which some attributed to commercial motivation. This is an example of ASA-ANSI and IEC WGs not working very well together to achieve harmonization between similarly purposed standards. The modified Zwislocki ear simulator, made originally by Knowles Electronics, is no longer available. In the most recent version of IEC 60318–4 (which replaces IEC 60711), the transfer impedance tolerances were loosened and the frequency range was extended from 100 Hz–10 kHz to 20 Hz–16 kHz.

Some models of current hearing aids have increased bandwidths, for example, for better sound quality when listening to music, thus creating the need for measurement equipment which reliably assesses the high-frequency performance of hearing aids.

Because of the lack of consistency of a resonance at 12 to 14 kHz in the IEC 60318–4 ear simulator response, there has been considerable concern within WGs as to whether the IEC 60318–4 ear simulator is suitable for making valid and repeatable measurements on wide-band hearing aids at frequencies above 10 kHz. Consequently, a new coupler is in development especially for this purpose.

3.3.6 Measuring Electroacoustic Performance up to 16 kHz: IEC TS 62866 (at the time of this writing, there was no corresponding ANSI document)

The effective internal volume of the coupler described in this technical specification is 0.4 cm^3, which does not produce a resonance in the frequency range below 16 kHz. Having high acoustic source impedance and small volume, the 0.4 cm^3 coupler produces about 14 dB higher output SPL at 1 kHz compared to the 2-cm^3 coupler. Initially, IEC TS 62866 has been formulated as a technical specification, rather than an IEC standard, to allow sufficient time for those in the field to gain experience using the 0.4 cm^3 coupler.

Thus far, laboratories that have utilized the 0.4 cm^3 coupler have found the tests results to be stable and representative enough that it has been suggested that the 0.4 cm^3 coupler may someday replace the 2-cm^3 coupler and the IEC 60318–4 ear simulator.

3.3.7 Measuring Hearing Aid Circuit Noise

ANSI S3.22, IEC 60118–0, and IEC 60118–7 specify an equivalent input noise level (EINL) measurement—calculation to express the amount of noise that would be present at the hearing aid input required to produce the noise output SPL from the hearing aid. This method normalizes for different hearing aid gain values and may be performed in a single, broadband calculation or in narrow-frequency bands, for example, one-third octaves (▶ **Fig. 3.3**), as specified in an annex of ANSI S3.22 and in additional optional test procedures in IEC 60118–0.

Different hearing aid wearers will vary in their ability to hear a given amount of circuit noise produced by a hearing aid, depending on the amount of their hearing loss and configuration of their audiogram. The ASA-ANSI S3/WG48 committee theorized that a given amount of hearing aid circuit noise might be heard by those with mild high-frequency hearing loss, and particularly those with steeply sloping or precipitous hearing loss, with normal hearing thresholds in the lower and middle frequencies. To determine whether the circuit noise produced by a hearing aid is audible and possibly objectionable for a wearer, a member of the S3/WG48 committee conducted a study to determine whether such a characterization was possible.[9] The results of his study, which makes intuitive sense, showed that for at least six of the eight subjects with moderate hearing loss, hearing aid circuit noise became audible at the level for which the one-third octave noise level is tangent to the audiometric curve, plotted in SPL and at about 10 dB above the audible noise level, the circuit noise begins to be objectionable. The study concluded that it would be useful for clinicians to have one-third octave noise data from hearing aid manufacturers.

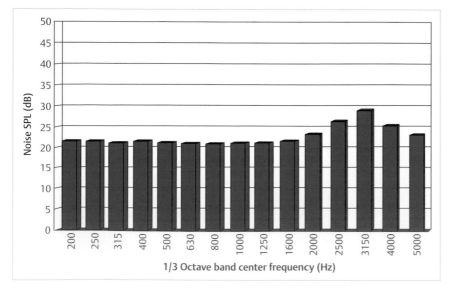

Fig. 3.3 Example of hearing aid output noise spectrum in one-third octave bands.

A related study was conducted at the National Acoustic Laboratories,[10] whose goal was to set acceptable limits of the EINL of hearing aids based on the sensation level of the internal noise output of hearing aids when used in accordance with the NAL prescription. The project concluded that no simple rule can be used since it was found that the acceptable maximum EINL criterion is nonlinear and variable over frequency, and can be relaxed as a function of the hearing aid gain for higher-gain hearing aids.

At the time of this writing, the S3/WG48 committee has abandoned this standardization effort due to the lack of consensus on how to set the volume control and programmable parameters for such measurements.

3.3.8 Measuring Hearing Aid Performance on Real Ears: ANSI S3.46(2013) and IEC 61669 (2015)

These ANSI and IEC standards are totally harmonized (the ANSI version coming first), and define terms that have been long used in practice to express real-ear hearing aid performance, including real-ear insertion gain (REIG), real-ear unaided response (REUR) and real-ear unaided gain (REUG), real-ear aided response (REAR) and real-ear aided gain (REAG), and real-ear occluded response (REOR) and real-ear occluded gain (REOG). The last revision of ANSI S3.46 (2013) added real-ear coupler difference (RECD), real-ear aided response with 85- or 90 dB SPL input level (REAR85 or REAR90), which has been called real-ear saturation response (RESR) previously, and the real ear to dial difference (REDD). Use of the ISTS for real-ear testing was also added in the most recent revisions of ANSI S3.46 and IEC 61669.

During the update process of ANSI S3.46, members of the ANSI S3/WG80 committee that formulated the standard found that including the RECD measurement was somewhat problematic because of the inconsistent techniques used to make this measurement in the field under the guise of the term "RECD." Two important issues for the RECD measurement that became apparent are the use by some of the HA-2 coupler configuration and different earmold plumbing terminations for the coupler and real-ear parts of the measurement, both of which do not conform to the essential definition and intent of the RECD. Use of different acoustical "plumbing," that is, an earmold substitute rather than the actual earmold and different tubing materials for the coupler and real-ear portions of the RECD calculation is not the way the RECD was originally defined. WG members were also concerned that high acoustic output impedance sources (e.g., insert earphones like the Etymotic Research ER-3A having a higher acoustic impedance than hearing aid receivers) are sometimes used to obtain the RECD for infants, which produces results not representative of the actual RECD obtained with a hearing aid. Because of such varying practices in the field, RECD values obtained for a specific hearing aid and wearer may be quite variable between facilities. As a result, an extensive Annex C with potential sources of errors in performing RECD measurements was added in the 2013 revision of ANSI S3.46, including common pitfalls, explanatory notes in the definition of RECD, and text to discourage certain practices such as the two provided above, and to clarify the definition of RECD. For the RECD calculation, ANSI S3.46 (2013) specifies use of the HA-1 coupling configuration with the actual tubing and earmold or ear tip that is used for the real-ear part of the measurement, and the same high-impedance sound source for both the coupler and real-ear measurements.

3.3.9 Testing Assistive Listening Devices (ALDs) or Hearing Assistive Devices/Systems (HADS) Including Wireless Hearing Aid Systems: ANSI S3.47 (2014)

ANSI S3.47 (2014) specifies terminology definitions and measurements for assessing the electroacoustic performance of HADS, that is, hearing devices using, at least partially, nonacoustic signal transmission methods that have varying physical configurations to amplify and/or improve the signal-to-noise ratio (SNR) of an acoustic signal. Examples of HADS include personal ALDs, hearing assistance technologies, auditory trainers, large-area assistive listening systems, telephone amplifiers, and alerting devices. The scope of this standard includes only HADS not worn entirely on the body that transmit directly to a person via earphones or a hearing aid. HADS are classified by transmission method, that is, hardwired or wireless, which includes radio frequency (RF) or near-field induction, audio-frequency induction, and infrared. Delivery via hearing aid includes direct electrical input (DAI), induction coupling through a telecoil in the hearing aid, or a built-in receiver, for example, an FM transceiver in the hearing aid. One possible application of the standard is measuring the input–output characteristics of a remote (companion) microphone system, for example, an FM transmitter on a teacher sending the teacher's voice to an FM receiver connected to a neckloop worn by the hearing aid wearer that relays a corresponding magnetic signal to a telecoil in a hearing aid.

Many hearing aids in the current marketplace incorporate both audio amplifiers and wireless transceivers. ANSI S3.47 (2014) recommends that the amplification of sounds picked up by a microphone internal to a hearing aid be tested by ANSI S3.22, and the wireless communication functionality with remote audio devices be tested according to ANSI S3.47. Since there is considerable overlap in functionality of HADS and hearing aids, many of the parameters tested according to ANSI S3.47 were taken from the ANSI S3.22 standard with appropriate test setup modifications for HADS testing. The ASA-ANSI S3/WG81 committee, which developed ANSI S3.47 (2014), had to create definitions early on that distinguished between hearing aids and HADS devices. Interestingly, one result of that effort was a consensus definition for a hearing aid that was subsequently included, for the first time, in the most recent draft revision of ANSI S3.22 (2014), after ANSI S3.22 had been in widespread use for nearly four decades.

3.3.10 Measuring Cellular Telephone Interference in Hearing Aids and Hearing Aid Immunity: ANSI C63.19 and IEC 60118–13

Because the amount of interference some digital wireless devices (WDs) caused in hearing aids, soon after the initial market introduction of digital cellular telephones over 20 years ago, standardization efforts to characterize the amount of interference produced by WDs and the immunity of hearing aids to the interference were begun by both national and international standards committees, and are still ongoing.

ANSI and IEC standardization efforts outside of the ASA standards organization resulted in ANSI standard C63.19 (developed in a subcommittee of Accredited Standards Committee C63, EMC, which is sponsored by IEEE). Concurrently, IEC developed and published IEC 60118–13. Both standards assess how much interference wireless devices such as mobile telephones cause in hearing aid audio processing. ANSI C63–19 specifies measurements for both RF emissions of WDs as well as hearing aid immunity to interference from WDs, whereas IEC 60118–13 assesses only hearing aid immunity to WD interference. At the time of this writing, both of these standards are being revised to take into account new wireless device technologies that are being incorporated into the latest smartphones in the marketplace.

Digital cellular telephones can cause two types of interference in hearing aids: (1) a crackling or buzzing sound produced by the modulated WD carrier frequency being demodulated in the hearing aid and (2) a magnetic interference in hearing aids that is caused by inductive energy at audio frequencies generated by the WD battery and display coming into the hearing aid telecoil. The amount of disruption caused by the interference produced in hearing aids by WDs is a function of how much annoyance and degradation it causes in speech intelligibility.[11,12] Certain types of RF modulation, for example, that produced by Global System for Mobiles (GSM) WDs, cause more annoyance for hearing aid wearers than others

such as Code Division Multiple Access (CDMA) WDs.[13] Studies generally agree that a 10 dB speech-to-interference ratio (SIR) is usable with major limitations, a 20 dB SIR is usable with minor limitations, and a 30 dB SIR provides normal use. Based on these SIR study results, measurements made in accordance with ANSI C63.19 result in an emission rating for phones and an immunity rating for hearing aids. When these two ratings are added, the result is a predicted degree of usability which can guide a hearing aid dispensing professional and hearing aid wearer in selecting a usable combination of hearing aid and wireless phone. For example, an M3 cellular telephone used with an M2 hearing aid results in a total rating of 5, which, according to ANSI C63.19 predicts normal use, whereas an M2 cellular telephone used with a M2 hearing aid predicts being usable. RF emission ratings for phones are also assigned for telecoil coupling mode and are given a T designation per the ANSI C63.19 standard. Recent tests conducted by the Hearing Industries Association (HIA) and Hearing Loss Association of America (HLAA) on several cellular phones have demonstrated that interference is more noticeable by hearing aid wearers when they use telecoil coupling to the WD than when they couple to the WD acoustically via their hearing aid microphones. Interference from WDs is generally worse when hearing aids are operating in induction pickup mode, as compared to microphone pickup mode, because there is so little differentiation between the baseband magnetic desired signal from the telephone (an audio signal not modulated by a high-frequency RF carrier signal) and the magnetic interference signal, which is frequently produced by the display and/or current drawn from the battery of the mobile phone. Unfortunately, improvements to increase hearing aid telecoil immunity have been very difficult to achieve because the interference signals are essentially the same as the desired audio signals from the telephone.

Initially, the IEC 60118–13 standard specified hearing aid immunity measurements to express the level of "bystander interference" from hearing aid wearers using cellular telephones in proximity, that is, spaced 2 m away from their hearing aids, and did not include measurements representative of what could occur if a hearing aid wearer was using a cellular telephone held in the normal use position at the ear. Since hearing aid wearers need to use mobile phones, it became obvious that a measurement reflecting the level of "user" interference was needed as well. The current revision of IEC 60118–13 standard includes measurements which are intended to reflect both bystander and user interference levels with the hearing aid.

By including RF filters in hearing aids, in microphones and in amplified telecoils, and with wire routing in hearing aids that minimizes interference, hearing aid immunity to RF emissions increased by about 30 dB over 10 years.[14] In the DELTA study, which was sponsored by the EHIMA, immunity to RF interference was measured for 350 hearing aids of varying styles from 11 hearing aid manufacturers using procedures specified in IEC 60118–13.

In 2005, hearing aid manufacturers, using the methods specified in ANSI C63.19, voluntarily agreed to label the immunity to WD interface for their hearing aids M2 or greater. Currently, WD manufacturers and carriers are attempting to meet an Federal Communications Commission (FCC) requirement for a certain percentage of phones to be hearing aid compatible and compliant with the ANSI C63.19 standard at the M3 and T3 or greater level.

3.3.11 Wireless Standards and Their Application to Hearing Devices

In general, wireless device test standards are concerned with two main areas under the general umbrella of electromagnetic compatibility: (1) immunity of an electronic device to electromagnetic interference and (2) the amount of electromagnetic radiation that is produced by a wireless device.

IEC standard 61000–4–3, entitled "Radiated, radio-frequency, electromagnetic field immunity test," is the broadly accepted test method across many industries for performing radiated RF immunity tests, that is, it contains methods for determining and expressing the degree to which RF interference signals affect the performance of an electronic device. It specifies methods that are required by both the European Union and United States for testing medical devices, including all hearing aids, because it is the specified test method in the general medical electromagnetic compatibility (EMC) standard, IEC 60601–1–2 and in the radio equipment, EMC standard ETSI EN 301 489–1.

Many of the standards referenced above that contain specifications for maximum power radiated from wireless devices were intended for such devices as mobile phones, which radiate much greater RF power than hearing aids.

In the United States, the FCC regulates the maximum amount of RF power that wireless devices are allowed to radiate at a distance. Specifically, the maximum RF power radiated from a wireless hearing aid at given distances and in certain frequency ranges must adhere to the stipulations of FCC Code of Federal Regulations (CFR) 47 Part 15. In setting these limits, the FCC was mindful of the safety concerns of humans absorbing RF-radiated emissions, which are expressed by the specific absorption rate (SAR). A SAR value is a measure of the maximum energy absorbed by a unit of mass of exposed tissue of a person using a wireless device. SAR is normally averaged either over the whole body or over a small volume. Specifically, for cellular phones, the FCC has set a maximum permissible SAR limit of 1.6 W/kg, averaged over the volume containing a mass of 1 g of tissue that is absorbing the most signal.

FCC requires SAR testing only for devices having output power greater than 60 mW/carrier frequency (in GHz). In contrast to cellular telephones, RF-radiated emissions from wireless hearing aids have typical peak output power in the microwatt range, or about 100,000 times less than cellphone output power. With reference to the FCC regulation above, if the wireless feature in a hearing aid was active 100% of the time, and all of this output power was absorbed by 1 g of tissue, it would still be about 25 times lower than the .08 W/kg limit averaged over the whole body.

As mentioned previously in this chapter, ANSI standard C63.19 contains recommended test methods for determining the amount of radiation of mobile cellular telephones. Both ANSI C63.19 and IEC 60118–13 reference IEC 61000–4–3[15] as part of their test methods, but both deviate significantly from it. ANSI C63.19 deviates mainly in the areas of test chamber, test position, and frequency sweeping requirements, while IEC 60118–13 deviates mainly in test chamber and test position requirements.

The FDA, which regulates hearing aids as medical products, is concerned about coexistence of wireless devices.[16] They note that many medical devices are authorized to operate as unlicensed devices under Part 15 of the FCC rules in the industrial, scientific, and medical (ISM) frequency bands, for example, 2.400–2.4935 GHz, which is heavily used by many communications and industrial products.

3.4 Test Equipment for Assessing Electroacoustic Hearing Aid Performance

At the time of this writing, a number of manufacturers make test equipment for assessing hearing aid performance, including microphones, couplers, ear simulators, and test fixtures. Products from these companies range from generalized test equipment, supporting accessories, and software that are used in acoustics laboratories but can also be used for hearing aid analysis, to dedicated testers for audiology clinics and hearing aid dispensing offices. Some examples of companies that manufacture technical hearing aid test equipment include Audio Precision, Bruel & Kjaer, G.R.A.S., Listen, and Rohde & Schwarz; companies that manufacture equipment for the clinical testing of hearing aid performance include Audioscan, Frye Electronics, Interacoustics, and Otometrics.

Some of the measurements that hearing aid test equipment can perform per the ANSI S3.22 and IEC 60118–0 and IEC 60118–7 standards include the following:

- Gain and output.
  - Output SPL response, full-on acoustic gain, frequency response, and effects of different battery impedance or battery voltage on gain and OSPL 90.
- Amplitude nonlinearities (acoustic distortions).
  - Harmonic distortion and intermodulation distortion.
- Internal circuit noise.
- Battery current.
- Induction pickup coil performanc.
  - Frequency response and harmonic distortion.
- AGC (amplitude compression).
  - Input/output characteristics for sinusoidal signals, and dynamic output for different speech signals at different levels.

A typical data sheet, resulting from a hearing aid analyzer's measurement, reports the electroacoustic performance of hearing aids in accordance with ANSI S3.22–2014 as shown in ▶ Fig. 3.4.

Representative examples of portable hearing aid analyzers that are intended for clinical/hearing aid dispensing use are shown in ▶ Fig. 3.5 and ▶ Fig. 3.6. Besides being able to perform the coupler-based tests automatically as specified in ANSI S3.22, IEC 60118–0 and IEC 60118–7, and the real-ear tests per ANSI S3.46 and IEC 61669, these two hearing aid analyzer examples have some interesting test capabilities.

The Frye FP35 Touch hearing aid analyzer shown in ▶ Fig. 3.5 has a special DIG FS signal to test frequency lowering in hearing aids. It can display the output frequency spectrum of a hearing aid with frequency transposition activated while presenting a single frequency pure tone to the hearing aid as shown in ▶ Fig. 3.7. This tone is set to 4,000 Hz by default, but can be changed by the operator to other frequencies, if desired.

The FP35 can measure the digital processing time differences between two hearing aids, as well as whether the output transducer phase shift is the same of two supposedly matched hearing aids for a binaural fitting.

The Audioscan Verifit 2 hearing aid analyzer shown in ▶ Fig. 3.6 reflects the hearing aid performance testing features the company has frequently pioneered, including Speech Mapping, in which the hearing aid output in a user's ear canal is measured with real speech and compared to the user's hearing loss and loudness discomfort level, all plotted on the same graph. The Verifit 2 extends the Speech Mapping feature to 16 kHz and has tests for verifying adaptive directionality, noise reduction, frequency lowering, and feedback suppression. The Verifit2 includes a "binaural test box" as shown in ▶ Fig. 3.6, which allows assessment of state-of-the-art hearing

aid features, such as volume control and programming synchronization for wireless binaural hearing aid fittings and verification of audio streaming functionality in wireless hearing aids.

Manufacturers of dedicated hearing aid analyzers typically have web sites that provide reference manuals, calibration and troubleshooting procedures, helpful supporting articles and videos on the general subject of hearing aid testing. The article of Ravn and Preves can be referred to for further information on hearing aid performance analysis equipment.[17]

The ANSI S3.22 and IEC 60118–7 quality control–related standards contain tolerances for test equipment accuracy. These tolerances define test limits for calibration parameters needed for hearing aid performance analyzers to meet the test equipment requirements in these standards. Included are sound source output SPL and test signal frequency response and harmonic distortion requirements, coupler microphone frequency response, ambient noise, and electromagnetic interference in the test space.

3.5 Coupler Configurations Used for Testing Hearing Aids and Transducers

ANSI S3.22 and IEC 60318–5 Simulators of human head and ear—Measurement of hearing aids and earphones coupled to the ear by means of ear inserts was adopted by ANSI as S3.55-Part 5, provide specifications for several coupler configurations (denoted by HA-X) and their use in assessing hearing aids and transducers. (Note: the term "earphone" pertains to a hearing aid receiver.) The HA series coupler configurations specified in S3.22, except the HA-1 type, incorporate an internal earmold simulator. The 2-cm^3 series coupler configurations used for hearing aid testing are the following:

3.5.1 HA-1 Coupler Configuration

The HA-1 allows direct coupling of an earmold of a postauricular (behind-the-ear [BTE]) hearing aid, a molded insert with an internal earphone, or a shell of an in-the-ear (ITE) hearing aid. Clay or putty is used to seal the earmold or shell into the coupler. The S3.22 standard recommends testing with the vent in the hearing aid closed. An example of a custom hearing aid mounted on an HA-1 coupler is shown in ▶ Fig. 3.8.

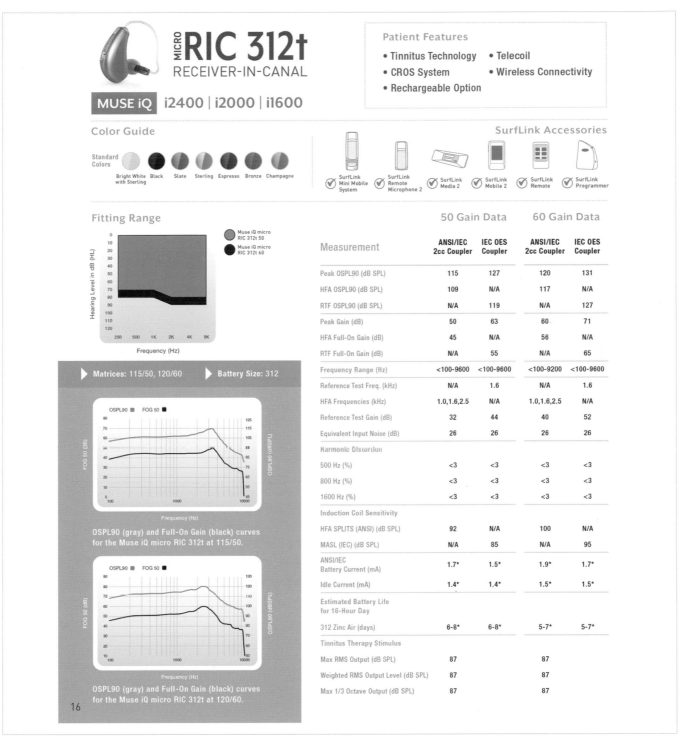

Fig. 3.4 Typical data sheet for hearing aids in accordance with ANSI S3.22–2014.

3.5.2 HA-2 Coupler Configuration

The HA-2 coupler is used for earphones (hearing aid receivers) with nubs such as an external receiver of a body-worn hearing aid. The HA-2 coupler configuration is sometimes used with an external tubing to connect an earphone in a hearing aid to an earmold or to an ear insert. For high-volume testing, the external tubing may be rigid for longer wear. Unless otherwise stated, the connecting tubing outside of the coupler has a length of 25 mm and an inner diameter of 1.93 mm (identical to standard No. 13 tubing). This length and diameter may be specified by the manufacturer and simulates the actual tubing used in practice. The earmold simulator in the HA-2 coupler has a 3-mm bore diameter, which may produce a high-frequency boost compared with an

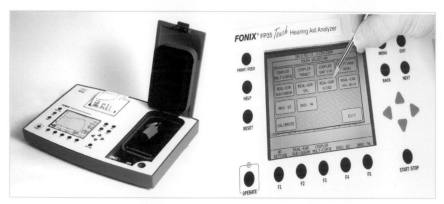

Fig. 3.5 Frye FP35 Touch hearing aid analyzer.

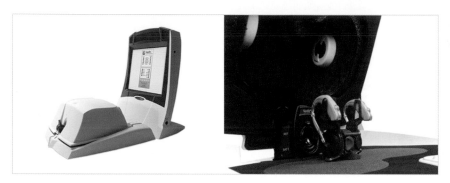

Fig. 3.6 Audioscan Verifit 2 hearing aid analyzer.

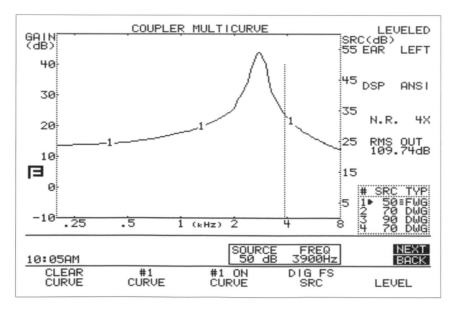

Fig. 3.7 Frye FP35 frequency shift test.

actual earmold with 2-mm bore diameter tubing.[18] A BTE hearing aid mounted on the HA-2 coupler configuration is shown in ▶ **Fig. 3.9**.

3.5.3 HA-3 Coupler Configuration

The HA-3 configuration is intended for testing modular ITE hearing aids and earphones and insert type receivers that do not have nubs. The entrance tubing maybe either flexible or rigid and, unless otherwise

stated by the manufacturer, has a length of 10 mm and a diameter of 1.93 mm (i.e., No. 13 tubing). An illustration of a receiver on the HA-3 coupler configuration is shown in ▶ **Fig. 3.10**.

3.5.4 HA-4 Coupler Configuration

The HA-4 configuration is a modification of the HA-2 coupler configuration to use extended tubing. Though seldom used in modern application, it was designed for testing postauricular or eyeglass

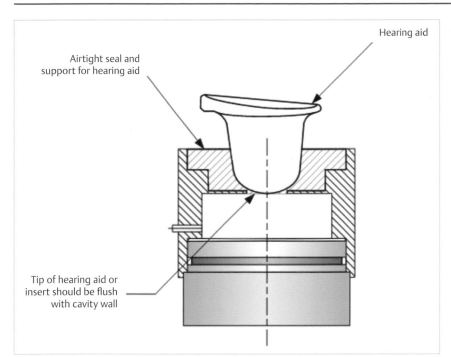

Fig. 3.8 HA-1 coupler configuration.

Hearing aid

Airtight seal and
support for hearing aid

Tip of hearing aid or
insert should be flush
with cavity wall

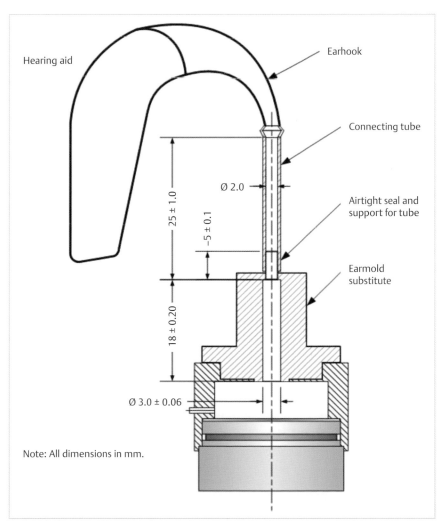

Fig. 3.9 HA-2 coupler configuration.

Hearing aid

Earhook

Connecting tube

Ø 2.0

Airtight seal and
support for tube

Earmold
substitute

25 ± 1.0

−5 ± 0.1

18 ± 0.20

Ø 3.0 ± 0.06

Note: All dimensions in mm.

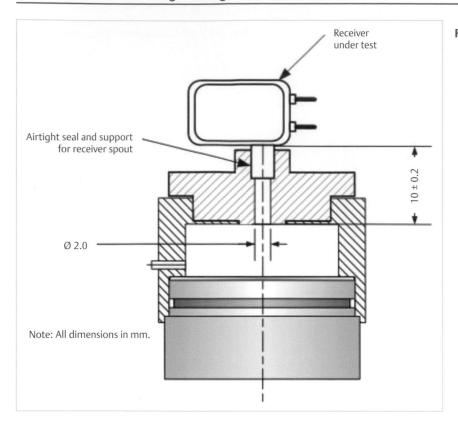

Receiver under test

Airtight seal and support for receiver spout

10 ± 0.2

Ø 2.0

Note: All dimensions in mm.

Fig. 3.10 HA-3 coupler configuration.

hearing aids in conjunction with a constant sound path bore from the hearing aid output through the earmold of 1.93-mm diameter. An illustration of a BTE hearing aid on the HA-4 coupler is shown in ▶ **Fig. 3.11** (The interested reader is referred to Lybarger for further information on couplers[18].

3.6 Predicting Hearing Aid Sound Quality with Electroacoustic Measures

A continuing goal of the ASA-ANSI S3/WG48 committee for standardizing hearing aid measurements has been to find objective measurements that correlate closely to subjective sound quality assessments of hearing aid–processed audio signals. With the proliferation of products that utilize compressed audio data such as MPEG-3, this has been a frequent topic of articles published, for example, by the Audio Engineering Society. The total harmonic distortion (THD) measurements specified in ANSI S3.22 are for quality control assessment, not for providing an indication of hearing aid–processed sound quality. Measures of intermodulation distortion (IMD) and difference frequency distortion have been shown to relate somewhat closer, but not completely, to perceived sound quality. Lee and Geddes showed that there is

a poor correlation between the perceived amount of THD and IMD and the perceived amount of distortion for music.[19]

Perceptual metrics of sound quality have been developed and used by the audio and telephone industries for many years. Some of these are purely subjective, employing five-category Mean Opinion Score (MOS) ratings obtained from subjective listening tests with different methods of audio processing and data compression. The Perceptual Speech Quality Measure (PSQM) and its replacement, the Perceptual Evaluation of Speech Quality (PESQ), which addresses listening quality,[20,21] are among the better known perceptual metrics that have been adopted by the International Telecommunication Union (ITU). An evaluation of the Perceptual Analysis Measurement System (PAMS), by members of the S3-WG48 working group, showed that sound quality had a good correlation to a percent of muted speech metric (speech activity). Additionally, the PAMS accounts for both listening quality and listening effort, which were not found to correlate well to subjective sound quality assessments. The Perceptual Evaluation of Audio Quality (PEAQ), which has been adopted as ITU standard BS.1387, is an objective method that employs a neural network together with several psychoacoustic parameters.

All of these sound quality measures estimate the amount of signal degradation using a (typically

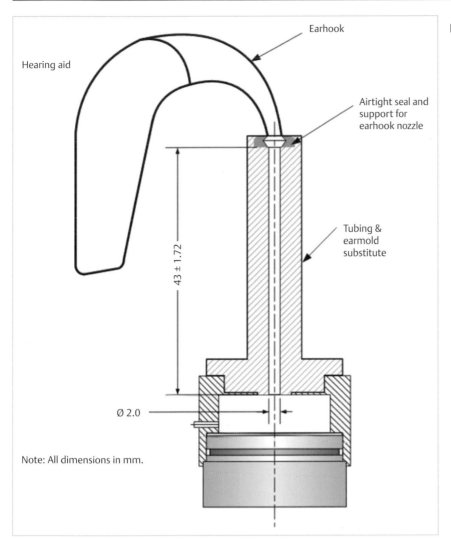

Fig. 3.11 HA-4 coupler configuration.

Earhook

Hearing aid

Airtight seal and support for earhook nozzle

Tubing & earmold substitute

43 ± 1.72

Ø 2.0

Note: All dimensions in mm.

unprocessed) baseline reference signal for comparison to the processed signal. Although these metrics can be considered for hearing aid–processed audio application, they may be useful only for speech signals, and they do not take into account the effects of spectral differences between the original reference signal and the processed hearing aid output signal. The Perception Model-based Quality estimation (PEMO-Q) objective method of predicting sound quality, advocated by Oldenburg University, has been proposed as a possible standard method.[22] The PEMO-Q method compares the unprocessed input signal to an internal representation of the processed hearing aid output signal, after passing both through a psychoacoustically based auditory model. Signal distortions below masked threshold levels are considered inaudible. Any perceptible differences are considered degradations of audio quality. However, before PEMO-Q can be used for hearing aid wearers, it needs to be modified to factor in the effects of hearing loss.

The Hearing Aid Sound Quality Index (HASQI), developed by Kates and Earhart, has recently shown to be a promising objective method of predicting hearing aid sound quality.[23] HASQI compares the hearing aid output to an unprocessed reference signal. The comparison comprises a cross-correlation of the time-frequency signal envelopes to measure how closely the processed envelope follows the original envelope, and short-time cross-correlations of signals within each auditory frequency band to measure temporal fine structure changes caused by the processing. The dominant term is the envelope cross-correlation because the spectral changes resulting from the long-term auditory excitation pattern and in the excitation pattern slope across frequency are less important than the envelope changes in calculating the overall quality index. HASQI is designed to predict listener subjective quality for a large number of different noises and distortions, not for a particular algorithm. The HASQI output represents fits of subjective data from normal-hearing and hearing-impaired listeners to a mathematical model. An auditory model that includes the middle ear, auditory filters, cochlear dynamics, neural firing rate adaptation, and normal or impaired auditory thresholds, is included as a "front end" of the calculations. HASQI version 2 can evaluate signals modified by hearing aid processing, including frequency lowering and imperfect acoustic feedback cancellation.[24,25]

3.7 Conclusion

Standards represent consensus opinions and practices, so generating and publishing a new standard or updating an existing standard requires considerable time. Therefore, standards development to assess new features incorporated in current hearing aids will always lag behind their market introduction. Most members of hearing aid–related ANSI-ASA and IEC standards committees work on developing standards after hours, apart from their actual jobs. Currently, significant efforts in achieving harmonization between corresponding ANSI and IEC standards are being made by these standards committees. Those manufacturing, utilizing, or otherwise having an interest in hearing device products should consider participating in the standards development process.

References

[1] ANSI. ANSI Essential Requirements: Due Process Requirements for American National Standards. New York, NY: American National Standards Institute (ANSI); 2008

[2] FDA. Code of Federal Regulations 21CFR801.420 Hearing Aid Devices: Professional and Patient Labeling. U.S. Food and Drug Administration (FDA); 2010

[3] ASACOS. ASACOS Rules for Preparation of American National Standards in Acoustics, Mechanical Vibration and Shock, Bioacoustics, and Noise. 6th edition of the ASACOS Editorial Guidelines, Acoustical Society of America Committee on Standards (ASACOS). ASA Standards Secretariat; 2003

[4] Preves D. Standardizing hearing aid measurement parameters and electroacoustic performance tests. In: Valente M, ed. Hearing Aids: Standards, Options, and Limitation. New York, NY: Thieme Medical Publishers; 1996:1–71

[5] Preves DA, Beck LB, Burnett ED, Teder H. Input stimuli for obtaining frequency responses of automatic gain control hearing aids. J Speech Hear Res. 1989; 32(1):189–194

[6] EHIMA. Testing Hearing Aids with a Speech-Like Signal. European Hearing Instrument Manufacturers Association; 2006

[7] Holube I, Fredelake S, Vlaming M, Kollmeier B. Development and analysis of an International Speech Test Signal (ISTS). Int J Audiol. 2010; 49(12):891–903

[8] Preves B, Burns T. Revised ANSI standard measures hearing aid directionality in 3D. Hear J. 2007; 60(1):45–49

[9] Agnew J. Perception of internally generated noise in hearing amplification. J Am Acad Audiol. 1996; 7(4):296–303

[10] Macrae JH, Dillon H. An equivalent input noise level criterion for hearing aids. J Rehabil Res Dev. 1996; 33(4):355–362

[11] Joyner K, Wood M, Burwood E, et al. Interference to Hearing Aids by the New Digital Mobile Telephone System, Global System for Mobile Communications Standard (GSM). Sydney, Australia: National Acoustics Laboratory; 1993

[12] Hansen M, Poulsen T. Evaluation of noise in hearing instruments caused by GSM and DECT mobile telephones. Scand Audiol. 1996; 25(4):227–232

[13] Levitt H, Kozma-Spytek L, Harkins J. In-the-ear measurements of interference in hearing aids from digital wireless telephones. Semin Hear. 2005; 26(2):87–98

[14] DELTA—Danish Electronics Light and Acoustics Technical-Audiological Laboratory. Improvement in Hearing Aid Immunity. Danish Electronics, Light & Acoustics Project No. A930005–1. Odense, Denmark: Technical-Audiological Laboratory for EHIMA; 2003

[15] IEC 61000–4–3, Electromagnetic compatibility (EMC)—Part 4–3: Testing and measurement techniques—Radiated, radio-frequency, electromagnetic field immunity test

[16] FDA. Radio Frequency Wireless Technology in Medical Devices. Guidance for Industry and Food and Drug Administration Staff. Document issued on August 14, 2013

[17] Ravn G, Preves D. Hearing aid-related standards and test systems Semin Hear. 2015; 36(1):29–48

[18] Lybarger S. The physical and electroacoustic characteristics of hearing aids. In: Katz J, ed. Handbook of Audiology. Baltimore, MD: Williams & Wilkins; 1985:849–884

[19] Lee L, Geddes E. Auditory perception of nonlinear distortion. Paper 4891 at the 115th convention of the Audio Engineering Society; 2003

[20] Rix A, Hollier M, Heksra A, Beerends J. Perceptual evaluation of speech quality (PESQ), the new ITU standard for end-to-end speech quality assessment. Part 1—Time delay compensation. J Audio Eng Soc. 2002; 50(10):755–764

[21]   Beerends J, Hekstra A, Rix A, Hollier M. Perceptual evaluation of speech quality (PESQ), the new ITU standard for end-to-end speech quality assessment. Part 2—Psychoacoustic model. J Audio Eng Soc. 2002; 50(10):765–778

[22]   Rohdenburg T, Hohmann V, Kollmeier B. Objective Perceptual Quality Measures (PEMO-Q) for the Evaluation of Noise Reduction Schemes. Oldenburg, Germany; University of Oldenburg, Medical Physics Group, D-26111; 2005

[23]   Kates J, Arehart K. The Hearing-Aid Speech Quality Index (HASQI). J Audio Eng Soc. 2010; 58:363–381

[24]   Kates J, Arehart K. The hearing aid speech quality index (HASQI) version 2. J Audio Eng Soc. 2013; 62:99–117

[25]   Kendrick P, Jackson I, Li F, Cox T, Faxenda B. Perceived audio quality of sounds degraded by non-linear distortions and single-ended assessment using HASQI. J Audio Eng Soc. 2015; 63(9):698–712

4 Hearing Aid Coupling: Theory and Application

James R. Curran, Dennis Van Vliet

4.1 Introduction

At first glance, the earmold appears to be the simplest and least complicated part of the hearing aid fitting. So much attention is paid to the electroacoustic performance of the hearing aid and to the selection of the correct frequency-gain response that the earmold often becomes a secondary and less important consideration. And yet, as will be seen, if chosen in error, it can cause the fitting to fail. It is clear that the configuration of the coupling plays a dynamic role in transferring sound to the ear; small changes in conformation, venting, depth of insertion, leakage, and other factors can have appreciable effects on the distribution of the amplified signal at the tympanic membrane. The purpose of this chapter and Chapter 5 is to cover these factors in a systematic and inclusive way so that clinicians, whether new to the subject or experienced, will acquire an appreciation of the topic leading to clinically appropriate decisions.

4.2 Connecting the Hearing Aid to the Ear

There is a wonderfully wide and perhaps perplexing variety of ways that a hearing aid can be linked to the human ear (▶ Fig. 4.1). Earmold laboratories and manufacturers have their own unique manner of crafting and describing their products and each offer different designs and materials. It will become evident, however, that there is a recognizable similarity in their use and application, no matter their apparent differences in appearance. More specifically, the similarities are intrinsically related to the acoustic effects their configurations (shapes) have on the amplified (or unamplified) signal in the real ear.

The first step in understanding and differentiating between the various coupling options is to consider

two (relatively separate) factors—first, the amount or degree of occlusion within the ear canal, and second, the type of retention in the outer ear (pinna).

Applicability across all fittings

The majority of the acoustic effects discussed in this chapter were discovered by systematically varying the configuration of solid behind-the-ear (BTE) custom earmolds. Much of the information that follows, therefore, is based on these observations. That being said, it is quite important to realize that these findings pertain to and influence the acoustics of all types of couplings, including custom receiver–in-the-canal (RIC) molds, custom hearing aid shells, thin-tube BTE custom molds, hollow custom molds, and stock silicone ear tips. In the text, where appropriate, each of the different types of couplings are treated separately to emphasize the universal application of the principles discussed or to illustrate any differences.

---

1. Occlusion, or lack of

The first and most defining characteristic of any coupling is how much it occludes the external auditory meatus (EAM) *medial to the concha meatal junction* (aperture) (▶ Fig. 4.2). That portion of the earmold/shell that lies within the EAM (variously termed the stem, stalk, or most usually, the canal) can be fabricated to provide differing degrees of occlusion or conversely, different degrees of unocclusion (openness). The terms *occluding* or *occluded* as used here refer to the earmold/shell acting to obstruct or prevent passage of all or a greater portion of unamplified sound into the ear canal. *Open, unoccluding,* and *unoccluded* refer to minimal, partial, or no obstruction to the passage of unamplified sound (▶ Fig. 4.3).

When using the terms *opening* or *venting* an earmold indicates a move toward an *unoccluding*

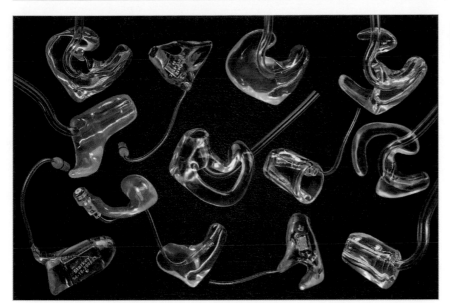

Fig. 4.1 Examples of various earmolds, each having a different appearance and shape. Courtesy of Starkey Hearing Technologies.

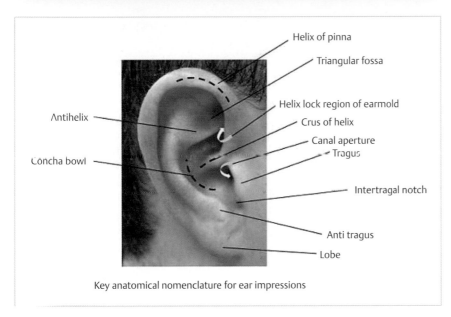

Helix of pinna

Triangular fossa

Helix lock region of earmold

Crus of helix

Antihelix

Canal aperture

Tragus

Concha bowl

Intertragal notch

Anti tragus

Lobe

Key anatomical nomenclature for ear impressions

Fig. 4.2 Key nomenclature of the external ear for communicating with earmold laboratories or hearing and manufacturers. Modified after Alvord et al.[1]

condition rather than the *occluding*. The ultimate unoccluded *open ear canal* fitting is typically achieved when a short section of tubing alone or receiver delivers amplification into the ear; the ultimate *occluded* fitting is when the ear canal is completely, tightly filled and the coupling is deeply inserted into the ear canal with no vent (▶ **Fig. 4.4a, b**).

As will become clear in succeeding sections, the conformation of the earmold medial to the aperture is the most important part of the earmold.[2] Differences in its configuration, that is, the degree that occlusion is present in the ear canal, or inversely, how unoccluding it is, can radically alter the acoustic signature of the signal at the eardrum. Additionally, too much occlusion may result in exacerbating the *occlusion effect* before an acceptable fitting has been accomplished.

Here it is important to not confuse the term *occlusion effect* with the terms *occluded* or *occluding*. The *occlusion effect* describes the disagreeable sound of a patient's own speaking voice that occurs when a too *occluding* earmold or shell *occludes* the patient's ear (see Chapter 4.2.10).

2. Retention

The second characteristic that describes an earmold is the manner in which the earmold/shell is retained in the cartilaginous portion of the external ear (pinna flange, auricle). Included here is the earmold material that is contained within the concha bowl, tragus, antitragus, intertragal notch, crus, helix, antihelix, and adjacent areas *lateral to the concha-meatal junction* aperture (▶ **Fig. 4.2**). The material within the pinna is intended to secure the

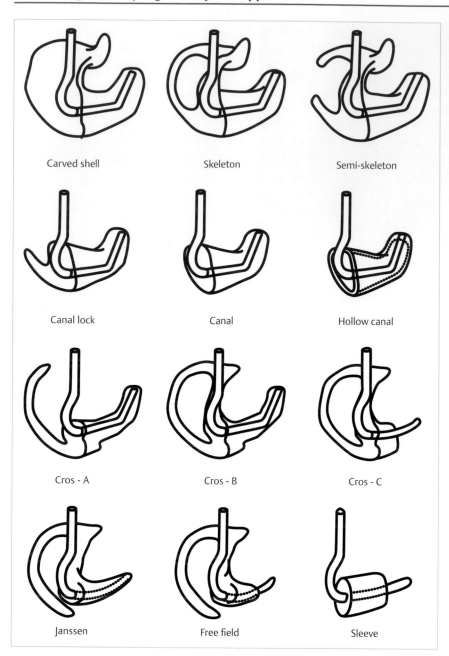

Fig. 4.3 This sketch of BTE earmolds depicts a range from occluding (two top rows) to unoccluding (two bottom rows). Note that the type of retention in the outer ear varies across earmolds from complete to minimal. Adapted with permission from Dillon.[3]

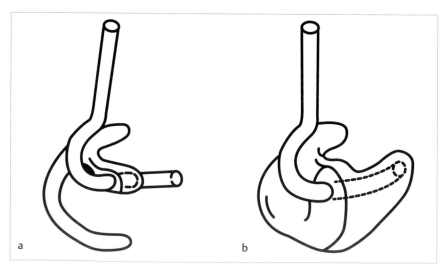

Fig. 4.4 **(a)** The earmold shown represents an unoccluding fitting, where the amplified sound is delivered through a tube only and the ear canal is left open. **(b)** The ear canal is completely filled with the earmold, a totally occluding condition.

The acoustic consequences of occluding the ear canal

The normal condition of the EAM is unoccluded. The natural amplification provided by the external ear apparatus provides a quantifiable high-frequency boost for the normal listener.[4,5] The more the ear canal is occluded, that is, plugged up with an earmold or shell, the further it is removed from its normal operating condition. Ear canal resonance, concha resonance, head and body baffle, and other pinna-related effects are essentially eliminated (►**Fig. 4.5**). The normal impedance condition that exists within an open ear as acoustic signals that are transmitted into the ear canal (and to the eardrum) is also disrupted by the occluding fitting.[6]

As a result, the patient with a hearing loss, when fitted with a partially or completely occluding coupling, is listening in an artificial condition. Not only is there a loss of some or all of the natural high-frequency gain of the external ear, but additional amplification must be provided by the hearing aid to overcome the hearing loss and minimize the effects of other factors (such as masking effects) that work against perception of important high-frequency signals.[3,7] When the earmold becomes more unoccluding or open (even incompletely), however, the external ear effects and the ear's normal impedance begin to be restored.[3,8,9,10,11,12]

earmold in place (►**Fig. 4.6**) and does not ordinarily affect the acoustics of the fitting.[1] However, too loose retention may have an effect on the amount of sound that leaks out of or passes into the ear canal, which may or may not be an undesirable outcome (see Chapter 4.2.8).

The appropriate amount of retention for a given fitting has been customarily related to the degree of hearing loss, that is, the greater the loss, the more retention, but this is a very tenuous generalization. Two other consequential factors operate here. First,

for reasons of appearance, it is always best to use the least amount of earmold material possible in the outer ear. The truth is, most folks are reluctant to advertise their hearing loss. As a rule, the less material that shows but still provides the proper amount of retention is the correct choice. Second, the conformation and plasticity of the pinna, as well as size and shape of the ear canal, plus the type of hearing aid fitted, will influence the type of retention needed.

4.2.1 Receiver-in-the-Canal Fittings

Moving the receiver from the hearing aid case and placing it in the ear canal necessitated the development of special earmold configurations. In RIC fittings, retention is primarily accomplished by a thin, stiff wire leading from the aid directly to the receiver (►**Fig. 4.7**). Various couplings are available for RIC aids to assist in assuring adequate retention, including the hollow mold, the embedded receiver mold, stock ear tips (►**Fig. 4.7**), and the helix mold (►**Fig. 4.8**).

4.2.2 Custom Hearing Aids

In custom hearing aids, the question of retention is always an overarching consideration in the case of in-the-canal (ITC), completely in-the-canal (CIC) and invisible–in-the-canal (IIC) fittings, but less so for in-the-ear (ITE) aids, for portions of the latter lie in the external ear, and usually provide adequate retention. Manufacturers employ well-defined computer-assisted protocols (algorithms, offsets, and style templates) in constructing ITC, CIC, and IIC aids to assure retention in the ear canal; occasionally, but not often, some ear canals defy attempts at resolution. Importantly, in custom hearing aid fittings (and

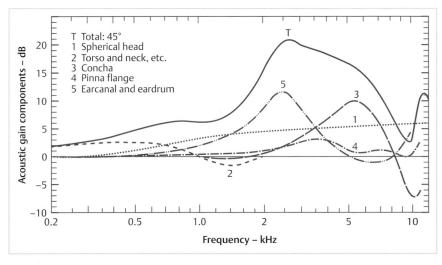

Fig. 4.5 The illustration shows the field to eardrum transfer function of the average normal unoccluded ear canal. The insertion of an occluding or partially occluding earmold subtracts all or part of these normally occurring external ear effects, and alters the impedance of the system. Adapted with permission from Shaw.[4]

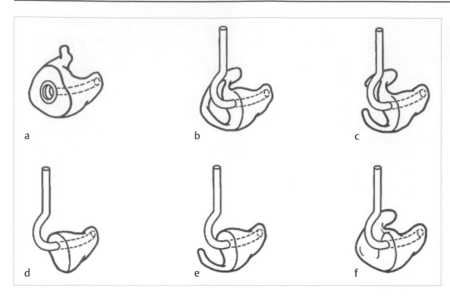

Fig. 4.6 All the earmolds in the illustration are identical in manner of occlusion; only the retention differs. Earmold laboratories often, but not always, describe their earmolds according to the manner of retention. Typical names would include **(a)** body aid earmold, **(b)** skeleton earmold, **(c)** semi-skeleton earmold, **(d)** canal earmold, **(e)** canal lock earmold, **(f)** shell mold. When ordering an earmold, the clinician ordinarily has the option of separately specifying both the amount of occlusion as well as the manner of retention. Adapted with permission from Valente and Valente.[13]

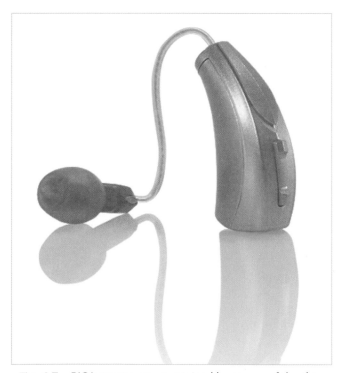

Fig. 4.7 RIC instruments are retained by means of the thin, stiff wire leading from the receiver to the coupling. Shown is a RIC aid with an attached unoccluding stock ear tip for insertion in the ear canal. Courtesy of Starkey Hearing Technologies.

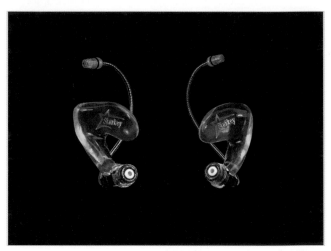

Fig. 4.8 Shown is an essentially open canal fitting (IROS) for RIC instruments, the "helix" earmold. Courtesy of Starkey Hearing Technologies.

4.2.3 Factors that Affect the Amplified Response

When a hearing aid is coupled to the human ear, the resultant response of the signal at the tympanic membrane is affected by certain elements in the transmission pathway in addition to that produced by the location of the microphone.[14,15,16] Each may only contribute minute amounts of influence, but if combined, the change may be consequential.[17,18] The list below summarizes some of the sources in the hearing aid's acoustic transmission pathway that can produce changes to the amplified spectrum.

1. The *diameter, length, and conformation of the vent* in an earmold/shell affect differentially the hearing aid's frequency-gain response and vent-related resonance, and determine

all other earmolds as well), an accurate, well-formed impression of the entire ear canal beyond the second bend, as well as the outer ear, is the first condition for assuring retention.

In summary, when specifying an earmold or any acoustic coupling (including custom hearing aids), the most important consideration is deciding the configuration of that portion of the coupling that lies within the EAM. Following this, the retention portion of the fitting is selected.

the amount of unamplified sound that reaches the eardrum.[19,20,21,22,23,24]

2. The *tightness (or looseness)* of the earmold/shell *(seal)* in the EAM affects gain and output (output sound pressure level [OSPL]) across frequency, especially at the low frequencies.[3,6,19,25,26,27]

3. The *depth of insertion* of the earmold or shell in the ear canal either increases (if deep) or decreases (if shallow) the overall sound pressure in the residual space/cavity between the earmold/shell tip and the tympanic membrane.[3,19] This is a well-known effect (Boyle's law) that states if the volume of a cavity is halved, SPL doubles, and if the cavity volume is doubled, SPL is reduced by half. Both the gain and output (OSPL90) increases or decreases.[28,29,30,31]

4. The overall *length and diameter of the tubing* following the receiver and the *conformation of the sound bore* of the earmold or custom hearing aid will affect the frequency-gain response.[3,13,18,32,33,34]

5. In BTE aids the hearing aid's frequency-gain response will be affected by the characteristics of the *ear hook* or by *specially constructed ear hooks* (see Chapter 4.3.1).[13,34,35]

In addition, but not under the control of the practitioner, individual *differences in the volume, compliance, and impedance* of the ear canal will affect the spectrum of the amplified signal at the plane of the tympanic membrane independent of depth of insertion of the mold/shell or leakage.[30,36,37,38,39]

The presence of all or some of the above five factors modifies the transmission of amplified signals from the receiver to the eardrum. For the modern practitioner, the most important are the first three above, venting, seal, and depth of insertion. However, all five should be appreciated, for there will be occasions where knowledge of the effects produced by one or another element of the transmission pathway will prove important in providing an appropriate fitting.

▶Fig. 4.9 is a famous illustration[32] showing an assortment of amplified responses that were obtained by modifying or altering the characteristics of the coupling for a single BTE hearing aid. Changes to the shape and dimensions of the tubing, ear hook, sound bore, and earmold altered the distribution of the acoustic signal at the tympanic membrane. This was important information until the 2000s, for clinicians did not have the advantage of today's digital fitting software to manipulate the hearing aid's frequency-gain response. Understanding the changes produced by earmold modifications became critically important to the successful practitioner.

The literature of the 1970s through the 1990s is flushed with articles and studies explaining and defining the effects of various coupling configurations.[2,6,19,21,27,32,33,34,40,41,42,43,44,45,46,47] The results of the studies made it clear that the coupling attached to the hearing aid is not just a passive link in the amplifying system, but has an active effect on performance.

If ▶Fig. 4.9 were to be redrawn today, nearly all of the response variants would be eliminated or be of limited clinical relevance, as they represent changes made to the ear hook and/or tubing and the earmold bore. These modifications, because of the passage of time and technological improvements, have less clinical utility today,[48] and are primarily of interest and are included for the acoustic principles they embody (see Chapter 4.3).

4.2.4 The Role of Vents

A vent can be defined as an opening of any size in an earmold/shell that connects the surrounding, ambient environment to the residual space/cavity/volume (i.e., the space between the termination of the mold/shell and the eardrum). A typical vent, for example, may take the shape of a defined,

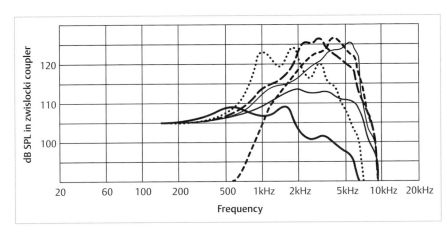

Fig. 4.9 Illustration shows the variety of response changes obtained on one hearing aid simply by altering the construction of the earmold. In the past, analog hearing aids afforded limited response modification capability. To augment adjustability, clinicians manipulated the earmold and associated parts to change portions of the frequency-gain response, as shown in the illustration. Today digital signal processing has eliminated the necessity to make similar adjustments, except in special circumstances. Adapted with permission from Killion.[32]

intentional passageway that starts at the earmold's outside surface through the residual space. Another kind of vent is the gap between the peripheral surface of an earmold or shell and the surrounding walls of the EAM that allows the passage of sound. Finally, a totally open or substantially unoccluding coupling represents another variation of venting.

That said, we might ask, how are vents used in the fitting of hearing aids? There are four different reasons for venting.

The first reason for venting is to reduce amplification in the low frequencies, and by contrast, elevate or maintain the high frequencies.

The first-fit option contained in manufacturers' fitting software or in prescriptive formulas provides an averaged prediction of the amplification required, and therefore, is only an approximation in the individual instance. Subsequent manipulation of the frequency-gain response is usually required in both the high and low frequencies; special care must be exercised to make sure that the lower frequencies are not overemphasized, for there is the possibility that the informational cues in the higher frequencies may be masked (obscured or diminished) by overly amplified low-frequency signals,[49,50,51,52] or result in an unpleasant or too loud listening experience. Later we will discuss another consequential reason for venting, resolving the occlusion effect, but in this discussion, we emphasize the effects and nature of venting as a powerful adjunct for adjusting the balance between low- and high-frequency gain.

4.2.5 Low-Frequency Transmission Loss

Many investigators examined in more detail the effects of venting in BTE hearing aid earmolds, and later, in RIC and custom hearing aids.[6,19,21,22,27,39,40,43,44,46,47,57,58,59,60,61,62,63,64,65] Most of the studies cataloged response changes as one or more variables in the coupling were altered, for example, vent diameter, vent length, vent shape and type, depth of insertion, slit leak, and dimensions of the ear canal. Some of the studies were performed on artificial couplers, either the 2-cm³ coupler or the occluded ear simulator.[66,67] Others used human subjects or were simulated by computer.[30,38,68,69,70,71,72,73,74]

All studies show essentially the same sequence of vent response change, that is, as the amount of venting (opening) is progressively increased, there is a concomitant reduction of amplification in the low frequencies affecting both gain and OSPL90 (▶Fig. 4.12). However, the vent response curves and/or the numerical values of attenuation

Early findings

Before the 1970s, the field had only a general idea of what happened as the shape of an earmold was altered. The average hearing aid specialist (dealer) of the time was wary of venting for it often led to acoustic feedback, but might install a small vent to make the fitting more comfortable if a person objected to the feeling of a closed earmold. In general, however, the field was underinformed about the acoustic consequences. The limited research available was usually performed on 2-cm³ couplers using body aids with external (button) receivers.[42,43,53,54,55,56] There was little information about earmolds for ear-level aids until the 1970s, when rigorously controlled studies began to appear.

Of particular interest was a remarkable study by McDonald and Studebaker[28] who used a laboratory-type probe microphone arrangement to measure the distribution of energy at the eardrums of human subjects fitted with various earmold shapes. Four earmold configurations were investigated, shown in ▶Fig. 4.10, and a swept pure tone signal was presented. The resultant responses across subjects were averaged to produce the tracings in ▶Fig. 4.11. With the hollowed out and shortened earmold (B), a drop of approximately 5 to 8 dB was observed across the frequency spectrum for frequencies up to about 2,500 Hz. Addition of a vent hole in the shortened, hollowed out earmold (C) produced appreciable low-frequency attenuation of the signal. Finally, the fourth earmold shape, a totally unoccluding earmold, showed a dramatic reduction in the low frequencies. This early study was arguably the first to graphically demonstrate the realistic effect of three defining variables on the amplified spectrum, that is, depth of insertion of the earmold into the canal, presence of an intentional vent, and complete unocclusion.

at each frequency reported are not identical and vary from study to study; each provides different data. The unique experimental circumstances of each study are responsible for producing the specific transmission loss data reported at each frequency, for example, see **Table 4.1** and **Table 4.2** for results on human subjects. Upon inspection, it is seen that one or more of the variables that affect transmission loss are at issue. For example, the amount of leak around the periphery of the molds or custom aids may or may not have been controlled, or the effect of different depths of insertion varied between subjects, or instead were based on a single, standardized length of canal/vent. In the individual patient, these factors will vary unpredictably and consequently

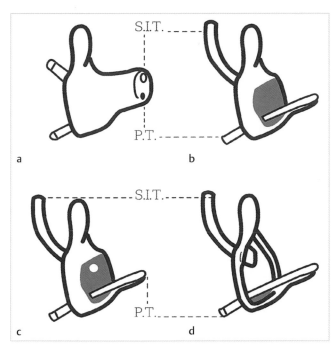

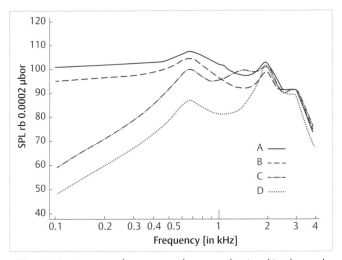

Fig. 4.11 Averaged response changes obtained in the real ear for the four different earmold configurations shown in ►Fig. 4.10. Adapted with permission from McDonald and Studebaker.[28]

Fig. 4.10 Using a probe microphone assembly, McDonald and Studebaker[28] investigated the changes in the real-ear response produced by four different earmold shapes. **(a)** Full mold, **(b)** shortened earmold with no vent, **(c)** shortened earmold with vent, **(d)** open mold (very large vent). Adapted with permission from McDonald and Studebaker.[28]

will affect the amount of low-frequency reduction differentially.

In addition, the results obtained on humans are usually averaged across subjects and therefore lack precise predictive value in the individual instance.[28,39, 46,63,64,65,68,69,75] As a result, when the manufacturer's fitting software or a prescriptive fitting program[76,77,78,79] provides or suggests vent sizes or types for certain hearing losses, the expected low-frequency attenuation in the real ear will vary to a greater or lesser degree from that predicted.[3,18,44,71]

This lack of specificity or precision should not be dismaying. The real merit of the studies is to afford an understanding of the *direction of change* that can be expected when a vent is modified from the occluding to the unoccluding condition. The goal is to understand the approximate effect of a given modification or vent, not to assume or predict a specific magnitude of transmission loss at a given frequency. In spite of lacking specific predictive data, experience shows if one thoroughly understands the probable progression of acoustic events that occur as an earmold or shell is vented or modified, the ability to accomplish a good fitting will not be handicapped. With practice, clinicians become intuitive and skilled in selecting a useful amount of venting/modification in a specific instance. (For instructions on how to perform physical modification of a vent, see Chapter 4.3.5).

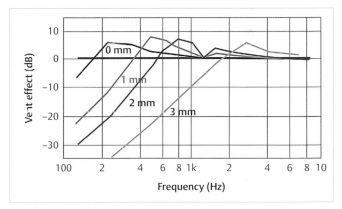

Fig. 4.12 Systematically increasing the diameter of a vent results in successive increases in the low-frequency attenuation (transmission loss). For comparison, see also ►Fig. 4.16a, b. The different amounts of attenuation shown at each frequency in the three figures (►Fig. 4.11, ►Fig. 4.16a, b) are the result of differences in the measurement conditions. Unless all conditions are equivalent, the absolute transmission loss values will not be the same. Adapted with permission from Kuk and Baekgaard.[8]

4.2.6 Selection of Vent Size

Although it is not possible to predict accurately the precise amount of low-frequency roll-off each time one chooses a certain vent diameter (or length), nevertheless, as we have seen, various sources in the literature provide best estimates detailing the effect of different-sized vents, for example, **Table 4.1** and **Table 4.2**. In light of this, are the vent tables and/or manufacturers' vent recommendations of any value? The answer is yes, especially for the beginning practitioner, for the tables, although not identical, do provide a general idea of the approximate transmission loss expected. The answer to the

How vents shunt low frequencies

The acoustic effect of a vent on the amplified spectrum is explained by the interaction of the impedance of the vent, which is an acoustic mass (inertance), and the impedance of the residual cavity (the space between the tip of the earmold/shell and the tympanic membrane), which is a compliance. The acoustic mass is directly proportional to the length of the vent, and inversely proportional to its cross-sectional area. The impedance of an acoustic mass is low for low frequencies, and rises as frequency increases. Compliance is directly proportional to the residual cavity volume. The impedance of a compliance decreases as frequency rises.

When the residual cavity volume is small, as when a deeply fitted, occluding earmold is present, the SPL in the residual cavity is high and the compliance is small. As the volume of the residual cavity increases, as with a short, vented earmold, SPL in the residual cavity falls, the compliance increases, and impedance increases particularly for low-frequency signals. Consequently, amplified low frequencies are met with the higher impedance of the residual cavity, and leave or escape easily through the vent that has low impedance for low-frequency signals. Since acoustic mass decreases as a vent is either shortened and/or is enlarged in diameter, a greater proportion of the amplified low-frequency signal will escape by comparison to fittings with longer, narrower vents.[5,19,47]

cise as any others in the literature, but are included for instructional purposes (see Chapter 4.3.7).

When fitting children, incidentally, we feel it is best to follow the venting suggestions that are included in the prescriptive fitting procedures specifically designed for them. Note, however, it is not unusual to find the size of the ear canals in a given child may be too small to allow the prescribed venting.

4.2.7 Real-Ear Measurements

Given the variability of vent-related low-frequency attenuation, the routine use of real-ear measurements (REM) is invaluable for assessing the specific effect of a given vent on the hearing aid's frequency-gain response. With REM the practitioner can monitor the real-ear aided response (REAR) as the earmold and/or vent is modified, as well as the interaction of the vent with the fitting software. Since it is not uncommon that the actual REAR response may be quite different from what is expected, the REM finding may provide an explanation for a patient's dissatisfaction or complaint.

Further, experience will be gained that will better enable correct clinical decisions as to vent size or earmold configuration in future fittings. To ensure reliability, however, it is important that the probe tube is adequately sealed in order to not conflate the obtained response (see Chapter 4.2.8).

4.2.8 The Influence of Slit Leak

Amplified sound proceeds from the hearing aid into the residual volume/cavity between the tip of the earmold/shell and the eardrum. At the eardrum, a greater amount of the amplified acoustic energy is absorbed, and a lesser amount is reflected back. The reflected sound will try to escape, either

question is also no, if the tables are taken as gospel. In a subsequent section we offer guidelines for selection of earmold/shell according to degree of hearing loss and also include a few suggestions for vent size. Our generalized vent recommendations are just as impre-

Table 4.1 Low-frequency transmission loss values (dB) obtained on human subjects with three different vent diameters for sealed and unsealed ITE aids.

Diameter	Frequency				
	200 Hz	500 Hz	1000 Hz	1500 Hz	2000 Hz
No sealing					
1.3 mm	−7.1 (3.1)	0.3 (2.9)	1.5 (0.7)	0.5 (0.6)	0.1 (0.5)
2.0 mm	−11.1 (3.9)	−0.9 (3.6)	1.9 (0.9)	0.7 (0.7)	0.2 (0.8)
3.0 mm	−21.9 (4.0)	−10.5 (3.2)	3.1 (2.8)	2.6 (1.7)	1.9 (0.9)
Sealing with E-A-R rings					
1.3 mm	−6.8 (2.2)	2.8 (1.3)	0.8 (0.6)	0.3 (0.4)	−0.2 (0.9)
2.0 mm	−12.1 (2.5)	2.2 (3.5)	1.7 (0.7)	0.6 (0.7)	0.3 (0.9)
3.0 mm	−25.0 (2.6)	−9.8 (3.2)	5.1 (2.0)	2.9 (1.4)	2.0 (0.7)

Notes: E-A-R rings, slipped over the instruments' canals, were used to prevent unintentional leakage. Disparities in transmission loss values are related to differences in sealing effectiveness and length of the vents. Values in parentheses represent standard deviations from the mean. Source: Adapted with permission from Tecca[64,65] and Valente and Valente.[13]

Table 4.2   Results obtained on human subjects fitted with either non-operating hollow custom ITE shells[39] or custom ITE hearing aids[64,65] showing progressive low-frequency roll-off as vent diameters were increased

Study	Instrument	Frequency (Hz)									
		200		500		1000		1500		2000	
1.0/1.3-mm vent diameter*											
Staurt et al.[39]	Shell[a]	−4.0	(4.0)	0.8	(3.7)	0.4	(0.9)	0.4	(1.4)	0.025	(1.0)
Tecca[64]	Hearing aid[b]	−7.1	(3.1)	0.3	(2.9)	1.5	(0.7)	0.5	(0.6)	0.1	(0.5)
2.0-mm vent diameter											
Staurt et al.[39]	Shell[a]	−13.2	(5.9)	−2.0	(4.0)	2.6	(2.7)	1.4	(1.4)	0.9	(0.9)
Tecca[64]	Hearing aid[b]	−11.1	(3.9)	−0.9	(3.6)	1.9	(0.9)	0.7	(0.7)	0.2	(0.8)
Tecca[65]	Hearing aid[c]	−15.8	(2.3)	−3.7	(4.5)	2.5	(1.4)	0.9	(1.2)	0.3	(1.0)
Tecca[65]	Hearing aid[d]	−13.9	(1.7)	0.6	(4.0)	1.3	(1.4)	1.1	(1.0)	1.0	(0.7)
3.0-mm vent diameter											
Staurt et al.[39]	Shell[a]	−18.3	(5.9)	−8.0	(2.9)	1.9	(3.6)	2.4	(1.6)	1.5	(1.1)
Tecca[64]	Hearing aid[b]	−21.9	(4.0)	−10.5	(3.2)	3.1	(2.8)	2.6	(1.7)	1.9	(0.9)

Note: Standard deviations of the mean are presented in parentheses.
[a] 14-mm vent length, n = 12. [b] 22-mm vent length with slit vent, n = 10. [c] 16-mm vent length, n = 10. [d] 22-mm vent length, n = 10.
*Tecca[64] utilized a 1.3-mm vent diameter, whereas the present study used a 1-mm vent diameter.
Notes: Differing attenuation values between studies are a function of differences in length of vent, amount of slit leak, and transmission properties of the individual ears.
Source: Adapted with permission from Stuart et al.[39]

through a vent if present, or around the circumference (periphery) of the earmold/shell. The escape of sound around the circumference of the earmold/shell canal has been termed *slit leak* by Lybarger.[6,27]

Acoustically, slit leak is essentially equivalent to that of an intentional vent.[3] *The greater the slit leak, the more amplification in the low frequencies is attenuated or reduced.* The degree of leak to the outside environment is dictated by the quality of the seal between the earmold/shell material and the surrounding ear canal tissue. Very tightly fitted earmolds or custom shells having long canals will present more of an obstacle to the escaping sound than loosely fitted molds or shells with short canals.[80] In the former instance, the tight seal may present such resistance to the escape of sound pressure that only a minimal amount of the amplified acoustic signal escapes to the outside.

In times past, too much slit leak and/or too large a vent would precipitate acoustic feedback easily. This was a serious problem for the practitioner attempting to attenuate low-frequency gain by increasing slit leak, either by enlarging/shortening the vent, or reducing the circumference of the canal. Often, feedback ensued before the appropriate frequency-gain response was achieved. Today, the advent of effective feedback cancellation algorithms has made this substantially less of a problem.

Importantly, low-frequency attenuation due to slit leak is additive to the low-frequency attenuation provided by intentional vents until total unocclusion is reached. Since the degree of seal and consequently the amount of slit leak is primarily

Parallel and diagonal vents

There are two basic types of vents used in custom earmolds: parallel and diagonal (side branch) (▶ Fig. 4.13). Each vent influences the shape of the REAR in a different manner: (1) *parallel* vents run the length of the earmold/shell and never intersect with the sound bore. Installation of these vents will maintain the high-frequency portion of the response, as shown in ▶ Fig. 4.14. By contrast, (2) if a *diagonal (side branch)* vent is installed, that is, a vent that intersects with the sound bore, there will be a roll-off in the high frequencies as well as the expected transmission loss in the low frequencies (▶ Fig. 4.14).[19,44,45] In situations when the type of vent has not been specified by the practitioner, a custom earmold may occasionally be returned from the earmold laboratory with a diagonal vent—not a desirable situation. In children, however, because of size constraints, a diagonal vent may be the only alternative. In these cases, the diagonal vent should terminate in the sound bore as close to the tip as possible to minimize the amount of high-frequency loss.[19] Fortunately, in custom aid shells and RIC earmolds, all intentional vents are parallel, so the frequencies above the vent-related resonance are maintained.

Another popular vent type, the external vent, a v-shaped groove along the bottom of the earmold/shell, is useful when an ear canal is so small that no room is available for standard intentional venting. The effect on the frequency-gain response is primarily an increase in low-frequency roll-off due to slit leak (▶ Fig. 4.15).

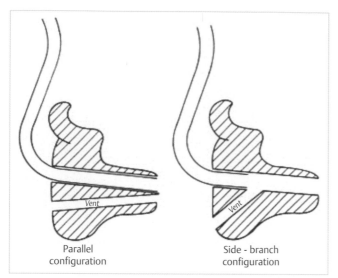

Fig. 4.13 Two types of vents, each having a different effect on the high frequencies. Adapted with permission from Cox.[19]

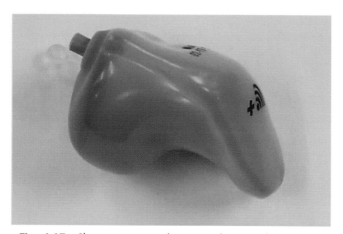

Fig. 4.15 Shows an external or "trench" vent that may be grooved on the exterior surface when enough room is not available in the custom earmold or hearing aid shell for installation of an interior intentional vent. Courtesy of Starkey Hearing Technologies.

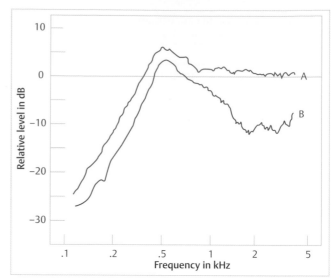

Fig. 4.14 Use of a parallel vent **(a)** will maintain the high-frequency response above the vent-related resonance, whereas a diagonal vent **(b)** will roll off the high frequencies. If a diagonal vent must be used, it should terminate as closely as possible to the tip of the earmold. Adapted with permission from Leavitt[81] and Studebaker and Cox.[46]

a function of how snug or not the custom earmold/shell fits within the ear canal medial to the concha-meatal junction, increasing earmold bulk in the pinna (e.g., using a built-up standard earmold) may not be of appreciable help in achieving a better seal.[2,82,83]

4.2.9 Vent-Associated (Helmholtz) Resonance

▶**Fig. 4.16a, b** shows graphs from two different sources illustrating the expected drop in the low frequencies as the vent diameter increases, but also showing sharp peaks in the response above the cutoff frequency. These peaks are vent-associated (*Helmholtz's*) resonances, where the length and diameter of the vent and the residual cavity (volume) interact to produce a resonance peak in the response.[19,46,47] The air contained within this vent/cavity system is set into sympathetic vibration at its resonant frequency by the passage of amplification through the earmold.[3,30] Vents with small diameters typically produce a resonance in the lower frequencies (200–800 Hz). As the vent is enlarged, shortened, or slit leak is increased, the resonance shifts to the higher frequencies, above about 800 to 1,000 Hz (▶**Fig. 4.12**).[3]

The response curves in ▶**Fig. 4.16a, b** and ▶**Fig. 4.12** (as well as many others reported in various studies on venting) were obtained under tightly sealed conditions, and/or on hard-walled couplers. If taken at face value, one might conclude that vent-related resonance peaks are present in the real ear as well, but this is not true in most instances.[19,25,26,47,57,66,67,84] Resonance peaks usually disappear or are substantially reduced in the average fitting due to slit leak and/or the damping effect of the surrounding ear canal tissue, and consequently, to a great degree, are not a concerning factor (▶**Fig. 4.17**).

However, on occasion a vent-related response peak may appear in the low frequencies in the REAR tracing of a hearing aid coupled to the ear with a tight, deep earmold with very small vent. If a vent-related resonance is suspected, its presence can be confirmed by obtaining the real-ear occluded response (REOR). If a resonance is present, the REOR will show a peak in the curve near that of the REAR. In some situations, the vent-related resonance maybe considered useful, in others, not, depending on the degree of the loss and the goal of the amplification.[19,26,63] If not

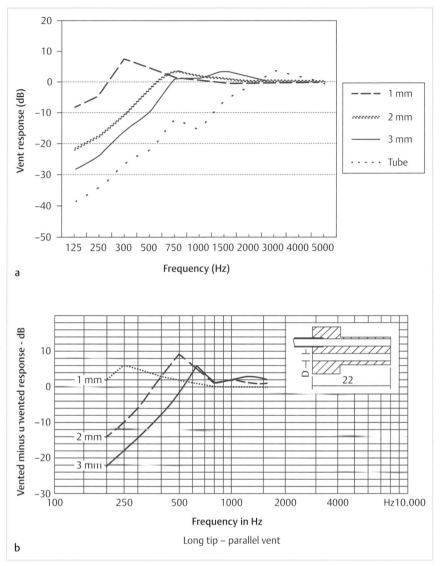

a

b

Long tip – parallel vent

Fig. 4.16 (a, b) Obtained on hard-walled coupler, both sets of curves depict the expected low-frequency attenuation as the vent diameter increases. The sharp peaks show where the vent's dimensions and the residual cavity interact to produce a vent-related (Helmholtz) resonance in the amplified signal. Adapted with permission from Yanz[85] and Lybarger.[27]

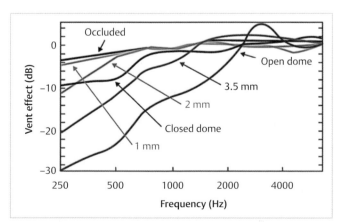

Fig. 4.17 The vent response curves shown in the illustration were obtained on real ears, showing substantially less presence of vent-related resonance peaks. The results are more representative of actual fittings than those shown in ▶**Fig. 4.16a, b**. The response curves are relative to a snugly fitted, entirely occluding earmold. Adapted with permission from Dillon.[3]

considered desirable, to reduce it, the vent or tip of the canal may be shortened slightly to increase slit leak (see Chapter 4.3.6).

An important concept reemphasized

Although most information on venting was obtained primarily on standard tube BTE earmolds, the principal thing to remember is that the acoustic effects are the same for any earmold/coupling condition. In other words, RIC earmolds, custom hearing aid shells, thin-tube BTE hearing aids, stock silicone ear tips, and hollow custom molds follow the same acoustic rules, that is, short, large diameter vents produce greater low-frequency attenuation than long, small diameter vents, and depth of insertion and slit leak effects are in play in all fittings.

4.2.10 The Second Reason for Using a Vent is to Overcome (Reduce) the Occlusion Effect

Resolving the occlusion effect is a fine-tuning issue commonly encountered in daily practice. When patients present with pure tone thresholds better than 30 dB HL (or even in some instances, 35–45 dB HL or better) in the low frequencies, between 250 and about 1,000 Hz, and are fitted with occluding earmolds or custom shells, they usually will complain that their own voice sounds hollow, echoey, boomy, or as if they are "speaking in a barrel." They are experiencing the occlusion effect.[3,70,86,87,88]

The hearing loss may be of any audiometric configuration (i.e., high-frequency, gently or abruptly sloping, flat, or rising), as long as the loss in low frequencies is not substantial. The patient may be a man or a woman (▶ Fig. 4.18).[89] Importantly, most patients will usually not adapt or become accustomed to the occlusion effect percept. In most cases, it will not simply disappear over time,[69] but a few patients, however, learn to tolerate it.

Investigators have attempted to quantify both the frequencies of occurrence and the magnitude of the SPLs of the occlusion effect in the residual cavity.[70,75,88,90,94,95,96,97] Studies show that occluded own-voice SPLs vary in amplitude between patients from as little as 5 to 10 dB to 20 to 25 dB or more, with peaks occurring at different frequencies, from 100

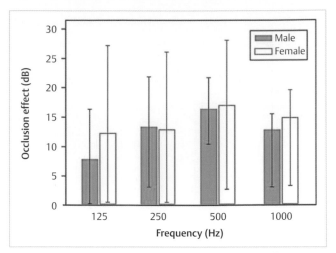

Fig. 4.18 The occlusion effect is not a respecter of gender, occurring in both men and women. In addition to the average results shown here (darkened bars), note the wide dispersion of results at each frequency, occasionally reaching a peak of 25 dB or more. Adapted with permission from Mueller et al.[98]

to 1,000 Hz.[69,88,90,94,97,98,99] It has been suggested that the variability of SPL levels and frequency peaks may be related to differences in the methods of measurement, the depth of earmold insertion, volume and compliance of the residual cavity, elasticity of the cartilaginous portion of the ear canal, the tightness/looseness of the coupling, or a combination of some or all of the above.[3,70,99,100,101]

4.2.11 Acoustic Mass (Inertance)

The acoustic mass of a vent can be calculated,[3] and is based on its diameter and length. As a vent becomes longer or narrower, acoustic mass increases. Conversely, a shorter, wider vent has less acoustic mass. Kuk et al,[70] measuring in real ears with slit leak and insertion depth controlled, showed a linear relationship between the acoustic mass of intentional vents and the objective, measured level of SPLs in the ear canal. They found that as vent diameters were successively increased, thereby reducing acoustic mass, the SPLs in the occluded ear canal decreased in an orderly, predictable manner (**Table 4.3**). Similarly, progressively shortening the vent in controlled increments also results in a sequential reduction of acoustic mass, and thus, successively lessened ear canal SPL levels.[69]

4.2.12 Subjective Perception of the Occlusion Effect

Although Kuk et al[70] showed that the acoustic mass of the vent was closely related to the SPL levels in the residual cavity, they also found that acoustic mass

---

Cause of the occlusion effect

When an individual produces a voiced sound, the vibrations within the vocal tract (larynx, nasopharyngeal column, etc.) are transmitted by bone conduction through the skull to the ear canal.[90,91,92] In addition, when talking, the movement of the mandibular condoyle causes minute displacements of the cartilaginous portions of the ear canal.[93] Together, these two sources of vibration set into motion air particles within the ear canal across the frequency spectrum. These self-generated acoustic vibrations are always present when a person vocalizes or talks, regardless of whether the ear canal is open or occluded.[88] In the case of an open, unoccluded ear canal, the patient's own voice is not perceived negatively because the sound leaks out into the environment. However, when the ear canal is occluded with an earmold/custom shell that *terminates in the cartilaginous portion*, the sound is trapped and unable to escape. The occluded ear canal becomes a resonant cavity, and the low-frequency SPLs, which have been boosted, pass into the cochlea because there is no other escape route available.[92,94]

Table 4.3 Vents with less acoustic mass will result in greater low-frequency transmission loss (dB) than vents having more mass

Vent size	Vent acoustic mass (Henrys)	Frequency (Hz)								
		250	500	750	1000	1500	2000	3000	4000	6000
Unvented, average fit		−4	−2	−1	−1	1	0	0	0	0
1 mm	26,700	−5	−2	−1	−1	1	0	0	1	1
2 mm	7,000	−11	−3	−1	−1	1	1	1	1	2
Closed dome		−10	−8	−3	−2	−2	−1	1	−2	0
IROS (ITE/ITC)	4,700	−16	−11	−4	−3	2	4	2	−1	0
3.5 mm	2,400	−21	−12	−6	−4	1	2	2	1	1
Janssen (ITE)	2,100	−23	−13	−3	−3	1	6	4	−1	1
Open dome	830	−30	−24	−16	−12	−8	−3	5	0	0

Notes: Vents with small diameters have greater mass than large-diameter (or unoccluding) vents. Numerical attenuation values shown are relative to tightly sealed earmold or shell.
Source: Adapted with permission from Dillon.[3]

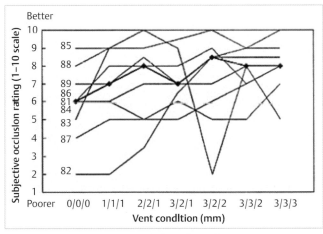

Fig. 4.19 Kuk et al found that the subjective perception of the occlusion effect (ordinate) was not systematically related to the amount of acoustic mass in the vent for subjects as the vent diameters increased from small to large (abscissa). Adapted with permission from Kuk et al.[70]

is not highly related in a systematic manner to the patient's *perceived amount of the occlusion effect* (▶ **Fig. 4.19**). Other investigators also have found fairly small or only modest correlations between objective measurements and subjective ratings of the occlusion effect,[69,102,103] or none at all.[94,104,105] At the extremes we know a very small, long vent will invariably elicit a judgment of a significant hollowness, while very short vents and those with diameters of 4 mm or larger usually serve to significantly reduce or eliminate it altogether.[3,59,69,96] Between those two extremes, it appears that the own-voice experience of occlusion is a subjective phenomenon and its relation to objective measurements is inconstant.[70,94,100,103]

Acoustic versus electronic reduction of low frequencies

All things being equal, is electronic/digital low-frequency reduction superior to or equivalent to that of installing a vent to attenuate low frequencies? Or to eliminate the occlusion effect? Hearing aid fittings that rely solely on low-frequency reduction by means of manufacturer's fitting software may not be successful if at the same time, an incorrect type or configuration of the earmold/shell has been selected and appropriate venting is disregarded.[20,71,106]

Here are two related situations where earmold/shell venting to reduce low frequencies is preferred to low-frequency reduction afforded solely by electronic means. First, if a too occluding earmold is fitted to a high-frequency loss, and the electronic fitting software is used to cut the low frequencies, the patient will hear amplified stimuli essentially through a high-pass filter, a counterproductive circumstance, especially if the patient's remaining hearing (in the low frequencies) is within normal limits.[107] The aid may produce an objectionable sound quality, and any normal hearing in the low frequencies will be eliminated; both may cause the patient to reject the aids.

Second, electronic low-frequency reduction alone will not alleviate the occlusion effect.[70,108,109] To reduce or eliminate the occlusion effect, increasing the venting is required. The occlusion effect is not related to the amplified signal transmitted through the hearing aid into the ear canal. *It is simply the presence of an occluding earmold or custom shell that gives rise to the unnatural, hollow sensation as the patent vocalizes.*

The conclusion is that it is impossible to predict *a priori* the level of perceived relief from the occlusion effect that a patient may experience when a given vent diameter/length is installed. Each patient has an individual, personal level of tolerance/acceptance of the hollow voice sensation. Further, it appears experienced listeners exhibit greater tolerance of the occlusion effect than new.[70] Although instrumentation and easily implemented techniques are available for measuring the properties (frequencies and SPL levels) of the occlusion effect,[88,99] in the end, it is the patient who decides whether or not the occlusion effect is disturbing. Relief from the annoying own-voice percept is obtained by systematically decreasing the mass of the vent, but examining a set of objective measurements cannot tell us when the SPL levels are reduced enough, although measurements may be valuable for record keeping.[97]

4.2.13 Methods for Resolving the Occlusion Effect

The most common and popular method for shunting a portion of the amplified low frequencies is to enlarge the venting in orderly steps to 3- to 4-mm diameter and greater. Or, if more convenient, by shortening the length of the vent. In the latter case, incidentally, there will be additional reduction of low frequencies occur due to an increase in slit leak.[3,19,27,70,81] Both methods assume familiarity with bench modification techniques, covered in a later section (see Chapter 4.3.5).

It has also been suggested that deeply inserted earmolds/shells that terminate beyond the cartilaginous section of the EAM, that is, in the ear canal's most sensitive area, the bony portion, also have the potential to provide some relief from the occlusion effect. The logic is sound, for the particle movements present in the cartilaginous portion of the canal are bypassed.[48,86,89,110,111] However, not only can it be challenging to take ear impressions deep down in the ear canal, many patients cannot tolerate the pressure or friction when the earmold/shell touches against the walls of the bony canal and in addition, patients may experience discomfort and loosening of the earmold/shell when speaking. For this reason, the canal tip is sometimes tapered to facilitate insertion and to minimize discomfort. However, by doing so, the chances of doing away with the occlusion effect becomes problematic. A lucky few, however, do manage to comfortably wear deeply fitted hearing aids or earmolds that terminate in the bony section, and they ordinarily become enthusiastic and satisfied patients.[3,35]

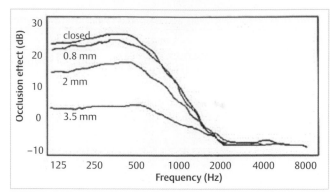

Fig. 4.20 Depicts the systematic reduction of the occlusion effect for one subject as vent diameter was increased. Adapted with permission from Sweetow and Pirzanski.[112]

In conclusion, the use of modification techniques to enlarge or shorten the vent is the preferred and most effective method for removing or decreasing the occlusion effect. The modification of the vent should proceed in small steps until resolution is achieved, as it is impossible to predict if a given vent dimension will be sufficient to reduce the occlusion effect (▶ **Fig. 4.20**).[3,39,69,70,88,102,106,118,119]

About "ampclusion"

Various investigators have proposed that the occlusion effect should more properly be termed *ampclusion*.[112,113,114] That is, they suggest the annoying own-voice percept is not solely or always caused by the occlusion effect, and may result from the distracting or newly experienced sound of amplification itself.[70,115] It is theorized that both factors, the hollow voice sensation and the unfamiliar sound of amplification (or overamplification), may manifest at the same time. However, one can determine if the patient is reacting to the occlusion effect rather than ampclusion. With the aid in place, turn it off and ask the patient to speak or phonate the vowel(ee) or read a passage. (In bilateral fittings, remove the contralateral aid.) If the annoying sensation is still present, gently break the seal of the aid, or pull it slightly out of the ear. If the sensation disappears or lessens as the aid is loosened, the culprit is the occlusion effect.[112]

In our judgment, and in agreement with others,[109,116,117] we have concluded that most of the hollow voice complaints, indeed, are primarily earmold/shell related and usually not, as has been suggested, caused by too much low-frequency gain, or by the new or unfamiliar sound of amplification. The latter problems, that is, those not related to occlusion, are customarily dealt with by software manipulation of the amplified signal and/or by counseling.[112,113,116]

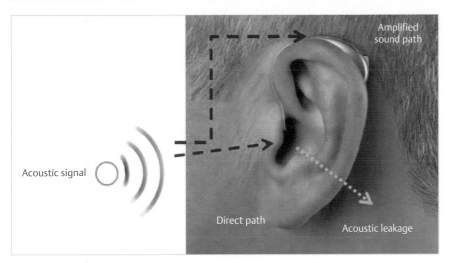

Fig. 4.21 Illustrates the simultaneous behavior of a vent; amplified and unamplified signals pass into the ear canal, and at the same time, some of the amplified signal escapes. Courtesy of Starkey Hearing Technologies.

4.2.14 The Third Use of Venting is to Allow Unamplified Speech and Other Signals into the Ear

Vents allow unamplified sound waves to pass into the ear canal as well as allowing, at the same time, low-frequency signals to escape (▶Fig. 4.21). The range of frequencies that pass into the ear through the vent is exactly the same as the range of frequencies that flow out of the vent; the upper limit of the range is defined by the vent-associated resonance.[3,120] Extremely large vents, say 4 mm or larger, or totally unoccluding fittings, may have vent-associated resonances that range from approximately 2,000 to 3,000 Hz and above.[3,69] Consequently, in large vent conditions, low-, mid- and many high-frequency sounds from the external environment will pass *into the ear unimpeded and essentially unchanged*, for most ear canal resonance, concha resonance, head and body baffle, and other pinna-related effects will be maintained (▶Fig. 4.5, ▶Fig. 4.22).[3,9,10,11,12] However, when the vent diameter begins to diminish or the vent is lengthened, the vent-related resonance shifts to a lower frequency. As a result, the range of transmitted frequencies through the vent is also reduced, diminishing the passage of unamplified mid- and higher-frequency signals into the residual cavity. When the diameter of a long vent is quite small, the vent itself also produces an impedance mismatch to the passage of mid- and, especially, high-frequency stimuli into the ear.[19]

However, low frequencies, which have longer wavelengths, will pass into the residual space of the ear canal even when there is the smallest of vents, or no vent at all. Unamplified low frequencies from the outside may slip into the residual cavity through the slit between the periphery of the earmold or custom shell and the surrounding walls of the ear.[19,57] We almost always can count on some unamplified

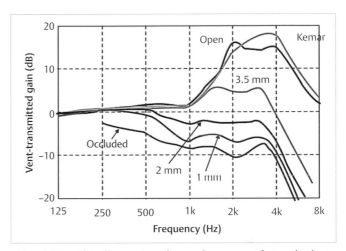

Fig. 4.22 This illustration shows the range of signals that pass through the earmold as the vent diameter varies in size from closed (occluded) to open. The completely open condition shows substantial increase in high-frequency gain and bandwidth due to the restoration of external ear effects. Adapted with permission from Dillon.[3]

low-frequency signals (if intense enough) entering the ear canal, even when the seal is extremely tight and the canal is very deep.[3]

4.2.15 Effects of Open Canal Fittings on Directivity and Noise Reduction Algorithms

It is well established that the directivity index (DI) of a directional microphone hearing aid will be compromised in large vented, open canal fittings by comparison to occluded, or small vent fittings.[87,121,122,123,124] In the presence of large vents, gain is rolled off in the low frequencies where the greatest amount of directional effectiveness is located. As a result, the patient receives little or no directional benefit in this region.

The origin of open canal amplification

The first known mention in the literature of open canal (unoccluding) amplification was by Harford and Barry[129] where they described using a tube instead of a closed earmold to deliver sound by means of a contralateral routing of signals (CROS) hearing aid into a patient's aidable ear in unilateral losses (▶ Fig. 4.23). Today's modern methods for control of feedback were unknown at the time, and the separation between the microphone and receiver in CROS aids substantially diminished the chance of feedback. Eventually, it was found in addition that CROS aids were useful for fitting bilateral, high-frequency losses, and even though the result was amplification for one ear only, the fitting was far more acceptable than, if as was the custom at the time, bilateral closed or small vent molds were used.[130,131,132,133,134,135,136] In fact, bilateral open canal ipsilateral routing of signals (IROS) tube fittings were also tried, but were restricted to mild losses because of acoustic feedback problems.[137]

The popularity of open canal amplification CROS fittings increased rapidly, for relief from the occlusion effect blended with normal hearing in the lows and excellent amplification in the high frequencies resulted in a degree of satisfaction not achievable with other types of fittings.[3,106,131] In the early 1970s, the records show that in some years CROS fittings accounted for nearly 20% of all head-worn aids.[138] By 1974, Harford and Dodds[139] estimated that CROS fittings comprised close to 40% of all recommendations in University audiology clinics. Eventually, open earmold amplification was discovered to be also useful for resolving flat or gently sloping losses in addition to high-frequency losses.[140]

However, the introduction and rapid rise in the popularity of custom ITE hearing aids in the late 1970s resulted in open canal and CROS fittings for high-frequency losses becoming almost forgotten. Today, because of active feedback cancellation strategies the popularity of open canal amplification has returned, for the number of patients with bilateral high-frequency losses that can be fitted successfully without feedback has expanded dramatically.[75,141,142,143]

However, directional hearing aids have a certain amount of directionality in the higher frequencies, above the vent-related cutoff frequency. Based on work in his laboratory, Ricketts[125] estimated that on the average, the DI is reduced by about half in open canal fittings as compared to closed. Magnusson et al[126] found that open canal fittings reduced the directional benefit by about 60% when compared to nonvented, closed earmolds. Despite the reduced directional effectiveness in unoccluded fittings, studies have found appreciable improvement in open fittings with directional microphone aids by comparison to performance with nondirectional microphone instruments.[87,126,127,128] Even the smallest amount of improvement in noise afforded by directional hearing aids warrants their being fitted whenever possible in both partially and totally open coupling conditions.[128]

In general, *adaptive noise reduction algorithms* have relatively little effect on improving speech clarity in open canal fittings.[3] The action of the digital reduction algorithm is relatively useless in the presence of large vents, for the low frequencies (usually noise related) are not amplified and therefore there is little or no possibility of electronic reduction of background noise. Magnusson et al[126] looked at the effectiveness of directional hearing aids combined with noise reduction algorithms in open canal fittings and concluded the open, unoccluded condition significantly reduces the advantages of both, compared to unvented, conventional earmolds. As expected, they did find some improvement in speech recognition in noise with directional hearing aids in the open mold condition, but suggested that adding noise reduction to directional aids offered little advantage in open canal fittings.

4.2.16 Phase Difference Effects

Whenever a very large vent is used, two things happen simultaneously. The appreciable venting produces a low-frequency transmission loss in the *amplified* signal as it is delivered from the hearing aid into the residual cavity. At the same time, *unamplified* sound from the surrounding environment passes through the large vent unimpeded and combines in the residual cavity with the amplification from the hearing aid (▶ Fig. 4.24). The amplitude of the incoming amplified signal produced by the hearing aid may be either less than, equal to, or greater than the unamplified vent transmitted signal at any frequency.

In modern hearing aids there is an average group processing delay of approximately 5 ms, that is, the signal takes about that long to travel through the digital circuitry of a given hearing aid.[144,145,146] The question is, in open canal fittings do the out-of-phase arrivals of the two incoming signal paths, the amplified and the unamplified, affect the spectrum of the combined signal? Or the perception of it by patients? It turns out that when one of the two sounds is 10 dB or greater than the other, the dominant signal will pass into the residual space with no change.[3] In large vent situations, the incoming unamplified, low-frequency signals from the environment are ordinarily the dominant signals and consequently, are not altered by the out-of-phase arrival times.[9,19] Similarly, in the higher ranges (from about 1,500 Hz and above), the amplified signal from the hearing aid is usually substantially

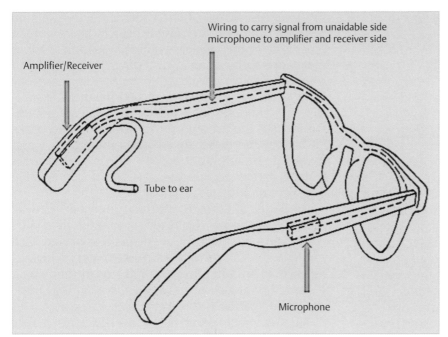

Amplifier/Receiver

Wiring to carry signal from unaidable side microphone to amplifier and receiver side

Tube to ear

Microphone

Fig. 4.23 Because feedback cancellation had not yet been invented, in early years the eyeglass CROS aid, shown in the illustration, allowed open canal amplification. The microphone was connected to the receiver by a wire through the eyeglass frame, and the separation between the two substantially reduced the chance of feedback. First used to fit patients with unilateral hearing loss, it soon expanded for use with patients having bilateral high-frequency losses. Adapted with permission from Staab.[147]

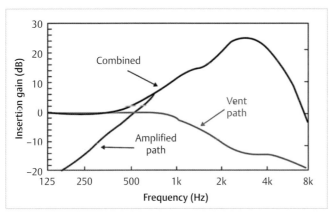

Fig. 4.24 The incoming unamplified signal passes through the vent, combining with the amplification provided by the hearing aid in the residual cavity to produce the spectrum shown by the dark line in the illustration. Adapted with permission from Dillon.[3]

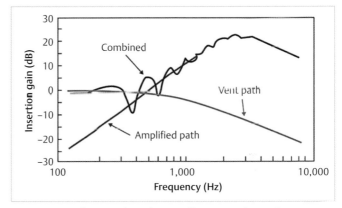

Fig. 4.25 The combined cancellation and reinforcement effects of the amplified signal and vent path signal due to phase and amplitude interactions may be observed when performing real-ear measurements, as above. These perturbations are essentially either absent or diminished during actual listening situations, and have little or no effect on perception of the amplified signal. Adapted with permission from Dillon.[3]

greater than any sounds coming though the vent. Here the dominant amplified signal will be directly transmitted to the eardrum without being affected in any way by the out-of-phase arrival times.[3,148]

However, whenever the amplified and vent transmitted unamplified sounds have nearly identical levels, cancellation and reinforcement effects may appear in a portion of the combined spectrum. If both signals are exactly equal in phase and amplitude, they are reinforced by about 6 dB; if the signals are 180 degrees out of phase, the amount of cancellation is about 10 dB. In reality, the two signal paths will rarely be equal in amplitude nor exactly 180 degrees in or out of phase, but rather will vary, because normally the source signals are constantly and rapidly changing

in amplitude and phase relationships.[3] In most situations, therefore, spectral notches and peaks due to cancellation and reinforcement will be substantially reduced or absent in the real ear. In other words, the effect on the combined signal, though it may be detected in REAR measurements, is more operative in theory than in practice (▶**Fig. 4.25**).[19]

In hearing aids with approximately 5 ms or less delay studies have shown that the out-of-phase arrival times of the two signals are occasionally discernible.[146] More importantly, however, the preponderance of evidence suggests there is generally little or no effect on acceptability by subjects with mild-to-moderate hearing loss.[148,149,150,151]

4.2.17 Achieving Insertion Gain Targets

Gain is increased by about 10 to 15 dB or more in the 2,000- to 3,000-Hz region in open canal fittings (compared to closed) because of the addition of the open ear effects (canal and concha resonance, head and pinna baffles, etc.) to the amplified signal (▶ Fig. 4.22).[3,35] Nevertheless, in some unoccluding, very large vent fittings, occasionally the desired amount of high-frequency gain needed to match targets may not be achievable before acoustic feedback occurs.[8,59,152] Reducing the vent's size will enable some restoration of gain in the high frequencies and increase amplification in the lows, and as well, the chance that the occlusion effect will also be enhanced. In adults, achieving a very good target match in the high frequencies at the expense of increasing the occlusion effect can be a poor bargain; resolving the occlusion effect and foregoing a perfect match is often the better option.[3] Fortunately, modern feedback cancellation algorithms permit increases in gain of approximately 15 to 20 dB,[125,153,154] providing a better chance of achieving approximate matches in the high frequencies without resorting to reducing the size of the venting.

4.2.18 Fourth Reason for Using Vents is to Provide Pressure Equalization or Circulation of Air in the Residual Cavity

Some patients with very severe or greater losses may experience discomfort (a sense of stuffiness) if fitted with totally occluding earmold/shells, and desire some sort of equilibration of pressure between the outside ambient atmosphere and the residual space.[22,61,106] Fine intentional vents (e.g., 0.04 mm) are sometimes drilled to alleviate the perceived pressure imbalance, or very small external "trench" vents can be grooved into the periphery of the earmold/shell (▶ Fig. 4.15). Although both maneuvers may provide relief, unfortunately, repeated plugging with earwax or debris may interfere with providing a permanent resolution of the complaint.

4.3 The Hearing Aid Transmission Line

4.3.1 Resonance Peaks

In standard-tube BTE hearing aids, the length and diameter of the ear hook, the earmold's tubing, and the bore and length of the earmold together form an acoustic transmission line from the hearing aid receiver to the termination of the earmold in the residual cavity (▶ Fig. 4.26). (A similar transmission line is present in thin-tube BTE fittings, but to a lesser degree, for the ear hook is absent.) Because ordinarily there is high impedance at the receiver end, and essentially lower impedance at the residual cavity and eardrum,[36,38,48] a series of (quarter) wavelength resonances (peaks) may occur in the system at about 1,000 Hz and odd multiples.[23,48] Although not a substantive issue in modern BTE fittings, the presence of transmission line peaks has been found to negatively affect intelligibility and the quality of amplification,[155,156] or if a peak is great enough, it may invade the patient's uncomfortable level, necessitating reduction of overall gain.[157,158]

Until the 1970s, there was really only one method available to reduce the resonance peaks in analog BTE hearing aids; hearing aid dispensers played with "lamb's wool," a type of cotton-like material, installing various amounts in vent holes or in the tubing to damp or smooth response peaks, a hit and miss, unreliable practice.

A better way to damp peaks in a BTE hearing aid's response was introduced in the late 1970s, involving placement of fused mesh damping elements of various impedances at certain locations in the ear hook, tubing, or earmold bore.[23,33,159,160] These dampers, each with different impedance values, act as simple resistances, smoothing out, and diminishing the resonance peaks (▶ Fig. 4.27). They are superior to lamb's

A contemporary perspective

Today, issues of resonant peaks are not a substantive issue in standard-tube and thin-tube BTE instruments and are essentially absent in RIC and custom instruments. Digital filtering is used at the manufacturing level to reduce or round off any peaks[161]; further, in digital signal processing (DSP) aids that feature a high number of independent channels, fitting software can be used to control the occasional peak.

In the 1980s, interest in response modification of the transmission line also led to the introduction of a series of special purpose "acoustically tuned" ear hooks by Killion and colleagues to manipulate various portions of the hearing aid's frequency-gain response.[33,34,162] Examples of the type of gain-frequency response variations they produce are shown in ▶ Fig. 4.9. Today their use is limited, but interested clinicians may obtain additional information by contacting Etymotic Research.

Further information about the use of dampers in ear hooks and tubing can be found in Dillon,[3] Mueller et al,[35] and Valente and Valente.[13] Additionally, BTE ear hooks with fused mesh dampers of various impedances already installed are available from some hearing aid manufacturers.

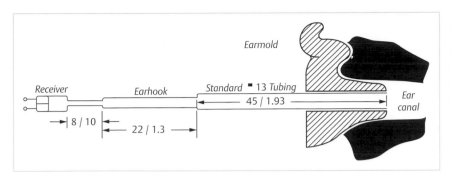

Fig. 4.26 Sketch of a BTE acoustic transmission line. Note systematic increases in the diameter of each successive element that provide the foundation for utilization of horn molds (see text; also ▶Fig. 4.28). Adapted with permission from Cox.[19]

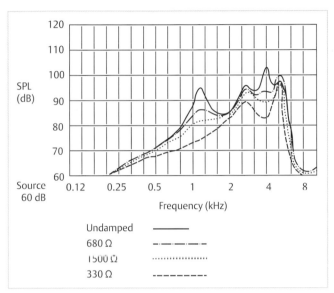

Fig. 4.27 Before the advent of digital signal processing, the clinician could reduce the resonance peaks in the amplified response of an analog instrument by installing dampers of different impedance values in the ear hook or tubing. Adapted with permission from Valente and Valente.[13]

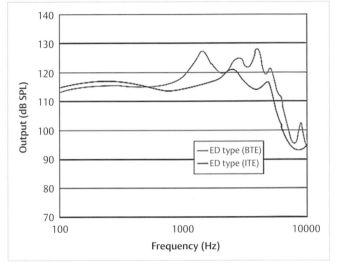

Fig. 4.28 Shows the response of the same receiver in both a BTE and ITE configuration. Note the lessening or absence of peaks in the ITE condition; the acoustic transmission line (ear hook, tubing, earmold) is nearly eliminated. Adapted with permission from Kuk and Baekgaard.[8]

wool, for they produce repeatable effects. However, whether located in the tubing, ear hook, or bore, caution is advised for they tend to quickly plug up with moisture and debris and need to be changed often.

Although manufacturers doctored the response of analog BTE hearing aids electronically and mechanically as best they could to minimize peaks,[33,48,163] it continued to be an issue until the introduction of custom hearing aids. The advent of custom hearing aids partially reduced the problem as shown in ▶Fig. 4.28. The acoustic transmission line in custom aids is appreciably shorter; consequently, most resonant peaks are shifted to higher frequencies, beyond the bandwidth of the instrument.[48]

4.3.2 Acoustic Horns

Killion introduced the use of the acoustic horn for use with custom BTE earmolds in the early 1980s.[7,32,48,160,164] During this period, the first wide-band receivers came on the market; as a result, use of a horn earmold for further increasing high-frequency gain and bandwidth became possible.[165] Horn earmolds are fabricated by systematically increasing the inside diameter of the transmission line starting at the receiver, through the ear hook and tubing, to the tip of the earmold (▶Fig. 4.29 and ▶Fig. 4.26). This acoustic horn structure decreases the mismatch between the impedance of the hearing aid's receiver system (source), and the impedance of the ear canal/middle ear system,[19] resulting in a better transmission of high-frequency signals at 3,000 Hz and above, a desirable outcome. ▶Fig. 4.30 shows the high-frequency boost obtained with various BTE horn mold constructions. Dillon[3] has suggested that this elegant horn concept may also be useful for boosting high-frequency signals when fitting thin-tube BTE hearing for they ordinarily have slightly less high-frequency bandwidth by comparison to standard-tube BTE hearing aids.[35,116,166]

A constriction located anywhere along the acoustic transmission line is called a "reverse" horn, and will cause a decided reduction of amplification in the high

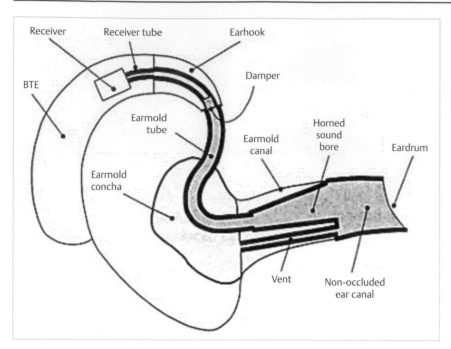

Fig. 4.29 The diagram illustrates the hearing aid transmission line culminating in an acoustic horn earmold. Installation of a damper, as shown in this diagram, is not required to produce useful horn formation. Adapted with permission from Pirzanski .[167]

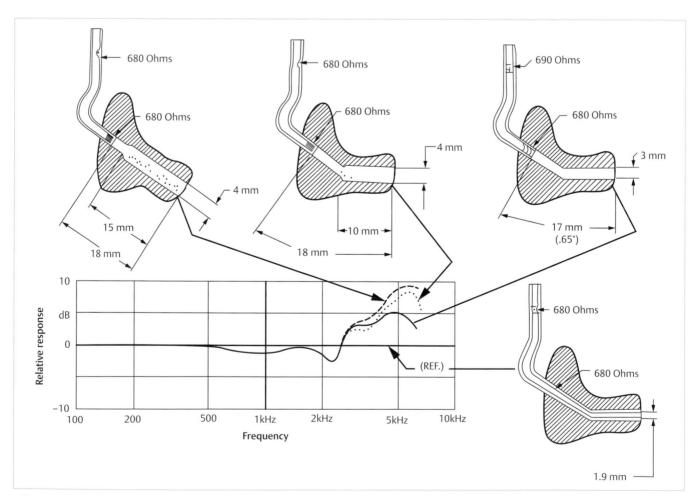

Fig. 4.30 Killion showed how small changes to an earmold's bore would result in increasing high-frequency transmission. Here again dampers were installed to reduce peaks, but if absent, do not negatively impact the horn effect. (see also ▶**Fig. 4.32**) Adapted with permission from Killion.[32]

frequencies rather than boosting it. For example, if when fitting a high-power BTE aid, a thick-tube (3.30-mm OD) is substituted for a standard tube (1.30-mm OD) to reduce vibration-induced feedback, forcing the thick tube into an earmold bore that has been drilled for a standard-size tube will produce an acoustic constriction and roll off the high frequencies.

A common form of reverse horn is shown in ►Fig. 4.31 where earmold tubing is pulled through

---

Limitations of the earmold horn effect

It is difficult to build earmolds with acoustic horns in custom hearing aids or RIC aids (and body aids, for that matter). The reason has to do with the short distance (transmission line) that follows the receiver to the end of the earmold. In BTE aids, the ear hook, earmold tubing, and earmold are long enough together to allow formation of an appropriate horn coupling apparatus. In custom hearing aids unless special steps are taken,[168] the receiver tube is insufficient in length to execute useful horn formation. Some earmold laboratories offer horn-like earmolds for use with RIC aids; be aware that any high-frequency boost that obtains will be above 5,000 to 6,000 Hz.[3]

At one time, most earmold laboratories offered preformed molded horns of various sizes, (e.g., the Libby horn,[169,170] Bakke horn, and the continuous-flow adaptor [CFA]), that could be ordered installed into a BTE custom earmold. However, their use is limited by the size of the patient's ear canal, a particular problem with young children, and have been discontinued by some earmold laboratories. As an alternative, the horn effect may be partially achieved by carefully grinding out and enlarging the sound bore in the earmold as deeply as possible (8–10 mm or greater), leaving enough of the earmold tubing in place (at least 5 mm) to prevent accidental detachment (►Fig. 4.32). [3,19,171]

---

to the tip of the earmold. The tubing through to the tip serves as a constriction in the acoustic transmission path before sound enters the residual cavity. Clinicians should be aware that drawing the tube through to the tip of a BTE mold will cause a constriction or "reverse" horn that, in consequence, will reduce some amount of high-frequency amplification, usually an unfavorable situation.[172,173]

4.3.3 Adjustable Venting Systems

Nearly all manufacturers and earmold laboratories provide sets of venting plugs or tubing inserts that can be fitted into the vent apertures of BTE earmolds, RIC ear-

molds, or custom hearing aid shells (►Fig. 4.33). The hollow tubes have different inside and outside diameters; the venting plugs have varying inside diameters. Known by different names, such as select-a-vents or variable vents, their primary use is to reduce the diameter of a preinstalled vent in order to control feedback in moderately severe to severe hearing losses.

At one-time, adjustable venting systems were recommended for modifying or adjusting the low-frequency portion of the amplified spectrum, but vent plugs especially have been found to be essentially ineffectual and unpredictable as response modification adjuncts.[19,21,27] Realistically, these venting systems are only useful for reducing feedback in moderate-to-severe losses. Adjusting and manipulating low-frequency gain in partially occluding and occluding couplings is more easily affected by using computer-mediated software and other forms of earmold modification.

4.3.4 Stock Ear Tips

Stock ear tips have a long history in the hearing aid industry, going back in various forms to before the 1930s (►Fig. 4.34). Their usage gradually diminished over the years after the introduction of custom earmolds, for the latter ensured better fit and better control over acoustic effects and feedback. With the advent of RIC and thin-tube BTE instruments, various manufacturers reintroduced sets of stock silicone ear tips (also variously termed preformed, prefabricated, disposable, instant-fit, modular earbuds, ear sets, or domes) designed to slip over the receiver of RIC hearing aids or onto the tubing of thin-tube BTE aids (►Fig. 4.35a, b). Incorporating graduated amounts of venting, from unoccluding to occluding, the ear tips are specifically intended to substitute for custom earmolds.

Open, vented, unoccluded stock ear tips are often used in open canal fittings as they are effective in resolving mild-to-moderate high-frequency, flat, or sloping losses (►Fig. 4.36).[141,142] Their plentiful use in these fittings is partially responsible for the rapid growth of RIC hearing aid fittings in the last decades.[115]

On the other hand, despite careful attention to selection and fitting, occluded stock ear tips, (those with no vents), intended for patients with moderate to moderately severe losses, vary in their sealing efficiency across subjects and under test–retest conditions, as do maximally occluded power domes intend for advanced hearing losses. ►Fig. 4.37 and ►Fig. 4.38).[68,174] Depth of insertion and degree of seal have the potential to change within the same patient each time the aid is removed and reinserted. It is conceivable, therefore, given the chance of variability of occluded and maximally occluding power ear tip fittings, that initial target matches may be compromised under normal wearing conditions.

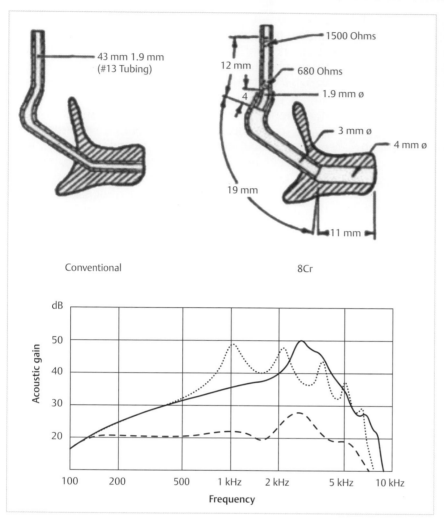

Fig. 4.31 Dotted line shows the frequency-gain response for a BTE hearing aid when the earmold tubing is pulled through to the end of the bore versus a horn mold. Note, approximately 10 dB greater gain at about 3,000 Hz with the horn earmold (8CR) as opposed to the "conventional" earmold with the tubing terminated at the end of the mold. Dampers were used to smooth out the response of the (8CR) fitting, but are unnecessary in modern digital BTE aids. (Adapted with permission from Killion.[33])

Stock ear tips versus custom earmolds

Occasional reports from the field indicate that some experienced practitioners have opted to fit custom earmolds for RIC and thin-tube BTE fittings rather than stock ear tips.[35,141,175] For these clinicians, the advantages of custom earmolds include the following:

1. Greater control of venting effects, the frequency-gain response, and target matching in a repeatable manner.
2. Custom earmolds resolve the problem of inserting and properly placing the ear tip for patients with dexterity issues.
3. Some ear canals develop a skin sensitivity with repeated insertion and removal of the stock ear tips, and/or to ear tip material.
4. Some consider the custom earmold fitting, by contrast to an off-the-shelf ear tip, to be a more professional approach to dispensing.

A final note: It is our observation that the increased usage of stock silicone ear tips in lieu of custom earmolds has resulted, unfortunately, in a reduction of the clinical experience required for accurate impression taking, especially in students and new practitioners. Certainly, excellence in dispensing and patient care necessarily requires a high degree of comfort and conversance with these skills, which are obtained only with commitment and repetition.

4.3.5 In-Office Bench Modifications

From time to time, there will be need for on-the-spot modifications to the couplings, for example, reducing or thinning the helix area, tapering or shortening the canal tip, altering the vent, or grinding and buffing down the exterior surface. The prime candidates, however, for in-office modification, are cases when relief from the occlusion effect is desired. There will be more than a few times in the busy practice where "opening" the fitting will provide an immediate resolution. As mentioned earlier, there are two basic bench modification procedures that are customarily recommended for unoccluding a custom earmold/

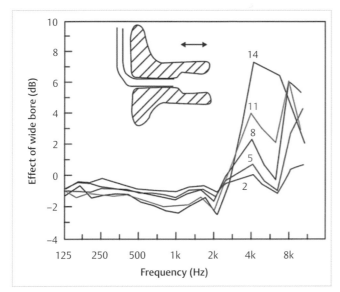

Fig. 4.32 Illustrates the high-frequency gain that can be achieved by simply drilling out (enlarging and lengthening) the bore in a BTE earmold to various depths (in millimeter). Adapted with permission from Dillon.[3]

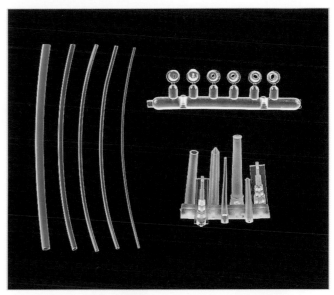

Fig. 4.33 Shows a variety of vent plugs and tubing inserts for use with custom hearing aids and custom earmold fittings. These adjustable vent systems can be useful for reducing feedback. The vent plugs are press fitted into the vent's external opening, and the hollow tubes are inserted into an existing vent path to decrease the vent's diameter. Courtesy of Starkey Hearing Technologies.

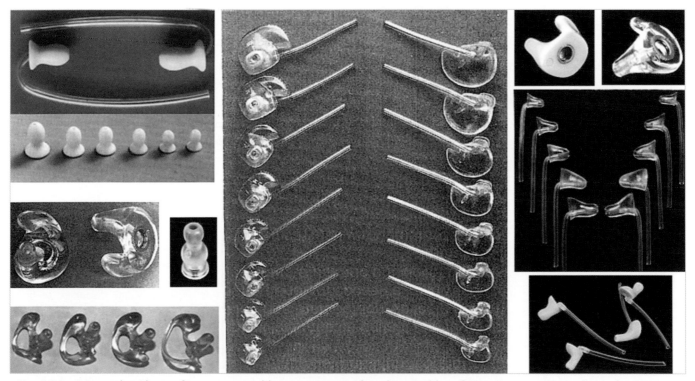

Fig. 4.34 Prior to the advent of custom earmolds, various types of stock earmolds or fitting tips were routinely used to connect the hearing aid to the ear. Their use has never entirely disappeared, witness the recent introduction of stock silicon ear tips for use with RIC and thin-tube BTE hearing aids. Adapted with permission from Staab.[147]

custom shell, (1) increasing the diameter of the vent, and, (2) shortening the length of the vent. Each will affect the low-frequency portion of the amplified spectrum by decreasing the vent's acoustic mass. (Recall that as the diameter of a vent is increased or as a vent is shortened, mass decreases accordingly, resulting in greater roll-off/attenuation in the low frequencies.)

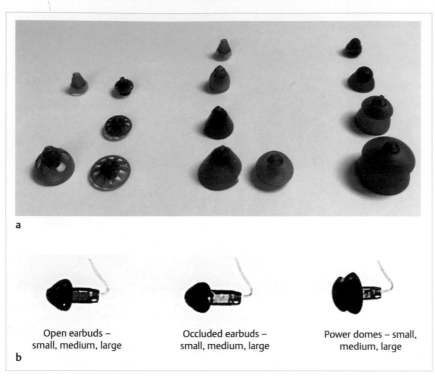

a

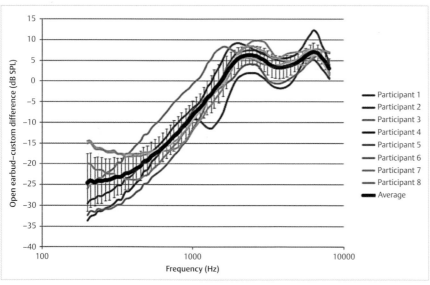

Open earbuds –
small, medium, large

Occluded earbuds –
small, medium, large

Power domes – small,
medium, large

b

Fig. 4.35   (a) Three basic versions (*left* to *right*) of typical stock ear tips: unoccluding (open), occluding (no vent), and maximally occluding (power or double dome). **(b)** Shows the ear tips installed on RIC receivers. Illustrations courtesy of Starkey Hearing Technologies.

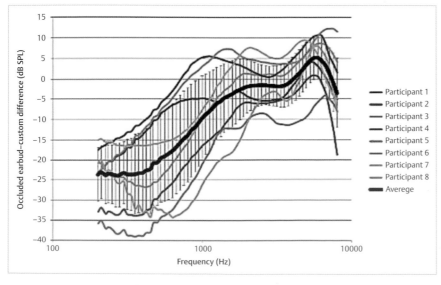

Fig. 4.36   The real-ear responses of eight subjects wearing unoccluding (open) stock ear tips showing acceptable reduction in the low frequencies for each subject. The solid line depicts the average response. A hole was installed in each ear tip into which the probe tube was tightly sealed to assure no additional slit leak. Adapted with permission from Coburn et al.[68]

Fig. 4.37   The real-ear responses of eight subjects wearing occluding (no vent) stock ear tips showing widely dispersed sealing across subjects. In some subjects, the low-frequency roll-off due to leakage was similar to that obtained with the unoccluding stock ear tips shown in ▶Fig. 4.35. A hole was installed in each ear tip into which the probe tube was tightly sealed to assure no additional slit leak. Adapted with permission from Coburn et al.[68]

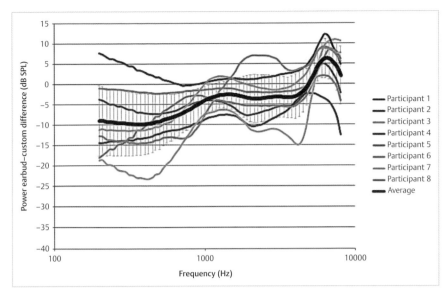

Fig. 4.38 Depicts the inconsistent sealing efficiency of maximally occluding (power dome, ultra or double dome) stock ear tips for eight subjects. A hole was installed in each ear tip into which the probe tube was tightly sealed to assure no additional slit leak. Adapted with permission from coburn et al.[68]

Shortening the vent

The recommended way to shorten the vent is to start from the tip of the canal, removing in small steps the material that surrounds the vent (▶ Fig. 4.39). The path of the vent in the aid is followed as it becomes exposed by grinding. Only a small amount of excess material from around the vent opening is removed at a time, followed in turn by buffing and polishing. The aid is then inserted in the ear for the patient to listen to and to evaluate the change in performance. The shortening steps are repeated as many times as necessary until the patient no longer perceives the occlusion effect (▶ Fig. 4.40). All surfaces should be smoothed and gently rounded to prevent irritation. The key idea is to proceed in small steps, repeatedly allowing the patient to listen after each modification (Curran,[176] see ▶ Fig. 4.40a, ▶ Fig. 4.40b, and ▶ Fig. 4.40c).

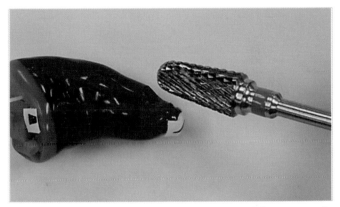

Fig. 4.39 Expose the vent by removing a small amount of material at a time, starting at the tip of the earmold or custom instrument. Courtesy of Starkey Hearing Technologies.

Most sources when discussing tactics for resolving the occlusion effect recommend increasing the vent's diameter to attenuate low frequencies. In our opinion, this maneuver, when properly accomplished, though highly effective, can be a difficult proposition. Enlarging the vent's diameter requires some skill when modifying a custom aid or a RIC aid with a custom-embedded mold to avoid accidentally drilling into the hearing aid or the receiver, and may take considerable time to accomplish.

Alternatively, shortening the vent to "open" up the fitting may be a simpler and quicker way to reduce the occlusion effect, and appropriate for use with custom BTE earmolds (including embedded RIC molds as well as standard- and thin-tube BTE molds) and custom hearing aids. As mentioned earlier, a short vent, besides having less mass, presents less resistance to the escape of sound around the periphery of the mold/shell than a longer vent, resulting in an increase in slit leak, which adds further low-frequency reduction to the signal.[3,19,27,70,81]

In addition to shortening the vent from the medial end of the earmold/shell, one might also shorten the vent from the lateral, exterior surface, but care must be taken to not affect retention properties, especially in canal aids. Further, in some ears, the elasticity of the skin at the aperture

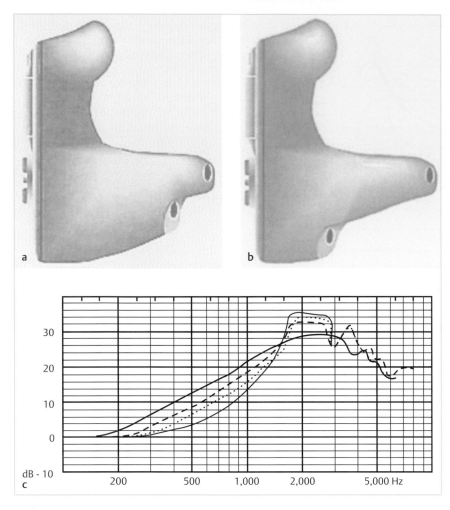

c

Fig. 4.40 **(a)** Shows a custom instrument with the vent shortened approximately 6 mm from the tip. Notice that the sides of the exposed vent have been smoothed and reduced. **(b)** Considerable shortening of the vent to about 15 mm from the tip. Proceed in a series of small steps, each time reinserting the aid to check the effect of the shortening on the occlusion effect. (Courtesy of Starkey Hearing Technologies). **(c)** Shows the results of vent shortening for the instrument shown in **(a)** and **(b)**. Notice a reduction in gain of approximately 10 to 12 dB in the 500- to 1,000-Hz range as the vent was successively shortened approximately 14 mm from the tip. Courtesy of Curran.[177,178]

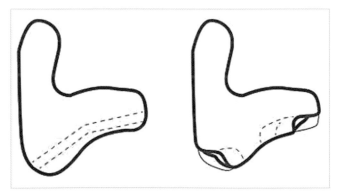

Fig. 4.41 Illustrates removal of material from both ends of the vent. The vent may be both shortened and also enlarged at the same time as needed. Adapted with permission from Dillon.[3]

may be such that it may droop and block the exterior vent opening if shortened. Finally, slightly increasing the diameter of the vent's bore at either the exterior lateral opening or the medial

end of the vent will also result in decreasing mass (▶ **Fig. 4.41**).

4.3.6 Modifying Custom Canal Hearing Aids

Some custom canal aids may have shorter canals (and, consequently, shorter vents) than full-shell ITE aids or fully occluding custom earmolds, and all things being equal, will likely have less acoustic mass and greater acoustic leakage by comparison. Because of these factors, vent shortening should be quite effective in reducing low-frequency output by comparison to custom aids or earmolds having longer canals (▶ **Fig. 4.42**).[59,60,65] However, if not satisfactory, there are other traditional methods for minimizing the occlusion effect: (1) tapering and/or shortening the tip (▶ **Fig. 4.43**) or (2) making a trench vent (▶ **Fig. 4.15**). Each maneuver will increase slit leak resulting in an increase of low-frequency transmission loss.

Importance of bench modification skills

It is the observation of the authors that instruction in the skills necessary for executing simple modifications to custom earmolds or custom hearing aids in the office has received less emphasis during the last decade. Use of off-the-shelf stock ear tips and computer-mediated fitting software has made fitting certain losses less of a problem than previously. However, the ability to perform simple on-the-spot modifications to custom earmolds or custom shells is not only clinically desirable and economical, it speaks directly to the practitioner's competence. Making the effort to learn and practice modification skills is especially important for the beginning clinician, for it makes the clinician a highly desirable colleague in any practice setting. For the interested audiologist desirous of further increasing bench skills, Starkey makes available an online *Modification Guide* that gives instructions with illustrations for accomplishing many modification techniques. It can be downloaded at https://starkeypro.com/pdfs/Hearing_Aid_Modification_Guide.pdf

In addition, articles by Curran[177,178,179] cover the equipment recommended and some details of the procedures described in this and other sections.

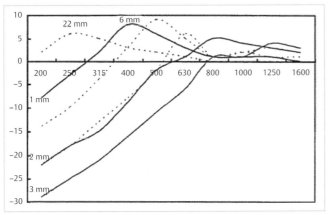

Fig. 4.42 The graph shows the effect of increasing the vent diameter in two earmolds, one with a short vent (6 mm), and the other with a long vent (22 mm). As expected, the vent-related resonance shifts toward the higher frequencies in both earmolds as the diameters of the vents increase. Note the 2-mm diameter short vent provides the same amount of attenuation in the low frequencies as the 3-mm diameter provides long vent. The conclusion is that given the same vent diameter, shorter vents afford greater low-frequency roll-off than longer vents. Adapted with permission from Kuk and Keenan.[59]

4.3.7 Suggestions for Earmold Selection

How does one make a decision about what kind or type of earmold/custom shell to fit? To provide some basic guidance, we divide couplings into three broad categories[10,11] according to the amount/degree of occlusion medial to the concha-meatal junction (aperture). Each category, in turn, is loosely related to the configuration and degree of loss shown by the patient's pure tone threshold audiogram at 250, 500, 750 (if available), and 1,000 Hz.

- Category 1 earmolds/shells are defined as open or almost entirely unoccluding.
- Category 2 earmolds/shells are both partially open and partially occluding.
- Category 3 includes earmolds/shells that are nearly or completely occluding, with either a small pressure relief vent or no vent.

▶**Fig. 4.44** shows an audiogram template that illustrates approximate ranges of the three coupling categories. By fitting the patient's low-frequency thresholds (250–1,000 Hz) into the template, one can gain a general idea of what category of earmold/custom shell may be suitable. **Table 4.4** summarizes the types of couplings available for the three categories.

4.3.8 Category 1 Fittings

Category 1 couplings, entirely or almost entirely unoccluding, incorporate very large venting in one form or another. They are capable of providing the greatest degree of low-frequency transmission loss, and at the same time allow a broad range of unam-

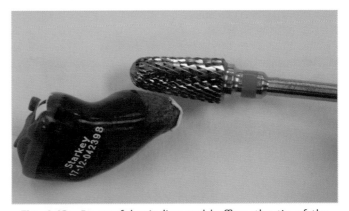

Fig. 4.43 By careful grinding and buffing, the tip of the earmold/shell may be shortened or tapered to increase slit leak, producing greater low-frequency roll-off. Courtesy of Starkey Hearing Technologies.

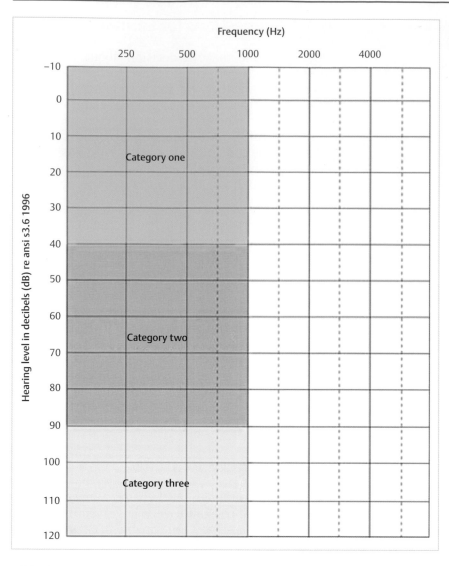

Fig. 4.44 By fitting the patient's low-frequency thresholds (250–1,000 Hz) into the template, one can gain a general idea of what coupling category may be suitable. Refer to **Table 4.4** for a summary of the types of fittings available in the three categories.

plified low-, mid-, and high-frequency sounds to pass into the residual cavity through the vent. To be considered a Category 1 fitting, the thresholds in the low frequencies, 250 to 1,000 Hz, should not exceed approximately 35 to 45 dB HL, as greater low-frequency loss usually will require greater occlusion (▶ **Fig. 4.44**). Category 1 fittings include mild, moderate, flat, or gently sloping losses as well as precipitously sloping high-frequency losses.

The coupling options available for Category 1 fittings include the following:

1. *Hollow earmolds.* The hollow earmold may be the most popular custom mold for RIC and BTE aids (▶ **Fig. 4.45a, b**).[69,180] Hollow molds ordinarily have a wall thickness of 0.07 to 1 mm and therefore a vent placed in the tip of a hollow mold will be the same length as the wall thickness. Hollow mold vents, therefore, will have substantially less mass than a similar diameter vent in a solid earmold. In addition, since hollow earmolds are often shorter than solid BTE earmolds, there is ordinarily more slit leak. Kuk et al[180] concluded the combination of less mass and greater slit leak in hollow molds provides markedly greater transmission loss in the low frequencies compared to solid molds with vents of the same diameter. They found, for example, that installation of a 1-mm vent in a hollow mold is roughly equivalent to a 3-mm vent in a solid custom earmold, and showed that hollow mold vents of 2 mm and above tend toward nearly complete unocclusion.

2. *RIC embedded earmolds.* In these fittings, the RIC receiver is *embedded* within the mold itself by the manufacturer. A Category 1 embedded mold with a very large vent is sometimes referred to as and IROS or biggest available vent (BAV) mold and the large vent will vary in size according to degree of loss, receiver size, and ear canal geometry (▶ **Fig. 4.46**).

Table 4.4 Coupling suggestions that may be appropriate for use in each of the categories defined in ▶ Fig. 4.44

	Standard tube Behind the Ear (BTE)	Thin tube Behind the Ear (BTE)	Receiver in the Canal (R1C)	Custom ITE, ITC, CIC
Category 1	Custom Free Field, IROS, tube	Custom Free Field, IROS, tube	Helix IROS	Largo vent, IROS, BAV,*** or manufacturer's decision**
	Custom Hollow, BAV Medium vent	Custom Hollow, BAV Medium vent	Custom Hollow, BAV;*** Custom embedded, BAV***	
		Stock eartip, unoccluded	Stock eartip, unoccluded	
		Stock sleeve	Stock sleeve	
Category 2	Custom Modifier* large vent	Custom Modifier* large vent	Custom Hollow, medium parallel vent*	Medium vent*, or manufacturer's decision**
	Custom short canal* medium vent	Custom short canal* medium vent	Custom embedded, medium vent*	
	Custom Hollow, parallel vent	Custom Hollow, parallel vent	Stock eartip, occluded	
		Stock eartip, occluded		
Category 3	Custom, deep canal, small vent	Stock eartip, power	Custom embedded, no vent"	Deep canal, no vent
	Custom, deep canal, no vent		Stock eartip, power	
	* Optional tube inserts	** Vent size based on space available		*** Biggest available vent

Notes: With the exception of Category 3, there is more than one option available for each type of hearing aid.
Source: Courtesy of Starkey Hearing Technologies.

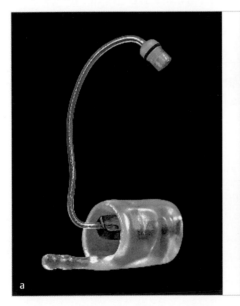
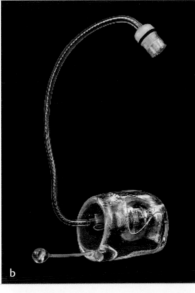

Fig. 4.45 Two versions of Category 1 RIC hollow earmolds: **(a)** Soft. **(b)** Hard. Courtesy of Starkey Hearing Technologies.

3. *Unoccluding (large vent) stock ear tips.* Used with both RIC instruments and thin-tube BTE hearing aids, these are often referred to as ear buds and include stock sleeves that can be slipped over the receiver for a completely open fitting (▶ Fig. 4.7, ▶ Fig. 4.35a, b).

4. *Custom BTE earmolds.* Used with standard-tube BTE or thin-tube BTE aids, they are

unoccluding molds, CROS molds, IROS molds, or Janssen molds, each having slightly different shapes (▶Fig. 4.3 and ▶Fig. 4.4a), and provide nearly total unocclusion.

5. *Custom hearing aids (including ITE, ITC, CIC, and IIC).* Routinely used in Category 1 fittings since their inception, they may be obtained by specifying an IROS or BAV vent (▶Fig. 4.47a, b). Each manufacturer has proprietary rules; therefore, vent sizes may differ according to degree of loss, the type of custom aid ordered, and size constraints.

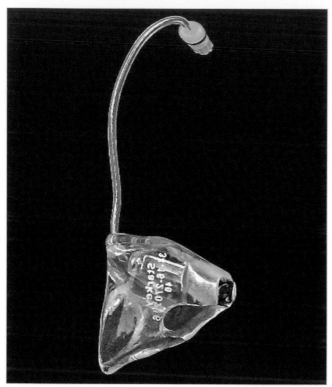

Fig. 4.46 A Category 1 embedded RIC earmold with a biggest available vent (BAV). Courtesy of Starkey Hearing Technologies.

However, more often than not, in most instances they provide adequate unocclusion.

4.3.9 Category 2 Fittings

▶Fig. 4.44 shows the approximate range of low-frequency audiometric thresholds for Category 2 fittings. These fittings represent a partially open and partially closed condition, providing both a certain amount of low-frequency gain as well as allowing some unamplified signals to pass into the ear through the vent, depending on the size of the venting. As the hearing loss becomes greater in the low frequencies, so does the need to increase the occlusion of the fitting; the balance begins to shift toward occlusion, but not entirely. They are indicated for gently sloping, flat, and irregular audiometric configuration from approximately 40 to 50 dB HL to about 75 to 85 dB HL in the low frequencies (250–750 Hz).

The coupling options available for Category 2 fittings are as follows:

1. *Hollow earmolds.* For use with RIC and thin-tube BTE aids, custom hollow molds can be ordered with a parallel vent (1–2 mm) that runs the length of the earmold; however, Kuk et al[180] found that hollow molds lose their effectiveness as the hearing loss becomes greater and more gain is needed. Adjustable tubing inserts are recommended (▶Fig. 4.45a, b).

2. *RIC embedded earmolds.* For moderate losses, 1.5- to 2-mm vents may be installed; for moderately severe losses, 1- to 1.5-mm vents (▶Fig. 4.48). These molds may require some form of wax mitigation at the end of the receiver spout.

3. *Occluding (no vent) stock ear tips.* Used with both RIC and thin-tube BTE

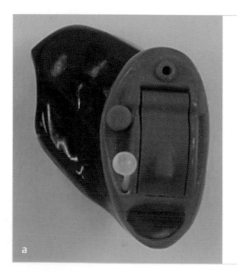
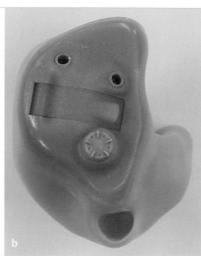

Fig. 4.47 **(a)** Shows BAV for Category 1 custom canal aids. **(b)** Typical IROS vent for Category 1 custom ITE. Each manufacturer has its own versions of venting for custom aids. Courtesy of Starkey Hearing Technologies.

instruments, no-vent (occluding) stock ear tips, often called earbuds, may vary considerably in sealing ability.[68] Slit leak may change each time the hearing aid is removed and replaced, affecting gain in the low frequencies (►**Fig. 4.47**, ►**Fig. 4.35a, b**).

4. *Custom earmolds.* Used with standard- and thin-tube BTE aids. For moderate losses, the so-called "modifier" earmold, that is, shortened, sometimes belled canal with

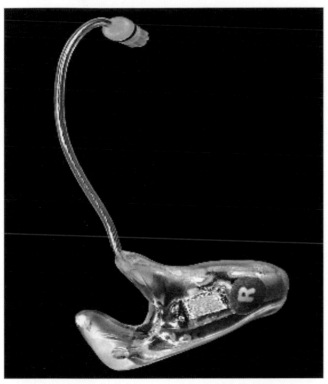

Fig. 4.48 A variation of a Category 2 RIC embedded (canal) earmold with 1.5-mm vent at bottom of mold. The bottom vent lends itself to shortening if less occlusion is desired, or tubing inserts can be used to provide greater occlusion. Courtesy of Starkey Hearing Technologies.

appreciable vents (2–4 mm) (►**Fig. 4.49a, b**). As the hearing loss becomes greater in the low frequencies, so does the need to increase the occlusion of the fitting; longer canals with smaller-diameter vents (1–2 mm) become desirable. Adjustable tubing inserts or vent plugs are recommended for use with Category 2 custom molds, either to increase occlusion (and gain) and/or decrease acoustic feedback.

5. *Custom hearing aids (including ITE, ITC, CIC, and IIC).* Routinely available with different vent sizes (►**Fig. 4.49a, b**). Each manufacturer has proprietary rules; the size of the vent that is installed is based on degree of hearing loss, the type of custom aid ordered, and size constraints. Adjustable tubing inserts are a recommended option in Category 2 custom hearing aid fittings, either to increase occlusion (and gain) and/or decrease acoustic feedback (►**Fig. 4.50**).

4.3.10 Category 3 Fittings

Category 3 fittings are indicated for flat or sloping losses of 85 to 90 dB HL (250–500 Hz) or greater (►**Fig. 4.44**). They can be described as either (1) a totally occluding (closed), deep canal earmold/ shell with a very small intentional vent, or (2) a totally occluding, very deep canal earmold/shell with no vent.

The coupling options available for Category 3 fittings are as follows:

1. *Custom BTE earmolds.* For use with standard- or thin-tube BTE aids, moderately deep to very deep, tightly fitted canals are recommended. Very small pressure relief vents (0.04 mm or less)

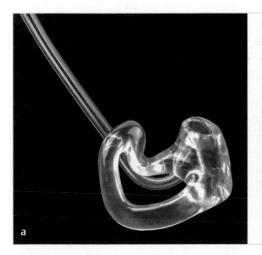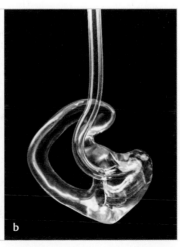

Fig. 4.49 (a, b) Two aspects of the Category 2 "modifier" BTE earmold. It features a short-to-medium hollowed out canal and short 2- to 4-mm vent. Adjustable vent plugs or tubing inserts are recommended (see►**Fig. 4.33**). Courtesy of Starkey Hearing Technologies.

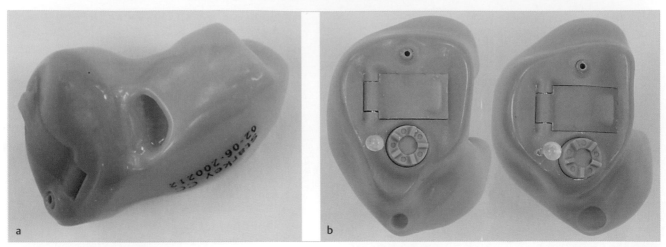

Fig. 4.50 **(a)** Shows example of venting for Category 2 custom CIC hearing aid. **(b)** Different size of vents are available for Category 2 custom ITE hearing aids according to need. Use of tubing inserts and/or bench modifications are recommended for opening or closing the vent. (see ▶ **Fig. 4.33**). Each manufacturer has its own versions of venting for Category 2 custom aids. Courtesy of Starkey Hearing Technologies.

Regions of transition

There is no absolute demarcation between Categories 1 and 2, nor between Categories 2 and 3, for the configuration of the threshold values reveal nothing about the physical properties of the ear and little consistent information regarding individual perception of occlusion.[30,39] For example, one patient may require additional low-frequency gain (a partially occluding Category 2 fitting), whereas another with nearly identical thresholds may be satisfactorily fitted with a more open, unoccluding coupling (Category 1).

When unsure, seasoned professionals will hedge their bet when ordering an earmold or custom aid, choosing an option then will allow bench modification of the vent or the earmold to a more open or closed condition as needed. For example, a Category 2 solid BTE custom earmold of medium depth and 2-mm vent may be easily converted in the office along a continuum leading to a nearly unoccluding Category 1 fitting by greatly enlarging or shortening the vent, and by shortening the canal length; a no vent hollow mold may be converted from occluding to unoccluding by installing a small vent and successively increasing the diameter in small steps.

may be installed depending on degree of loss. Care should be taken to assure appropriate retention properties without extreme bulkiness; skeleton and shell configurations are useful recommendations (▶ **Fig. 4.51a, b**).

2. *RIC embedded earmolds.* The largest available receiver is embedded in a solid, deeply inserted earmold to provide the needed gain and output; variously referred to as an absolute power (AP) or ultra power (UP) fitting. Very small pressure relief vents (0.04 or less) are available (▶ **Fig. 4.52**). These molds may require some form of wax mitigation at the end of the receiver spout.

3. *Maximally occluding power domes/ear tips.* Can be used with RIC and thin-tube BTE aids; sealing properties may vary when the ear tip is removed and reinserted(▶ **Fig. 4.35a, b**).[68]

4. *Custom hearing aids (including ITE, ITC, CIC, and IIC).* Have been routinely available for Category 3 fittings since their inception. Occasionally, but not often, an ear canal may be too small to accommodate a high-power canal aid, necessitating a half shell or a full ITE instead. Each manufacturer has proprietary rules based on degree of hearing loss, the type of custom aid ordered, and size constraints.

4.4 Conclusion

Coupling the hearing aid to the ear not only provides mechanical security for the device, it also functions to shape the transmitted acoustic spectrum. This chapter emphasized the impact the

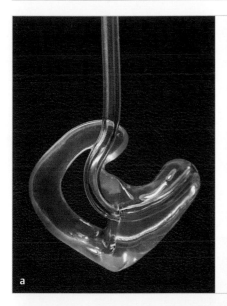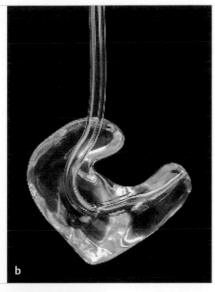

Fig. 4.51 **(a)** Shows a Category 3 deep insertion BTE skeleton earmold with a small vent. **(b)** Shows a Category 3 deep insertion BTE shell earmold with no vent. Courtesy of Starkey Hearing Technologies.

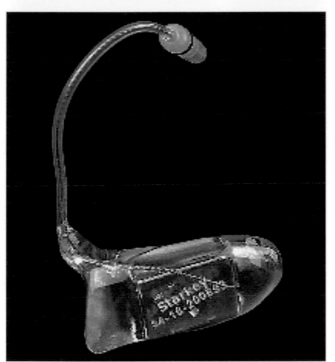

Fig. 4.52 Shows variation of a Category 3 RIC deep canal large receiver embedded earmold (absolute power [AP], ultra power [UP]) for very advanced hearing losses. Courtesy of Starkey Hearing Technologies.

configuration of the coupling has on the acoustic characteristics of the amplified signal. We pointed out the various factors that should be accounted for when selecting a coupling, and documented the extensive assortment of fittings and options at the clinician's disposal. With a good grasp of this information, the practitioner is able to predict with some certainty the effect of the coupling chosen, but more importantly, has at disposal a wide variety of alternatives for resolving any issues and problems that may arise.

There is certainly science involved in providing the right fitting, but just as importantly, there is also art. Learning and developing the skills of acoustic modification is a value-added proposition leading to quick and successful resolution of problems, and providing a sense of personal accomplishment.

In the same way as a chain is no better than its weakest link, each element in the transmission pathway, including the coupling, must be optimally executed for the hearing aid to perform as intended. Whether a custom earmold, a custom ITE, a BTE, or a RIC is selected, the coupling and its conformation is a critically important factor for delivering the desired signal. Choosing the appropriate type and structure from the many alternatives available can be challenging, but the eventual success of the fitting may weigh in the balance.

4.5 Acknowledgements

The authors would like to thank the following for their kind assistance in preparing this chapter: Andrea Pociecha, Courtney Coburn, Elizabeth Galster, Jason Galster, Mary Leisses, Allison Grimes, David Preves, Wayne Staab, Brian Kaspari, and Chris Marxen. Illustrations were provided by Chris Bracke, photos by Hieu Nguyen, Jacques De Lange, and the authors.

References

[1] Alvord LS, Morgan R, Cartwright K. Anatomy of an earmold: A formal terminology. J Am Acad Audiol. 1997: 8: 100–103

[2] Kuk FK. Maximum usable real-ear insertion gain with ten earmold designs. J Am Acad Audiol. 1994; 5(1):44–51

[3] Dillon H. Hearing aid earmolds, earshells and coupling systems. In: Dillon H, ed. Hearing Aids. 2nd ed. Turramurra, Australia: Boomerang Press; 2012:127–169

[4] Shaw EAG. The external ear. In: Keidel WD, Neff WD, eds. Handbook of Sensory Physiology. New York, NY: Springer-Verlag; 1974:455–485

[5] Wiener FM, Ross DA. The pressure distribution in the auditory canal in a progressive sound field. J Acoust Soc Am. 1946; 18:401–408

[6] Lybarger SF. Ear molds. In: Katz J, ed. Handbook of Clinical Audiology. Baltimore, MD: Lippincott & Wilkins; 1972:603–623

[7] Killion MC. Principles of high fidelity hearing aid amplification. In: Sandlin RE, ed. Handbook of Hearing Aid Amplification, Vol. I. Boston, MA: Little Brown; 1988a:45–79

[8] Kuk F, Baekgaard L. Hearing aid selection and BTEs: choosing among various "open ear" and "receiver-in-canal" options. Hear Rev. 2008; 14(3):22–36

[9] Mueller HG, Ricketts TA. Open canal fittings: ten take home tips. Hear J. 2006; 59(11):24–39

[10] Sullivan RF. An acoustic coupling-based classification system for hearing aid fittings, Part I. Hear Instrum. 1985a; 36(9):25

[11] Sullivan RF. An acoustic coupling-based classification system for hearing aid fittings, Parts II, III. Hear Instrum. 1985b; 36(12):16

[12] Yanz JL, Olsen L. Open-ear fittings: an entry into hearing care for mild losses. Hear Rev. 2006; 13(2):48–52

[13] Valente M, Valente LM. Earhooks, tubing, earmolds and shells. In: Valente M, Hosford-Dunn H, Roeser RJ, eds. Audiology Treatment. 2nd ed. New York, NY: Thieme Medical Publishers; 2008:36–71

[14] Lybarger SF, Barron FE. Head-baffle effect for different hearing-aid microphone locations. J Acoust Soc Am. 1965; 38:922

[15] Preves DA. Real-ear gain provided by CIC, ITC, and ITE hearing instruments. Hear Rev. 1994; 1(7):22–24

[16] Sullivan R. Custom canal and concha hearing instruments: a real ear comparison. Hear Instrum. 1989; 40(4):23–24

[17] Byrne D. Theoretical prescriptive approaches to selecting gain and frequency response of a hearing aid. Monographs in Contemporary Audiology. 1983; 4(1):1–39

[18] Cox RM. Combined effects of earmold vents and suboscillatory feedback on hearing aid frequency response. Ear Hear. 1982; 3(1):12–17

[19] Cox RM. Acoustic aspects of hearing aid-ear canal coupling systems. Monographs in Contemporary Audiology. 1979; 1(3):1–44

[20] Kuk FK. Perceptual consequence of vents in hearing aids. Br J Audiol. 1991; 25(3):163–169

[21] Lybarger SF. Earmold venting as an acoustic control factor. In: Studebaker GA, Hochberg I, eds. Acoustical Factors Affecting Hearing Aid Performance. Baltimore, MD: University Park Press;1980:197–217

[22] Lybarger S. Earmolds. In: Katz J, ed. Handbook of Clinical Audiology. 3rd ed. Baltimore, MD: Lippincott & Wilkins; 1985:885–910

[23] Valente M, Valente M, Potts LG, Lybarger EH. Options: earhooks, tubing, and earmolds. In: Valente M, ed. Hearing Aids: Standards, Option, and Limitations. New York, NY: Thieme Medical Publishers; 1996:252–326

[24] Westermann S. Ear canal resonances. In: Sandlin R, ed. Textbook of Hearing Aid Amplification. 2nd ed. San Diego: Singular Publishing Group Thomson Learning; 2000:369–410

[25] Curran JR. Earmold modification effects. Hear Rev. 1978; 29(12):14

[26] Ely W. Electroacoustic modifications of hearing aids. In: Bess FH, Freeman BA, Sinclair JS, eds. Amplification in Education. AG Bell: Washington, DC; 1981:316–341

[27] Lybarger SF. Controlling hearing aid performance by earmold design. In: Larson VD, Egolf DP, Kirlin RL, Stile SW, eds. Auditory and Hearing Prosthetics Research. New York, NY: Grune and Stratton; 1979:101–132

[28] McDonald FD, Studebaker GA. Earmold alteration effects as measured in the human auditory meatus. J Acoust Soc Am. 1970; 48(6)–1366

[29] Chasin M. The acoustics of CIC hearing aids. In: Chasin M, ed. CIC Handbook. San Diego, CA: Singular Publishing Group; 1997:69–81

[30] Kates JM. Acoustic effects in in-the-ear hearing aid response: results from a computer simulation. Ear Hear. 1988; 9(3):119–132

[31] Mueller HG, Hall JW. Boyle and his famous law. In Audiologists' Desk Reference. Vol. II. San Diego, CA: Singular Publishing Group; 1998:304

[32] Killion MC. Problems in the application of broadband hearing aid earphones. In: Studebaker GA, Hochberg I, eds. Acoustical Factors Affecting Hearing Aid Performance. Baltimore, MD: University Park Press; 1980:219–26

[33] Killion MC. Earmold options for wideband hearing aids. J Speech Hear Disord. 1981; 46(1):10–20

[34] Killion MC. Recent earmolds for wideband OTE and ITE hearing aids. Hear J. 1984; 8:15–18

[35] Mueller HG, Ricketts T, Bentler R. Ear impressions, earmolds, and associated plumbing. In: Mueller H, Ricketts T, Bentler R, eds. Modern Hearing Aids. Pre-fitting Testing and Selection Considerations. San Diego, CA: Plural Publishing; 2014:281–321

[36] Gilman S, Dirks DD, Stern R. The effect of occluded ear impedances on the eardrum SPL produced by hearing aids. J Acoust Soc Am. 1981; 70(2):370–386

[37] Gilman S, Dirks DD. Acoustics of ear canal measurement of eardrum SPL in simulators. J Acoust Soc Am. 1986; 80(3):783–793

[38] Larson VD, Egolf DF, Cooper WA. Application of acoustic impedance measures to hearing aid fitting strategies. In: Studebaker GA, Bess FH, Beck LB, eds. The Vanderbilt Hearing-Aid Report II. Parkton, MD: York Press; 1991:165–174

[39] Stuart A, Allen R, Downs CR, Carpenter M. The effects of venting on in-the-ear, in-the-canal, and completely-in-the-canal hearing aid shell frequency responses: real-ear measures. J Speech Lang Hear Res. 1999; 42(4):804–813

[40] Courtois J, Johansen PA, Larsen BV, Christensen PH, Beilin J. Open molds. In: Jensen HJ, ed. Hearing Aid Fitting, Theoretical and Practical Views, Thirteenth Danavox Symposium. Stockholm: Almqvist & Wiksell; 1988:175–200

[41] Dillon H. Earmolds and high frequency response modification. Hear Instrum. 1985; 36(12):8–12

[42] Lybarger SF. The earmold as a part of the receiver acoustic system. Canonsburg: Radioear Company; 1958

[43] Lybarger SF Livonia MI. Earmold acoustics. Audecibel. National Hearing Aid Society. 1967:9–19

[44] Lybarger SF. Earmolds. In: Katz J, ed. Handbook of Clinical Audiology. 2nd ed. Baltimore, MD: Williams & Wilkins; 1978:508–523

[45] Studebaker G. The acoustical effect of various factors on the frequency response of a hearing aid receiver. J Audio Eng Soc. 1974; 22:329–334

[46] Studebaker GA, Cox RM. Side branch and parallel vent effects in real ears and in acoustical and electrical models. J Am Audiol Soc. 1977; 3(2):108–117

[47] Zachman TA, Studebaker GA. Investigation of the acoustics of earmold vents. J Acoust Soc Am. 1970; 47(4):1107–1115

[48] Killion MC. Earmold acoustics. Semin Hear. 2003; 24(4):299–312

[49] Danaher EM, Osberger MJ, Pickett JM. Discrimination of formant frequency transitions in synthetic vowels. J Speech Hear Res. 1973; 16(3):439–451

[50] Danaher EM, Pickett JM. Some masking effects produced by low-frequency vowel formants in persons with sensorineural hearing loss. J Speech Hear Res. 1975; 18:261–271

[51] Danaher EM, Wilson MP, Pickett JM. Backward and forward masking in listeners with severe sensorineural hearing loss. Audiology. 1978; 17(4):324–338

[52] Trees DE, Turner CW. Spread of masking in normal subjects and in subjects with high-frequency hearing loss. Audiology. 1986; 25(2):70–83

[53] Burkhard MD, Corliss LR. Responses of earphones in ears and couplers. J Acoust Soc Am. 1954; 26:679–685

[54] Dalsgaard SC, Johanssen PA, Chisnall LG. On the frequency response of earmolds. J Audit Technol. 1966; 5:126–139

[55] Ewertsen HW, Ipsen JB, Nielsen SS. On acoustical characteristics of the earmould. Acta Otolaryngol. 1957; 47(4):312–317

[56] Sandberg LE, Nielson SS. Acoustic characteristics of insert-earphone versus external earphone. Acta Otolaryngol. 1967; 64(2):179–186

[57] Dillon H. Allowing for real ear venting effects when selecting the coupler gain of hearing aids. Ear Hear. 1991; 12(6):406–416

[58] Courtois J. Binaural IROS fitting of hearing aids. In: Dalsgaard SC, ed. Earmoulds and Associated Problems, Seventh Danavox Symposium. Stockholm: Almqvist & Wiksell; 1975:194–234

[59] Kuk F, Keenan D. How do vents affect hearing aid performance? Hear Rev. 2006; 13(2):34–42

[60] Lau C. Clinical performance of standard and extra small CICs. Hear Rev. 1998; 5(4):22

[61] Lybarger SF. Sound leakage from vented earmolds. In: Dalsgaard SC, ed. Earmolds and Associated Problems, Seventh Davavox Symposium. Stockholm: Almqvist & Wiksell; 1975:260–270

[62] Macrae J. Acoustic modifications for better hearing aid fittings. Hear Instrum. 1983; 34(12):8–11

[63] Stuart A, Stenstrom R, MacDonald O, Schmidt MP, MacLean G. Probe-tube microphone measures of vent effects with in-the-canal hearing aid shells. Am J Audiol. 1992; 1(2):58–62

[64] Tecca JE. Real-ear vent effects in ITE hearing instrument fittings. Hear Instrum. 1991; 42(12):10–12

[65] Tecca JE. Further investigation of ITE vent effects. Hear Instrum. 1992; 43(12):8–10

[66] Preves DA. Effects of earmold venting on coupler, manikin, and real ears. Hearing Aid J. 1977; 9:43–47

[67] Studebaker GA, Cox RM, Wark DJ. Earmold modification effect measured by coupler, threshold and probe techniques. Audiology. 1978; 17(2):173–186

[68] Coburn S, Rosenthal J, Jensen KK. Acoustic variability of occluded earbuds in receiver-in–the-canal hearing aid fittings. Starkey Hearing Technologies. Poster presented at Scientific and Technology meeting, American Auditory Society, Scottsdale, AZ; 2014

[69] Kiessling J, Brenner B, Jespersen CT, Groth J, Jensen OD. Occlusion effect of earmolds with different venting systems. J Am Acad Audiol. 2005; 16(4):237–249

[70] Kuk F, Keenan D, Lau CC. Vent configurations on subjective and objective occlusion effect. J Am Acad Audiol. 2005; 16(9):747–762

[71] MacKenzie K, Browning GG. The real ear effect of adjusting the tone control and venting a hearing aid system. Br J Audiol. 1989; 23(2):93–98

[72] Burnett ED, Beck LB. A correction for converting 2 cm³ coupler responses to insertion responses for custom in-the-ear nondirectional hearing aids. Ear Hear. 1987; 8(suppl 5):89–94

[73] Mason D, Popelka GR. Comparison of hearing-aid gain using functional, coupler, and probe-tube measurements. J Speech Hear Res. 1986; 29(2):218–226

[74] Egolf DP. Techniques for modeling the hearing aid receiver and associated tubing. In: Studebaker GA, Hochberg I, eds. Acoustical Factors Affecting Hearing Aid Performance. Baltimore, MD: University Park Press; 1980:279–319

[75] Flynn MC. Opening ears: the scientific basis for an open ear acoustic system. Hear Rev. 2003; 10(5):34–37

[76] Dillon H. NAL-NL1: a new prescriptive fitting procedure for non-linear hearing aids. Hear J. 1999; 5(4):10–16

[77] Seewald RC, Cornelisse LE, Ramji KJ, Sinclair ST, Moodie KS, Jamieson DG. DSL for Window: A software implementation of the desired sensation level for fitting linear and wide-dynamic–range compression hearing instruments: user's manual. London, Ontario, Canada: Hearing Health Care Research Unit; 1997

[78] Byrne D, Dillon H. The National Acoustic Laboratories' (NAL) new procedure for selecting the gain and frequency response of a hearing aid. Ear Hear. 1986; 7(4):257–265

[79] Scollie S. DSL version v5.0: Description and early results on children. http://www.audiologyonline.com/articles/dsl-version-v5-0-description-599. Accessed January 19th, 2018

[80] Hellgren J, Lunner T, Arlinger S. Variations in the feedback of hearing aids. J Acoust Soc Am. 1999; 106(5):2821–2833

[81] Leavitt R. Earmolds: acoustic and structural considerations. In: Hodgson WF, ed. Hearing aid assessment and use in audiologic rehabilitation. 3rd ed. Baltimore, MD: Williams & Wilkins; 1986:71–108

[82] Pirzanski CZ. Earmold acoustics and technology. In: Sandlin RE, ed. Textbook of Hearing Aid Amplification. 2nd ed. San Diego, CA: Singular Publishing Group; 2000:137–169

[83] Pirzanski CZ, Chasin M, Klenk M, Maye V, Purdy J. Attenuation variables in earmolds for hearing protection devices. Hear J. 2000; 53(6):44–50

[84] Dirks DD, Kincaid GE. Basic acoustic considerations of ear canal probe measurements. Ear Hear. 1987; 8(suppl 5):60–67

[85] Yanz JL. Panelists challenge "conventional wisdoms" on hearing aid design. Hear J. 2006; 59(3):38–44

[86] Killion MC, Wilber LA, Gudmundsen GI. Zwislocki was right. A potential solution to the "hollow voice" problem. Hear Instrum. 1988; 39(1):28–30

[87] Kuk F, Keenan D, Ludvigsen C. Efficacy of an open-fitting hearing aid. Hear Rev. 2005; 12(2):26–32

[88] Revit L. Two techniques for dealing with the occlusion effect. Hear Instrum. 1992; 43(12):16–18

[89] Mueller HG, Ebinger KA. CIC hearing aids: potential benefits and fitting strategies. Semin Hear. 1996; 17(1):61–81

[90] Goldstein DP, Hayes CS. The occlusion effect in bone conduction in hearing. J Speech Hear Res. 1965; 8:137–148

[91] Khanna SM, Tonndorf J, Queller JE. Mechanical parameters of hearing by bone conduction. J Acoust Soc Am. 1976; 60(1):139–154

[92] Tonndorf J. Bone conduction. In: Tobias JV, ed. Foundations of Modern Auditory Theory. New York, NY: Academic Press; 1972

[93] Zemlin WR. Speech and Hearing Science. 4th ed. Needham Heights, MA: Allyn and Bacon; 1998

[94] Fagelson MA, Martin FN. The occlusion effect and ear canal sound pressure level. Am J Audiol. 1998; 7(2):50–54

[95] Fulton B, Martin L. Drilling a vent often falls to give relief from occlusion Hear J. 2006; 59(7):44–45

[96] Kampe ST, Wynne MK. The influence of venting on the occlusion effect. Hear J. 1996; 49(4):59–66

[97] Killion MC. The "hollow voice" occlusion effect. In: Jensen JH. ed. Hearing Aid Fittings: Theoretical and Practical Views, 13th Danavox Symposium. Copenhagen: Stougaard Jensen; 1988b

[98] Mueller HG, Bright KE, Northern JL. Studies of the hearing aid occlusion effect. Semin Hear. 1996; 17(1):31–32

[99] Stender T, Appleby R. Occlusion effect measures: are they all created equal? Hear J. 2009; 62(7):21–24

[100] Carle R, Laugesen S, Nielsen C. Observations on the relations among occlusion effect, compliance, and vent size. J Am Acad Audiol. 2002; 13(1):25–37

[101] Pirzanski CZ. Diminishing the occlusion effect: clinician/manufacturer factors. Hear J. 1998; 51:66–79

[102] Vasil KA, Cienkowski KM. Subjective and objective measures of the occlusion effect for open-fit hearing aids. J Acad Rehabilitative Audiol. 2006; 39:69–82

[103] Vasil-Dilaj KA, Cienkowski KM. The influence of receiver size on magnitude of acoustic and perceived measures of occlusion. Am J Audiol. 2011; 20(1):61–68

[104] Biering-Sørensen M, Pedersen F, Parving A. Is there a relationship between the acoustic occlusion effect and the sensation of occlusion? Scand Audiol. 1994; 23(2):111–116

[105] Sweetow R, Valla A. Effect of electroacoustic parameters on ampclusion in CIC hearing instruments. Hear Rev. 1997; 4(9):8–12

[106] MacKenzie K, Browning GG, McClymont LG. Relationship between earmould venting, comfort and feedback. Br J Audiol. 1989; 23(4):335–337

[107] Cox RM, Alexander GC. Acoustic versus electronic modifications of hearing aid low-frequency output. Ear Hear. 1983; 4(4):190–196

[108] Lundberg G, Ovegård A, Hagerman B, Gabrielsson A, Brändström U. Perceived sound quality in a hearing aid with vented and closed earmould equalized in frequency response. Scand Audiol. 1992; 21(2):87–92

[109] Mueller HG. There's less talking in barrels, but the occlusion effect is still with us. Hear J. 2003; 56(1):10

[110] Staab WJ, Finlay B. A fitting rationale for deep fitting canal hearing instruments. Hear Instrum. 1991; 42(1):6–10

[111] Staab WJ, Martin RL. Taking ear impressions for deep canal hearing aid fittings. Hear J. 1994; 47(11):19–28

[112] Sweetow RW, Pirzanski CZ. The occlusion effect and the ampclusion effect. Semin Hear. 2003; 24(4):333–334

[113] Kuk F, Ludvigsen C. Ampclusion management 102: a 5-step protocol. Hear Rev. 2002; 9(9):34

[114] Painton SW. Objective measure of low-frequency amplification reduction in canal hearing aids with adaptive circuitry. J Am Acad Audiol. 1993; 4(3):152–156

[115] Laugesen S, Jensen NS, Maas P, Nielsen C. Own voice qualities (OVQ) in hearing-aid users: there is more than just occlusion. Int J Audiol. 2011; 50(4):226–236

[116] Kuk F, Peeters H, Keenan D, Lau C. Ampclusion management 103: high frequency hearing loss. Hear Rev. 2005; 12(4):74–75

[117] Mueller HG. CIC hearing aids: what is their impact on the occlusion effect? Hear J. 1994; 47(11):29–35

[118] Grover BC, Martin MC. Physical and subjective correlates of earmould occlusion. Audiology. 1979; 18(4):335–350

[119] Kiessling J, Margolf-Hackl S, Geller S, Olsen SO. Researchers report on a field test of a non-occluding hearing instrument. Hear Rev. 2003; 56(9):36–41

[120] Chung K. Challenges and recent developments in hearing aids. Part II. Feedback and occlusion effect reduction strategies, laser shell manufacturing processes, and other signal processing technologies. Trends Amplif. 2004; 8(4):125–164

[121] Bentler RA, Wu YH, Jeon J. Effectiveness of directional technology in open-canal hearing instruments. Hear J. 2006; 59(11):40–47

[122] Freyaldenhoven MC, Plyler PN, Thelin JW, Nabelek AK, Burchfield SB. The effects of venting and low-frequency gain compensation on performance in noise with directional hearing instruments. J Am Acad Audiol. 2006; 17(3):168–178

[123] Ricketts T. Directivity quantification in hearing aids: fitting and measurement effects. Ear Hear. 2000; 21(1):45–58

[124] Ricketts T, Henry P. Low-frequency gain compensation in directional hearing aids. Am J Audiol. 2002; 11(1):29–41

[125] Mueller HG. A candid round table discussion on open-canal hearing aid fittings. Hear J. 2009; 62(4):19–26

[126] Magnusson L, Claesson A, Persson M, Tengstrand T. Speech recognition in noise using bilateral open-fit hearing aids: the limited benefit of directional microphones and noise reduction. Int J Audiol. 2013; 52(1):29–36

[127] Klemp EJ, Dhar S. Speech perception in noise using directional microphones in open-canal hearing aids. J Am Acad Audiol. 2008; 19(7):571–578

[128] Valente M, Mispagel KM. Unaided and aided performance with a directional open-fit hearing aid. Int J Audiol. 2008; 47(6):329–336

[129] Harford E, Barry J. A rehabilitative approach to the problem of unilateral hearing impairment: the contralateral routing of signals (CROS). J Speech Hear Disord. 1965; 30:121–138

[130] Curran JR. Understanding and using CROS fittings and open-canal amplification. Hearing Dealer. 1971; 8:22–23

[131] Dunlavy AR. CROS: The New Miracle Worker. Audecibel 1970;141–148

[132] Green DS, Ross M. The effect of a conventional versus a nonoccluding (CROS-type) earmold upon the frequency response of a hearing aid. J Speech Hear Res. 1968; 11(3):638–647

[133] Harford E. Innovations in the use of the modern hearing aid. International Audiology. 1967; 6:311–314

[134] Harford E. Recent development in the use of ear-level hearing aids. Maico Audiological Series. 1968; 5:10–13

[135] Kaspar EA. The non-occluding mold. Hearing Dealer. 1967; 17(2):12–13

[136] McClellan ME. Aided speech discrimination in noise with vented and unvented earmolds. J Aud Res. 1967; 7:93–99

[137] Berland O. No-mold fitting of hearing aids. In: Dalsgaard SC, ed. Earmoulds and Associated Problems, Seventh Danavox Symposium. Stockholm: Almqvist & Wiksell; 1975:173–193

[138] Annual Industry Statistics, (1965–1980, December) The National Hearing Aid Journal

[139] Harford E, Dodds E. Versions of the CROS hearing aid. Arch Otolaryngol. 1974; 100(1):50–57

[140] Harford ER, Fox J. The use of high-pass amplification for broad-frequency sensorineural hearing loss. Audiology. 1978; 17(1):10–26

[141] Johnson EE. Practitioners give high marks for user benefit to open-canal mini-BTEs. Hear J. 2008; 61(3):19–20

[142] MacKenzie DJ. Open-canal fittings and the hearing aid occlusion effect. Hear J. 2006; 59(11):50–56

[143] Taylor H. Real-world satisfaction and benefit with open-canal fittings. Hear J. 2006; 59(11):74–82

[144] Dillon H, Keidser G, O'Brien A, Silberstein H. Sound quality comparisons of advanced hearing aids. Hear J. 2003; 56(4):30–40

[145] Agnew J, Thornton JM. Just noticeable and objectionable group delays in digital hearing aids. J Am Acad Audiol. 2000; 11(6):330–336

[146] Stone MA, Moore BCJ. Tolerable hearing aid delays. II. Estimation of limits imposed during speech production. Ear Hear. 2002; 23(4):325–338

[147] Staab WJ. Hearing aid evolution VI—hearing aid coupling. http://hearinghealthmatters.org. Accessed January 19th, 2018

[148] Zakis JA, Fulton B, Steele BR. Preferred delay and phase-frequency response of open-canal hearing aids with music at low insertion gain. Int J Audiol. 2012; 51(12):906–913

[149] Stone MA, Moore BCJ, Meisenbacher K, Derleth RP. Tolerable hearing aid delays. V. Estimation of limits for open canal fittings. Ear Hear. 2008; 29(4):601–617

[150] Bramsløw L. Preferred signal path delay and high-pass cut-off in open fittings. Int J Audiol. 2010; 49(9):634–644

[151] Groth J, Søndergaard MB. Disturbance caused by varying propagation delay in non-occluding hearing aid fittings. Int J Audiol. 2004; 43(10):594–599

[152] Aazh H, Moore BCJ, Prasher D. The accuracy of matching target insertion gains with open-fit hearing aids. Am J Audiol. 2012; 21(2):175–180

[153] Merks I, Banerjee S, Trine T. Assessing the effectiveness of feedback cancellers in hearing aids. Hear Rev. 2006; 13(4):53–57

[154] Ricketts T, Johnson E, Federman J. Individual differences within and across feedback suppression hearing aids. J Am Acad Audiol. 2008; 19(10):748–757

[155] Davis LA, Davidson SA. Preference for and performance with damped and undamped hearing aids by listeners with sensorineural hearing loss. J Speech Hear Res. 1996; 39(3):483–493

[156] van Buuren RA, Festen JM, Houtgast T. Peaks in the frequency response of hearing aids: evaluation of the effects on speech intelligibility and sound quality. J Speech Hear Res. 1996; 39(2):239–250

[157] Byrne D, Christen R, Dillon H. Effects of peaks in hearing aid frequency response curves on comfortable listening levels of normal hearing subjects. Aust J Audiol. 1981; 3:42–46

[158] Teder H. Smoothing hearing aid output with filters. Hear Instrum. 1979; 30(4):22–23

[159] Carlson EV, Mostardo AF. Damping element. U.S. Patent 3930560. Washington, DC: U.S. Patent and Trademark Office; 1976

[160] Killion MC. Transducers, earmolds and sound quality considerations. In: Studebaker GA, Bess F, eds. The Vanderbilt Hearing-Aid Report. Upper Darby, PA: Monographs in Contemporary Audiology; 1982:104–11

[161] Killion MC. Myths that discourage improvements in hearing aid design. Hear Rev. 2004; 11(1):32

[162] Killion MC, Wilson D. Response modifying earhooks for special fitting problems. Audecibel; 1985:28–30

[163] Killion MC, Papalias CW, Becker AJ. Electronic damper circuit for a hearing aid and a method of using the same. U.S. Patent No. 5. Washington, DC: U.S. Patent and Trademark Office; 1998

[164] Killion MC, Berlin C, Hood L. A low frequency emphasis open canal hearing aid. Hear Instrum. 1984; 35(8):30

[165] Knowles HS, Killion MC. Frequency characteristics of recent broad band receivers. J Audiol Tech. 1978; 17:86–99

[166] Alworth LN, Plyler PN, Reber MB, Johnstone PM. The effects of receiver placement on probe microphone, performance, and subjective measures with open canal hearing instruments. J Am Acad Audiol. 2010; 21(4):249–266

[167] Pirzanski CZ. Issues in earmold fitting and troubleshooting. Seminars in Hearing. 2003; 24(4):355–364. DOI: 10.1055/s-2004-815547

[168] Preves DA. Stepped bore earmolds for custom ITE hearing aids. Hear Instrum. 1980; 31(10):24

[169] Libby ER. A new acoustic horn for small ear canals. Hear Instrum. 1982a; 33(9):48

[170] Libby ER. In search of transparent gain insertion aid responses. In: Studebaker GA, Bess FH, eds. The Vanderbilt Hearing Aid Report. Upper Darby, PA; 1982b:112–123

[171] Pirzanski C. Earmolds and hearing aid shells: BTE styles, materials and acoustic modifications. Hear Rev. 2006; 13(8):26–28

[172] Ricketts TA, Bentler RA. Impact of "standard" earmold on RECD. Am J Audiol. 1995; 4(1):43–45

[173] Skinner MW. Hearing Aid Evaluation. Englewood Cliffs, NJ: Prentice-Hall; 1988

[174] O'Brien A, Keidser G, Yeend I, Hartley L, Dillon H. Validity and reliability of in-situ air conduction thresholds measured through hearing aids coupled to closed and open instant-fit tips. Int J Audiol. 2010; 49(12):868–876

[175] Rose DE. The return of the earmold. Hear Rev. 2006; 13(9):14–19

[176] Curran JR. A forgotten technique for resolving the occlusion effect. Starkey Innovations 2012;2(2):19–24

[177] Curran JR. Practical modification and adjustments of in-the-ear and in-the-canal hearing aids, Part 1. Aud Today 1990a;2(1):27–28

[178] Curran JR. Practical modification and adjustments of in-the-ear and in-the-canal hearing aids, Part 2. Aud Today 1990b;2(3):23–25

[179] Curran JR. Practical modification and adjustments of in-the-ear and in-the-canal hearing aids, Part 3. Aud Today 1991;3(1):24–26

[180] Kuk F, Keenan D, Lau CC. Comparison of vent effects between a solid earmold and a hollow earmold. J Am Acad Audiol. 2009; 20(8):480–491

Suggested Reading

Ballachanda BB. Theoretical and applied external ear acoustics. J Am Acad Audiol. 1997; 8(6):411–420

Bryant MP, Mueller HG, Northern JL. Minimal contact long canal ITE hearing instruments. Hear J. 1991; 42(1):12–15

Curran JR. The discovery of open canal amplification. Starkey Innovations. 2011; 1(2):22

Fiene H. Acoustic device. U.S. Patent 2312534 A. Washington, DC: U.S. Patent and Trademark Office; 1943

Flynn M. Maintaining the directional advantage in open fittings. Hear Rev. 2004; 11:32–36

Jespersen CT, Groth J. Vent is designed to reduce occlusion effect. Hear J. 2004; 57(10):44–45

Juneau RP. NAEL: fitting facts. Part I: the ear impression. Hear Instrum. 1983; 34(3):6–7

Lantz J, Jensen OD, Haastrup A, Olsen SO. Real-ear measurement verification for open, non-occluding hearing instruments. Int J Audiol. 2007; 46(1):11–16

Macrae J. Acoustic modification of hearing aids. Hear Instrum. 1985; 36(12):13–15

Strom JR. Otoscopic tip element and related method of use. U.S. Patent 7354399 B2. Washington, DC: U.S. Patent and Trademark Office; 2008

5 Hearing Aid Coupling: Techniques and Technologies

James R. Curran, Dennis Van Vliet

5.1 Introduction

In this chapter, we consider concepts and practices that are equally as important for achieving fitting success as those discussed in the previous chapter. The competent practitioner is expected to be adept and comfortable with the methods and techniques available for examining the ear, dealing with anomalies, and taking excellent impressions. Efficient accomplishment of these practical steps undergirds and is necessary for delivering satisfactory rehabilitative outcomes.

5.2 Preparation and Initial Inspection of the Ear

The physical examination of the ear should occur as the history is being taken. Any history of disease that may affect hearing and life experience such as noise exposure and trauma to the ear is important to note. Of specific concern is past medical treatment including surgery in and around the ear, susceptibility to infection from diabetes or conditions suppressing the immune system, and treatment with any medication or a medical condition that reduces blood coagulation. These facts combined with a thorough hearing evaluation are important not only to help with diagnosis, but also are important for protecting the patient and clinician from injury, infection, or other unintended consequence as a result of the examination and treatment.

Observing infection control protocols is part of best practice and of critical importance. Specific measures are beyond the scope of this chapter. For the interested reader, refer to *Guide to Infection Prevention for Outpatient Settings*,[1] and review ear-specific practices developed by industry experts such as Bankaitis.[2] An important component of the skills necessary for diagnosis and treatment of hearing loss is familiarity with the nomenclature required to identify the associated anatomy. Alvord et al[3] offered formal terminology for the external ear to facilitate communication with earmold laboratories and manufacturers (▶ **Fig. 5.1**).

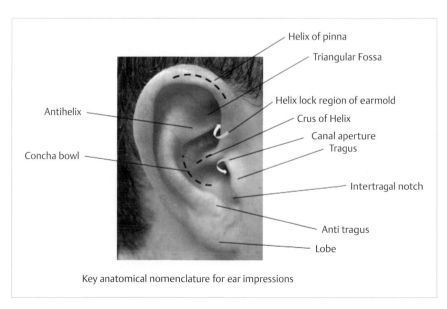

Key anatomical nomenclature for ear impressions

Fig. 5.1 Key nomenclature of the external ear for communicating with earmold laboratories or hearing aid manufacturers. Modified after Alvord et al.[3]

A complete examination includes visualization of the external ear, the ear canal, and the tympanic membrane. An examination of the ear canal requires adequate light, a proper viewing angle, and may require manipulation of the cartilaginous portion of the ear canal by lifting or pulling back the pinna to bring the entire canal and tympanic membrane into view. A number of light sources suitable for ear inspection are available, and are discussed below. Failing to fully inspect in and around the ear may cause one to miss a condition such as the rare, but well-documented postauricular fistula.[4]

5.3 Head Mirror

Invented in the mid-1800s, the head mirror, once in common use by general practitioners, was eventually largely replaced by headlamps, otoscopes, and less cumbersome light sources, but remains in use in some ENT and audiology practices today.[5] The *head mirror* is a concave mirror designed to be mounted to a head band with the mirror facing outward, and a viewing port centered in front of the eye of the examiner. The light source is behind the patient, directed at the examiner (▶ **Fig. 5.2a, b**). Reflected light is concentrated by the concave shape of the mirror and may

be directed into the area to be examined. The hole in the mirror allows for binocular viewing in the direct line of the reflected light.

5.4 Headlamp and Loupe

Headlamps provide a convenient, hands-free light source for examination. The illumination is most useful if the beam that is cast by the lamp can be focused in a small diameter to avoid reflected light from the surrounding tissue so as to not impair the view. Head-worn lamps are often paired with magnifying loupes for improved viewing. Binocular viewing capability is desirable for ear block placement and cerumen management because proper depth perception allows for more precise control. Binocular loupes paired with a central, focused light source offer excellent visibility for examination, cerumen management, and safe ear impressions (▶ **Fig. 5.3a, b**).

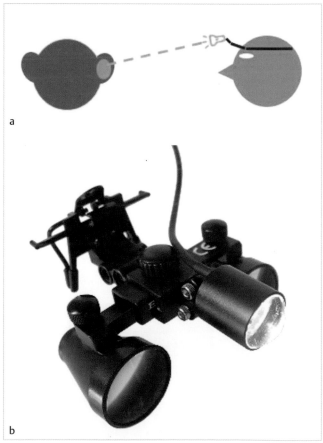

Fig. 5.3 **(a)** The diagram depicts use of a headlamp. **(b)** Shows a flip-up binocular loupe with attached light source. Available with or without headband or attachment to eyeglasses, and with or without a headlamp, the loupes provide excellent magnification and depth of field.

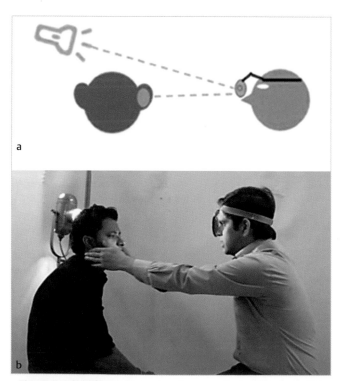

Fig. 5.2 **(a)** Shows the setup for use of a head mirror. **(b)** Shows the head mirror reflecting the light from behind the patient, providing well-lighted binocular viewing.

5.5 Otoscope

Reportedly initially described by Guy de Chauliac in his *Chirurgia Magna* in 1363,[6] the first instrument was designed for viewing ear and nasal passages. Refinements over the following centuries, including conical specula, improved power supplies, optics, and light sources, have provided continuous performance improvements. Sunlight and flame light sources evolved to incandescent lamps which were followed by halogen bulbs and eventually to light-emitting diodes (►Fig. 5.4a); a brightness of greater than or equal to 100 foot-candles is recommended.[7] Carbon dry cell batteries have been followed by a succession of improved power sources following developments in consumer electronics. In the years after 2010, lithium ion rechargeable cells have continued to receive attention for research and application in most portable rechargeable electronic devices, including the otoscope[8]; (►Fig. 5.4b).

5.6 Video Otoscope

A video otoscope serves a similar purpose to an optical otoscope, but provides the clinician with an enlarged view of the ear canal and tympanic membrane by displaying the image on a handheld or remote monitor, and allows still or video images to be captured (►Fig. 5.5a, b). The design of the video otoscope allows the inspection vantage to be deeper in the ear than good-quality standard optical otoscopes, yielding a far better field of view. Beyond the inspection of the ear canal, the video otoscopes provide an excellent opportunity for documentation, student training, patient education, and transparency for the care patients are receiving from the clinician.[9]

5.7 Ear Light

Used to assist in the placement of blocking material in the ear, standard ear lights are simply clear plastic probes capping the end of a penlight that take advantage of the fiberoptic characteristics of the plastic cap to provide a concentrated light source. Commercially available lighted cerumen curettes also can be used to assist placing cotton or foam blocks (►Fig. 5.6a–c).

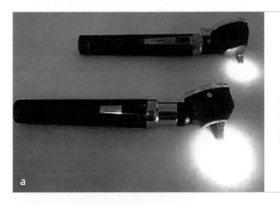
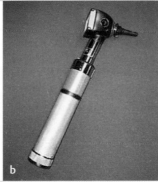

Fig. 5.4 **(a)** Illustrates the difference between incandescent versus light-emitting diode illumination. **(b)** Shows an example of a standard optical otoscope for clinic and field use; Welch Allyn 25020 otoscope head with 71000-C rechargeable handle.

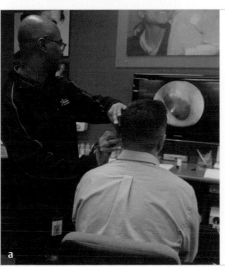
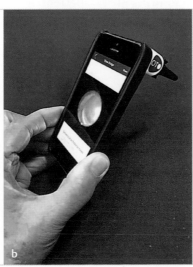

Fig. 5.5 **(a)** Shows clinician using a video otoscope to examine the ear. The image of the ear canal and tympanic membrane is enlarged and displayed on a video monitor. (Courtesy of Starkey Hearing Technologies). **(b)** Illustrates the *Cellscope Oto*, an accessory that can be easily attached to a smart phone and together with a dedicated app can serve as a mini video otoscope.

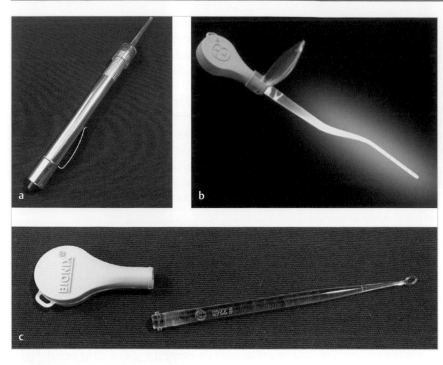

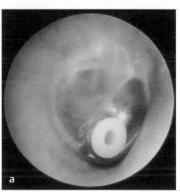

Fig. 5.6 Three versions of ear lights. **(a)** Standard, typical ear light with plastic probe attached. **(b)** Bionix illuminated placement probe with magnifier. **(c)** Curette with light source used for removing cerumen; single use curettes in different styles are available.

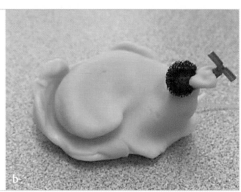

Fig. 5.7 **(a)** Shows tympanostomy tube in place in the tympanic membrane. It is important to assure secure placement of the dam or block to prevent passage of the impression material to the tympanic membrane or into the middle ear. **(b)** An impression from a pediatric patient with the foam block improperly placed. The impression material flowed by the block, and adhered to ventilation tube (*blue*). When the cured impression was removed, the tube was pulled out of the tympanic membrane.

5.8 The Ear Examination

One purpose of the patient history and ear examination is to discover any conditions that may present complications contraindicating ear impressions, hearing aid, or earplug usage. The most common complication is the presence of cerumen that is either occluding the ear canal, or nonoccluding but occupying space, preventing a proper ear impression. Cerumen must be sufficiently cleared from the ear canal before proceeding with ear impressions. Cerumen removal techniques are a topic beyond the scope of this chapter, requiring a solid knowledge base and skill development. For the interested reader, refer to Roeser and Wilson[10] for a more complete discussion. In addition, excellent color photographs of a wide variety of ear canal and eardrum conditions can be found in Sanna et al.[11]

Ears that have altered anatomy as a result of disease, surgery, or congenital anomalies need extra care and planning to avoid injury or discomfort. For example, *tympanostomy* tubes or perforations as a result of injury or disease present a danger to the patient if impression material migrates up against the eardrum or into the middle ear (▶ Fig. 5.7a, b). In the latter event, potentially complicated middle ear surgery is required to remove the material, with associated risks to the patient.[12]

Patients with a history of *mastoidectomy* where the ear canal has been reconstructed or other surgical alterations of the ear canal present a challenge. The resultant cavity is typically much larger than the entrance to the ear canal (aperture) (▶ Fig. 5.8). As a result, any impression material placed too deep in the cavity would be impossible to remove without discomfort and likely injury. When taking an impression, the cavity must be carefully packed with blocking material so that the impression material flows no farther into the cavity than the narrowest part prior to the enlarged section (▶ Fig. 5.9a, b).[13]

5.9 Bony Exostoses

Benign ear canal growths such as exostoses offer challenges for ear impressions and medical management.[14] The lesions should be isolated from impression material by packing the ear canal with blocks lateral to the growth to prevent impression material from surrounding the tissue. Following proper blocking of the ear canal, impressions may be taken as usual (▶Fig. 5.10).

Beyond observable anatomical issues other situations that are of concern prior to obtaining ear impressions include the following.

5.10 Anticoagulant and Antiplatelet Medication

When patients are taking medication to reduce blood clotting, they may be more susceptible to bruising, for-

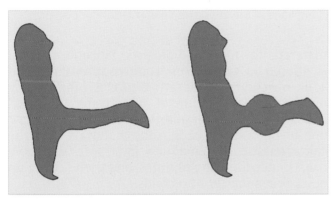

Fig. 5.8 Cross-section diagram of a normal ear canal configuration (*left*) and a greatly enlarged canal (*right*) due to either a congenital anomaly or following surgery that leaves a much wider recess or void medial to the aperture.

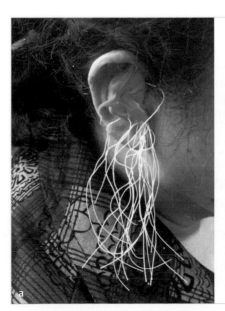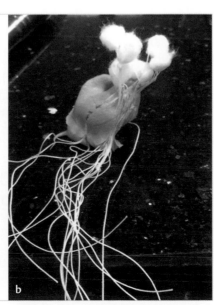

mation of hematomas, and bleeding. Even with careful technique, cerumen removal or taking of an ear impression may cause these complications to occur. If immediate medical care for complications is not available in the practice setting, a decision to defer treatment, or to refer the patient to a facility where proper treatment is available on call may be considered for these patients.[15] As always, patients should be given all the information they need to make an informed decision about their treatment before proceeding.

5.11 Active Infection

Patients with active otitis externa, bleeding or draining ears, and ear canals that are swollen are poor candidates for impressions and cerumen management, and should be referred for medical care. Audiologic treatment should be deferred until the patient is medically cleared. Best practices, as well as Federal Regulations require medical referral when these medical issues are present.[16] When a referral for swim or shower plugs is received for a patient under medical management for a tympanic membrane perforation or tympanostomy tube, in the absence of an obvious active infection and swelling of the ear canal, impressions are routinely appropriate after careful placement of ear dams.

5.12 The Ear Impression

The following sections discuss the history of ear impressions, the current state of the art in practice, and emerging technology. There have been changes in material and process, and new methods are on the horizon.

Fig. 5.9 (a, b) In order to prevent impression material from migrating into a large void medial to a narrow isthmus or the aperture, it may be necessary to pack it fully with a large number of blocks. This patient had undergone radical mastoid surgery with extensive ear canal reconstruction.

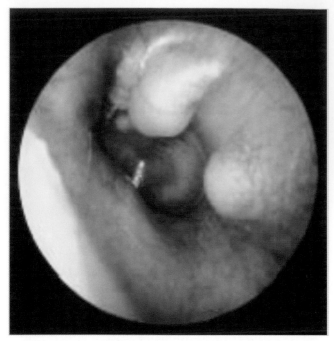

Fig. 5.10 Exostoses present as bony growths covered by a thin layer of tissue that can be sensitive. The ear canal should be carefully packed.

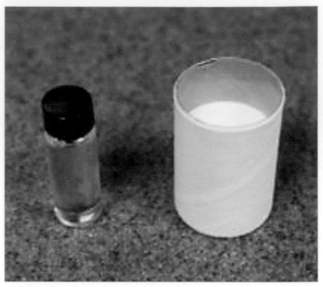

Fig. 5.11 Less used than formerly, liquid and powder impression material (methyl methacrylate) may be useful when the time between the taking of the impression and fabricating the earmold is short enough that drooping or shrinkage of the impression material does not occur.

Knox Brooks, a California Hearing Aid Specialist who followed his father in the hearing aid business in 1949, noted that obtaining impressions with plaster of Paris was standard practice in the 1930s and early 1940s, but was reportedly used reluctantly because it was cumbersome and dangerous; the plaster would easily break upon removal, and the material could become uncomfortably warm as it set up. He reported it was also very common at the time to use stock molds and modify them in the office for a reasonable fit (K. Brooks, personal communication, 2016).

A powder (polymer) and liquid (monomer) mixture (methyl methacrylate) became the impression material of choice in the 1950s; it is economical and involves straightforward mixing and handling in order to produce acceptable impressions (▶ Fig. 5.11). Shrinkage of the cured impressions over time and inability to maintain a stable shape (caused by temperature variations) are common complications and consequently have resulted in diminished popularity, but are still preferred by some practitioners. There is a rare, but known tendency for acrylic polymers to be a skin sensitizer for contact dermatitis.[17] As a result, when methyl methacrylate is to be used with patients, the history should include questioning about allergies to similar materials.

Silicone impression materials became available in the 1980s, are more expensive, but are stable and accurate. They have become the preferred materials for most audiologists. Silicone material is offered in two forms, condensation-cure, and addition-cure. Condensation-cure is prepared by mixing a small amount of an activator (catalyst) into a base material; addition-cure is a two-part, one-to-one ratio mix. Silicone materials have the characteristic of remaining in a soft, workable consistency for a few minutes, and then setting up quickly in a matter of seconds.

Silicone impression material is available in bulk, single application packaging, or in cartridges. Bulk or single application condensation-cure silicones and powder and liquid material are designed to be hand mixed in a cup (or on a clean surface, with clean hands), and then placed in a syringe and introduced into the ear by depressing the syringe plunger. When addition-cure silicone cartridges are used, the material is delivered using a mechanical device with a pistol grip (the gun) and a ratcheted lever to advance the plungers, forcing the material through a mixing cannula to assure proper blending (▶ Fig. 5.12a–c).

5.13 Skill Development: Taking the Ear Impression

Preparation for and the taking of ear impressions is addressed in general terms in best practice guidelines[18,19] with specific skills training left to "tribal knowledge" passed down from instructors, clinical supervisors, and earmold and hearing aid manufacturers. For reference, a good, specific professional practice guideline is available from the College of Audiologists and Speech-Language Pathologists of Ontario.[27]

The manual dexterity skills required for ear impressions are some of the most demanding we face as audiologists. Safety of the patient is of utmost importance in this procedure. A basic rule to keep in mind is that any time an instrument is placed in the ear canal, (otoscope, ear light, curette, syringe, etc.) the hand holding the instrument should be braced against the head of the patient so that if the patient moves, the hand and the instrument follows the movement, reducing the chance of injury. If resting the hand on the head isn't possible, the gap from the head to the hand may be "bridged" with the other hand (▶ Fig. 5.13).

5.14 Ear Dams and Blocks

The terms dam or block are used interchangeably in this discussion as they refer to the same item (▶ Fig. 5.14a–c). Commercially prepared blocks are available in cotton or foam. Some clinicians prefer to prepare their own from cotton with fine thread or floss to aid in retrieval from the ear canal, and others have developed effective techniques for trimming the foam blocks to comfortably and safely rest in the ear canal.

With either type of block, the technique used to insert the block and to verify that the block is properly placed and secure in the canal is of critical importance. The ear canal tissue is very sensitive from about the first bend to portions more medial. The instruments used for inspection and for guiding the ear dam into place should be kept away from the canal walls as much as possible to keep the patient comfortable and to avoid injury. Here it is important to recall the many illumination and magnification options that are available. A highly illuminated and magnified visualization of the ear canal is very important for facilitating appropriate positioning of the block.

The "feel" of the progress of the ear block must be monitored as it is inserted into position in the canal. A slight change in resistance may be caused either by the block being too large, simply reaching a point of narrowing in the canal, or by reaching the eardrum. Candidates for deep impressions must be selected carefully. If the ear canal is very narrow, or has a narrow section that opens up to a larger volume near the eardrum, deep impressions may be contraindicated because of the danger of patient injury or discomfort upon removal (▶ Fig. 5.15).

Visual inspection alone is insufficient to determine if the block is secure in position; it should be followed by direct but gentle palpation with a curette, or ear light around the full lateral surface of the block to confirm that there are no areas or voids beyond the dam that yield to light pressure. These voids, impossible to discover without palpation, can lead to an imperfect block, and allow impression material to migrate. When the material does flow around the dam, a "blow-by" incident has occurred (▶ Fig. 5.16).

If the impression material contacts an intact eardrum, its presence is usually not much of a problem, but removing the impression is. An uncomfortable vacuum can occur with removal, causing discomfort and may result in a hematoma injury on the eardrum or canal adjacent to it (▶ Fig. 5.17). Retrieval of any impression, deep or shallow, should be slow and gentle, making sure to break the vacuum by gently rotating and wiggling the impression as it is being removed. When taking a deep impression especially,

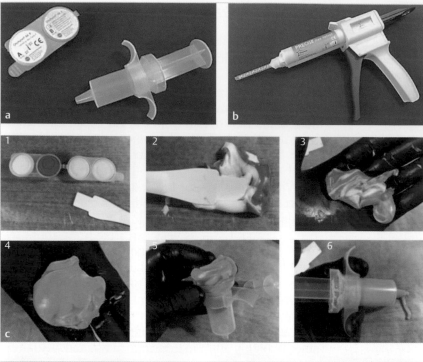

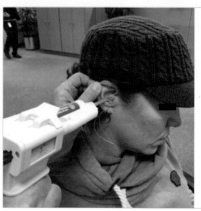

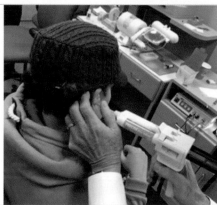

Fig. 5.12 **(a)** Shows a typical impression syringe, used with hand-mixed silicone and/or powder and liquid impression materials. **(b)** Depicts an impression gun with the addition-cure silicone impression cartridges ready for injection. **(c)** Silicone impression material must be quickly and thoroughly mixed for proper curing; proper hygiene is required whenever hand mixing. Here, equal parts of premeasured addition cure material (1) are mixed with a spatula (2) or by hand (3) until the material is a uniform color (4). The mix is placed in a hand syringe (5). A small amount of the material is expelled to relieve any air pockets at the nozzle of the syringe (6) and to evaluate the texture of the material prior to introducing the mix into the ear.

Fig. 5.13 Two views of proper bridging showing the clinician's fingers in contact with the patient's head. Note that the hand forming the bridge remains in constant contact with the impression gun throughout the procedure. As illustrated, a bridge may be formed while simultaneously manipulating the pinna to straighten the ear canal. A similar process is used with a syringe.

many clinicians apply a thin coat of lubricant to facilitate removal, prior to taking the impression.

Make it perfect

The perfect impression terminates beyond the second bend of the ear canal, even if a shallow earmold or shell will be fitted; it is necessary for the earmold/shell technician to be able to visualize the entire canal in order to place the sound outlet and vent properly.

5.15 Inserting the Impression Material

The force used to deliver the impression material is dependent on the skill and judgment of the clinician. Keep the tip of the syringe submerged within the impression material while filling the ear canal, and slowly

retract it as the impression material is expressed. Fill the outer ear with the remaining material, even if a canal aid is being ordered. If the approach angle is not proper, or the feed of the material is too feeble, the impression will likely be of poor quality and need to be retaken.

The ear impression is without a doubt one of the most challenging things we do as audiologists and the skills to safely take an impression can only be learned by practice and repetition. Although we have emphasized the issues involved in impression taking, the beginning practitioner should not be overawed or hesitant, for with practice, the technique will soon become routine and straightforward.

5.16 Open or Closed Jaw?

The ear canal is a dynamic part of the body that changes to a different degree depending on the individual. A relaxed jaw position is often recommended for impressions because the result is essentially an average of the size of the movements the canal will typically make. An open-jaw impression, depending on the anatomy of the individual, will often yield a tighter impression because the canal in many individuals enlarges as the jaw is opened.[28] Observing the ear canal during jaw movement may be helpful in making the decision for an open or closed jaw impression, especially if the patient has a known fit complication (e.g., excessive feedback while talking, chewing, etc.).

outer ear. Then, while holding (but not pulling) the string or thread, and at the same time grasping the impression, begin to break the seal between the impression and the canal walls while lifting up and/or pulling down on the pinna. Ask the patient to open and close the jaw. Gently lift, wiggle, or slightly rotate the impression, all the while maintaining slow and steady removal pressure. Do not force the removal and be not in a hurry; removal is a gradual proposition that requires patience and responds better to slow and easy rather than to quick and jerky (▶ Fig. 5.18).

Suppliers offer silicone impression material with a variety of characteristics

Color: The two-part mixtures are provided in contrasting colors to allow the adequacy of the mix to be assessed. The colors are often brand specific, and have little significance across manufacturers.

Viscosity: Silicone materials are available with a range of viscosities. A less viscous, or more fluid material may be better for a small ear, or for a very deep impression to allow the material to easily flow into the ear canal. A highly viscous, or stiffer material may be necessary to provide pressure to open collapsed soft tissue in an ear canal, or to push away excessive hair in the canal that cannot be trimmed away prior to the impression.

Shore: Shore refers to the rigidity of the cured impression; the lower the number the softer the material. It may be desirable to use a softer cured impression material for insertion very deep into the bony portion of the ear canal, but this is based on clinician preference and beliefs rather than strong evidence. It is important to remember that different suppliers offer different characteristics in their material and it is beneficial to become familiar with the properties of a particular material before using it on a patient. (The viscosity of many popular impression materials can be found in the Starkey Modification Guide, downloaded at https://starkeypro.com/pdfs/Hearing_Aid_Modification_Guide.pdf).

Cotton or foam?

Both cotton and foam blocks are designed to protect the ear from the ear impression material flowing into areas where it is not intended to go. Cotton is generally more comfortable for the patient, but should be modified by trimming, fluffing, and flattening out to allow it to be an effective block. Foam has the property of filling voids because of its natural elasticity. However, foam blocks can be too abrasive for some ears, causing discomfort when rubbing against the canal wall, especially if the chosen size is too large. Importantly, very deep ear impressions that terminate at a greater distance past the second bend must be handled carefully, for the bony portion of the ear canal is quite sensitive, and often contraindicate the use of a foam block. For these impressions, a properly prepared and sized cotton block may be the better alternative than foam to keep the impression material away from the tympanic membrane. The preference for cotton or foam is clinician-dependent. There are strong opinions offered in favor of one or the other, yet little evidence is available suggesting that one is superior to the other.

5.18 Taking the Impression, Step by Step

Following the history and examination of the ear, when the clinician is satisfied that it is safe and appropriate to proceed, the patient must be counseled about what to expect, be ready for the impression, and give consent to proceed. A suggested workflow is as follows:

- Counsel the patient about the purpose of the impression, and the process that will follow, including a description of the sensations that the patient will experience.

5.17 Removal of the Impression

As mentioned earlier, removing the cured impression is always done slowly to allow for a gradual release of any negative pressure on the eardrum. The first step is to gently separate the impression material from the curves and crevices of the

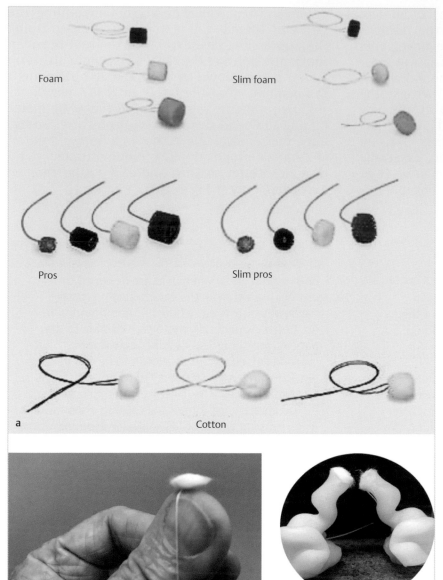

Fig. 5.14 **(a)** Cotton and foam blocks are available from suppliers in convenient packs and are available in a variety of sizes and configurations. Here cotton and foam blocks are illustrated in standard and slim configurations. The slim blocks take up less space in the ear canal and can be used when deeper impressions are desired. Image courtesy of Oaktree Products. **(b)** Shows a cotton block fluffed and flattened out prior to insertion. **(c)** Two perfect impressions showing no voids, delivery of impression material beyond the second bend, and a filled-in external ear.

- Obtain consent to proceed.
- Arrange the seating of the patient and clinician so that the patient's ear is at the clinician's eye level. Avoid stooping or bending. A comfortable seated position for the patient and clinician is preferable.
- Ensure that adequate lighting and the tools and supplies necessary for the impression are organized and accessible.
- Carefully inspect the instruments to be used for the ear impression. The syringe should be clean and free of cracks, or sharp edges. If using an impression gun, the mechanical operation should be smooth, and the mixing cannula should be firmly attached to the cartridge.
- Place the block in place, using proper technique to avoid discomfort to the patient, and ensuring that it is secure with no voids. Assess position and placement with otoscopy and palpation.

- Prepare the impression material as directed by the material manufacturer. Do not use outdated supplies as they may not set up properly. The impression materials are designed to be used within a specific temperature range. If the materials have been in a hot delivery truck, for example, they should be allowed to return to room temperature before using.
- Gently grasp the top of the pinna and pull up or back to assist in viewing the ear canal.
- Position the syringe or gun cannula so that the tip is around the first bend and directed at the ear dam. The hand holding the syringe or gun must be adequately braced against the head.
- The progress of the silicone through the cannula should be observed to ensure that proper mixing is taking place. Keep the tip of the syringe or cannula embedded in the fluid

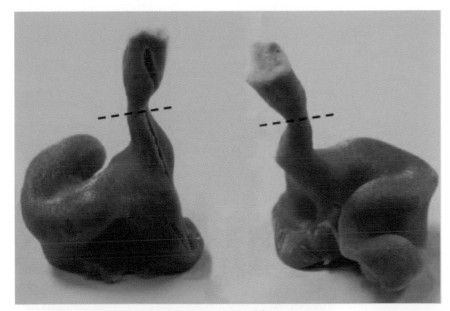

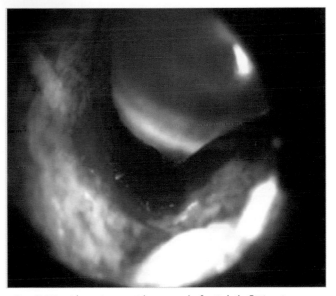

Fig. 5.15 These illustrations show anatomy that is unsuitable for a deep ear impression due to the very narrow isthmus before the medial, much larger area of the canal adjacent to the tympanic membrane. Proper procedure for ears with similar narrowing is to block the canal at the dashed line to prevent the material from progressing. Removal of the impressions pictured created a minor injury and discomfort for the patient.

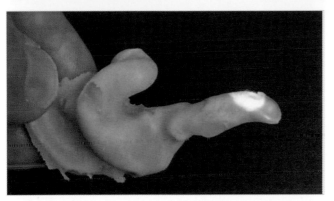

Fig. 5.16 This impression was the result of a poorly placed, unmodified block, or by improper technique in injecting impression material. The result was a "blow-by" impression that allowed the material to reach the tympanic membrane.

Fig. 5.17 Abrupt or rapid removal of a tightly fitting impression may result in a hematoma on the tympanic membrane.

material, backing it out slowly as the ear fills with the material.

- Proceed with the injection of the material at a firm and steady flow rate that allows the material to reach the block and fill the ear canal completely. After completely filling the canal, fill in the antihelix, triangular fossa, and helix. Proceed then to fill in the concha and intertragal notch. To assure excellent fitting earmolds and shells, a completely filled in and covered external ear is as a desirable element.

- Resist the impulse to smooth and flatten out the exterior surface of the impression. In fact, this maneuver has good probability of distorting the impression, leading to an inaccurate fit.

- Allow the impression material to set up. Test the cured material by depressing an edge with

a fingernail. If a line persists in the material, wait until fingernail pressure leaves no mark before removing.

- Prepare to remove the impression by asking the patient to open and close her or his jaw, and move the impression slightly by releasing the helix and concha bowl from the impression first.

- Ask the patient to tell when a pressure release is noted. Once the release of the vacuum is noted, the impression may be slowly rotated out of the ear.

- It's not over! Ask the patient how the ear feels, look in the ear for any areas of concern, and inspect the impression for defects, voids, and suitability for the product desired.

Syringe or impression gun?

Skilled practitioners are capable of making good-quality impressions with either the syringe or the mechanical gun. Some clinicians find the impression gun more cumbersome to manage and properly brace. On the other hand, the proper force applied
to the plunger of a syringe requires a little experience to achieve good results. Some large practice institutions have adopted the dual cartridge-gun combination to minimize the chance of inexact mixing and to standardize the method of delivery of material. Usually, however, the choice of syringe or gun is up to the clinician who is normally in the best position to judge which is the best for the patient and for the clinician.

5.19 Allergic Reactions

Silicone impression materials are generally hypoallergenic and very few individuals exhibit allergic reactions to an impression with silicone material. The acrylic powder and liquid mix materials do occasionally create allergic reactions that range from mild redness and itching to blistering and weeping of the skin. In practice, clinicians are often warned by users if they have had an allergic reaction in the past. Other than by discovery in the history or by patient report, there is no way to predict if a patient will have a reaction to the chemicals in the impression materials. When a reaction does occur, depending on the reaction, a medical referral may be necessary for treatment.

5.20 Fabrication of the Custom Shell or Earmold

5.20.1 Original Investment Method

The traditional method for fabricating earmolds and shells is still used by some manufacturers either as a business choice, or in an individual instance where a quickly fabricated product is necessary. In the traditional method, the ear impression is immersed in a casting medium. The impression is then removed, leaving a cavity that is a perfect negative representation of the original impression; this is called the investment (▶**Fig. 5.19a–c**). The desired material of the finished earmold/shell is introduced into the investment and allowed to cure. The final shell or earmold is then hand-shaped and detailed into the finished product.

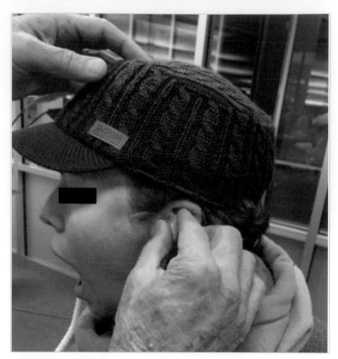

Fig. 5.18 Instructing the patient to open and close jaw during the impression removal may help to break the seal and relieve any vacuum pressure. Here, the helix is loosened and the impression will be slowly rotated and wiggled out of the ear canal.

5.20.2 Digitizing the Process

In the past two decades, the fabrication of shells and earmolds has been digitized using 3D CAD modeling and printing processes. The ear impression, obtained in the field with standard procedures, is either scanned in the field and the information is electronically transmitted with the order, or the impression is shipped and scanned at the earmold laboratory or by the manufacturer. The scanning of the impression produces an exact "point-cloud" digital image that can be stored in the computer and digitally manipulated and shaped by a skilled operator into the desired shell or mold style, type, and configuration (▶**Fig. 5.20**). The completed image of the newly modeled earmold or shell is translated into instructions that are then sent to a 3D printer which fabricates the shell or mold. (▶**Fig. 5.21a**).

A computer-controlled ultraviolet light (UV) beam traces a shape in a photosensitive liquid matrix of acrylic, forming a layer of cured acrylic. Additional layers of cured acrylic are built on the first, culminating in a shape that follows the 3D modeling file. The 3D printing processes substantially reduce the

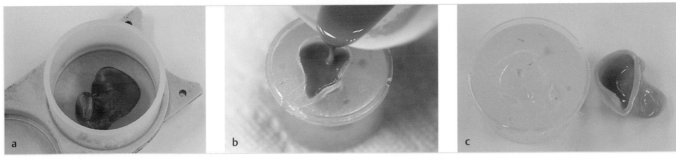

Fig. 5.19 **(a)** The ear impressions are deposited in containers, and a liquid colloidal material is poured in. The impressions are retrieved from the colloidal gel after it has set, leaving a cavity (investment) that is a reverse duplicate of the impression. **(b)** Methyl methacrylate shell/earmold material is poured into the investment, and allowed to cure. **(c)** After curing, the shell/earmold material is removed from the investment for further processing.

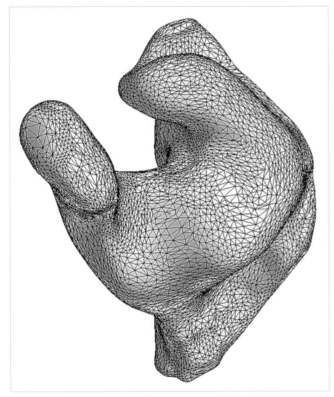

Fig. 5.20 The impression is scanned at thousands of points yielding an exact digital representation (point cloud) that is stored in the computer.

A wide range of materials is available, but medical grade silicone for soft molds, and UV cured acrylics for hard molds or shells are the most popular currently. Hard acrylic material is easy to modify in the office, easy to clean, and very durable. It is typically thought to be contraindicated in pediatric cases or for individuals engaged in contact sports because of the risk of physical injury in the event of a mechanical blow to the head. It has been suggested that soft materials are better for severe to profound losses because they have some capacity to flex with movement of the ear canal and allow a tighter fit when desired. Research has not proven this hypothesis, however. In a review of relevant research, Pirzanski[29] noted the following:

"In general, all these data indicate that earmold fit and acoustic seal are not enhanced by the use of soft materials. Rather, the accuracy of the earmold fitting is determined by the impression-taking technique, the viscosity of the impression material, and the parameters of the molding process.[29]"

5.21 Future Developments

3D scanning of impressions to create a digital image for fabrication of a mold or shell has been used since the early 2000s (C. Marxen, personal communication, 2016). The technology has now evolved to the point that techniques for direct scanning of the entire ear canal are being actively developed. The goal is to create a less invasive method for obtaining the ear impression. The benefit for the patient and clinician will be a quicker, more comfortable, and accurate process. The benefit for the manufacturer will be more consistent impressions, and integrated electronic transmission of demographic as well as anatomical information for manufacturing. As of this writing, it

labor time to fabricate shells and molds, reduce worker exposure to dust and chemicals, and allow intricate shaping of internal cavities not possible with fabrication by hand(▶ **Fig. 5.21b**).

5.20.3 Earmold Materials

The simple way to look at earmold materials is to think of them as either hard and rigid, or flexible.

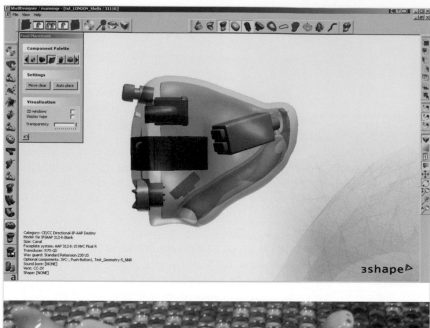

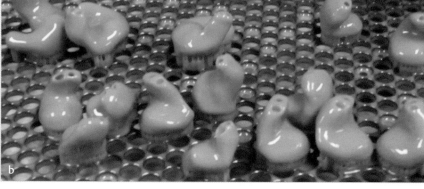

Fig. 5.21 **(a)** From the digitized representation of the impression, software programs are used to model either an earmold or shell. The computer screenshot shown here depicts an ITC aid in its projected form complete with proposed positioning of the components within the aid. This virtual representation becomes the guide for the assembly technician when fabricating the product. **(b)** Using modern 3D printing, the earmold or shell is fabricated, layer by layer, from photosensitive liquid acrylic resin.

is not clear what techniques will be adopted but clinicians are keenly interested and will likely adopt the technology as it becomes available and affordable.

5.22 Conclusion and Summary

In this chapter and Chapter 4, we have discussed the many factors and considerations of the coupling that impact the total amplified signal. As with so many clinical activities, which may seem complicated and difficult in the beginning, with practice becomes routine and well ordered.

At bottom, the foundation for a good and proper fitting is the impression. Take complete ownership of the entire fitting process; become an expert in taking the impressions, devoting to it the time and careful attention it deserves. Whenever possible, we suggest rejecting the temptation to skip over a custom fitting in lieu of fitting stock ear tips. Although they have their place, it is our judgment that they ordinarily should be considered as second choice options.

These chapters were written with the newly emerging audiologist in mind, and emphasis has been placed on presenting the information to facilitate easy assimilation. Those clinicians who become conversant with the information and the necessary skills discussed will be able to provide the very highest level of successful hearing aid fittings and service to their patients when entering into a clinical setting.

5.23 Acknowledgements

The authors would like to thank the following for their kind assistance in preparing this chapter: Andrea Pociecha, Courtney Coburn, Elizabeth Galster, Jason Galster, Mary Leisses, Allison Grimes, David Preves, Wayne Staab, Brian Kaspari, and Chris Marxen. Illustrations were provided by Chris Bracke, photos by Hieu Nguyen, Jacques De Lange, and the authors.

References

[1] Guide to infection prevention for outpatient settings: minimum expectations for safe care, v 2.3. (2016, September). https://www.cdc.gov/infectioncontrol/pdf/outpatient/guide.pdf. Accessed 22nd January, 2018

[2] Bankaitis AU. Infection control: getting your practice compliant with OSHA standards. Audiology Practices. 2011; 2(2):22–27

[3] Alvord LS, Morgan R, Cartwright K. Anatomy of an earmold: a formal terminology. J Am Acad Audiol. 1997; 8(2):100–103

[4] Choo JC, Shaw CL, Chong YC S. Postauricular cutaneous mastoid fistula. J Laryngol Otol. 2004; 118(11):893–894

[5] Roberts-Grey G. Is there still a place for the head mirror? ENT Today. http://www.enttoday.org/aran-iconic-tool-is-there-still-a-place-for-the-head-mirror/2/. Accessed January 19th, 2018

[6] Feldman H. Die Geschichte der Ohr-Specula Laryngorhinootologie. 1996; 75(5):311–318

[7] Johns Hopkins University. (2002). A view through the otoscope. Retrieved from he-aap/Committees-Councils-Sections/Section-on-infectious-diseases/Documents/monograph.pdf. https://www.aap.org/en-us/about-thool of Medicine. Accessed January 19th, 2018

[8] Pillot C. Battery market development for consumer electronics, automotive, and industrial: materials re& trends. http://www.rechargebatteries.org/wp-content/uploads/2015/01/Avicenne-marpdf 0. Accessed January 19th, 2018

[9] Sullivan RF. Video otoscopy in audiologic practice. J Am Acad Audiol. 1997; 8(6):447–467

[10] Roeser RJ, Wilson PL. Cerumen management. In: Hosford-Dunn H, Roeser RJ, Valente M, eds. Audiology: Practice Management. 2nd ed. New York, NY: Thieme; 2000:273–290

[11] Sanna M, Russo A, De Donato G. Color Atlas of Otoscopy. New York, NY: Thieme; 1999

[12] Algudkar A, Maden B, Singh A, Tatla T. Inadvertent insertion of hearing aid impression material into the middle ear: case report and implications for future community hearing services. Int J Surg Case Rep. 2013; 4(12):1179–1182

[13] Wynne MK, Kahn JM, Abel DJ, Allen RL. External and middle ear trauma resulting from ear impressions. J Am Acad Audiol. 2000; 11(7):351–360

[14] Kemink JL, Graham MD. Osteomas and exostoses of the external auditory canal—medical and surgical management. J Otolaryngol. 1982; 11(2):101–106

[15] Institute for Safe Medication Practices. (2015). High alert medications—warfarin. http://www.consumermedsafety.org/tools-and-resources/medication-safety-tools-and-resources/high-alert-medications/warfarin-coumadin. Accessed 22nd January, 2018

[16] American Speech-Language Hearing Association. (2008).0 Practice Portal. Hearing Aids for Adults. http://www.asha.org/PRPSpecificTopic.aspx?folderid=8589935381&section=Key_Issues#The_Hearing_Aid_Fitting_Process. Accessed January 19th, 2018

[17] Pemberton MA, Lohmann BS. Risk assessment of residual monomer migrating from acrylic polymers and causing allergic contact dermatitis during normal handling and use. Regul Toxicol Pharmacol 2014;69 (3):467–475. http://www.sciencedirect.com/science/article/pii/S0273230014000956. Accessed 22nd January, 2018

[18] American Academy of Audiology. Guidelines for the audiological management of adult hearing impairment. Audiology Today. 2006; 18(5):32–36

[19] American Speech-Language Hearing Association. (2016).0 Practice Portal. Hearing Aids for Adults. http://www.asha.org/PRPSpecificTopic.aspx?folderid=8589935381&section=Key_Issues#The_Hearing_Aid_Fitting_Process. Accessed 22nd January, 2018

[20] Timeline of casting technology. (2014). The Free Library. http://www.thefreelibrary.com/Timeline+of+casting+technology.-a019043906. Accessed 22nd January, 2018

[21] Bremner M. The Story of Dentistry. New York and London: Dental Items of Interest Pub Co., Inc; 1958

[22] Guerini V. A History of Dentistry. Philadelphia and New York: Lea and Febiger; 1909

[23] Berger KW. The Hearing Aid: Its Operation and Development. 3rd ed. Livonia, MI: National Hearing Aid Society; 1984

[24] Frederick HA. Acoustic device. U.S. Patent No. 1,601,063. Washington, DC: U.S. Patent and Trademark Office; 1926

[25] Wengel A. Hearing aid device. U.S. Patent 2192669. Washington, DC: U.S. Patent and Trademark Office; 1940

[26] Bergman M. On the Origins of Audiology: American wartime military audiology Audiology Today. 2002; 1:1–28

[27] College of Audiologists and Speech Language Pathologists of Ontario. (2005, 2014). Preferred practice guidelines for ear impressions. Toronto, Ontario, Canada.http://www.caslpo.com/sites/default/uploads/files/PPG_EN_Ear_Impressions.pdf. Accessed 22nd January, 2018

[28] Pirzanski CZ. Issues in earmold fitting and troubleshooting. Semin Hear. 2003; 24(4):355–364

[29] Pirzanski CZ. Earmolds: are soft materials superior? Hear J. 2001; 54(7):36–42

6 Audio Signal Processing for Hearing Aids

Ayasakanta Rout

6.1 Introduction

Nearly all hearing aids dispensed today have digital signal processing (DSP) at their core. The rapidly developing field of hearing aid signal processing has come a long way since the introduction of the first commercial body-level digital hearing aid, the Nicolet Project Phoenix, in the 1980s. Prior to the launch of commercially available digital hearing aids numerous research prototypes of hearing aids incorporating digital technology was reported in the 1970s. Levitt[1] presents a summary of early developmental milestones in DSP hearing aids. While the Nicolet Phoenix was not a commercial success, it paved the way for rapid miniaturization and development of ear-level digital hearing aids. The first commercial ear-level DSP hearing aids were launched by two manufacturers in 1996. As with any new groundbreaking technology, the new digital hearing aids introduced a high level of excitement and opened up opportunities for research and development.

From a clinical perspective, a hearing aid that could be programmed using a computer and a visual graphical interface was extremely desirable. To address this issue, hearing aid manufacturers introduced analog programmable hearing aids in the late 1980s. These hearing aids used analog components that were controlled by a digital chipset and provided some of the potential benefits of digital hearing aids, such as memory for storing parameter settings, the ability to modify settings of the hearing aid easily and with greater precision than earlier analog hearing aids, and convenient selection of appropriate parameter settings for different listening situations. The first reported commercial programmable hearing aid was introduced by Dalhberg Miracle Ear in 1988, soon followed by products from Bernafon and Siemens. Additional features such as data logging were available in programmable hearing aids in the following years (▶ Fig. 6.1).

The challenges and design constraints in developing digital hearing aids are extensive. For universal acceptance by patients the hearing aid must be small, the signal processing has to be almost in real time, and all this accomplished with a battery supplying 1.4 V. This chapter is written with the clinician in mind to provide an introduction to DSP in hearing aids and the challenges associated with such a complicated task.

6.1.1 Difference between Analog and Digital Signal Processing

Analog signal refers to a continuous representation of the signal over time, also described as "in the time domain." When a vibratory source sets air molecules into motion, a sound wave propagates as a continuous event. Such a sound wave can be plotted as a continuous signal on a XY plot (called a waveform). When a microphone picks up that sound wave, the diaphragm of the microphone vibrates continuously and generates an electrical voltage fluctuation that corresponds to the original sound wave. Hence, the electrical voltage can also be plotted as a continuous representation of the sound wave. As long as there is no distortion, an analog signal represents the purest form of the original sound. In analog hearing aid technology, the electrical voltage from the microphone is amplified as a continuous ongoing signal. An advantage of such a technique would be to achieve loud sounds easily.

However, the listening needs of hearing aid users are complex. We need hearing aids to suppress unwanted sounds, manage amplification without audible oscillations (whistling feedback), and amplify speech to a comfortable level while making loud sounds tolerable among many other desirable features. Consequently, this is a difficult task to perform with an analog circuit

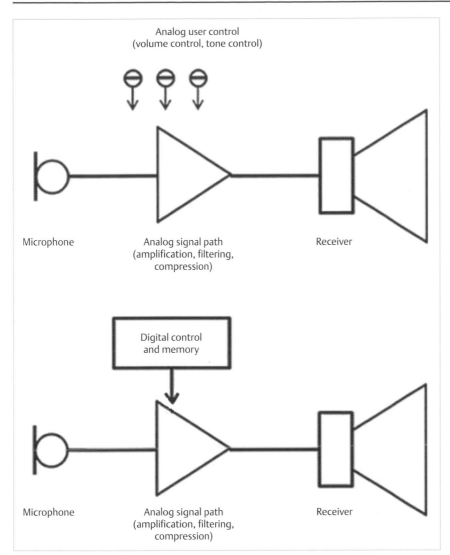

Fig. 6.1 Block diagrams of an analog hearing aid (*top*) and an analog programmable hearing aid (*bottom*).

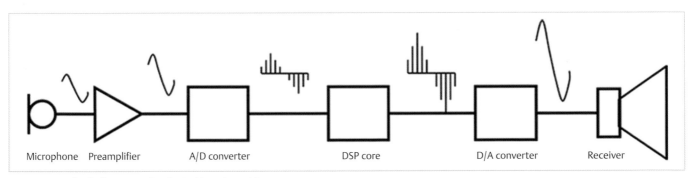

Fig. 6.2 Block diagram of a digital hearing aid.

in real time with the size constraints of ear-level hearing aids. DSP on the other hand, offers a different strategy by chopping up the analog signal into millions of discrete data points and processing all the data effectively to apply several mathematical rules to achieve the desired sound output. There are four general components of DSP in hearing aids (▶ **Fig. 6.2**).

1. Front end: Picks up the sound from the microphone and converts the analog voltage to digital samples.
2. DSP core: Applies signal processing rules to the incoming sound. Typically, there are multiple DSP cores in an advanced digital hearing aid.

3. Output stage: Converts the digitized signal back to analog format that the ear can perceive.
4. Wireless connectivity: Modern digital hearing aids offer connectivity to several audio, video, and wireless devices as well as data exchange between a pair of hearing aids.

6.1.2 Digital Signal Processing Basics

The first step in DSP involves converting the analog signal into a series of discrete data points. In order to accurately represent the original analog signal, the front end of the hearing aid needs to "sample" the waveform frequently (sampling rate) to record the amplitude at those points. It is also important for the amplitude of the sampled data point to be recorded as precisely as possible. This is referred to as quantization or bit resolution.

6.1.3 Sampling Rate

Digitization of an audio signal results in a set of data points representing the amplitude of the signal at a certain interval. The rate at which one samples the analog signal is often referred to as the sampling rate or sampling frequency (f_s). The unit for sampling rate is Hertz (Hz). A sampling rate of 10,000 Hz indicates that the analog waveform is "sampled" 10,000 times every second resulting in 10,000 data points. ▶ **Fig. 6.3** shows the waveform of an analog signal (a sine wave in this case) and ▶ **Fig. 6.4** shows sampling of the same analog signal.

Only the sampled data points are used by the DSP to reconstruct the original waveform. An appropriate sampling rate is determined based on Nyquist's rule that requires the minimum sampling frequency to be at least twice of the highest frequency of interest. In hearing aid–related applications, most speech information is present below 10,000 Hz. Based on Nyquist's rule, the minimum sampling rate required is 20,000 Hz. Otherwise, an audible error known as *aliasing* will be introduced into the signal (▶ **Fig. 6.5**). If the original signal contains frequencies higher than 10,000 Hz, and we sample the input with 20,000 Hz sampling rate, the high frequencies will be distorted and represented as unwanted low frequencies. This results in unpleasant sound quality.

Another important concept worth considering is called anti-aliasing filtering. Simply stated, this is a low-pass filter at the input stage of the hearing aid. The cutoff frequency of the low-pass filter matches the highest frequency that the sampling

frequency can faithfully process without aliasing. The anti-aliasing filter is designed to not allow any high-frequency signals to enter the hearing aid that cannot be handled by the hearing aid.

In many cases, it might be advantageous to use a much higher sampling rate than the bare minimum. Such a technique is called oversampling (see Chapter 6.1.5 for a description).

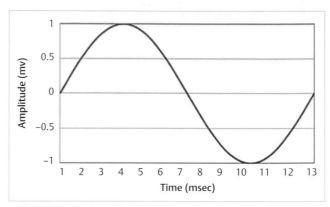

Fig. 6.3 Analog waveform of a sinusoid signal. Analog refers to continuous representation of the signal.

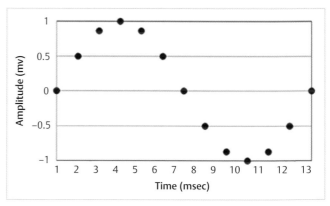

Fig. 6.4 The analog signal in ▶ **Fig. 6.3** is sampled at discrete intervals (every 1 second) and the amplitudes at the sampled points are plotted.

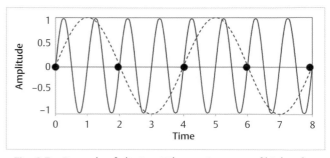

Fig. 6.5 Example of aliasing. When a sine wave of higher frequency (solid line) is sampled at less than twice the frequency, a lower-frequency signal (dashed line) can be misrepresented.

6.1.4 Bit Resolution (Quantization)

Another parameter that affects the sound quality of a digital hearing aid is the *bit resolution*—or the number of bits used to store information about each sample. One bit (derived from the term binary digit) is a word length that is similar to a decimal digit. However, while a decimal digit can be represented by 10 states (0 through 9), a binary digit can only be represented by two states: 1 or 0. For example, a two-bit binary number has four ($2^2 = 4$) states and a three-bit number has eight ($2^3 = 8$) states and so forth. ▶ **Table 6.1** illustrates a comparison of increasing the number of bits (word length) and the corresponding binary codes for real numbers. Since a two-bit system has only four states, the highest number that can be represented by such a system is three (0, 1, 2, and 3). In comparison, a four-bit system can represent 16 numbers (0–15).

As we discussed earlier, an analog signal is represented continuously with a precise value of the amplitude. However, a DSP cannot measure the amplitude of the signal at any given point with an infinite precision. Consequently, each sampled value is rounded to a nearest whole number. A sufficient number of bits must be available to represent both the largest and the smallest signal amplitudes. If too few bits are available to represent the signal, it leads to quantization errors—imprecision in the representation of the signal in the case of low-signal levels, and

distortion (clipping) with high-signal levels. The distortion resulting from poor bit resolution is perceived as a static noise or other forms of unpleasant sound quality, also referred as quantization noise. As the bit resolution increases, the difference between the digitized sample and the original signal becomes increasingly smaller, and the level of the quantization noise is decreased (▶ **Fig. 6.6**).

The quantization noise decreases by 6 dB per bit with the increase in bit resolution. For example, a 16-bit process can result in a 96 dB reduction in quantization noise. This reduction in noise should not be confused with the digital noise reduction described in Chapter 6.1.15. The 96 dB in a 16-bit system here refers to "how far below" the noise floor of the A/D converter is compared to the maximum output of the system. In the audio signal processing literature, this is often referred to as the input dynamic range or the headroom. The audio recordings in compact discs (CDs) use 16 bits at 44.1 kHz sampling while DVD audio recordings offer a higher-quality signal with 24 bits at 96 kHz. Currently, most advanced digital hearing aids in the market digitize the signal that is equivalent to 16 to 20 bits at 20 kHz sampling frequency.

It is obvious from the preceding section that a good hearing aid needs to have a good front end to convert the analog signal into cleaner digital data. However, each additional bit requires increased space and power consumption. Neither of these two options is desirable in a good hearing aid. During

Table 6.1 Decimal system and binary digits. The whole integers are converted into 2-, 3-, and 4-bits word length

	2 bits ($2^2 = 4$ states)	3 bits ($2^3 = 8$ states)	4 bits ($2^4 = 16$ states)
0	00	000	0000
1	01	001	0001
2	10	010	0010
3	11	011	0011
4		100	0100
5		101	0101
6		110	0110
7		111	0111
8			1,000
9			1,001
10			1,010
11			1,011
12			1,100
13			1,101
14			1,110
15			1,111

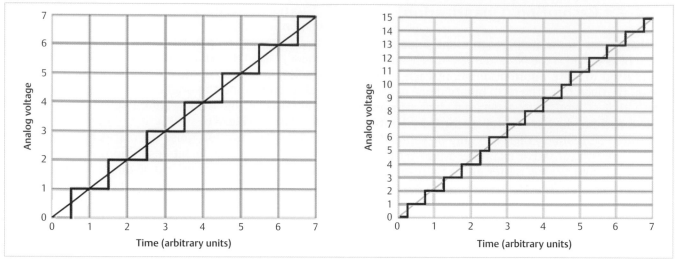

Fig. 6.6 Example of bit resolution and quantization error. The two panels illustrate the difference when the same linear line is quantized using a 3-bit (*left*) and 4-bit resolution. The deviation of the quantized signal from the original line is less for the higher-bit resolution.

the last two decades hearing aid design engineers have adopted a novel 1-bit analog-to-digital (A/D) converter instead of the traditional approach described above. This technique is referred to as delta-sigma (Δ-Σ) converter in signal processing language.

6.1.5 Delta-Sigma (Δ-Σ) Analog-to-Digital Converter

Before we understand how delta-sigma technique works in hearing aids, it is important to understand another concept called oversampling. As we discussed earlier, Nyquist's rule dictates the sampling frequency to be at least twice of the highest frequency of the signal. What is the consequence if the signal is sampled at a frequency that is much higher than that recommended by the Nyquist rule? Regardless of the sampling rate, the overall energy level of the noise generated is the same. When we increase the sampling rate, the highest frequency that can be accurately represented by the system is increased. As a result, the quantization noise is spread out over a wider frequency band. In fact, for every doubling of sampling frequency, the noise floor of the A/D processor decreases by approximately 3 dB. Once we manage to spread the quantization noise over a wide frequency range, a low-pass filter can be applied to discard the unwanted frequencies and achieve a desirable signal-to-noise ratio. The sampling rate in case of oversampling is typically higher than 1 MHz, several hundred times more than the speech frequencies. ▶**Fig. 6.7** shows a hypothetical scenario of decreased quantization noise as a result of oversampling.

The delta-sigma converter employs a very high sampling rate; the amplitude at each sampled point is represented in a 1-bit code (either a 0 or 1). There are two functional components in a Δ-Σ converter—a modulator and a decimation filter. The modulator converts the incoming voltage to a rapid series of pulses. The pulses can be represented as 1-bit signals. As we learned earlier, a 1-bit system has only two states ($2^1 = 2$). In this case, the two states are 0 or 1. The resulting pulse stream can represent a complex time-varying signal-like speech.

The output from the modulator is a very high-frequency signal. The original input signal (e.g., speech) is embedded in this high-frequency pulse train. At this point, the pulse stream is very noisy. The decimator filter is applied to recover the original digitized signal from the high-frequency pulse stream by low-pass filtering the output of the modulator (▶**Fig. 6.8**). Modern delta-sigma converters offer high resolution, low power consumption, and low cost, making them a good analog-to-digital converter choice in digital hearing aids. Finer details and architecture of Δ-Σ converters are beyond the scope of this chapter. Baker[2,3] provides a detailed technical description of how Δ-Σ converters work.

6.1.6 Digital Signal Processing Core

Once the analog-to-digital conversion process is completed, the digitized signal (data stream) is processed by the DSP core of the hearing aid chip. The DSP core is responsible for analysis and classification of the signal as well as implementation of the signal processing algorithms programmed in the hearing

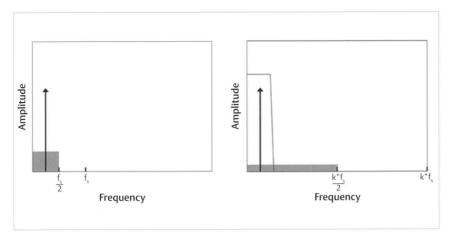

Fig. 6.7 Hypothetical example of oversampling. When we oversample at a rate much higher than required by Nyquist's rule, the noise floor is spread over a broad frequency band. Applying a low-pass filter removes some of the noise yielding better signal-to-noise ratio.

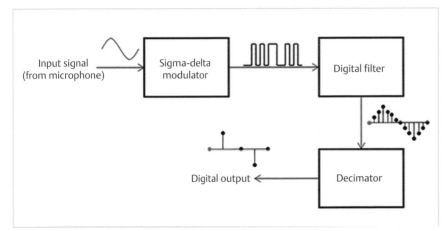

Fig. 6.8 Operational flow diagram of a delta-sigma converter. Adapted from Baker.[2]

aid. Signal processing algorithms can be as simple as applying gain at specific frequencies or complex approaches such as advanced noise reduction algorithms. A good digital hearing aid needs to have an accurate signal analysis and acoustic classification algorithm. The incoming signal is analyzed for amplitude (intensity), temporal modulation (is it fluctuating or steady state), loop gain (probability of audible feedback), and other parameters to determine which algorithms to engage in the DSP. The signal classification is done simultaneously in real time within each frequency band of the hearing aid.

The signal processing algorithms use millions of mathematical operations to achieve the desired parameters. For example, if the clinician programs a 6 dB gain at a certain frequency, the DSP algorithm achieves the gain by multiplying the digitized data by a factor of 2. Similarly, a multiplication by a factor of 4 results in 12 dB gain.

Another common operation within the hearing aid is filtering. A filter is a system that removes some components or modifies some characteristics of a signal. Filters are used for dividing the input into frequency bands, and implementing the signal processing algorithms such as noise reduction and feedback cancellation. A low-pass filter allows low frequencies to pass through while impeding higher frequencies. High-pass filters allow high frequencies to pass through. Similarly, a band-pass filter allows only a certain band of frequencies while attenuating the rest. A band-reject filter (notch filter) is designed to reject a narrow band of frequencies. We discussed the use of low-pass filtering to avoid aliasing in the input stage of the hearing aid. Band-pass filters are used to create individual frequency bands within which the signal processing algorithms operate. In addition to these basic filter types based on frequency response, today's advanced digital hearing aids have numerous complex adaptive filters working simultaneously to process the signal.

Filtering can be viewed as a form of smoothing. The speech signal consists of many fluctuations in the time domain. The rapid fluctuations are from the high-frequency components while the slow varying fluctuations are from the lower frequencies. If this rapidly fluctuating signal is sampled and each sample is averaged with samples before and after, the resulting output will be a signal which is smoother in its fluctuations (i.e., the rapid variations are removed). When we remove the rapid fluctuations in the time domain, we remove the high frequencies in the frequency domain. This is an example of a simple low-pass filter.

There are two basic classes of digital filters—finite impulse response (FIR filters) and infinite impulse response (IIR filters). Both classes of filters can be implemented to give any frequency response we want (low-pass, band-pass etc.). The primary difference between a FIR filter and an IIR filter is how the delay is implemented. Advantages and limitations of both types of filters are summarized in ▶ **Table 6.2**. A proper implementation of the filter can result in smooth frequency response and an acceptable processing delay, both of which are important considerations in hearing aid design.

6.1.7 Finite Impulse Response or Nonrecursive Filters

Two common filter types are described in the next sections: such filters are used in the creation of hearing aid channels, in which amplitude compression and a variety of other signal processing may be performed. An example of a FIR filter is shown in the block diagram in ▶ **Fig. 6.9**. The incoming signal is delayed and added back to the original signal at a given moment. Also notice that the signal is being multiplied by a constant factor (b). If we were to calculate the average of the two signals (original and delayed), then the value of b would be 0.5. Similarly, we can use any factor as a multiplier in the filter. The figure shown below represents one part of the FIR filter. If we were to be averaging more data points, then there would be a corresponding number of delays and additions in the circuit. FIR filters can be designed to be very consistent in frequency response (low distortion) which is highly desirable in a good hearing aid. However, that comes with a high computational cost. It is also worth pointing out that any filter comes with an inherent delay, called group delay or processing delay. Long processing delays can result in perceivable change in the sound quality.[4] Consequently, there is a trade-off between computational expense and filter characteristics. The reader is referred to Kates[5] and Levitt[6] for more in-depth explanation of filter design in digital hearing aids.

6.1.8 Infinite Impulse Response or Recursive Filters

IIR filters are designed by adding successive outputs back to the original signal (▶ **Fig. 6.10**). It might seem as though IIR filters require more calculations to be performed, since there are previous output terms in the filter expression as well as input terms. In fact, the reverse is usually the case. An IIR filter generally requires a much lower-order filter (and therefore less computational expense) than the equivalent nonrecursive (FIR) filter. IIR filters are commonly implemented in feedback cancellation algorithms.

Table 6.2 Advantages and limitations of FIR and IIR filters

	Advantages	Limitations
Finite impulse response filter (FIR)	• Smooth frequency response (less distortion)	• Longer processing delay at all frequencies compared to IIR • Computationally more expensive than IIR
Infinite impulse response filter (IIR)	• Requires less computational power (easier to implement) • Shorter processing delay	• Possible distortion in frequency response

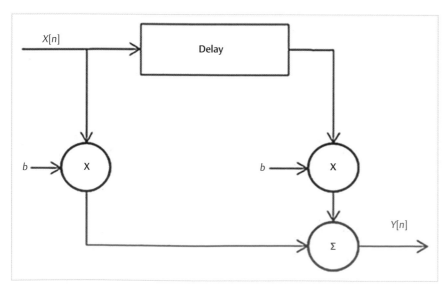

Fig. 6.9 Block diagram of a finite impulse response (FIR) filter.

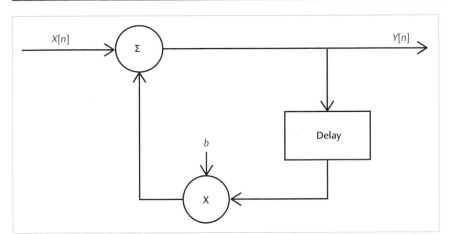

Fig. 6.10 Block diagram of an infinite impulse response (IIR) filter.

6.1.9 Digital-to-Analog (D/A) Conversion

One of the advantages of converting the analog signal to digital data is the convenience of DSP. Once we have the digital data, we can apply multiple mathematical operations to process the signal efficiently. However, the listener does not hear the digital data stream. The digital data stream is converted back to analog signal in the final step of hearing aid processing. This process is called digital-to-analog conversion or D/A conversion.

The D/A conversion process is very similar to the delta-sigma conversion we discussed earlier. As you may recall, the modulator in the delta-sigma converted is responsible for changing the analog signal into a series of high-speed pulse train. In the D/A conversion, the opposite process happens where the high-speed pulses are converted back to analog signal. In engineering terms, this process is called pulse width modulation (PWM) technique. The resulting analog signal is very noisy. A low-pass filter is applied to remove the unwanted high-frequency components to form the desired output. Because of the space constraints in designing a hearing aid, a clever technique is employed where the receiver itself acts a low-pass filter. Many hearing instrument manufacturers have marketed such a technique as digital receiver or directly driven digital receiver.

6.1.10 Hearing Aid Chip Design and Development

The rapid developments in hearing aid signal processing can primarily be attributed to the developments in chip design—in this case, the word "chip" refers to the computer chip that manages all DSP. Every 3 to 5 years major hearing aid manufacturers launch a new platform that is faster and more efficient than the previous-generation technology. In this section, an overview of the chip development process is presented with the clinician in mind.

Gordon Moore, the co-founder of Intel predicted in 1965 that the number of transistors per square inch on an integrated circuit will increase exponentially in the future. That prediction has held true for 50 years. When the earliest commercially available integrated circuits were marketed, they were rather large in size and extremely slow in computing capability. As the silicon fabrication techniques advanced, the number of transistors per square inch exponentially increased. ▶Table 6.3 lists examples of different processors and their transistor counts. Another important number is the fabrication process node which simply refers to the distance between neighboring transistors. The shorter the distance, the more transistors can be packaged onto a chip. Current hearing aid chips are fabricated with 65 nanometer process which is comparable to many advanced computer chips from only a few years ago. It is worth pointing out that the hearing aid chip, while not as powerful, requires far less power and is significantly smaller in size compared to that of a computer or smartphone. ▶Table 6.4 lists examples corresponding to three micro units of length.

Chip development for hearing aids is very challenging because it has to process signal almost in real time in a tiny package and an extremely limited power supply. In addition to these design constraints, hearing aid manufacturers introduce new platforms every 3 to 5 years. There is a chip design approach called system-on-a-chip (SoC), that can integrate several different components of the hearing aid processing on one very small chip. However, it is not possible to upgrade any single feature without building an entirely new chip. For example, if a hearing aid manufacturer wants to upgrade the wireless compatibility on their instruments, in a SoC design, the entire chip needs to be redeveloped (in material science language it is call re-spinning). This process is expensive and time consuming. To be nimble in the development process, today's advanced hearing aids have multiple chips. It is common to have six to eight chips in a premium-level hearing

Table 6.3   List of computer processors and their transistor counts in comparison to hearing aid chips

Processor	Year	Transistor count	Fabrication process node
Intel 4004	1971	2,300	10,000 nm
Intel Pentium	1993	3,100,000	800 nm
Intel Pentium 4	2002	55,000,000	130 nm
Advanced hearing aid chips	**2016**	**~ 65,000,000**	**65 nm**
Intel Core 2 Duo	2006	291,000,000	65 nm
Apple A7 chip	2013	1,000,000,000	28 nm
Apple A8 chip	2014	2,000,000,000	20 nm

Table 6.4   Micro units: making sense of scale

Micro units		Example
Millimeter (mm)	10^{-3} m (one thousandth of a meter)	Height of a 312 battery = 3.6 mm Diameter of a 312 battery = 7.9 mm
Micrometer (μm)	10^{-6} m (one millionth of a meter)	Diameter of human hair ≈ 100–200 μm Atmospheric dust particles ≈ 1–5 μm
Nanometer (nm)	10^{-9} m (one billionth of a meter)	Hearing aid transistor = 65 nm Diameter of a Carbon atom ≈ 0.2 nm

aid (individual chips for wireless, analog front end, power management etc.). The reader is referred to a technical note (TND6092/D, 2014) from ON Semiconductor[7] for a detailed description of chip design in modern hearing aids.

6.1.11 Signal Processing Architecture

Hearing aid manufacturers have recently introduced hearing aids that can be upgraded from a mid-level to a premium-level technology. How do they do it? The answer lies in the signal processing platform architecture of the hearing aid chip. The DSP architecture can be designed as a closed platform where all the features are permanently built in. This approach is extremely efficient in power management (low battery consumption). However, if the manufacturer wants to update certain signal processing algorithms, the entire chip needs to be redesigned; for this reason, most companies have moved away from this design.

Another approach to solving the nonflexibility of a closed platform is to develop a programmable architecture. This is not as energy efficient as the closed platform, but it gives the engineers flexibility to update several signal processing algorithms. The hearing aids that allow clinicians to do in-clinic technology-level

upgrades are built on this architecture generally called open-programmable architecture. The obvious limitation of programmable architecture is increased battery consumption. However, with clever design the hearing aid battery drain can be improved significantly.

6.1.12 New Developments in Platform Design

In order to achieve faster processing in a smaller chip, the manufacturers have adopted multicore architecture in chip design. Multicore simply refers to two or more processing cores on the same chip. These individual processors carry out different operations simultaneously resulting in efficient signal processing. Another advantage of multicore architecture is that the chip does not overheat and consumes less power.[8]

Major hearing instrument manufacturers develop their chips in-house which allows for innovation and miniaturization specific to hearing aid design. This is a very expensive process. As we have observed in recent years, mergers and acquisitions by major manufacturers allow for codevelopment of chips. A less common approach to chip development in hearing aids is to use standard core processors, which can be customized for hearing aid signal processing.[7]

6.1.13 Digital Signal Processing Algorithms in Hearing Aids

As we discussed earlier, one of the benefits of DSP is the ability to implement complex algorithms on a very small processor. Signal processing algorithms constitute the "brain" of the hearing aid. Often manufacturers market their products at different technology levels (e.g., premium vs. mid) according to the level of sophistication of the signal processing algorithms. A high-end hearing aid can have multitudes of features such as amplitude and frequency compression, adaptive directionality, digital noise reduction, feedback cancellation, wind noise reduction, binaural synchronization, and transient noise reduction among others. Detailed implementation and operational architecture of each of these algorithms is beyond the scope of this chapter. The reader is referred to Holube et al[9] and Kates[5] for further information on hearing aid signal processing algorithms.

The platform architecture of an advanced hearing aid is shown in ▶**Fig. 6.11**.[10] It can be seen on the flow diagram that certain algorithms such as speech enhancement, noise reduction, and wind noise management are implemented on the outputs of each individual microphone. The two microphone signals are then combined and other signal processing algorithms such as compression and expansion are engaged. This particular hearing aid splits the input signal into 64 different frequency channels. Most manufacturers use FIR filters at the front end so that all filters have linear phase and the same processing delay (group delay). Uniform group delay is important because in binaural hearing the listener uses small interaural time differences (ITDs) between ears to assist with localization of sounds; for this reason, the processing delay from all microphones, on both ears, should be identical.

6.1.14 Frequency Bands versus Channels

The two terms, bands and channels, are often misunderstood and used interchangeably in clinical audiology. However there is a difference in terms of signal processing. A hearing aid *channel* can be defined as a range of frequencies that is created by a digital filter or series of digital filters within the hearing aid. In addition to compression, most signal processing features such as digital noise reduction, feedback suppression, and multichannel directionality operate on a channel-by-channel basis. *Bands* can be defined simply as the number of adjustment "handles" provided

in the programming software for gain manipulation.[11] The hearing aid architecture shown in ▶**Fig. 6.11** has 64 channels for signal processing but the clinician adjusts 16 gain handles in the fitting software for prescribing appropriate gain. While the more channels allow for a finer scale signal processing, it is not essential that more channels improve speech intelligibility.

6.1.15 Digital Noise Reduction in Hearing Aids

Speech understanding in the presence of background noise continues to be one of the most challenging situations for hearing aid users. Hence noise reduction has remained a primary focus of hearing aid design and development process. Each generation of new platform introduces a more advanced noise reduction compared to the previous chip. A generic approach to digital noise reduction will be presented in this section.

Before trying to separate noise from speech, it will be beneficial for us to understand what are some of the acoustic parameters that separate these two signals. We can analyze the signals in three domains:
1. Spatial domain
2. Temporal domain
3. Spectral domain

6.1.16 Noise Reduction in Spatial Domain

For the purpose of our discussion noise will be defined as an unwanted acoustic signal and speech is the signal of interest. In many environments the hearing aid user turns toward the direction of the signal of

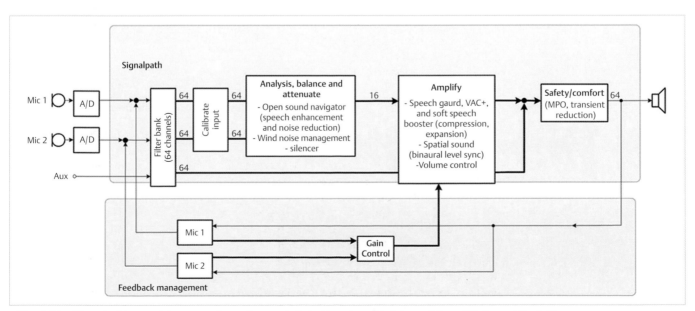

Fig. 6.11   The platform architecture of an advanced digital hearing aid. Adapted from Weile and Bach.[10]

interest. In such a scenario, there exists a spatial separation (directional source of the wanted vs. unwanted signal) between the speech and noise. Multi-microphone directional systems have been used in hearing aids for decades to selectively attenuate signals arriving from certain directions. More advanced forms of multi-microphone–based systems, generally referred as adaptive directionality, are standard in all premium- and mid-level hearing aids.

In order to create an adaptive directional system we need at least two microphones. There is a time difference when a signal arrives at the two microphones. This difference (typically in the order of a few microseconds) is commonly referred as external time delay. If a sound is originating from the back of the hearing aid, it reaches the rear microphone first, and continues on to reach the front microphone a few microseconds later. If a delay of a few microseconds introduced to the signal from the rear microphone, then both signals will arrive at a summing point in the hearing aid signal processing at the same time. This delay is called internal time delay. The ratio of the external and internal time delays determines the sensitivity of the directional microphone system. In fact, theoretically it is possible to change the internal delay every few milliseconds to obtain a different sensitivity pattern of the microphone. A popular way of representing the sensitivity pattern of a directional

system is called polar patterns. A block diagram of an adaptive directional system is shown in ▶ **Fig. 6.12**.

6.1.17 Noise Reduction in Temporal Domain

Speech and noise are time-varying signals and they can be differentiated in terms of how rapidly each signal fluctuates in time. ▶ **Fig. 6.13** shows the time waveform of a sentence spoken in quiet (top panel) and the waveform of a sample of random noise generated by a machine. The speech signal is modulated at a slow rate, while the noise is modulated at a faster rate. The rate of modulation is called modulation frequency which is a measure of the number of fluctuations per second. Different acoustic units yield different modulation frequencies. For example, we can expect 10- to 12 phonemes uttered per second in conversational speech yielding a modulation frequency of 10 to 12 Hz. Similarly, syllables yield a modulation frequency of 5 Hz.[9] We can also notice that the depth of modulation is much higher in the speech signal compared to that of the noise. Modulation depth is typically expressed in percent. For example, 100% modulation depth refers to the quietest parts of a sentence where there were gaps or pauses. Finally, the amplitude of the noise remains relatively steady over a long time window. Based on these differences several noise reduction algorithms

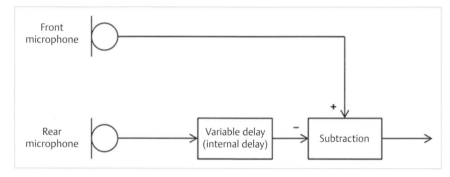

Fig. 6.12 Block diagram of a generic adaptive directional microphone system. The output of the rear microphone is delayed and subtracted from the front microphone signal. In a more advanced system, the output of each microphone is split into multiple channels and the internal delay in each channel varied to obtain different polar patterns. For an in-depth description of adaptive directional systems the reader is referred to Kates.[5]

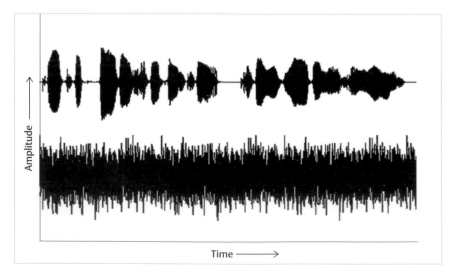

Fig. 6.13 Waveforms of speech (*top*) and random steady-state noise (*bottom*).

have been developed for use in hearing aids. Temporal modulation-based noise reduction is a term commonly used to refer to these algorithms.

We can apply mathematical rules to classify the incoming signals as either fast modulating or slow modulating. A slow modulated signal with greater depth will be classified as speech while rapidly fluctuating signals that remain steady over a long period will be classified as noise. The noise reduction algorithm then applies gain reduction based on speech versus noise classification. The modulation spectra of speech and noise are shown in ▶Fig. 6.14 and ▶Fig. 6.15, respectively. The modulation rate peaks at around 3 to 4 Hz for the spoken sentence, while the noise yields a faster modulation rate around 32 to 64 Hz.

Gain reduction as a function of modulation frequency and modulation depth is shown in ▶Fig. 6.16 and ▶Fig. 6.17, respectively. These figures were adapted from the work of Powers and colleagues.[12] In these examples, maximum gain reduction of 9 dB is applied for noise reduction based on modulation frequency. The gain reduction is more aggressive (12 dB) for modulation depth of

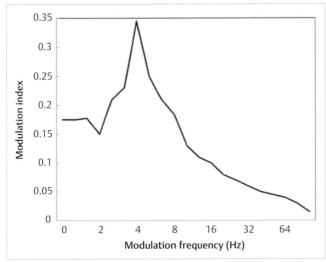

Fig. 6.14 Modulation spectrum of speech (single sentence). Modulation index (a measure of the depth of modulation) is plotted on the Y-axis. Modulation frequency peaks around 4 Hz in this speech sample. Adapted from Powers et al.[12]

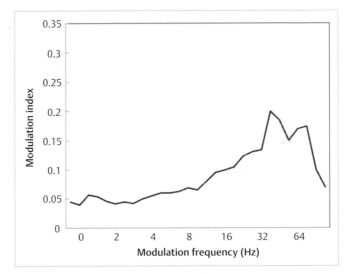

Fig. 6.15 Modulation spectrum of jet engine noise. Modulation index (a measure of the depth of modulation) is plotted on the Y-axis. Modulation frequency peaks around 32 to 64 Hz in this speech sample. Adapted from Powers et al.[12]

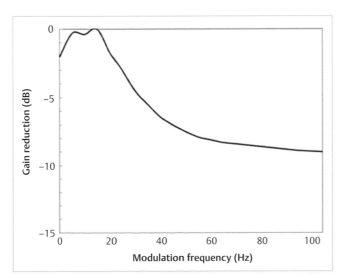

Fig. 6.16 Gain reduction for different modulation frequencies. In this example, maximum gain reduction of 9 dB is applied at modulation frequencies above 64 Hz. Note that no gain reduction is applied below 16 Hz. Adapted from Powers et al.[12]

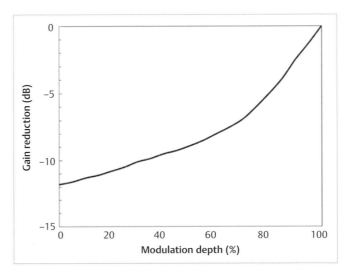

Fig. 6.17 Gain reduction for different modulation depth. In this example, maximum gain reduction of 12 dB is applied for steady-state signals (modulation depth near 0%). Note that no gain reduction is applied for modulation depth close to 100%. Adapted from Powers et al.[12]

0%. This indicates that this particular algorithm is more confident of reducing gain when there is an ongoing steady-state signal (e.g., a computer hum or a steady engine noise). It is important to note that each manufacturer applies different sets of rules for gain reduction in their algorithms. Currently, the maximum gain reduction for steady-state signals ranges from 9 to 20 dB.

Temporal modulation-based noise reduction is implemented within each channel of the hearing aid. If the hearing aid's filter bank splits the incoming signal into 64 channels, then the signal within each channel is analyzed for modulation rate and depth. Hence, increasing the number of channels can theoretically help to "clean up" the noise on a finer scale. However, there is a computational cost of implementing more channels in a small chip. As of this writing many premium-level hearing aids offer 16 to 64 channels for noise reduction. It should be noted that there is no evidence to suggest that a greater number of channels increases the effectiveness of noise reduction. For an in-depth description of digital noise reduction, the reader is referred to Bentler and Chiou,[13] Chung,[14] Kates,[5] and Holube et al.[9]

6.1.18 Limitations of Temporal Modulation-Based Noise Reduction

The temporal modulation characteristics are used to identify speech and noise as long as the noise is a steady-state signal; however, in real-life situations, noise may also be a single or group of talkers. These real-world noisy environments are not easily detected as noise by a temporal modulation-based algorithm. Additionally, in environments where speech is mixed with a steady-state background noise, the hearing aid noise reduction algorithms "default" to classifying this combined signal as speech. In real life, this situation is encountered frequently. So, the effectiveness of a temporal modulation-based algorithm may be reduced in many real-life scenarios.

6.1.19 Noise Reduction in Spectral Domain

Can we separate speech from noise in the spectral domain? This has been a time-honored clinical approach in audiology to "reduce the gain at low frequencies" as a method of noise reduction. There are two assumptions here: (1) noise is predominantly present at low frequencies, and (2) mid- and high frequencies are more important for speech intelligibility. The latter assumption is validated by decades of research on speech intel-

ligibility index. The first assumption is not entirely true since the spectra of different noise types show peaks at different frequencies. Additionally, when the unwanted signal is speech, the spectrum matches with the spectrum of the speech signal we want to hear. In such a scenario, we end up with a compromise by reducing the gain at low frequencies—some noise can be attenuated but the frequencies that are most important for speech intelligibility are not attenuated.

Frequency-specific gain reduction is seldom used in modern hearing aids but has historically complemented temporal modulation-based approaches. Currently, available noise reduction algorithms may have speech preservation logic that limits gain reduction at mid frequencies (typically around 1,000–4,000 Hz region). This conservative approach indicates the underlying difficulty in separating speech from noise.

6.1.20 Adaptive Wiener Filter-Based Noise Reduction in Hearing Aids

Wiener filter is a spectral subtraction approach where a known spectrum of the unwanted signal (i.e., noise) can be subtracted from the noisy speech to yield a cleaner speech sample.[15] Wiener filter can work well in off-line noise reduction algorithms (e.g., hiss reduction from old music samples) when the spectrum of the noise can be estimated ahead of time. However, this is not possible in hearing aids. The signal processing happens in real time in hearing aids and the type of noise changes considerably depending on the environment. Adaptive Wiener filter-based approaches in hearing aids estimate the noise spectrum by analyzing gaps in speech. The spectrum of the estimated noise is then subtracted from the incoming signal. Such an approach is implemented in commercially available hearing aids. Adaptive Wiener filtering is usually most effective when the signal-to-noise ratio is positive. These methods of noise reduction have been shown to improve the acceptance of background noise and reduce the subjectively reported annoyance of background noise.[16]

6.1.21 Feedback Cancellation

Feedback continues to be one of the most undesirable consequences of amplification. When an amplified signal leaks out from the hearing aid and reenters the microphone, the additional gain makes the output even higher and the process repeats. As a result, an acoustic loop is formed. When the gain of this loop gets sufficiently high, the system becomes unstable. This leads to audible oscillations or acoustic feedback. ▶ Fig. 6.18 shows a schematic representation of a possible external feedback path leading to a loop. The route which the amplified signal travels back to the microphone is called the feedback path. The goal of feedback cancellation, therefore, is to break this feedback path. Several approaches are available today to suppress feedback in hearing aids.

There have been two main approaches to feedback cancellation in hearing aids: notch filtering and phase cancellation. Notch filtering works by removing a narrow band of frequencies around the feedback. This technique used to be the standard in the early days of digital hearing aids. While this approach was able to suppress feedback, the removal of a frequency band resulted in poor sound quality. Additionally, this approach was not adaptive to changes in feedback path, meaning that the occurrence of feedback was more likely than might be experienced with more modern approaches. Newer feedback cancellation approaches based on phase cancellation were introduced in early 2000s. A schematic diagram of phase cancellation is shown in ▶ Fig. 6.19. When a feedback path is detected, the phase cancellation algorithm mimics the feedback and creates a clone of this signal. Within the hearing aid DSP, this clone is subtracted from the amplification path, therefore breaking the loop. Phase cancellation approach is capable of suppressing the feedback effectively as long as the feedback loop is stable. However, in real-life situations the hearing aid user changes the feedback path due to head movements, chewing, wearing a hat, or picking up the phone to talk. These changes happen rapidly and unpredictably. In order to intercept the rapid changes in feedback path, we need a feedback cancellation algorithm that can act within a few milliseconds. There is a trade-off with such fast-acting systems. These algorithms can mistakenly engage

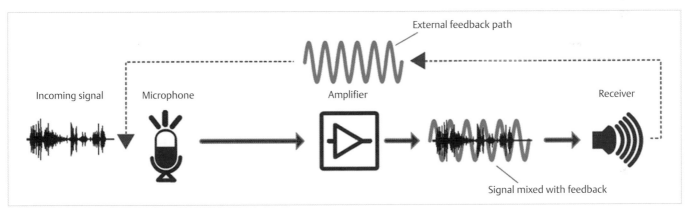

Fig. 6.18 External feedback path of a hearing aid. When the output of the hearing aid leaks out and gets picked up by the microphone, the process results in a loop. The gain in this loop becomes unstable and results in audible oscillations (feedback). Adapted from Banerjee.[17] © 2006 by Starkey Hearing Technology.

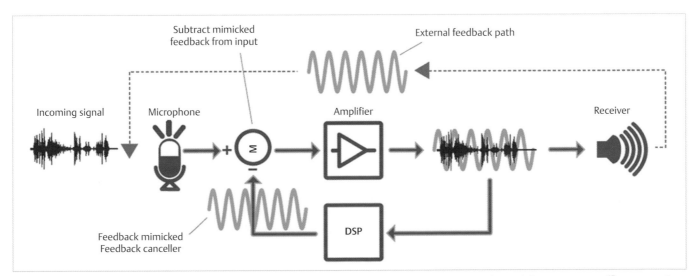

Fig. 6.19 General principle of phase cancellation approach to feedback suppression. Adapted from Banerjee.[17] © 2006 by Starkey Hearing Technologies.

in phase cancellation when there are tonal signals in the environment. This false alarm by the phase cancellation algorithms is called entrainment.

A great deal of research and development has focused on dynamically modelling the feedback path. The reader is referred to Kates[5] for an in-depth technical description of feedback cancellation approaches in hearing aids. Chalupper and colleagues[18] describe a multidimensional approach to modelling the dynamic feedback path. In commercial literature such an approach is described as adaptive phase cancellation system combined with a transient frequency shift.

What is frequency shifting? When a feedback loop is established and the gain becomes unstable, the algorithm shifts the frequency of the feedback by a small amount. By briefly shifting the frequency breaks the feedback loop and it helps to suppress the feedback. Some manufacturers shift the frequency by 25 Hz[18] and others shift the frequency by 10 Hz,[19] while others introduce random and pseudo-random jitter to the frequency shift. Frequency shifting can potentially reduce sound quality. So, it is important to minimize frequency shifting.

The tremendous popularity and success of open-fit hearing aids can largely be attributed to effective feedback cancellation algorithms. This allows the clinician to address issues of comfort (no need to fit tight earmolds) and occlusion (low frequencies are attenuated in an open-fit hearing aid). While feedback cancellation algorithms are generally effective, there is a large variability across manufacturers.[20]

6.1.22 Wind Noise Reduction

Wind noise is generated in hearing aids due to the turbulence of airflow over the microphone ports. When there are more obstructions in the path of airflow (e.g., body of the hearing aid, pinna, head), there is increased turbulence. This results in overloading of the microphone. The hearing aid user perceives the wind as a fluctuating noise and speech intelligibility is greatly reduced under such circumstances. Simple physical modification to the hearing aid can result in reduced wind noise. For example, by placing a microphone cover over the inlet ports prevents the turbulent wind from directly impinging on the microphone's diaphragms. Certain hearing aid styles such as invisible in the canal (IIC) hearing aids can potentially "protect" the microphone from being exposed to wind noise. For the vast majority of hearing aid wearers wind noise is a challenging situation.

Modern hearing aid algorithms address the wind noise problem by exploiting the very nature of turbulent airflow at the two microphone inlets. Turbulence is random by nature. Hence the input at the two microphone ports is more likely to be uncorrelated for wind. Conversely, when speech signal arrives at the two microphone inlets, the input at the two ports will exhibit greater correlation. This signal correlation can be used as a test for wind noise.

In addition to the correlation approach, wind noise can be reduced in the spectral domain. The spectrum of wind noise is dominant at low frequencies with most of the energy below 300 Hz.[21,22] High-pass filtering the input to exclude the low frequencies below the peak of the wind noise spectrum offers another approach to noise reduction. Kates[5] argues that twin microphone directional systems have an inherent advantage for wind noise reduction. When two correlated signals are summed, the output increases by 6 dB. Summing two uncorrelated signals can yield a gain of 3 dB. Since the speech signal is correlated and the wind noise is uncorrelated, there is a built-in 3 dB signal-to-noise ratio advantage with the two-microphone directional system. Additionally, low-frequency roll-off in the directional system can attenuate more wind noise. All the above-mentioned techniques are used in combination in today's hearing aids.

6.1.23 Frequency-Lowering Algorithms

Patients with steeply sloping high-frequency hearing loss pose unique challenges in hearing aid gain prescription. First, the hearing aid's receiver may not be capable of providing a high gain at the highest frequencies. Second, high gain makes the hearing aid vulnerable to acoustic feedback. Third, there is evidence to support that there is limited benefit to high-frequency gain when the hearing loss is severe.[23] Several signal processing techniques are available in hearing aids to provide audibility to the high-frequency sounds. A generic term, *frequency lowering* is often used to describe these approaches. There are three main frequency-lowering techniques available in hearing aids today.

Frequency transposition: Transpositions aims to improve audibility for high-frequency sounds by moving an entire band of frequencies to a lower-frequency region. This results in a narrow spectrum with no energy at the high frequencies. The transposed frequency components are superimposed on existing signals.

Frequency compression: Frequency compression narrows the output bandwidth of the hearing aid by mapping the high frequencies to progressively lower frequencies. This yields a narrow bandwidth, but unlike transposition, none of the frequency components are superimposed on another band. Additionally, a cutoff frequency is defined, below which the hearing aid output is not at altered by the frequency compression algorithm.

Frequency translation: The above two techniques restrict the bandwidth of the signal and could introduce noticeable change in sound quality. Frequency replication technique addresses this problem by retaining the original bandwidth and "searching" for high-frequency speech sounds (e.g., /s/ and /sh/). When these sounds are detected, a frequency-lowered version of the sound is added at a lower frequency. The frequency-lowering effect only occurs when the high-frequency energy of interest is present.

Acoustically, these approaches can provide improved access to high-frequency speech sounds. However, perceptually there seems to be individual variability in preference for frequency-lowered sound quality. The reader is referred to Simpson[24] and Alexander[25] for in-depth descriptions of different frequency-lowering approaches and their patient benefits.

6.1.24 Wireless Technology

Wireless technology has been in existence in our field for a long time including induction loop systems, FM and infrared systems. The new types of wireless technology in hearing aids has changed the way hearing aids communicate with each other in a pair, and with other devices such as smart phones and external audio sources. ▶Fig. 6.20 shows the functional block diagrams of a digital hearing aid with wireless functionality. Current wireless technology can be classified in two categories based on the distance within which they can transmit the signal: near-field and far-field transmission.

Near-field refers to short transmission distances (typically < 1 m). These systems are based on near-field magnetic induction (NFMI). NFMI is quickly and relatively easily implemented in hearing instruments, as the technology is similar to telecoil. There is no need to develop specially designed antennae to implement NFMI technology. This is the primary reason hearing aid manufacturers adopted NFMI as the wireless technology in the beginning. There are limitations to this approach. Since the near-field signal can only travel up to 1 m, it is not possible to wirelessly communicate across greater distances such as receiving direct audio signal from the TV. Therefore, hearing aids using NFMI technology must also use an intermediate gateway device to communicate with distant sources. The gateway device communicates with the audio source (e.g., TV adapter) via Bluetooth technology and translates the Bluetooth signal into electromagnetic signal. This electromagnetic signal is broadcasted by the loop of the gateway device

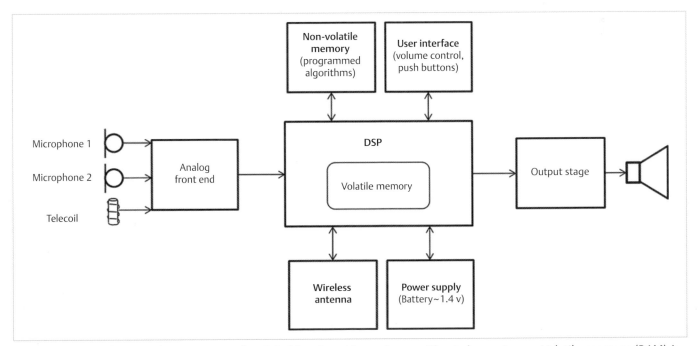

Fig. 6.20 Main functional components of a digital hearing aid are shown with wireless antenna. Volatile memory (RAM) is integrated on the main DSP chip. It does not store its contents when the hearing aid is powered down. A nonvolatile memory in the form of electrically erasable programmable read-only memory (EEPROM) is on a separate chip where the algorithms, fitting parameters, and data logs are stored. When a hearing aid is programmed in the clinic, the programming information is stored in the nonvolatile memory. This data do not get erased when the hearing aid is powered down. It can be written over multiple times (as in case of reprogramming or fine tuning a patient's hearing aid) Adapted from ON Semiconductor Technical Note.[7]

which is typically worn around the patient's neck. The NFMI antenna picks up the magnetic signal similar to the principle in which induction loop systems work. The transmission frequency in NFMI systems falls in the range of 10 to 14 MHz.

The main advantage of an NFMI system is the ease with which it can be designed and low power consumption. Another advantage is with communication between a pair of hearing aids (left and right side). Since the transmission frequency is relatively low, the signal can go around the head with relative ease and the two hearing aids can maintain communication. As discussed elsewhere, a pair of hearing aids exchanges data at a fast rate to synchronize several parameters between the two hearing aids. However, there are limitations to this approach. First, the gateway device is an additional piece of equipment that some patients might object to wearing. Second, Bluetooth protocol can result in significant transmission delays often ranging from 40 to 125 ms. Longer audio delays can potentially introduce audio–video asynchrony while watching television.

Far-field wireless technology uses radio frequencies (RFs) to broadcast signals over a longer distance, typically, 7 to 9 m (23–30 ft). This eliminates the need for a gateway device around the patient's neck. Since there is no intermediary device and no need for translating one language to another, the transmission delay from the sound source (e.g., TV) to the hearing aid is minimal.

Different RFs can be used to broadcast the signal. Standard protocols in the United States use 900 MHz RF to broadcast, while the European Union uses 868 MHz. This is problematic on two counts: compatibility issues for the patient and the manufacturer. Furthermore, these RFs require specially designed antennae that are rather large for hearing aids. Another option is to use a universally available RF. Currently, 2.4 GHz is used to directly communicate between the hearing aid and other devices capable of communicating at that frequency. The 2.4 GHz technology has some limitations as well. Power consumption to run 2.4 GHz radio is much higher. Therefore, the hearing aid battery life will be significantly diminished when the patients stream audio from the TV or listen music from the phone. The 2.4 GHz signal does not propagate well around the human head, making it poorly suited for ear-to-ear communication.

Recent innovations have resulted in hearing aids that use a dual-radio solution. This approach packs two separate antennae into a small hearing aid. ▶ Fig. 6.21 shows the functional blocks of the chip with separate integrated circuits (ICs) and the two radios. Advantages and limitations of NFMI and RF technologies are summarized in ▶ Table 6.5.

6.1.25 Hearing Aids "Made for iPhone"

The 2.4-GHz RF allows direct communication between a hearing aid and an iPhone or any other compatible iOS device. Currently, any Apple device

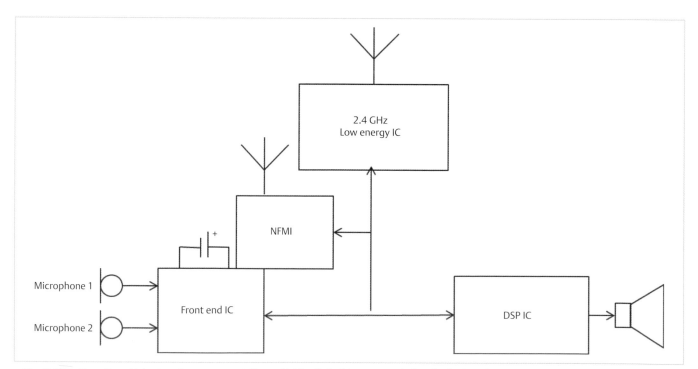

Fig. 6.21   Functional blocks of a commercially available digital hearing aid chip (Velox) with separate integrated circuits and the two radios (TwinLink). Adapted from Weile and Bach.[10] © 2016 Oticon A/S.

Table 6.5 Summary of advantages and limitations of NFMI and RF technology

	Advantages	Limitations
NFMI (hearing aid to gateway device)	• Ease of implementation, existing RF chips, simple antenna design • Low frequency means easier ear-to-ear communication • Low power consumption	• Short transmission distance (less than 1 m) • Requires a streaming device for all media, phone, and programming connectivity • May encounter interference with magnetic sources (cochlear implants)
Bluetooth (sound source to gateway device)	• Can be implemented using existing technology. No need to design special antenna within the hearing aid	• Bluetooth for audio streaming introduces a delay (often > 100 ms) that is likely to cause audio–video synchrony problems while watching television
RF 900/868 MHz	• Does not require a "gateway device" for media connectivity • Long-distance signal transmission • Relatively low power consumption • Low latency (processing delay) from source to listener • No echo problems and no lip synchronization issues when watching TV	• Requires a specially designed antenna • Requires a streaming device for Bluetooth connectivity • 900-MHz band is limited to use in certain areas including United States, Greenland, and some eastern Pacific Islands • 868-MHz band is limited to use in EU.
RF 2.4 GHz	• Does not require a "gateway device" • Long-distance signal transmission (up to 9 m) • Robust and reliable connections • High transmitted data capacity: bandwidth, stereo, low distortion • Low latency (delay) • Worldwide applicable	• Requires a specially designed antenna • Cannot propagate over physical barriers (e.g., human head) • Relatively high power consumption
Combined NFMI and RF	• NFMI allows better ear-to-ear communication • RF eliminates the need for a gateway device	• Need complex antenna design and space constraints

Abbreviations: EU, European Union; NFMI, near-field magnetic induction; RF, radio frequency.

running on iOS 7 or later is compatible with the made for iPhone hearing aids. The first "made for iPhone" hearing aids were introduced in 2014. This opened exciting opportunities for the hearing aid user as well as the manufacturers. This direct connection eliminates the need for accessories and introduced a number of custom-designed hearing aid apps that allow the patient to control the hearing aid through the iPhone. A hearing aid user can benefit from direct connectivity to iPhone by the following:

- Audio streaming from iPhone without any intermediary device: the hearing aid user can stream music, directly connect to a phone call, or stream the audio of YouTube videos directly to the hearing aid.
- Custom hearing aid app: Apps developed by hearing aid manufacturers can be used to control and personalize the hearing aid with an iPhone.
- Finding misplaced hearing aids: the hearing aid app can help locate the hearing aids by showing a stronger signal as the two devices are brought closer to each other. If the hearing aid's battery dies or the hearing aid is turned off, the app can show the location where the hearing aid and iOS device were last connected.

- Geo-tagging: the hearing aid user can tag a geographic location (e.g., library or coffee shop) and set specific settings for that location. When the user returns to that location at a later time, the hearing aid automatically engages the stored settings for that location.

The made for iPhone technology gives the hearing aid design engineers a whole new world in signal processing. The main challenges in hearing aid signal processing are imposed by the limited power supply and the small packaging of the chip. By connecting wirelessly to the iPhone, it is possible to run complex signal processing algorithms within the iPhone and send the output to the hearing aid for further processing. You may recall that Apple's A8 chip has 2 billion transistors compared to 65 million transistors in an advanced hearing aid. The added processing power can help implement many complex signal processing algorithms that were deemed impossible until now. It is also possible to make the hearing aid a part of a home network where several compatible devices are programmed to function synchronously. For example, when a hearing aid user powers up the hearing aid for the first time in the morning, it can send a signal to a compatible coffee maker within the home network to start brewing coffee. With the advent of new technologies, it is quite possible to see more innovations in the area of connectivity.

6.2 Future Directions in Hearing Aid Signal Processing

6.2.1 Advanced Acoustic Scene Classification

Currently, hearing aids can classify different acoustic scenes into four to eight distinct environments. The hearing aid analyzes the incoming signal and matches the parameters with preset static values to determine a certain acoustic scene (e.g., speech in quiet, speech in noise, machine noise, wind noise, music, etc.). At the current level of technology, most acoustic scene analyzers are designed to be "conservative" in their classification. It might be possible to use more dynamic approaches to accurately classify different environments. It is also expected that these advanced signal processing schemes can automatically "learn" and adapt the hearing aid's amplification based on the user's listening environments.

6.2.2 Wireless Connectivity

As discussed in the previous section, hearing aids in the near future will not be an isolated device any more. Rather, the hearing instrument will be a device as a part of a secured wireless network. As a result of this convergence of hearing aids and other wearable devices, we can expect to see an explosion of combination devices referred as "hearable technology" in the very near future. Such devices could be an attractive option for individuals with hearing loss who are reluctant to wear a traditional hearing aid.

Other applications of advanced wireless connectivity may include parallel signal processing using the hearing aid and an external processor such as an iPhone. The superior processing speed and battery capacity of the iPhone can be used to execute computationally expensive algorithms external to the hearing aid. Similarly, many useful mobile applications (apps) such as foreign language translation can be directly interfaced to the hearing aid.

The above-mentioned directions in future developments in hearing aid signal processing are based on the current and projected evolution of technology. There are several new areas that might dictate completely new signal processing strategies. For example, when hair cell regeneration becomes a viable treatment for humans, it is unclear if the current signal processing approaches are going to be applicable for a newly regenerated system. Recent research on recovery of function after hair cell regeneration shows limited improvements in perception of sound in birds.[26] There are several clinical trials underway to evaluate different pharmaceutical agents for treatment of hearing loss, most are aimed at sudden hearing loss and the degree of recovery cannot be predicted at this time. While these are exciting developments, the repaired auditory system might require a different set of signal processing (e.g., compression and expansion) algorithms in the future.

References

[1] Levitt H. A historical perspective on digital hearing AIDS: how digital technology has changed modern hearing AIDS. Trends Amplif. 2007; 11(1):7–24

[2] Baker B. How delta-sigma ADCs work, part 1. Analog Application Journal. 2011a; 3Q:13–16

[3] Baker B. How delta-sigma ADCs work, part 2. Analog Application Journal. 2011b; 4Q:5–7

[4] Stone MA, Moore BCJ. Tolerable hearing-aid delays: IV. effects on subjective disturbance during speech production by hearing-impaired subjects. Ear Hear. 2005; 26(2):225–235

[5] Kates JM. Digital Hearing Aids. San Diego, CA: Plural Publishing; 2008

[6] Levitt H. Digital hearing aids: a tutorial review. J Rehabil Res Dev. 1987; 24(4):7–20

[7] ON Semiconductor. Solving the hearing aid platform puzzle: seven things hearing aid manufacturers should think about [Technical note # TND6092/D]. http://www.onsemi.com/pub/Collateral/TND6092-D.PDF. Accessed June 10, 2016

[8] Chai L, Gao Q, Panda DK. Understanding the impact of multi-core architecture in cluster computing: a case study with intel dual-core system. IEEE International Symposium on Cluster Computing and the Grid

[9] Holube I, Puder H, Velde TM. DSP hearing instruments. In: Metz MJ, ed. Sandlin's Textbook of Hearing Aid Amplification. San Diego, CA: Plural publishing; 2014:221–293

[10] Weile JN, Bach R. The VeloxTM platform [technical white paper]. http://www.oticon.global/professionals/evidence. Accessed December 11, 2016

[11] Galster J, Galster EA. The value of increasing the number of channels and bands in a hearing aid. Audiology Online. http://www.audiologyonline.com/articles/value-increasing-number-channels-and-826. Accessed Jun 5, 2016

[12] Powers T, Holube I, Wesselkamp M. The use of digital filters to combat background noise. Hear Rev. 1999; 3(suppl):36–39

[13] Bentler R, Chiou LK. Digital noise reduction: an overview. Trends Amplif. 2006; 10(2):67–82

[14] Chung K. Challenges and recent developments in hearing aids. Part I. Speech understanding in noise, microphone technologies and noise reduction algorithms. Trends Amplif. 2004; 8(3):83–124

[15] Boll S. Suppression of acoustic noise in speech using spectral subtraction. IEEE Trans Acoust Speech Signal Process. 1979; 27(2):113–120

[16] Ricketts TA, Hornsby BW. Sound quality measures for speech in noise through a commercial hearing aid implementing digital noise reduction. J Am Acad Audiol. 2005; 16(5):270–277

[17] Banerjee S. Active feedback intercept: a state-of-the-art algorithm [white paper]. https://starkeypro.com/pdfs/technical-papers/WTPR9634-EE-ST.pdf. Accessed June 10, 2016

[18] Chalupper J, Powers TA, Steinbuss A. Combining phase cancellation, frequency shifting, and acoustic fingerprint for improved feedback suppression. Hear Rev. 2011; 18(1):24–29

[19] Callaway SL. Feedback shield LX and feedback analyzer: reinventing feedback management for the next generation of hearing aid [white paper]. http://www.oticon.global/professionals/evidence. Accessed December 10, 2016

[20] Ricketts T, Johnson E, Federman J. Individual differences within and across feedback suppression hearing aids. J Am Acad Audiol. 2008; 19(10):748–757

[21] Larsson P, Olsson P. Detection of Wind Noise in Hearing Aids [Master's Thesis]. Lund, Sweden: Lund Institute of Technology; 2004

[22] Raspet R, Webster J, Dillon K. Framework for wind noise studies. J Acoust Soc Am. 2006; 119: 834–843

[23] Hogan CA, Turner CW. High-frequency audibility: benefits for hearing-impaired listeners. J Acoust Soc Am. 1998; 104(1):432-41

[24] Simpson A. Frequency-lowering devices for managing high-frequency hearing loss: a review. Trends Amplif. 2009; 13(2):87–106

[25] Alexander J. Frequency lowering ten years later—new technology innovation. Audiology Online. http://www.audiologyonline.com/articles/20q-frequency-lowering-ten-years-18040. Accessed May 14, 2017

[26] Ryals BM, Dent ML, Dooling RJ. Return of function after hair cell regeneration. Hear Res. 2013; 297:113–120

7 Fundamentals of Real-Ear Measurements

John Pumford, David Smriga

7.1 Introduction

Recommendations for audiologic best practice universally include the measurement of a hearing aid when placed in the patient's ear canal. These in situ measurements are commonly and interchangeably referred to as probe microphone or real-ear measurements (REMs). Measurement of the hearing aid response is the only objective means of confirming hearing aid performance and should be a part of every hearing aid fitting. In the absence of these measurements, it is impossible to be confident about the level of sound delivered to the patient's eardrum. To state this differently, a measurement must be made in order to document what is audible to the patient with hearing loss.

It is estimated that between 30 and 40% of practicing clinicians in the United States routinely use REMs.[1] The exact rationale for this low uptake of REMs is unclear, however, anecdotally some have attributed it to the expense of the equipment, perceived complexity of the procedure and the associated time required to complete REM. Thankfully, manufacturers offer REM systems at a variety of price points to address any perceived financial obstacles. Furthermore, equipment has advanced to provide more user friendly interfaces and automated procedures to assist with completion of REM in a timely fashion.

A REM should not be confused with the hearing aid response shown on the screen of modern programming software. These displays are estimates of the hearing aid response derived from average data that include residual ear canal volume, earmold venting, microphone location, and properties of the hearing aid receiver. While the developers of hearing aids attempt to generate an accurate prediction, measurement of the hearing aid response should be preferred and regarded as the gold standard.

This chapter introduces hardware required for REM and describes fundamental measures that might be considered at the time of hearing aid fitting and subsequent fine tuning of the hearing aid response.

7.1.1 Hardware used for Real-Ear Measurements

A wide range of real-ear measurement systems are available in the market from a number of manufacturers (▶Fig. 7.1, ▶Fig. 7.2, ▶Fig. 7.3). These units range from basic, inexpensive models with relatively few features that evaluate core audibility requirements to high-end, fully loaded products that contain additional tests, signals, and hardware that also facilitate efficient verification of adaptive features (e.g., noise reduction, directionality, interdevice communication) found in modern hearing instruments. A number of these verification systems are of the dedicated real-ear only variety, whereas others offer both real-ear and test box measurement capability. Systems also vary in terms of their ability to integrate with other clinical devices such as audiometers and hearing aid fitting software, ranging from stand-alone options to modular and/or PC-enabled platforms. Portability options are also offered depending on the needs of the individual clinician to conduct verification in more than a single office location. Despite the

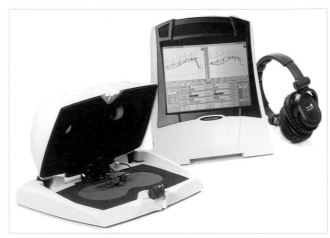

Fig. 7.1 Example of a desktop, verification system offering test box and real-ear capability.

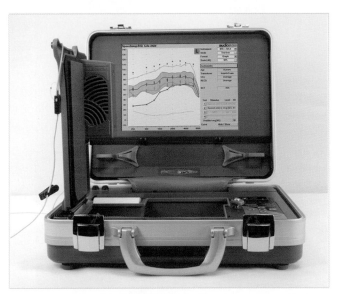

Fig. 7.2 Example of a portable verification system offering test box and real-ear capability.

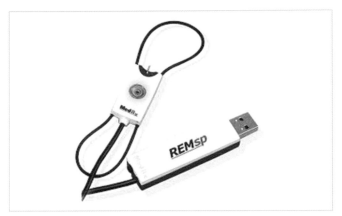

Fig. 7.3 Example of a PC-enabled verification system offering real-ear capability.

range in capability and price, each REM system can be expected to offer the core components listed below in some form or fashion.

Loudspeaker: REM requires the generation of various test signals to support the evaluation method of interest. As such, a loudspeaker is required to generate these signals. The loudspeaker capability can vary, from REM systems that leverage computer speakers should they be integrated into a separate computer to those that use dedicated loudspeakers integrated into the REM system itself. In some cases, these speakers are used to support both test box and REM testing depending on the positioning of the speakers (e.g., lid of test box open or closed); whereas in other cases, there are separate speakers that are solely dedicated for either real-ear or test box measurement. A number of real-ear manufacturers also provide the ability to connect external loudspeakers for various purposes through external speaker connections. For instance, a separate loudspeaker can be attached to external stands to provide the ability to assess directional microphone performance by presenting signals from loudspeakers positioned in front of and behind the listener. Alternatively, should a clinician desire the flexibility to position the patient in a different test location away from the REM hardware (e.g., to avoid sound field reflections, provide more test space), an external loudspeaker can be used in place of the internally integrated speaker and mounted via a number of methods such as speaker stands, speaker brackets, or swing arms. The loudspeaker options can vary by REM manufacturer and as such, the clinician would be well served to confirm with the manufacturer whether or not

the equipment provides the capability they require. Minimally, clinicians should confirm that the loudspeakers proposed for use offer a smooth frequency response and provide sufficient output to support testing with signals of interest without concerns for distortion or test signal artifacts.

7.1.2 Probe Module

To facilitate measurement in the ear canal, a number of manufacturers provide a probe module that contains both the reference and probe microphones involved in testing, along with a mechanism for attaching the apparatus to the patient (▶Fig. 7.4, ▶Fig. 7.5). Some systems separate the probe microphone and reference microphone (sometimes referred to as a monitor or regulating microphone) and offer them as two distinct components that require separate attachment to the patient. As with the discussion on loudspeakers, the manner in which the probe module is executed can vary by manufacturer. At its core, the probe module provides a housing that conveniently addresses the need to locate the probe microphone and any probe tube attached to it, along with the reference microphone near the ear canal.

Beyond providing a containment mechanism for the probe and reference microphones, probe modules also typically provide a mechanism that supports connection of the apparatus to the patient. For instance, some systems provide a retention cord and cord tightening mechanism to facilitate connection of the probe module to the outer ear near the patient's ear canal. Other systems offer ear hooks, sometimes in combination with Velcro attachments, headbands, or neck-worn housings. The physical connection of the probe module and its associated microphones to the measurement system can vary across manufacturers as well, with some offering a wireless connection whereas others offer a wired approach.

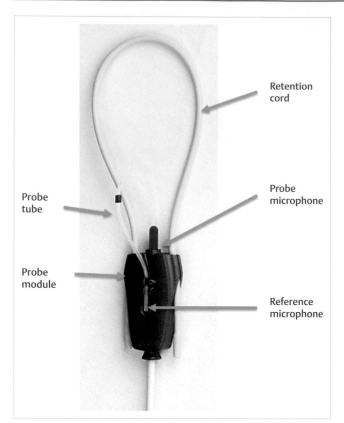

Fig. 7.4   Probe module containing both the probe and reference microphones with probe tube attached.

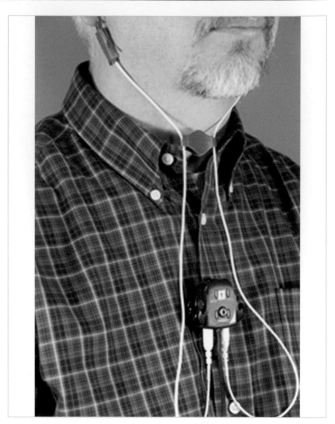

Fig. 7.5   Probe modules and associated cables connected to patient in preparation for clinical testing.

Various forms of clips and lanyards may also be provided to assist with attaching the measurement hardware to the patient and maintaining their position throughout testing.

7.1.3 Probe Microphone

The probe microphone measures sound in the ear canal via the probe tube that is attached to it. While theoretically one would desire to place the probe microphone at the measurement location of interest (i.e., at or near the eardrum), in practice, this approach would lead to a multitude of issues across patients, including microphones plugged with cerumen and infection control issues. As such, the probe tube was designed as a virtual method of moving the measurement microphone down into the ear canal while avoiding the costly and problematic issue of damaged and contaminated microphones that would have occurred had the microphone been placed in situ. That said, as will be described later, to ensure the acoustic effects introduced by the probe tube are eliminated from the assessment so that we are only measuring the effect of interest, probe tube calibration is required.

7.1.4 Reference Microphone

The reference microphone serves the purpose of ensuring proper sound field calibration so that the desired signal level/spectrum is provided at the measurement point. In systems with active, concurrent sound field calibration, ongoing measurements made by the reference microphone will result in the REM system adjusting the loudspeaker level across frequencies as needed to ensure that the requested signal level is accurately and consistently provided. Essentially the reference microphone is the standard against which the loudspeaker signal is compared[2] and helps to overcome the impact of patient movement and poor environmental/test conditions on the measurement results and ensure a consistent input. That said, there are limitations in terms of what can be addressed via the reference microphone. The clinician should be mindful of general measurement considerations (e.g., distance to measurement speaker, environmental noise) during REM to increase the likelihood of a valid result. These considerations will be discussed further in a later section of this chapter. The reference microphone is typically located such that it resides just below the lobule/ear lobe, close to the opening of the ear canal. While this location works well for most applications, it can create issues during the verification of open fittings should the reference microphone remain active throughout testing as amplified sound may leak from the ear canal and combine with the direct sound field path, leading to inaccurate sound field calibration. Methods for addressing this potential sound field calibration issue and measurement artifact with open fittings are discussed later in this chapter.

7.1.5 Probe Tube

The probe tube facilitates measurement of the signal of interest without requiring the probe microphone to be placed down into the ear canal. Probe tubes are typically manufactured of silicone material with dedicated dimensions designed for a particular manufacturer. As such, it is recommended that replacement probe tubes be used that are specifically designed for the equipment in question. Probe tubes may also provide adjustable measurement markers/rings that can be used to assist with probe tube placement in the ear canal based on the relative location of the marker to anatomical landmarks (e.g., the intertragal notch) or preexisting earpieces, earmolds, or hearing aids. During use, the probe tube is attached to the probe microphone and inserted into the ear canal. Probe tubes should be replaced for each patient and never reused. Beyond the infection control issues, reuse of probe tubes can lead to costly damage to the probe microphones to which they are attached should debris or cerumen transfer from the end of the probe tube connection to the probe microphone. It has been noted in the literature[3,4] that probe tubes can be trimmed and reused at the same appointment with the same patient should they become plugged with cerumen. Should this approach be taken, it becomes imperative that the clinician recalibrate the probe tube/microphone to account for the altered acoustic characteristics of the shortened probe tube so that any subsequent mathematical corrections applied by the measurement system accurately captures the effects of the "new" probe tube dimensions.

7.1.6 Test Signals

REM systems provide a number of measurement signals, including but not limited to warble tones, noises, environmental sounds, and speech. In addition, most systems provide the ability to select a "live" signal mode whereby the measurement system simply acts as a spectrum analyzer and does not deliver a test signal itself. In these cases, an external sound source of interest to the clinician is generated. As will be described later, while use of a noncalibrated live signal can offer some face validity and can prove helpful in counseling, there are

significant limitations in terms of their repeatability and potential for generalizability outside of the test environment in question. As such, calibrated speech test signals are generally recommended given their repeatability, consistency, and accuracy for assessing many clinical questions of interest, particularly as it relates to target matching for prescriptive fittings where a specific input signal level and spectrum is required. For this reason, REM systems typically identify those test signals that are designed specifically for target matching, often times only generating fitting formula targets when those specific signals are generated by the equipment. The use of real speech signals also addresses potential concerns regarding the misinterpretation of "simulated speech signals" via the adaptive features in hearing aids as noise or feedback. As a result, the clinician can have increased confidence that any verification measures conducted would reflect performance of the device with real speech inputs in the patient's real-world listening environment.

Depending on the question of interest and the purpose behind the testing, there can be value in a number of other test signals beyond speech. For instance, for assessment of maximum output capabilities of hearing systems, narrow-band tone bursts are typically recommended and a number of companies offer signals designed specifically to evaluate this important component during hearing aid fitting. Further, with adaptive feature evaluation, some systems offer specific test signals for evaluating noise reduction, directional microphones, and frequency lowering, just to name a few. Even magnetically generated test signals are now available in many REM systems to assess telecoil and induction loop performance with modern hearing instrument systems. Beyond the integrated test signals, some REM systems also provide clinicians with the ability to use their own recorded test signals within the test equipment. For instance, a USB connection containing recorded stimuli can be used to facilitate verification with the sound file of interest. Refer to the manufacturer specifications regarding the requirements for uploading user-defined stimuli should this option be available in the equipment in question. More details regarding applications for various stimuli in REM procedures will be described later in this chapter.

7.1.7 Display Options

An assortment of monochromatic and color screen display options are available in modern REM systems to facilitate observation of test results and support patient counseling. In some implementations, the screen display consists of a dedicated, integrated

LCD, typically with multiple color options for each measurement captured to facilitate easier identification and discussion of test results. For other REM systems, a separate computer monitor or display is required, particularly for those implementations that are integrated into computers. In addition, REM systems can offer the option of attaching secondary screen displays, either as a sole display option or in addition to the integrated offering to support a variety of counseling and viewing requirements across clinical practices. For instance, some clinicians will wall mount a larger monitor in addition to an integrated display to allow patients and family members to more easily view findings and support any counseling interactions that may be desired relative to a smaller integrated screen.

To facilitate easier workflow patterns when using programming software, a number of REM manufacturers support "on-top mode" capability, whereby the REM measurement screen and hearing aid fitting software reside on the same monitor. Simply toggling and/or resizing the displays for both applications can facilitate more efficient verification patterns. In some cases, this capability is offered via installation of remote console software whereby the fitting computer connects via networking capability to a separate REM system, whereas in computer-enabled systems without separate dedicated monitors this capability is offered as part of the integration capabilities of the system.

With ongoing advancement in consumer electronics, some systems also now support the use of VNC-viewer applications which enable viewing and operation of REM equipment on Apple products such as iPads or even iPhones. A simple download of a free VNC application and subsequent connection to the network address of any network-enabled REM system facilitates this operation and provides additional flexibility based on the needs of the fitting professional.

7.1.8 Monitor Headphones

One option provided with some REM systems that supports verification and fitting of hearing systems is monitor headphones. These devices can be worn by the clinician and used to listen in to any measurement being conducted, be it on the patient's ear or in the test box (for systems offering test box capability). Monitor headphones can assist with multiple aspects of verification, including but not limited to device troubleshooting, identifying sound quality issues, confirming proper function of user controls, and any paired devices. Depending on the REM system in question, flexibility is also offered for the clinician

to adjust the gain level of the monitor headphones and to determine which ear/channel of the system is being delivered to the binaural headphones.

7.1.9 Test Box

A number of REM systems also provide a sound-treated test box (▶**Fig. 7.6**) to facilitate various electroacoustic measurements, be it of a quality control nature (i.e., comparison to manufacturer's ANSI specifications), general adaptive feature verification (e.g., noise reduction, directional microphones), or to facilitate simulated REMs based on coupler-based testing. Depending on the manufacturer in question, the test box can be offered either as an integrated component with the REM capability of the platform, or as a separate accessory to the system. For those offering test box capabilities, there are wide ranging options in terms of the tests that can be completed given variability in the hardware contained within them and their associated measurement software platforms. Depending on the system in question, one could anticipate finding test box features that facilitate evaluation of battery drain via various battery pills, telecoils via integrated magnetic loops, directional microphones via various test box speakers, simulated REM via the combination of coupler measurements, and the addition of the real-ear-to-coupler difference (RECD; as

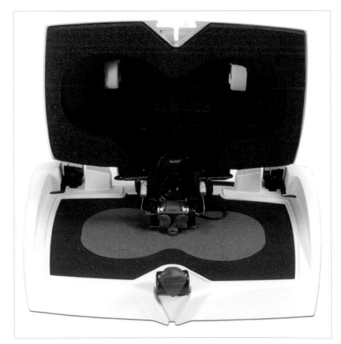

Fig. 7.6 An example of a verification system test box providing dual coupler and reference microphones for simultaneous measurement of two hearing aids, multiple speakers for directional testing, integrated magnetic loop for telecoil testing, and battery drain connection.

will be described later in this chapter). Hardware associated with coupling various systems in the test box can vary but typically involves provision of HA-1 (ITE) or HA-2 (BTE) 2cc couplers, putty to facilitate attachment of these devices to the couplers, a reference microphone (to monitor and control signal levels generated by the test box speaker) and a coupler microphone (to measure the output of the device in question after it is attached to the coupler/coupler microphone). With more recent systems, positioning tools are provided to facilitate placing the hearing instruments in the proper orientation in the test box, along with adaptors to allow connection of receiver-in-the canal (RIC) or slim tube devices without putty. Given the advent of modern amplification systems claiming extended bandwidth amplification, more recent verification systems also offer 0.4-cc couplers to facilitate extended bandwidth verification by bringing the output of any measured device above the measurement microphone noise floor.

7.1.10 Printing Options

Printing capability can vary across REM systems from those that offer integrated printers, to those that rely solely on externally connected or networked printers. Portable systems have included integrated printers to facilitate record keeping in remote applications, however external printer capability via direct connection or networked printers are also available with this category of REM equipment as well. The capabilities of the system in question to support any external printer and its associated drivers should be determined with the manufacturer in question given changing technological capabilities. Beyond direct printing from the measurement system platform, other software platforms that integrate with the REM equipment can also be used in certain cases to offer print capabilities. For instance, NOAH modules provided by various manufacturers can provide printing capabilities for any stored data. Screen capture technology is also offered with some networked systems whereby the current screen displayed on the equipment can be printed directly to a web browser. Other options provided in the market include printing test displays to connected USB storage devices in various image formats. All told, various printing options are available to support the documentation needs of the fitting professional.

7.1.11 Data Storage

To further support record keeping requirements, REM systems provide a number of data storage capabilities. For computer integrated systems, client records can typically be stored locally on the computer system in question for later review as needed. The storage of verification data can also be supported via the use of manufacturer-specific NOAH modules which attach any retrieved measurements to the client's file for later review. Data storage also facilitates the later transfer of client data to the measurement equipment at a future visit to expedite the fitting and verification process without the need to reenter data. External data storage can also be facilitated via transfer of measurements to USB devices and/or to a network folder for any networked verification system. Data storage and transfer capabilities vary by product and the interested reader is advised to contact the manufacturer directly for specific details for the device in question.

7.1.12 Networking

Networking capability is provided in modern REM systems to facilitate the transfer and storage of data and generally support full integration of the measurement equipment into clinical practice. As with previously described REM system features, networking capability can vary from one manufacturer/product to another, ranging from wired-only platforms to those providing both wired and wireless networking. REM systems typically provide a user-friendly automated networking procedure to assist with setup. Once enabled and activated, networking capability can facilitate a number of previously mentioned REM system features including remote operation, tele-audiology applications, printing flexibility, and data storage.

7.2 Methodology for Real-Ear Measurements

Decades of research have supported the perspective that REM is a valid, repeatable, and accurate approach for determining the level of amplified sound provided by a hearing instrument across frequencies to the eardrum of a patient. That said, to leverage the full potential of this objective measurement tool, there are a number of factors that clinicians should keep in mind when performing REMs.

7.2.1 Probe Tube Calibration

One of the first steps typically performed when conducting REM is probe tube calibration. As previously mentioned, the probe microphone is not physically located in the ear canal; the probe tube serves as an extension to it. Probe tube calibration is designed to account for the acoustic effects that the probe tube introduces as sound travels through it to the probe microphone. In essence, the probe tube calibration procedure makes the probe tube "acoustically invisible" to the measurement system by mathematically removing the tubing/resonance effects that occur as sound travels down the probe tube to the probe microphone. These tubing effects can be observed on the typical calibration screen shown in real-ear equipment. Thankfully, the system stores the calibration information and mathematically removes these effects automatically, so no further consideration is needed on the part of the clinician to account for them. Given the calibration values will be applied to all subsequent REMs, careful and accurate probe tube calibration is particularly important to increase the probability of valid REM.

Probe tube calibration can be conducted as frequently as desired. Depending on the system used, there are often options provided to store the calibration curves for various lengths of time (e.g., daily or weekly calibration intervals) at which point the REM system will prompt the clinician for a new calibration should additional testing be attempted. Typically, each probe tube supplied by a manufacturer is of the same physical dimensions and as such each probe tube calibration should be equivalent. That said, best practice procedures from a number of manufacturers dictate that probe tube calibration should be repeated if a probe module is replaced or if a probe tube with different dimensions than that used previously is installed. Given the unknown potential for integrity issues across probe tubes and/or measurement microphone drift in the modules, a case can be mode for routinely conducting probe tube calibration whenever a new probe tube in used (e.g., prior to testing with each patient).

REM involves two measurement microphones—the probe microphone and the reference microphone. The calibration procedure involves a comparison between the flat frequency response of the reference microphone and the probe microphone with the probe tube attached to it. Depending on the measurement system in question, probe tube calibration procedures may vary. That said, the process generally includes the following steps:

1. Select the probe tube calibration test on your equipment.
2. Press the enlarged end of a new probe tube as far as it will go into the recessed opening at the top of the probe module.
3. Position the open end of the probe tube in front of the reference microphone inlet and press it between the posts designed to hold the probe tube in this calibration location (▶ Fig. 7.4).

4. Hold the probe module 15 to 90 cm (6–36 in) away from and directly in front of the sound field loudspeaker with the reference microphone facing the loudspeaker (▶ Fig. 7.7).
5. Select "calibrate" on your equipment.

Note: With most systems, the distance of the probe tube calibration from the measurement speaker is inconsequential and does not relate to the position of the patient during testing. Calibration of the sound field for patient testing to ensure the proper signal level is delivered to the measurement point is a separate process.

Following calibration, the displayed measured curve provided by many measurement systems can be compared to the gold standard curve provided by your manufacturer in their documentation (▶ Fig. 7.8). To decrease the likelihood of an inaccurate measurement and to assist clinicians, a number of REM systems will flag an inaccurate probe tube calibration based on known tolerance/measurement boundary conditions. Audiologists should refer to the specific probe tube calibration procedure for the measurement equipment they are using to obtain system-specific instructions and learn what to expect in terms of the probe tube calibration curves and associated troubleshooting.

7.2.2 Otoscopic Examination

As with any clinical procedure involving the placment of devices into the ear canal, otoscopic examination is imperative prior to (and during) the process of REM. This procedure serves to identify any preexisting conditions that might impact the measurement (e.g., cerumen, TM perforation), document any pathological issues that may require medical referral, and ultimately aid with insertion of the probe tube. If the ear canal is occluded or cerumen is located in an area that may affect probe tube placement and potentially plug the probe tube, the cerumen should be removed prior to REM. Further, visualization of the ear canal can

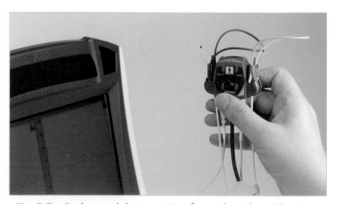

Fig. 7.7   Probe module in position for probe tube calibration.

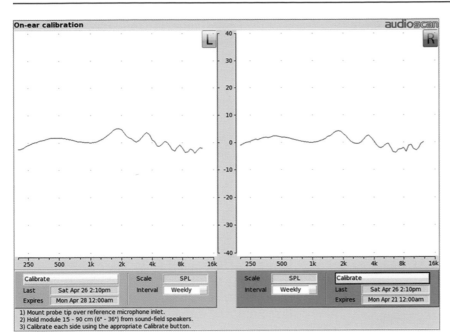

Fig. 7.8 Typical probe tube calibration curves from a real-ear measurement system.

assist with probe tube placement in the ear canal and ultimately assist with ensuring close proximity of the end of the probe tube to the eardrum to facilitate sufficient high-frequency measurement accuracy.

7.2.3 Positioning the Patient

For accurate REM results to be obtained, proper patient positioning is key. Given the nature of the sound field measurement being performed, it is understood that sound reflections from nearby surfaces (including the clinician) can cause large measurement errors if they are not appropriately controlled. Further, room/environmental noise can impact measurements, increase test time and impact hearing instrument processing, and therefore should be minimized to the extent possible during testing. In this regard, ANSI s3.46–2013[5] recommends positioning the patient and loudspeaker at least twice the "working distance" from the nearest reflective surface to minimize the likelihood of these effects contaminating the measurement. So, for example, if the distance between the patient and the loudspeaker for REM is 0.5 m, the nearest reflective surface should be 1 m away according to these recommendations. Obviously meeting these requirements can prove quite challenging in some clinical test rooms given their small dimensions, so moving the patient closer to the loudspeaker is typically the best solution.

Loudspeaker distance and azimuth considerations as it relates to REM accuracy have been evaluated by a number of researchers.[6,7] It has been noted as being particularly noteworthy as it relates to the substitution method of sound field equalization whereby the reference microphone is not actively monitoring and accounting for any changes in the sound field characteristics in the delivery of input signals to the measurement location. As it relates to loudspeaker azimuth, two choices have been documented as providing acceptable measurement accuracy: 0-degree azimuth (i.e., loudspeaker directly in front of patient) and 45-degree azimuth (i.e., loudspeaker at an angle to the ear of the patient on the side being evaluated), while 90-degree azimuth (i.e., loudspeaker directly to the side of the patient, facing the ear to be tested) has been reported as resulting in significant variability/errors and should generally be avoided.[6,8] Considerations regarding the elevation of the speaker relative to the test position should also be considered. For instance, placement of the loudspeaker too low (i.e., pointing at the stomach) could result in input signals that are lower than anticipated in the higher frequencies, impacting results, conclusions, and leading to inappropriate programming decisions.[3] As such, most REM systems recommend placement of the REM speaker at a vertical azimuth of 0 degree (i.e., ~ ear level height) to ensure the requested input signal level and spectrum is delivered to the hearing aid microphone.

Guidelines, as it relates to patient distance from the sound field speaker, attempt to strike a compromise between the desired measurement accuracy and patient comfort. Should the distance of the patient to the loudspeaker be too close, measurement results may be impacted by distortions in the sound field,[9] not to mention negatively impinge on the physical space of the patient. Alternatively, should the patient distance relative to the loudspeaker be too great, the REM system may be unable to deliver the requested signal level to the measurement point. As such, movement of the patient closer to the REM loudspeaker can minimize the likelihood of speaker overdriven issues and is a useful troubleshooting technique should such an error occur during REM.

While reported guidelines can vary across systems, typical recommendations regarding patient positioning to minimize the negative impact of environmental factors in the test space include the following:

1. Choose a quiet location and position the patient and the sound field speaker at least 1.5 m (5 ft) away from hard surfaces.
2. Position the client directly in front of, and facing (0-degree azimuth), the sound field speaker at a distance of 0.45 to 90 cm (18–36 in) from the center of the head.

Note: ANSI S3.46–2013[5] indicates ambient noise in the test environment should be at least 10 dB lower than the signal used in REM to ensure minimal effect on test results.

It should be noted that, depending on the verification procedure being conducted, there are cases where these positioning guidelines, particularly as it relates to loudspeaker azimuth, are modified. For instance, with CROS/BiCROS fittings, the loudspeaker location is moved within a range of +/− 90 degrees relative to the front of the patient depending on the verification stage as will be described later in this chapter. In a similar vein, with the front-to-back method (FBR) of evaluating directional microphone performance, the loudspeaker is positioned at 0- or 180-degree azimuth relative to the patient depending on the stage in the measurement. As previously noted, clinicians should review the documentation associated with their particular REM system to ensure they follow manufacturer recommended guidelines as it relates to patient positioning during the verification procedure in question.

7.2.4 Probe Tube Placement Techniques

Proper probe tube placement in the ear canal is crucial if accurate REM is to occur. In this regard, typical placement recommendations aim at resulting in a terminal probe tube location that is sufficiently close to the eardrum to provide an accurate assessment of sound pressure level across the frequency range of interest, particularly in the higher frequencies. Procedures aim to overcome issues with standing waves in the ear canal, whereby the reflected sound energy off of the eardrum combines and interacts with the incident sound wave at a distance equal to one-fourth the wavelength of the signal. Guidelines typically attempt the following:

1. Result in placement of the probe tube within approximately 5 mm of the eardrum so

that the high-frequency components of the response are accurately measured. As Dirks and Kincaid[10] illustrated, the closer the end of the probe tube is to the eardrum, the more accurate the high-frequency measurement becomes. Placement within 5 mm has been deemed clinically appropriate as it will generally result in an estimate within 2 dB of the SPL value at the eardrum up to 8 kHz. With the advent of modern REM systems with extended bandwidth measurement capability beyond 8 kHz, placement closer than this will result in improved high-frequency measurement accuracy. Clinically, the goal would be to strike an appropriate compromise between a location that is close enough to the eardrum to provide the desired high-frequency measurement accuracy while avoiding patient discomfort by contacting the eardrum.

2. Achieve a probe tube placement that is approximately 5 mm beyond the medial end of the earpiece to avoid "near-field effects." This general requirement relates to concerns regarding the validity of SPL measures in the transition zone from the sound bore to the ear canal. As ANSI S3.46–2013[5] indicates, however, this recommendation may not be required or met for deeply inserted hearing instruments. In that regard, research[11] has shown that conventional probe tube placement is not necessarily required for accurate REM with deeply fitted instruments such as CICs. As a result, clinicians can still achieve their measurement accuracy goals and avoid contact of the eardrum in cases where there is insufficient residual distance between the end of the hearing instrument and the eardrum to achieve the recommended location.

To assist with proper placement of the probe tube relative to the eardrum, there are a number of clinically available methods that can be used. Regardless of the procedure followed, otoscopy, clinical judgement, safety, and common sense should remain at the forefront of clinical probe tube placement techniques.

Visually-Assisted Positioning Technique

The visually-assisted positioning technique involves placement of the probe tube a constant insertion depth beyond the tragus or intertragal notch based on consideration of typical ear canal anatomy to result in a termination point that is within approximately 5 mm of the eardrum. Guidelines regarding how far to insert the probe tube vary depending on the age and gender of the patient. For instance, the

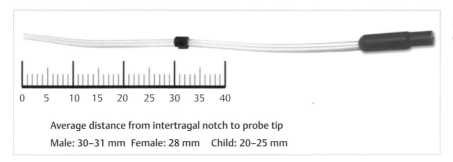

Fig. 7.9 Typical probe tube showing associated probe tube positioning marker.

Average distance from intertragal notch to probe tip

Male: 30–31 mm Female: 28 mm   Child: 20–25 mm

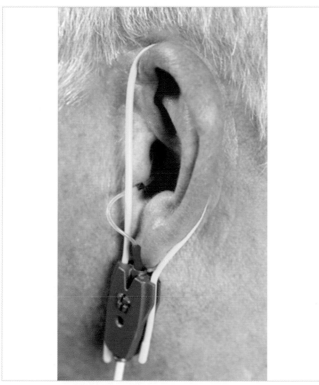

Fig. 7.10 Probe module and probe tube placement using the visually assisted positioning technique.

General guidelines regarding probe tube insertion depths to achieve measurement accuracy within 2 dB of the true value at the eardrum up to 8 kHz are as follows:

• Adult males = Insert probe tube 30 to 31 mm past the intertragal notch
• Adult females = Insert probe tube 28 mm past the intertragal notch
• Children = Insert probe tube 20 to 25 mm past the intertragal notch

For modern systems providing extended bandwidth high-frequency measurement capability up to 12.5 kHz, adding 2 mm to these guidelines would result in closer placement of the probe tube to the eardrum and an improvement of high-frequency measurement accuracy beyond 8 kHz. Research[12] evaluating extended bandwidth measurement has determined that it can be performed with suitable accuracy and repeatability with deeper insertion depths having significantly less variability and being more predictive of the level at the eardrum than shallower insertion depths. Overall, these guidelines are based on average anatomical dimensions and may not necessarily apply to each patient. In some cases, placement deeper than the guidelines may be possible whereas in other cases shallower placement may be required to avoid contact with the eardrum. As such, it is generally recommended that the clinician stop inserting the probe tube prior to achieving alignment of the marker with the intertragal notch, conduct otoscopy to determine the residual distance between the end of the probe tube and the eardrum, and then proceed accordingly with probe tube insertion should residual distance remain.

Geometrical Positioning Technique

Geometrical positioning involves use of the patient's earmold or hearing aid to assist with probe tube placement. Specifically, the outer ridge of the earmold or hearing instrument that corresponds with the location of the intertragal notch is identified. Given this location is not always apparent, clinicians may find it helpful to insert the hearing aid or earpiece into the ear canal

typical adult male presents with an ear canal length of 25 mm and a typical distance from the ear canal opening to the intertragal notch of 10 mm. Thus, inserting the end of the probe tube 30 mm past the intertragal notch should result in a placement that is within 5 mm of the eardrum for the average adult male. Adult females typically have relatively shorter ear canals, thereby resulting in a different insertion depth recommendation. Given the great variability in ear canal anatomy in pediatric clients, insertion depth guidelines are wider ranging and the use of a constant insertion depth approach is not generally recommended. To assist with this placement approach, the clinician can use the previously described markers found on most probe tubes (or gently create a mark on the tube using a pen) at the appropriate distance from the end of the probe tube, inserting the probe tube until this marker approximates the intertragal notch (▶Fig. 7.9, ▶Fig. 7.10).

prior to attempting this technique to identify appropriate landmarks. Once this location has been identified, lay the probe tube along the inferior portion of the hearing aid or earpiece and extend the open end of the tube 5 mm beyond the tip of the earpiece (▶ Fig. 7.11). It should be noted that this distance may need to be reduced for deeply fitting devices or with pediatric patients where there is insufficient residual distance to accommodate this positioning without contacting the eardrum. The probe tube is then marked where it aligns with the previously identified outer edge of the earmold or faceplate of the hearing aid and then inserted into the ear canal until the mark on the probe tube is at the intertragal notch. It should be noted that the extent to which this insertion depth is appropriate will also depend on the length of the earpiece in question. For instance, with earpieces having a shorter length canal (e.g., not beyond the second bend), it is likely that the probe tube will not be close enough to the eardrum to accurately assess the high frequencies.

Acoustical Positioning Technique

With the acoustical positioning technique, the clinician is leveraging the concept of standing waves in the ear canal to determine proper probe tube placement. Initially, the clinician selects a narrowband 6-kHz signal to be presented from the REM system loudspeaker at a level of approximately 70 dB SPL. With the patient positioned in front of the test system per manufacturer specifications, the probe tube is slowly advanced into the ear canal and the location of the greatest notch (or reduction in the response) at 6 kHz is identified. Confirmation of the minimum location can be assessed by moving the probe tube in further until the response at 6 kHz once again begins to rise. Based on standing wave theory and the anatomy of the typical adult male ear canal, it can be predicted that this notch will occur when the end of the probe tube is approximately 15 mm from the eardrum. The clinician would then simply advance the probe tube approximately 10 mm further to reach a location approximately 5 mm from the eardrum with the average adult male. In practice, this approach can be quite challenging as acoustic reflections from objects near the patient's ear (i.e., clinician's hand) while the tube is moved will impact the response. As such, ANSI s3.46–2013[5] recommends that the clinician's hand be moved away from the ear and reference microphone upon approaching the minimum response so as to increase the likelihood of an accurate response. In an attempt to automate this process, some REM systems provide a software-driven probe tube placement tool that leverages this concept of acoustical positioning, whereby the clinician is asked to actively monitor the

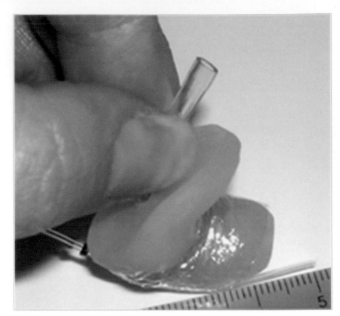

Fig. 7.11   Probe tube marker setting using the geometrical positioning technique.

response of a curve on the screen and/or wait for an indication by software when the desired location is obtained.

Acoustically Assisted Positioning Technique

With the acoustically assisted positioning, the probe tube insertion depth recommended by the visually assisted technique is first used as a basis of determining probe tube placement. Once the marker has approached the intertragal notch, the clinician then leverages the approach described in the acoustical positioning technique to determine the proper probe tube location. That is, per ANSI s3.46–2013,[5] the clinician would then measure a response in the ear canal while presenting a narrow- or broadband signal and note the response measured in the frequency region of interest (e.g., 6 kHz). The probe tube is then advanced 2 mm and the response is remeasured using the same input level. Should no change occur in the response relative to the previous measurement, this location is used as the probe tube measurement point. Otherwise, the clinician once again moves the tube forward 2 mm and remeasures, repeating these steps until such time as no change is observed in the frequency region of interest.

In summary, while manufacturer guidelines regarding probe tube placement can vary, general principles are as follows:

1. Conduct otoscopy to assess status of the ear canal, presence of any notable ear canal debris (e.g., cerumen), and aid with positioning of probe tube given patient ear canal anatomy.

2. Attach a new probe tube on the probe module.

3. Attach the probe module/housing to the patient.

4. Hang the probe module on the patient's ear, ensuring that the reference microphone is facing outward away from the face.

5. Adjust the positioning of the probe module on the ear such that the housing is snug against the head and under the ear lobe. Use any provided clips or retention devices to take up the slack in any cables to ensure the module position is maintained should the patient move.

6. Carefully slide the probe tube into the ear canal. If using a marker ring, insert the probe tube until the marker ring approaches the intertragal notch. Using otoscopy, determine if the probe tube is within approximately 5 mm of the eardrum and adjust placement as necessary.

Pearls: Clinical Tips to Assist with Probe Tube Placement ✔

- **Use the probe module retention cord as a method of holding the probe tube in place.** Friction as the probe tube is passed around the front of the cord can help hold the probe tube in place when hearing aids or earpieces are inserted or removed from the ear canal.

- **Use lubricant.** Placing a dollop of lubricant (e.g., Oto-Ease, OtoFerm) along the middle portion of the probe tube can help maintain position of the probe tube in the ear canal, and more easily allow other items to pass over the tube without creating friction that might move it. Lubricant along the tube (or when added to any earpiece inserted into the ear canal) can also help minimize the likelihood of feedback due to slit leak venting caused by the probe tube.

- **Use the housing of your measurement equipment as a ruler should you not have one handy for setting probe markers.** Many measurement systems provide either a ruler mounted on their equipment, or guidelines regarding the dimensions of their probe modules such that probe tube markers can be set by aligning the probe tube alongside the housing.

- **Consider simultaneous insertion of the probe tube and the earpiece.** This technique has proven valuable with pediatric patients[13] and/or with less cooperative patients who are less likely to remain still during probe tube/earpiece insertion. Using this approach, the probe tube is extended approximately 2 to 5 mm beyond the medial end of the earpiece and wrapped with moisture guard or a similar material to attach it to the earpiece. The earpiece and probe tube are then inserted simultaneously. The accuracy of this approach is obviously dependent on the length of the earpiece in question.

7.2.5 Sound Field Equalization

To ensure the appropriate input signal level and frequency spectrum is delivered to the measurement point, REM systems provide a number of methods for calibrating the test environment via sound field equalization. ANSI s3.46–2013[5] outlines a few methods of sound field equalization: the substitution method, the modified pressure method with stored equalization, and the modified pressure method with concurrent equalization as will be described below.

Substitution Method

In this approach, the sound field equalization is conducted without the patient near the measurement location (i.e., with the patient absent). Following calibration of the sound field with only the reference microphone located at the test location, the center of the patient's head is subsequently placed in the test location previously occupied by the reference microphone. Should the patient move from the calibrated position, or the test environment change, the sound field equalization process would need to be conducted once again to ensure the appropriate signal level/spectrum is delivered to the test location. Using this approach, the signal ultimately delivered to the test location with the patient in place would be altered by diffraction of sound off of the head and body and by external ear resonances.[8] As such, REM manufacturers specify the method of sound field calibration they are using as an input to fitting formula algorithms on their systems, so that target generation is appropriate for the assumed input signal.

Modified Pressure Method with Stored Equalization

With this sound field equalization approach, the patient is placed in the test location with the reference microphone on their ear per manufacturer's specifications. A calibration stimulus (e.g., broadband noise) is delivered to the test location by the measurement system and the output/frequency response of the system speaker is measured and stored. This sound field transform is subsequently applied to all test signals delivered from the REM speaker to ensure that the correct signal level/spectrum is delivered to the test location. Clinically, this sound field equalization approach is typically used with hearing aids having significant venting (i.e., open fittings) to address issues with amplified sound leaking from the ear canal during testing to an active reference microphone, thereby contaminating the sound field calibration process. As such, the modified pressure method with stored equalization is typically performed with the patient's hearing aid(s) in place on the ear and muted or turned off. Most REM systems will provide a process whereby an automated procedure guides the user through this calibration approach once an "open-fit" hearing aid style is selected. As with the substitution method, this approach calibrates a single location in space, and as a result, the calibration procedure needs to be updated whenever there is a change in the patient location or test environment.

Modified Pressure Method with Concurrent Equalization

As with the modified method with stored equalization, the concurrent equalization approach involves placement of the patient in the test location with the reference microphone on the ear. In contrast, however, the reference microphone with the concurrent approach remains active throughout the verification process, monitoring the sound pressure level received at the test location and adjusting the loudspeaker signal level and spectrum accordingly when needed to ensure a consistent signal is maintained. In this way, aspects of the environment that can destructively or constructively interfere with the loudspeaker signal as it travels to the measurement location (e.g., background noise, reflections, standing waves) can be accounted for and controlled to ensure the hearing aid receives a consistent input test signal. The fitter can then have increased confidence that any differences measured from one test occasion to another reflect true differences, not error created by variability in the input test signal from one test to another. Typically, this ongoing sound field evaluation and subsequent adjustment of the signal level/spectrum occurs during the presentation of a calibration stimulus (e.g., broadband noise) that is periodically generated during the test procedure while the selected test stimulus (e.g., speech) is played. It is therefore imperative that the test environment remain quiet and representative of the patient's subsequent test position during the presentation of the calibration stimulus. Clinically, the concurrent equalization approach provides many advantages for sound field equalization as it is forgiving of patient movement and does not require a recalibration process as is the case with the stored or substitution methods to ensure the correct signal level/spectrum is delivered to the test location throughout testing. That said, as previously described, concurrent equalization can result in test errors due to incorrect sound field calibration (and resulting incorrect input signal characteristics) with open-fit devices.

Simultaneous Bilateral REM Considerations

With the advent of REM systems that allow for simultaneous measurement of both hearing aids in the ear canal, additional considerations regarding proper sound field calibration have arisen. Essentially, the challenges relate to ensuring that the requested input signal level and spectrum is delivered to two measurement locations (i.e., both hearing aids) from a single sound source—the REM system sound field speaker. As sound travels from the loudspeaker, the possibility arises that the signal level will be asymmetrically altered by diffraction of sound off of the patient's head/body, reflections off of material near the patient (e.g., the clinician, walls, shelving) or environmental noise—resulting in input signals that are not equivalent at both hearing aid microphones. This is less of a concern with sequential monaural measurement since, as previously described, the reference microphone dedicated to the test ear in question will serve to ensure the loudspeaker delivers the correct signal level to the ear/device being evaluated. However, with simultaneous bilateral (sometimes referred to as binaural) measurements the question becomes how to adjust a single sound source to account for any bilateral sound field differences that may be present. As fitting formula targets require precise input signal level and spectrum characteristics, it is important to ensure that any sound field asymmetry in test signal delivery is properly accounted for so that proper programming decisions are made. Stated simply, the input level received by the hearing aid determines the output of that device and verification decisions will be impacted accordingly. What may appear to be an under- or overfitting relative to target may simply represent an incorrect input signal. A number of approaches are used by REM systems to determine the delivered signal level during simultaneous bilateral measurements and account for any asymmetry in input signal level/spectrum received at the measurement point. These approaches include averaging the difference between reference microphones or allowing the clinician to select one reference microphone as the basis for sound field calibration for all bilateral measurements. Both of these approaches involve accepting an unknown level of error as the input signal received at each device may not be equivalent and may vary from the requested level and/or spectrum. Results can vary and, depending on the non-uniformity of the sound field, can be quite different from measurements taken sequentially with ear-specific sound field calibration. To assist with these considerations and ensure the proper input signal is provided during simultaneous bilateral REM, some verification systems measure and compare the

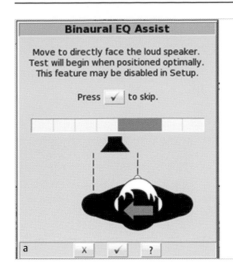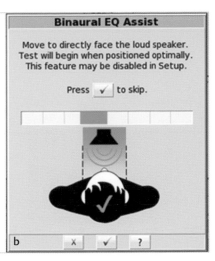

Fig. 7.12 Example of a REM system patient positioning tool automatically generated to address identified differences in input signal level characteristics between ears during simultaneous bilateral measurements **(a)**; and following patient repositioning to equate the sound field across ears at the reference microphone **(b)**.

reference microphone levels across ears and generate patient positioning tools should an asymmetry condition exist to provide the clinician with the opportunity to address it (▶ **Fig. 7.12a, b**).

7.3 Real-Ear Measurement Terminology and Measurement Types

7.3.1 Understanding Acronyms

To increase comprehension of various REM terms and their associated procedures, the reader should be aware of the manner in which various real-ear acronyms are constructed. First, real-ear terms typically begin with the letters "RE", which refers to the phrase "real-ear." These first two letters tend to be followed by two additional letters which refer to the specific measure being conducted (e.g., A = aided; U = unaided). Should the real-ear term end with the letter "G", the term refers to "Gain" and it is a difference measurement, where the input level used to generate the response is subtracted from the absolute output level measured across frequencies. Should the real-ear term end with the letter "R", the term refers to "Response" and it is an absolute value measure of output in SPL. In other words, there is no consideration of the input level used to generate the measured response. The relationship between acronyms ending in "R" and "G" is demonstrated for one measurement type in ▶ **Table 7.1**.

7.3.2 What, How, and Why

There are various types of real-ear measurements that can be performed depending on the question of interest during verification, with each having an associated acronym as outlined below. The following section, adapted from Pumford and Sinclair,[14] defines a number of commonly encountered REM terms, outlines how the associated procedures are conducted and touches on various applications for their use in clinical practice.

What Is It? (REUR/REUG)

Real-Ear Unaided Response (REUR)
Formal definition (per ANSI s3.46–2013)[5]

- SPL as a function of frequency, at a specified measurement point in the ear canal, for a specified sound field, with the ear canal unoccluded.

Informal definition

- The SPL, across frequencies, measured in the open (unaided) ear canal for a given input signal.

Real-Ear Unaided Gain (REUG)
Formal definition (per ANSI s3.46–2013)[5]

- Difference in decibels between the SPL, as a function of frequency, at a specified measurement point in the ear canal and the SPL at the field reference point, for a specified sound field, with the ear canal unoccluded.

Informal definitions

- The gain provided by the pinna and the ear canal with head diffraction effects as measured in the open ear canal. Subtract the input signal level from the REUR across frequencies to obtain the REUG.

- The natural amplification of the patient's open ear canal.

Table 7.1 Example of relationship between real-ear measurement acronyms using "G" (gain) and "R" (response)

Acronym	Frequency (kHz)								
	0.25	0.5	0.75	1	2	3	4	6	8
REA**R**	65	72	75	80	83	85	88	75	71
– Input	60	60	60	60	60	60	60	60	60
REA**G**	5	12	15	20	23	25	28	15	11

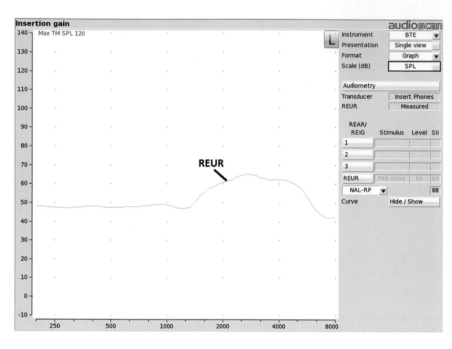

Fig. 7.13 Example of a real-ear unaided response (REUR) measurement, obtained with a 60 dB SPL pink noise signal.

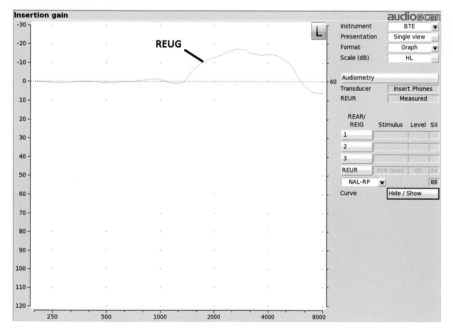

Fig. 7.14 Example of a real-ear unaided gain (REUG) measurement, obtained with a 60 dB SPL pink noise signal.

An example of a typical REUR/REUG is shown in ▶ **Fig. 7.13**, ▶ **Fig. 7.14**. The average adult will exhibit a primary peak in their REUG around 2,700 Hz of 17 dB with a secondary peak in the 4,000 to 5,000-Hz region of approximately 12 to 14 dB.[8] However, individual REUGs can vary substantially from person to person depending not only on typical anatomical variants, but also aspects such as eardrum perforations or surgical ears.

How Is It Measured? (REUR/REUG)

1. Conduct otoscopic examination.
2. Place probe tube into open ear canal to appropriate depth (e.g., within 5 mm of eardrum).
3. Place patient at appropriate distance/azimuth from loudspeaker (e.g., 0.5 m/0 degree).
4. Select desired input level and test signal type*.
5. Present and record the measurement (▶ **Fig. 7.13** and ▶ **Fig. 7.14**).

*As previously described, there are various considerations regarding test signal types and levels. Minimally one would want to ensure that the test signal is above the room noise floor, within a range that would be typical of hearing aid verification, and below a level that would potentially cause listening discomfort for the client.

Why Measure It? (REUR/REUG)

The REUR/REUG is typically used as the first step in the process when fitting to real-ear insertion gain (REIG) targets, and is subtracted from the real-ear–aided response (REAR) as will be described later. Depending on the REM system in question, the REUG will be automatically calculated and displayed on the fitting screen by automatically subtracting the input level used during the test which can facilitate troubleshooting of the result. Depending on the REM system implementation, the REUR/G can also be used in the SPL-o-gram approaches of hearing aid fitting (e.g., Desired Sensation Level [DSL] method), whereby the measured values are used to convert sound field audiometry from dB HL to dB SPL at the eardrum. A number of systems apply average REUG values to convert dB HL sound field audiometry to dB SPL at the eardrum values. In these cases, it is important that the loudspeaker azimuth specified in the REM system reflects that used during the hearing assessment as REUGs will vary depending on sound source location. When conducted on an SPL-o-gram screen, the REUG can also prove valuable in the candidacy process with open fit products by allowing the clinician to assess audibility of low-frequency sound without a hearing instrument in place. REUR results have also been documented as useful indicators of certain ear canal or middle ear abnormalities (e.g., eardrum perforations) based on their documented impact on the frequency response of the measurement.[4,8]

What Is It? (REAR/REAG)

Real-Ear–Aided Response (REAR)
Formal definition (per ANSI s3.46–2013)[5]

- SPL as a function of frequency, at a specified measurement point in the ear canal, for a specified sound field, with the hearing aid (and its acoustic coupling) in place and turned on.

Informal definition

- The frequency response of an activated hearing aid for a particular input signal measured in the ear canal.

Real-Ear Aided Gain (REAG)
Formal definition (per ANSI s3.46–2013)[5]

- Difference in decibels, as a function of frequency, between the SPL at a specified measurement point in the ear canal, and the SPL at the field reference point, for a specified sound field, with the hearing aid (and its acoustic coupling) in place and turned on.

Informal definitions

- The gain of an activated hearing aid across frequencies for a particular input signal measured in the ear canal.

How Is It Measured? (REAR/REAG)

1. Conduct otoscopic examination.
2. Place probe tube into open ear canal to appropriate depth (e.g., within 5 mm of eardrum; beyond sound bore of earpiece). *Note: If REAR/REAG is being used for insertion gain purposes, ensure the probe tube remains in the same location used for the REUR/REUG.*
3. Insert hearing aid into client's ear canal, being sure to maintain probe tube location.
4. Place patient at appropriate distance/azimuth from loudspeaker (e.g., 0.5 m/0 degree).
5. Turn hearing aid on at desired programmed settings. *Note: If significant venting (e.g., open-fit device), first calibrate sound field using "stored calibration" with hearing aid in place and turned off or muted prior to testing.*
6. Select desired input level and test signal type*.
7. Present and record the measurement (▶ **Fig. 7.15** and ▶ **Fig. 7.16**).

*As previously described, there are various considerations regarding test signal types and levels. Minimally one would want to ensure that the test signal is above the room noise floor, within a range that would be typical of hearing aid verification and below a level that would potentially cause listening discomfort for the client. For insertion gain approaches, the same input signal characteristics should be used for both the REAR and REUG should your system not

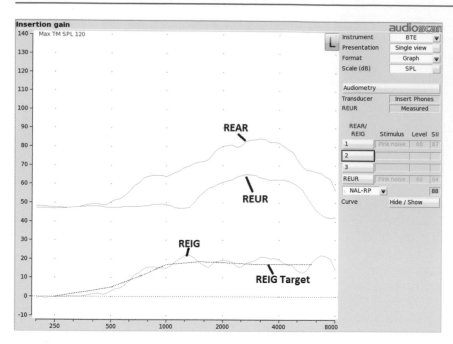

Fig. 7.15 Example of a real-ear aided response (REAR) measurement, obtained with a 60-dB SPL pink noise signal. Also shown is the previously measured real-ear unaided response (REUR) measurement, along with the resulting real-ear insertion gain (REIG) values and the REIG target.

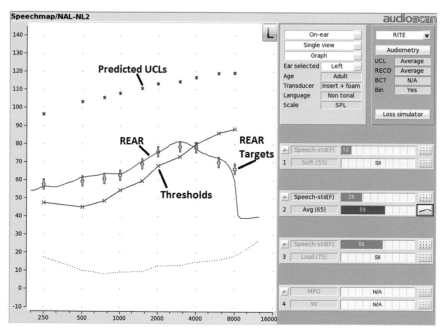

Fig. 7.16 Example of a real-ear aided response (REAR) measurement on a SPL-o-gram or Speechmap screen, obtained with an average speech input level. Also shown are the REAR targets generated by the prescriptive formula for that particular input level (+), the patient's thresholds (X), and the predicted UCLs for the patient (*).

automatically account for input signal differences across the two stages of the process.

Why Measure It? (REAR/REAG)

The REAR/REAG has been traditionally used as a reference for hearing aid fitting approaches that use the real-ear insertion gain (REIG) approach (i.e., REAG – REUG = REIG). More recently, this measurement has been used as the primary tool for hearing aid verification for a variety of prescriptive methods, particularly DSL. As will be described later in the chapter, when used in combination with the SPL-o-gram format, the REAR

quickly provides information regarding the suitability of hearing aid output relative to a patient's dynamic range (i.e., threshold to uncomfortable loudness levels), in addition to the traditional considerations regarding proximity to fitting formula targets.

What Is It? (REIG)

Real-Ear Insertion Gain (REIG)
  Formal definition (per ANSI s3.46–2013)[5]

- Difference in decibels, as a function of frequency, between the REAG and the REUG taken with the same measurement point and

the same sound field conditions. Previously called the real-ear insertion response (REIR).
Informal definition

- The amount of gain provided by the hearing instrument alone calculated by subtracting the REUG from the REAG across frequencies or by subtracting the REUR from the REAR across frequencies.

Note: ANSI s.3.46–2013[5] does not define the term REIR since the calculation of insertion gain is a difference measurement. Recall that a difference measure involves the calculation of gain and therefore is a term ending in "G."

How Is It Measured? (REIG)

1. Conduct an REUR as described above.
2. Conduct an REAR as described above, ensuring the same sound field conditions and probe tube placement location as the REUR.
3. Subtract the REUR from the REAR or subtract the REUG from the REAG. REM systems will perform this subtraction automatically and plot the resulting REIG on the screen for you.
4. Adjust the hearing aid programming so that the REAR (REAG) and thus the resulting calculation of the REIG provides the closest match to the target REIG across frequencies (▶ Fig. 7.15).

Why Measure It? (REIG)

The primary application of the REIG is to determine suitability of a hearing instrument setting relative to the REIG target prescribed by the selected fitting formula for the input level in question. In the absence of a theoretical target, the calculation of REIG becomes rather meaningless.[4,8] The REIG approach does present with some limitations relative to the SPL-o-gram (REAR only) methods, including the absence of a frame of reference regarding the impact of target mismatches on audibility and/ or implications relative to a patient's uncomfortable loudness levels (i.e., lack of dynamic range visibility). In addition, insertion gain approaches inherently assume a sound field audiogram given their inclusion of the open ear (i.e., REUG) in their target calculation. As the calculation approach is influenced by the individual nature of the patient's REUR/REUG, unusual REUGs containing valleys or dips in the high frequencies can impact the perceived suitability of a hearing aid fitting relative to target—not to mention the ability in some cases

to achieve the target in question. Questions related to the appropriate REUG to consider in the calculation has led some REM systems to recommend using only average REUG values for REIG calculation unless the audiometric assessment was performed using sound field speakers. Specifically, measured REUGs should only be used when thresholds were obtained in sound field as the individual REUG was then part of the assessment and therefore should be considered in target calculation. In cases with other hearing assessment transducers (e.g., headphones, insert phones), it is indicated that the average REUG provided by the fitting formula developers should be used because the individual REUG was not involved in the assessment.

What Is It? (REOR/REOG)

Real-Ear–Occluded Response (REOR)
Formal definition (per ANSI s3.46–2013)[5]

- SPL as a function of frequency, at a specified measurement point in the ear canal, for a specified sound field, with the hearing aid (and its acoustic coupling) in place and turned off.

Informal definition

- The SPL across frequencies for a hearing aid that is turned off for a particular input signal measured in the ear canal.

Real-Ear–Occluded Gain (REOG)
Formal definition (per ANSI s3.46–2013)[5]

- Difference in decibels, as a function of frequency, between the SPL at a specified measurement point in the ear canal and the SPL at the field reference point, for a specified sound field, with the hearing aid (and its acoustic coupling) in place and turned off.

Informal definition

- The difference in decibels, across frequencies, between the signal level measured in the ear canal and the input signal with the hearing aid on the ear and turned off. Subtract the input signal level from the REOR across frequencies to obtain the REOG.

How Is It Measured? (REOR/REOG)

1. Conduct otoscopic examination.
2. Place probe tube into open ear canal to appropriate depth (e.g., within 5 mm of

eardrum; beyond sound bore of earpiece). *Note: If REOR/REOG is being used for comparison to REUR/REUG, ensure the probe tube remains in the same location for all measurements.*

3. Insert hearing aid into client's ear canal, being sure to maintain probe tube location.
4. Ensure the hearing aid is muted or turned off.
5. Place patient at appropriate distance/azimuth from loudspeaker (e.g., 0.5 m/0 degree).
6. Select desired input level and test signal type*.
7. Present and record the measurement (►Fig. 7.17).

*While the input signal level and type can vary during this measurement, it is usually more meaningful if the same test signal characteristics are used for both the REOR/G and the REUR/G.

Why Measure It? (REOR/REOG)

A primary purpose for conducting the REOR/REOG is to assess venting characteristics.[4,8] That is, this measurement can prove helpful in determining whether or not the vent is performing as anticipated by allowing certain frequencies to pass through it to the eardrum. For example, we would anticipate that the REOR/REOG would approximate the REUR/REUG for the same ear canal if the earpiece under test is truly "open" in its venting characteristics (►Fig. 7.17). Conversely, in occluded fittings we would anticipate that the REOR/REOG would deviate significantly below the REUR/REUG, where at most frequencies the REOG would be negative in value (i.e., where negative gain is a loss). In the authors' experience, the simple selection of an earpiece labelled as "open" by a manufacturer does not necessarily result in an open fit (e.g., if a large-diameter earpiece results in a folding of excess material in the ear canal). As such, the use of REOR/G can assist with the proper selection of venting for any earpiece such that the desired venting characteristics (e.g., open fitting) are provided. To the extent that venting can occur via slit leaks of sound around the outside of an earpiece, the REOR/G can also be used in an attempt to document the tightness of a fitting. The REOR/G has also been mentioned as a method of documenting any vent-associated resonance in the ear canal that might introduce undesired acoustic effects.[4,8] While venting is often used to address concerns regarding occlusion, Bentler et al[4] point out that the REOR/G does not measure the occlusion effect and is a poor predictor of occlusion unless it is similar to the REUG (i.e., where an open ear canal would likely preclude the occlusion effect). Measurement of the occlusion effect will be described later in this chapter.

What Is It? (RECD)

Real-Ear-to-Coupler Difference (RECD)
Formal definition (per ANSI s3.46–2013)

- Difference in decibels, as a function of frequency, between the SPL produced near the tympanic membrane in an occluded ear canal by a coupled sound source having a high

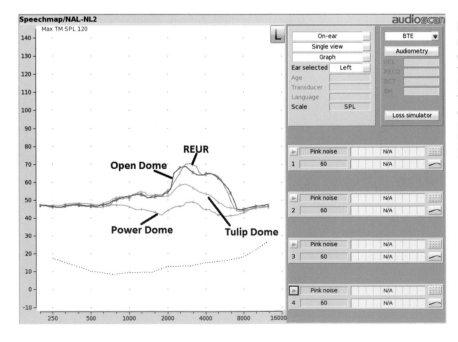

Fig. 7.17 Example of real-ear occluded response (REOR) measurements for various device venting conditions. Shown is the previously measured REUR, along with REOR measurements for an open dome, tulip/closed dome, and a power/occluding dome. Note the reduction in the measured response relative to the REUR as the venting is gradually decreased and the ear canal becomes more occluded.

acoustic impedance (see ANSI/ASAS1.1) and that produced in the HA-1 configuration of the 2-cc earphone coupler by the same coupled sound source.

Informal definition

- Difference in decibels across frequencies, between the SPL measured in the ear canal and in a coupler, produced by a transducer generating the same input signal.

The RECD is a term that was not defined in the previous ANSI s3.46–1997 REM standard although it has been used in the fitting and verification of hearing instruments for many years. With the introduction of ANSI s3.46–2013,[5] RECD was standardized and specifically defined to include use of an HA-1 coupler reference and a high-impedance sound source. This specific request resulted from evidence suggesting that use of an HA-2 reference could result in different RECD values for the same ear depending on the impedance of the sound source used in the measurement. The reader interested in learning more regarding the considerations related to sound source and coupling impedance effects on RECD measurements is referred to Annex C of ANSI s3.46–2013.[5]

How Is It Measured? (RECD)

A number of REM manufacturers have implemented automated RECD measurement procedures that walk the clinician through the various steps involved. Check with the manufacturer regarding the specific steps to be used with their equipment. The procedure outlined below reflects the general principles followed when conducting the RECD.

1. Conduct coupler measurement (▶ **Fig. 7.18**):
   a. Attach a signal generator/RECD transducer to the RECD signal jack.
   b. Attach the coupler* to the coupler microphone.
   c. Attach the RECD transducer to the coupler.
   d. Generate the signal**.
   e. Store the coupler measurement. *Note: Most measurement equipment will store the coupler response automatically. Some equipment will also flag measurement errors relative to the expected coupler response for troubleshooting.*

*The coupler used for the coupler portion of the measurement can vary by manufacturer. In some cases, an HA-2 2-cc BTE coupler is used to facilitate easy attachment of the RECD transducer and a mathematical HA-2 to HA-1 transform is used to provide values in an HA-1 format. In other cases, an HA-1 2-cc ITE coupler or a 0.4-cc coupler with a rubber adaptor cap is used to facilitate easy attachment of the RECD transducer. Please check with the manufacturer for your system-specific setup.

**While the input signal level and type can vary for this measurement, typically the manufacturer provides a specific broadband signal for this procedure that is sufficiently loud enough to be above the noise floor but at a comfortable loudness level for the patient.

2. Conduct REM (▶ **Fig. 7.19**):
   a. Conduct otoscopic examination.
   b. Place probe tube into open ear canal to appropriate depth (e.g., within 5 mm of eardrum; beyond sound bore of earpiece to be inserted)*.

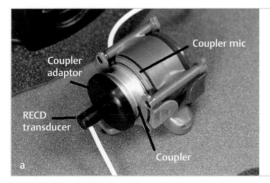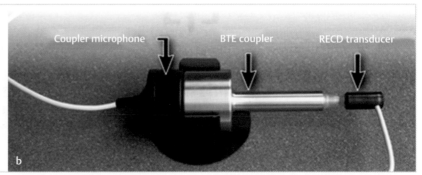

Fig. 7.18 Example setups for the coupler portion of the real-ear to coupler difference measurement using a 0.4-cc coupler (for wideband RECD measures) **(a)**; and using a 2-cc HA-2 (BTE) coupler (for traditional RECD measures) **(b)**. The coupler values are automatically transformed by the REM system to an HA-1 reference.

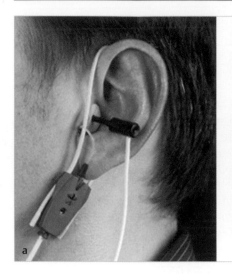
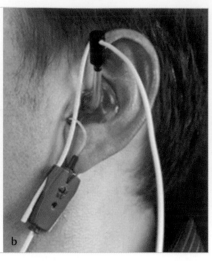

Fig. 7.19 Example setups for the real-ear portion of the real-ear to coupler difference measurement using a foam tip (**a**); and an earmold (**b**).

c. Attach the RECD transducer to a standard foam ear tip (or patient's earmold tubing or earpiece).

d. Insert foam ear tip (or earmold**) into the ear, being careful not to move the inserted probe tube. *Note: the lateral portion of the foam ear tip should be flush with the outer entrance of the ear canal per the depth used for audiometry.*

e. Generate the same signal used with the previous coupler measurement.

f. Store REM. *Note: Most measurement equipment will store the real-ear response automatically.*

g. Subtract the stored coupler response from the REM to produce the RECD. *Note: Most measurement equipment will calculate the RECD for you and plot the results relative to age-appropriate average values to facilitate troubleshooting. Some systems will also flag invalid REMs for troubleshooting.*

*Simultaneous insertion of the probe tube and the earpiece has been proposed as an alternative technique in certain pediatric cases and found to provide acceptable measurement accuracy. Further details regarding this technique can be found in Bagatto et al.[13]

**As a traditional RECD is not designed to capture vent effects, it is recommended that any vent present on an earmold be plugged medially should one be present.[15]

An example of a measured RECD is presented in ▶**Fig. 7.20a**. As can be seen, given the 2-cc volume of the coupler used in this case, the smaller volume of the individual ear canal results in a higher SPL measurement than the 2-cc coupler for the same signal, and thus the subtraction of the real-ear response

from the coupler response results in a positive RECD value. We also see that the measured RECD values are somewhat higher across frequencies than the age-appropriate average reference. In ▶**Fig. 7.20b**, we see an example of a wRECD (wideband RECD measurement) provided by one manufacturer to facilitate extended bandwidth verification. Given the reduced coupler volume used in the measurement (i.e., 0.4 cc), the measured coupler response is higher than the 2-cc response. As a result, the measured real-ear response is at some frequencies lower and generally closer to the coupler response resulting in a calculated wRECD that provides negative values at some frequencies. It is therefore important to keep in mind the characteristics of the coupler used during the procedure to determine whether or not the obtained RECD values make sense. In this respect, the age-appropriate average values provided by the REM system are a useful tool in combination with the general tips provided in the box on the next page. Regardless of the coupler used, most modern REM systems will convert the measurements mathematically to an HA-1 reference and provide these values in a table to facilitate use in other measurement systems or fitting software applications. Studies[16,17] evaluating the wRECD have revealed comparable test–retest reliability and measurement accuracy as the standard 2-cc coupler approach with the added benefit of additional data for the extended high frequencies beyond 8 kHz.

Why Measure It? (RECD)

The RECD is a powerful tool that is used for essentially two primary applications in the hearing aid fitting process: (1) audiometric conversion of dB HL

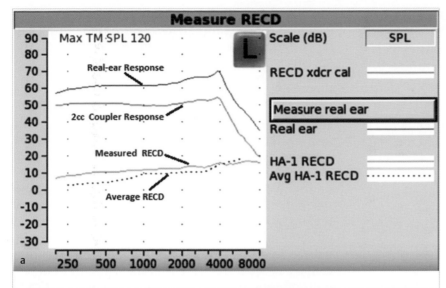

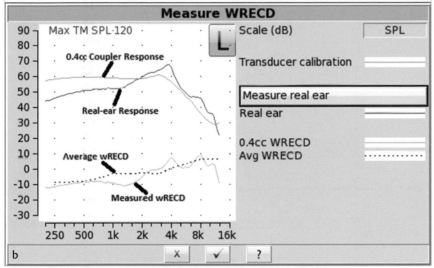

Fig. 7.20 (a) Example of a completed RECD measurement screen showing the measured real-ear response, the previously measured 2-cc coupler response, the automatically calculated measured RECD (i.e., real-ear curve–coupler curve), and the age-appropriate average RECD. (b) Example of a completed wRECD measurement screen showing the measured real-ear response, the previously measured 0.4-cc coupler response, the automatically calculated wRECD (i.e., real-ear curve–coupler curve), and the age-appropriate average wRECD.

insert earphone data to dB SPL values at the eardrum; and (2) the prediction of REMs using test box/coupler-based simulated REMs. While age-appropriate averages are available for both foam tip and earmold coupling types,[19] enough individual variability exists within any given age group, including adults,[20] to reinforce the benefit of individually measuring the RECD whenever possible.

For the purposes of audiometric conversion, the RECD is in essence adjusting the 2-cc calibration values used with insert earphones and capturing the impact of the patient's ear canal on what was delivered to the eardrum during audiometry. The specific calculation applied at each audiometric frequency is as follows:

$$\text{dB HL threshold} + \text{RECD} + \text{RETSPL} = \text{Real-ear SPL threshold}$$

Where: RETSPL = reference equivalent threshold sound pressure level, or the calibrated level of sound that should be produced by the audiometer across frequencies for a particular coupler reference (e.g., 2-cc coupler).

Given the RECD provides a 2-cc coupler reference as well, we can essentially personalize the calibration by factoring in the RECD to determine the level of sound delivered to the eardrum during audiometry across frequencies. Thankfully these transforms are conducted automatically within the REM system for the SPL-o-gram methods (e.g., DSL) that require this data. Studies [21] have shown this audiometric transform approach to be valid and repeatable. With an accurate determination of the true level at the eardrum during audiometric testing, the fitting formula can then provide a more accurate prescription for the patient.

Arguably the most useful application of the RECD is in the prediction of real-ear output when hearing aid measurements are made in the test box. As shown by Seewald et al,[22] given the RECD allows us to know

Pearls: RECD Troubleshooting ✔

For the benefits of the RECD to be realized, the measurement needs to be accurate and truly reflect the acoustic signature of the individual ear canal. To improve the likelihood of obtaining an accurate RECD measurement, most manufacturers provide an age-appropriate RECD reference on the measurement screen that can be used as a comparison to the measured values. As outlined by Bagatto,[18] there are general RECD trends that should be considered to increase the likelihood of an accurate measurement and to help decide whether or not the individually measured RECD is valid including the following:

Reduced low-frequency values

Possible cause: Venting.
Resolutions: Let foam tip expand completely; select larger foam tip and/or insert foam tip more deeply; remove and reinsert earpiece, use earmold lubricant along outside of earpiece, and/or place along middle of probe tube; plug vent medially if using vented earmold.

Possible cause: Perforation of eardrum, surgical ear.

Resolutions: None, RECD measurement valid as you are measuring a larger-volume cavity than the typical ear canal.

Reduced high-frequency values

Possible cause: Probe tube too shallow.
Resolutions: Remove earpiece and reinsert probe tube more deeply following clinical guidelines.
Possible cause: Using earmold for real-ear portion of measurement.
Resolutions: None, RECD measurement valid as earmold tubing rolls off high frequencies given longer length relative to tubing within a standard foam ear tip.

Large negative values across frequencies

Possible cause: Probe tube plugged, pinched or dislodged from real-ear module.
Resolutions: Remove and reinsert probe tube after checking tube for blockage and conducting otoscopy to check for possible obstructions. Replace probe tube and/or check connection with real-ear module/probe microphone. *Note: if plugged probe tube is trimmed and reused, please ensure you recalibrate the probe tube.*

Possible cause: Incorrect probe module selected in software.

Resolution: Confirm desired on-ear module matches the screen/ear selected in measurement system.

Possible cause: Measurement module and/or RECD transducer disconnected.

Resolution: Check and confirm your measurement module and RECD transducer are plugged in and connected to the system.

---

the difference between output in the real ear and in a coupler for the same signal, hearing aid output can be accurately predicted within a few decibels. The specific calculation applied at each audiometric frequency for real-ear prediction is as follows:

Coupler SPL (or gain) + RECD + MLE = predicted real-ear SPL or gain

Where: MLE = the microphone location effect of the hearing aid style under test or the transformation of sound as it travels from source to the hearing aid microphone.

It is well established[23,24] that various hearing aid microphone locations can enhance certain frequency regions by varying amounts due to diffraction of sound off of the head/body and by resonances from the external ear. To properly predict on-ear performance from coupler-based test box measurements, many REM systems offering test box verification will automatically add in the appropriate MLE to the input test signal based on the hearing aid style selected on the measurement screen.

The ability to predict the real-ear performance of a hearing aid via test box measurements is traditionally thought of as solely beneficial for pediatric applications. However, simulated REM facilitated by use of the RECD provides a number of benefits that apply to all age groups including the ability to preset hearing aids without the patient being present, reducing the amount of cooperation and time needed from the patient during the fitting process and minimizing the impact of extraneous noise on the measurement as all fitting is conducted under the tightly controlled acoustic conditions of the test box. The reader interested in learning more about the use and applications of the RECD is advised to refer to Bagatto et al[19] or Scollie.[25]

What Is It? (REDD)

Real-Ear to Dial Difference (REDD)
    Formal definition (per ANSI s3.46–2013)[5]

- Difference in decibels, as a function of frequency, between the SPL produced near the tympanic membrane by an audiometric sound source and the hearing level indicated by the audiometer driving the sound source.
  Informal definition

- Difference in decibels, across frequencies, between the SPL measured in the real ear and the audiometer dial setting that produced it.

How Is It Measured? (REDD)

The presence of an automated REDD procedure can vary across REM systems so check with your manufacturer for details specific to your equipment. The procedure outlined below reflects the general principles followed when conducting an REDD.

1. Conduct otoscopic examination.
2. Place probe tube into open ear canal to appropriate depth (e.g., within 5 mm of eardrum, beyond sound bore of earpiece).
3. Place the same earphones used during the audiometric assessment* over the patient's ears, being careful not to move the inserted probe tube.
4. Set the audiometer dial setting to a desired frequency (e.g., 250 Hz) and present a continuous 70 dB HL tone from the audiometer.
5. Measure the output in the ear canal.
6. Subtract the audiometer dial setting (e.g., 70 dB HL) from the REM (e.g., 80 dB SPL) at the measurement frequency (e.g., 250 Hz) to obtain the REDD for the frequency.
7. Continue and repeat the same process until the REDD values have been obtained at all desired audiometric frequencies.

*As noted by ANSI s3.46–2013,[5] the REDD is specific to the audiometer and sound source used in its measurement. Thus, if the REDD procedure is to result in an accurate conversion of the patient's dB HL audiometric data to ear canal SPL, you must use the same audiometer and sound source (e.g., headphones) as used during the patient's hearing test.

Why Measure It? (REDD)

The REDD is used to convert audiometric information (e.g., thresholds and UCLs) from dB HL to dB SPL as would be required when using an SPL-o-gram approach. As you may recall from the previous section, the RECD can also be used to conduct audiometric conversion from dB HL to dB SPL with insert earphones. As such, the REDD is typically considered in cases where headphones were used during audiometry. Given the increasingly common use of insert earphones and the challenges associated with locating the REM system and the audiometer/headphones close enough to one another to perform the measurement, the REDD is rarely conducted.[3,4] Studies evaluating the use of the REDD have shown it to be accurate within approximately 2.3 dB of the true real-ear SPL (i.e., the level that would have been measured at the eardrum had a probe tube been placed there during audiometry).[21]

What Is It? (REAR85/90)

Real-Ear–Aided Response for 85 or 90 dB Input (REAR85/90)
Formal definition

- SPL, as a function of frequency, at a specified measurement point in the ear canal, for a sound field at 85- or 90 dB SPL with the hearing aid (and its acoustic coupling) is placed and turned on, with the gain adjusted to full-on or just below feedback.

Informal definition

- The frequency response of an activated hearing aid, measured in the ear canal, with an input signal SPL of 85 or 90 dB. Also, may be described as an REAR at 85- or 90 dB SPL which may be loud enough to operate the hearing instrument at its maximum output level.

How Is It Measured? (REAR85/90)

1. Conduct otoscopic examination.
2. Place probe tube into open ear canal to appropriate depth (e.g., within 5 mm of eardrum, beyond sound bore of earpiece).
3. Insert hearing aid into client's ear canal, being sure to maintain probe tube location.
4. Place patient at appropriate distance/azimuth from loudspeaker (e.g., 0.5 m/0 degree).
5. Turn hearing aid on and set user gain control to the highest position before feedback or to the projected use setting. *Note: If significant venting (e.g., open-fit device), first calibrate sound field with hearing aid in place and turned off or muted prior to testing.*
6. Select an input signal of 85- or 90 dB SPL*. *Note: some systems provide a signal specifically designed for this test purpose (e.g., labelled MPO). Check with your manufacturer for details specific to your system for this test.*
7. Present and record the measurement (▶**Fig. 7.21**).

*Given the potential for high sound levels in the ear canal, it can be useful to preset the maximum output of the hearing instrument in the coupler (using the RECD to predict real-ear output) to avoid exceeding uncomfortable loudness levels. Alternatively, some REM systems provide a "maximum output SPL" parameter whereby you can select an ear canal SPL value that should not be exceeded and which will result in the signal stopping should it be exceeded. The patient's measured or predicted SPL values provided on the SPL-o-gram screen can be used to determine these values if desired.

*REAR85/90 values can vary depending on the input signal type used with narrow-band signals (e.g., pure tones, warble tones) typically providing a better estimate of worst case possible maximum output versus broadband signals.[26] As such, most REM systems

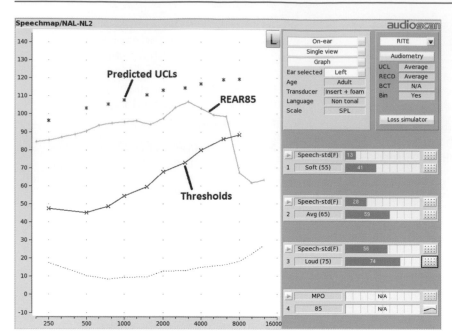

Fig. 7.21 Example of a real-ear aided response 85 (REAR85) measurement.

provide dedicated narrow band, short-duration signals designed specifically for assessing maximum output characteristics of the device under test. Check with your manufacturer for more details.

Why Measure It? (REAR85/90)

The primary purpose of the REAR85/90 is to document the maximum SPL that the hearing aid is capable of delivering to the user's ear for loud sounds. As it is possible that the input levels used during the test will not saturate the hearing aid, the former term of real-ear saturation response (RESR) that was sometimes associated with this procedure is no longer used. The information obtained during this measurement serves three primary purposes as it relates to documentation of the maximum output capabilities of the hearing aid: (1) to ensure that amplified signals do not exceed the uncomfortable listening levels of the patient during everyday use; (2) to ensure that amplified signals do not reach a level that could potentially damage a patient's residual hearing; and (3) to ensure that there is sufficient headroom in the hearing instrument (i.e., ensure MPO is not too low or overly restrictive) to allow for appropriate audibility, loudness perception for loud sounds, and to avoid saturation/distortion of louder sounds as they are processed by the hearing aid. As noted above, given the possibility of discomfort or trauma during the REAR85/90 for inappropriately high MPO settings, consideration should be given to either presetting the REAR85/90 via the use of simulated REMs (i.e., RECD-enabled coupler-based predictions) or acti-

vating the "maximum TM SPL" feature on the REM system to disable the input signal should the SPL at the eardrum exceed a predetermined level. The interested reader can refer to Hawkins[27] for more details regarding hearing aid output limiting considerations.

7.4 Assessment of Hearing Aid Signal Processing Features and Form Factors

7.4.1 Frequency Lowering

Frequency-lowering (FL) technology is designed to improve the audibility of high-frequency sounds when this is not possible via conventional amplification. Typically, the approach is applied in cases of precipitous high-frequency hearing losses where audibility cannot be provided, be it due to feedback or the gain limitations of the hearing aid. FL can be implemented via a number of different techniques (e.g., frequency compression, transposition, translation, and composition) with each having a unique impact on the amplified signal. Despite any implementation differences, each FL approach has a common goal of moving high-frequency input signals down to a lower-frequency output region where the individual may be better able to access them. Readers interested in a review of the rationale and evidence for FL are referred to Mueller et al[28] or Scollie et al[29] for more details.

While FL implementation methods may differ across manufacturers, the verification approach remains the same regardless of the technology as will be outlined in the protocol below. That is, verification of FL is designed to ensure audibility of high-frequency input signals when it cannot be provided via conventional amplification.[30] Implicit in this philosophy is the recommendation from current clinical guidelines[31] that the clinician maximize the aided output bandwidth prior to activating FL via use of a validated prescriptive method. Only after the best possible fitting is provided without FL does the clinician proceed to document audibility of high-frequency speech cues (e.g., /s/) to determine the need for activation of FL technology. As described by Glista et al,[30] completion of a standard verification protocol without FL allows for determination of the maximum audible output frequency (MAOF) range which is used as a target region for the /s/ signal. The MAOF range spans the frequency region between where the upper peaks of average speech cross the patient's threshold and where the long-term average speech spectrum (LTASS) crosses threshold (▶ **Fig. 7.22**).

REM systems typically provide a number of signals for use with FL technology. As a general rule, these signals are designed to provide fitters with a method for observing the movement of high-frequency input signals to a lower output frequency region. Since this can be difficult to do with broadband input signals where the lowered signal overlaps with existing lower-frequency energy, verification systems have provided a variety of narrow band (i.e., /s/, /sh/) or filtered (i.e., one-third octave bands of speech centered at 3,150, 4,000, 5,000, 6,300 Hz) signal types to overcome this issue. Evidence gathered by Scollie et al[29] has supported the value of using prerecorded calibrated speech signals of /s/ and /sh/ as the preferred approach for verification

of FL devices to assess audibility and spectral separation of these important high-frequency cues.

Some approaches for verification of FL technology have considered the use of "live voice" /s/ or /sh/ signals in spectral analysis mode to determine FL settings. While this method does provide some face validity, it is problematic in that the input signal is not calibrated and can vary from one presentation to another. As such, it becomes difficult to determine, for example, whether or not a change in the output spectrum is due to variability in the input signal or if it is in fact due to a programming change. To avoid potential errors in decision making, use of a calibrated, recorded input signal is preferred.

7.4.2 Fitting Protocol

General FL fitting guidelines, based on the approach outlined by Scollie et al[29] and Glista et al[30] include the following:

1. Turn the FL feature "OFF" and verify the hearing aid relative to fitting formula targets per the typical approach. The goal is to ensure the widest audible bandwidth of speech and the ability to match targets from the device gain/output capabilities alone. In some cases, FL is not required as audibility is provided without the feature.

2. Turn the noise reduction (NR) in the hearing aid "OFF." The test signals to be used (i.e., /s/ and /sh/) are noise-like in nature and could engage the NR, thereby giving an underestimation of the true audibility of these phonemes in running speech.

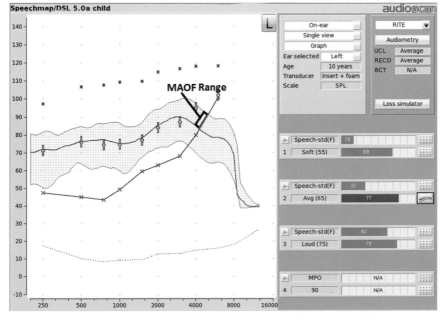

Fig. 7.22 Example of a real-ear aided response measurement for average speech, showing the MAOF range (i.e., region between where the peaks of average speech cross threshold and where the long-term average speech spectrum [LTASS] of average speech crosses threshold).

3. Play the /s/ signal (65 dB SPL) and determine whether this signal is audible. If /s/ is audible, FL is not required and verification is complete. If /s/ is not audible, FL should be activated and the settings determined following the steps listed below.

4. Turn FL "ON" at the default setting provided by the manufacturer.

5. Play the /s/ signal (65 dB SPL) and fine tune the FL settings until the upper shoulder of the signal is audible and within the "maximum audible output frequency range"* using the weakest setting possible.

6. Optionally** play the /sh/signal (65 dB SPL) to determine audibility for this phoneme and sufficient frequency separation from /s/. If overlapping is evident, the listener may not be able to differentiate these two phonemes or other sounds and fine tuning may be required.

7. Turn the NR in the hearing aid "ON" to default setting again.

8. Perform a listening check and consider whether or not the sound quality/distinction of /s/ and /sh/ in speech are acceptable.

9. At the fitting and follow-up, consider the listener's responses and outcome measures*** regarding the perceived sound quality and ability to distinguish /s/ and /sh/ in real-world listening.

*To assist with the fitting process, some REM systems provide guidance via an "MAOF range highlighter" where the region between where the peak of average speech and the LTASS of average speech crosses the patient's threshold is identified.

**Given step #5 naturally results in the minimal FL strength setting necessary for audibility of /s/, it could be argued that the maximum possible separation from /sh/has already been provided.

***Various outcome measures are available that would be deemed appropriate for assessing the impact of FL. The interested reader is referred to Scollie et al[29] for more information.

7.4.3 Case Example

An initial fitting to a prescriptive target was conducted using calibrated speech at multiple input levels. The REAR for average speech shown in ►Fig. 7.22 represents the maximum audible bandwidth possible with FL turned off and the MAOF range is highlighted. Subsequently NR was disengaged and the /s/ signal was presented. As can be observed in ►Fig. 7.23, the /s/ signal was not audible and did not fall within the MAOF range indicating that this patient was a candidate for FL with this device. FL was subsequently engaged on the instrument at the default setting for the manufacturer and the /s/ signal was presented once more. FL was fine-tuned until the upper shoulder of the /s/ was placed within the MAOF range as shown in ►Fig. 7.24. Technically, this approach would result in meeting the goal of providing the minimal setting of FL required to provide audibility of high-frequency cues while minimizing the potential for sound quality artifacts and confusion errors due to overlap with other high-frequency phonemes. That said, as an additional option, the /sh/ signal was presented to document the level of audibility for this signal and the amount of overlap/frequency separation from /s/ as shown in ►Fig. 7.25. As can be observed, both signals are indeed audible and there are spectrum differences. ►Fig. 7.26 represents an example of a stronger FL setting available in this device. Note the progressively greater movement of /s/ into the lower-frequency region. Complaints related to sound quality and confusion errors for high-frequency speech cues could result from overly aggressive FL settings—aspects that can be avoided through the proper implementation of FL verification protocols such as those outlined above.

7.4.4 Open Fittings

Open fittings represent a popular dispensing choice for many clinicians. The demand and associated success of open fit products relates in part to their potential to address the sound quality complaints of many hearing aid wearers, particularly "own voice" issues due to the occlusion effect as will be described later. Improvements in feedback cancellation technology have also enabled the use of open fittings with more individuals having higher gain requirements. That said, REM continues to represent a valuable tool to ensure that any additional useable gain translates into appropriate gain characteristics across frequencies for the hearing aid wearer.

Verification of open-fit products follows the same general steps and procedures used with minimally vented hearing instruments. However, given the additional amount of vented amplified sound present during REM with open fittings, special considerations are required for sound field calibration. As previously described in this chapter, the reference microphone serves to document the sound level at the measurement location and adjust the signal delivered by the loudspeaker to ensure the appropriate input level/spectrum is provided during testing. With open fittings, amplified sound from the hearing aid can leak

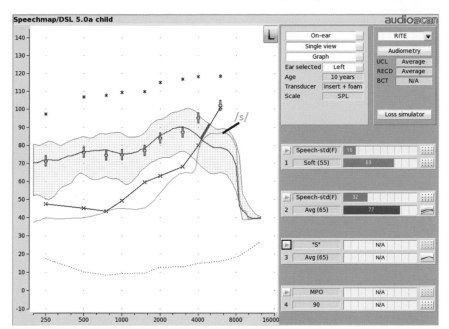

Fig. 7.23 Example of the previously measured LTASS for average speech and an aided response of the /s/ signal without frequency lowering activated. Note that the /s/ signal is not within the MAOF range and is not audible indicating candidacy for frequency lowering.

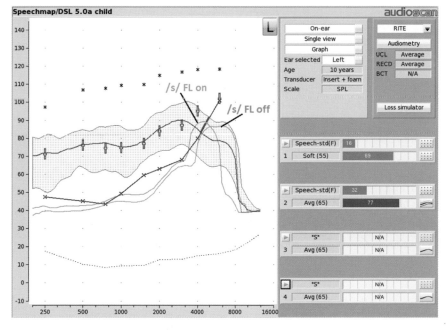

Fig. 7.24 Example of the previously measured LTASS for average speech and aided response measurements for the /s/ signal, both with and without frequency lowering activated. Note that with FL on and adjusted, the /s/ signal has been moved down in frequency relative to FL off setting and is now audible within the MAOF range.

out of the ear canal and contaminate the reference microphone measurements. This outflow of amplified sound is particularly problematic in cases where the modified pressure method with concurrent equalization is used (i.e., the reference microphone is active during testing as previously described). The reference microphone will measure a higher sound pressure level than it would have had less venting been present as it is now measuring vented amplified sound from the open ear canal. The control loop of the system will subsequently lower the loudspeaker signal level, thereby reducing the input to the hearing aid microphone and the measured real-ear output will be reduced as a result. The net effect of this

error is that you may underestimate the true amount of gain/output provided by the hearing aid and inappropriately program more gain into the device than required. As described by Bentler et al,[3,4] this potential error increases as the high-frequency gain of the hearing instrument increases, with some reports showing errors on the order of 5 to 10 dB or more.[32]

To address this measurement artifact, it is recommended that the stored modified pressure equalization approach previously described in this chapter be used when verifying open fittings. With this approach, the reference microphone will be disabled during the verification procedure and any outflow of amplified sound from the ear canal will not impact

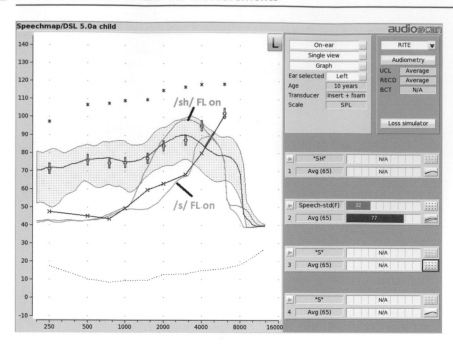

Fig. 7.25 Example of the previously measured LTASS for average speech, the aided response for the /s/ signal with FL on and adjusted to provide audibility within the MAOF range and the aided response for the /sh/ signal with the same FL setting. Note that both the /s/ and /sh/ signals are audible with different spectrums.

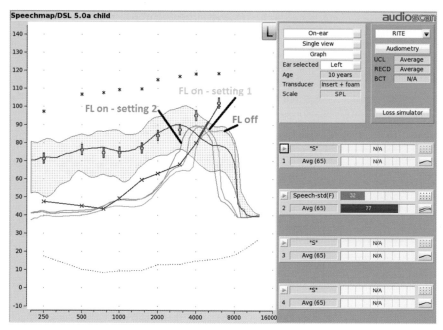

Fig. 7.26 Example of the previously measured LTASS for average speech and a range of FL strength settings and their impact on the aided /s/ signal. As shown, the aided /s/ signal for the "off" setting is not audible, setting 1 provides audibility within the MAOF range, and setting 2 depicts a stronger setting that provides additional audibility but could be considered stronger than needed to meet fitting goals while minimizing sound-quality issues and overlap with other high-frequency phonemes.

the loudspeaker signal. Provided the patient does not move from the previously calibrated test location, you can be assured you are delivering the correct input level/spectrum to the hearing aid microphone.

7.4.5 Fitting Protocol

A general protocol for open-fit verification is outlined below:

1. Conduct otoscopic examination.
2. Enter audiometric data and select fitting formula of choice per typical verification.
3. Place probe tube into ear canal and insert hearing aid per typical approach verification.

4. Turn off or mute the hearing aid.
5. Click on the test signal and store the equalization when prompted.*
6. Turn on or unmute the hearing aid.
7. Conduct verification for multiple input levels to target as you would with any hearing instrument.

* Note: the activation of stored equalization can vary across systems, but typically involves first selecting a hearing aid/venting type of "open" from an on-screen dropdown list. This selection will typically result in the system prompting you to store equalization when a test signal is first introduced (►**Fig. 7.27**). As you are using "stored equalization," should the

patient move from the previous calibrated position at any point during testing, you will need to reequalize the sound field to ensure the proper signal level is delivered to the new measurement location. Refer to your manufacturer's literature for details specific to your system.

7.4.6 Case Example

▶ Fig. 7.28 shows the results of verification conducted with an open-fit product using the protocol outlined above. To highlight the importance of proper sound field calibration and the potential error introduced by not applying stored equalization with this type of fitting, REARs for average speech are shown for the exact same hearing aid settings with the exact same ear canal with (1) the reference microphone active (i.e., concurrent equalization) and (2) with the reference microphone disabled (i.e., stored equalization). As can be noted, the concurrent equalization approach under these conditions resulted in a measurement that was approximately 5 dB lower in the 3,000-Hz frequency region than the stored equalization approach. Clinically, this measurement artifact might lead the fitter to increase gain needlessly if they are under fitting their target criteria or conversely lead them to maintain gain when they are overamplifying relative to target. Clearly, it is important that the proper input level and spectrum for the associated fitting formula target is delivered to the hearing instrument. As described above, stored equalization with open fittings makes it more likely that accurate conclusions and resulting programming decisions will be made.

Controversial Point: Simulated REM (Test Box Measures) and Open Fits

While simulated REMs that leverage the RECD to predict real-ear performance using test box measures have been shown to offer significant value, this approach can be problematic with open fittings. Accurate real-ear simulation via test box measures of venting that considers both the direct sound path (i.e., sound that travels down the vent to the eardrum) and the indirect path (i.e., amplified sound that is delivered by the hearing aid) has proven quite elusive. While efforts are no doubt underway to tackle this challenge, the authors are not aware of any method to accurately simulate on-ear vent effects via test box measures in a clinical verification system at the present time. As result, a number of REM systems offering test box capabilities disallow simulated REM with open fits and only offer the option to verify this hearing aid configuration on the ear.

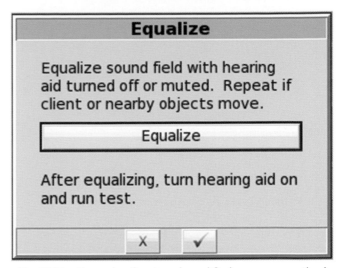

Fig. 7.27 Example of a stored modified pressure method equalization prompt provided by one manufacturer upon beginning REM with an open-fit device.

Pearls: Open Fittings and Noise Management Features ✔

The value of directional microphone processing and noise reduction (NR) with open fittings is sometimes questioned given the amount of unprocessed environmental sound that travels directly down the vent to the eardrum. While it is the case that the audible impact of adaptive features in the low frequencies is reduced, adaptive noise management features such as directional microphones and NR still have the potential to offer patient value in the mid-to-high frequencies where the amplified signal is dominant. REM tests of directional microphones and NR provide an excellent way to document the performance of these features under the vent conditions in question, demonstrate their behavior with your patients and inform counseling.[33]

7.4.7 Occlusion Effect Testing

The occlusion effect has been defined as the low-frequency enhancement in loudness of bone conducted sound due to occlusion of the ear canal.[34] Clinically, this issue typically manifests itself as a complaint regarding the unnatural sound of the hearing aid wearer's voice (echoes, sounds hollow) or the sounds of chewing food. These complaints can be particularly problematic for those with relatively normal-to-mild low-frequency hearing losses where sufficient venting is not provided. The effect results from the acoustic energy created by the vibration of the walls of the ear canal from

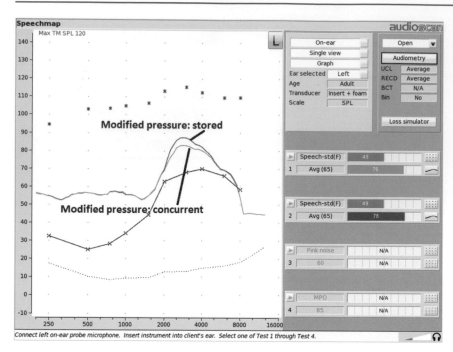

Fig. 7.28 Example of REARs for average speech for the same patient, using the same open-fit hearing aid at the exact same settings for the modified pressure method "stored" equalization approach; and the modified pressure method "concurrent" equalization approach. Note that the concurrent equalization measurement is lower than the stored equalization due to contamination from vented amplified sound during the calibration routine.

bone conducted sound being trapped in the ear canal.[34] Typically, this bone conducted energy vents from the ear canal when it is open during vocalization or when eating, however, the presence of a hearing instrument, particularly one without sufficient venting can result in a portion of this energy being trapped in the ear canal and perceived by the patient. Readers interested in a more detailed discussion of the occlusion effect are referred to Mueller et al.[35]

As complaints related to own voice issues may also relate to the provision of excessive low-frequency amplification, it can sometimes be difficult to determine which approach to utilize to address a patient's concerns—venting adjustments, programming changes, or some combination thereof. Thankfully, REM systems provide effective and easy-to-use tools to determine the presence of occlusion and inform clinical decision making.

Methods for measuring the occlusion effect can vary depending on the REM system in question, with the choice of either a dedicated occlusion effect test and/or a spectrum analysis mode (sometimes activated via a "live speech" mode). While it is not necessarily required for all fittings, should a patient report issues that might be associated with occlusion (e.g., sound of own voice, plugged feeling), occlusion effect testing is a quick and easy way to assess the presence of occlusion and the impact of any venting modifications designed to address it.

7.4.8 Fitting Protocol

The general procedure for conducting occlusion effect testing using the traditional/spectral analysis (or live speech) mode is outlined below.

1. Conduct otoscopic examination.
2. Place probe tube into open ear canal to appropriate depth (e.g., within 5 mm of eardrum, beyond sound bore of earpiece).
3. Activate the spectral analysis or live speech mode on your test equipment.
4. Have the patient vocalize the sound /ee/* and maintain it at a moderate level (~ 70–80 dB SPL) long enough for you to record the measurement. Some REM systems monitor and display the SPL level at the reference microphone during the measurement which can be used to ensure consistency in vocal level during all stages of the procedure. Alternatively, an inexpensive sound level meter could be used.
5. Insert hearing aid into client's ear canal, being sure to maintain the probe tube location.
6. Ensure the hearing aid is muted or turned off.
7. Have the patient once again vocalize the sound /ee/ and maintain it at the same level as the previous open-ear recording. Store the measurement.
8. Compare the two measurements and determine the extent to which they vary

from one another. The degree to which the occluded (hearing aid off) measurement is greater than the open ear canal measurement represents the magnitude of the occlusion effect (▶Fig. 7.29).

*Vocalizing the closed vowel /ee/ is typically preferred as the first formant is around the frequency of the maximum occlusion effect (~ 300 Hz), resulting in a higher SPL in the vocal tract and more low-frequency energy for assessing the occlusion effect than open vowels such as /ah/.

For those verification systems that incorporate a dedicated occlusion effect test, the general procedure followed is quite similar to the traditional/spectral analysis mode outlined above. The primary differences relate to the calculation convenience offered by the system simultaneously comparing and subtracting the level of sound measured from the reference microphone (measuring sound outside the ear canal) and the probe microphone (measuring sound inside the ear canal) to calculate the occlusion effect. In contrast to the spectral analysis technique, only one measurement is needed as the calculation does not require an initial open ear baseline response for comparison purposes. The extent to which the probe microphone measures a higher value than the reference microphone represents the level of occlusion present. Some systems will automatically subtract

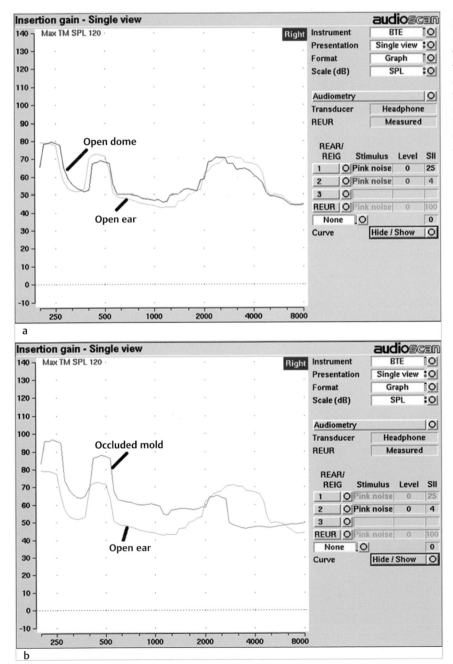

Fig. 7.29 Example of spectral analysis mode measurement of the occlusion effect for one patient with (a) an open dome relative to the previously measured open ear condition; and (b) an occluded mold relative to the previously measured open ear condition. As can be observed, more energy is trapped in the ear canal (occlusion effect) for the occluded vent condition relative to the open vent condition.

the C-weighted overall sound level measured by the two microphones in question and plot an occlusion effect bar that is color coded based on the difference. As can be observed in ▶Fig. 7.30, for the same patient, as the level of venting is progressively decreased from an open dome to a power dome, the occlusion effect bar progressively increases in size and changes in color to suggest an increased likelihood of complaints related to the occlusion effect (i.e., more energy trapped in ear canal for the same vocal effort). When considered in tandem with any patient reports of sound quality issues that may relate to occlusion, the clinician could use this test to assess whether or not additional venting is required or if the solution to the patient's own voice issues may instead require an alternative approach such as programming changes or counseling.

7.4.9 CROS/BiCROS

The management of patients presenting with an unaidable unilateral hearing loss (sometimes referred to as single-sided deafness) can be quite challenging. A method traditionally used to address this issue is the contralateral routing of signal (CROS) or the bilateral CROS (BiCROS) device. Both approaches attempt to provide increased awareness of sound originating from the side of the unaidable ear (i.e., aim to overcome the head-shadow effect). Typically, this goal is achieved by placing a microphone/transmitter on the unaidable ear that transfers all sound wirelessly to a hearing aid/receiver on the better ear. Implementation and fitting approach differences between the CROS and BiCROS relate to the level of residual hearing in the "better ear." Specifically, CROS fittings are typically provided to patients with normal hearing in their better ear. As such, only a single microphone is required on the unaidable ear and the aim of the CROS fitting is not to amplify sound, but simply to transfer sound from the unaidable side of the head to the better ear so as to minimize the head-shadow effect.[36] The fitting goal then relates to ensuring acoustic transparency (i.e., matching the REUG of the better ear). Alternatively, the BiCROS fitting is used with patients presenting with hearing loss in the better ear. As such, a microphone is also placed on the better ear side to provide awareness of sound originating from that side and additional amplification is required for the combined signal received by the better ear. The amount of amplification can be determined by using a prescriptive formula (e.g., NAL-NL2, DSLv5), as would be done with a traditional hearing aid fitting for the hearing loss present on the better ear.

While there are verification protocol differences between CROS and BiCROS devices, there are some common principles to keep in mind as outlined by Dillon,[36] Tecca,[37] Mueller and Hawkins,[38] and Pumford[39]:

1. The probe tube should always be located in the ear canal of the better ear.
2. The loudspeaker is positioned within a range of +/−90 degrees relative to the front of the patient depending on the stage in the fitting process.
3. The reference microphone should be located on the same side of the patient as the loudspeaker* (to ensure a consistent input signal during all stages of the measurement).

*To assist with this requirement, some REM systems provide binaural probe modules, whereby either the left or right reference microphone can be activated depending on the stage of testing via a "CROS" device dropdown menu. If the reference microphone cannot be separated from the measuring probe microphone, it should be deactivated and the substitution method should be used to calibrate the sound field. Please refer to your system-specific user guide for more details.

A general test protocol for conventional^ CROS and BiCROS hearing instruments as described by Dillon,[36] Tecca,[37] and Pumford[39] is outlined below.

^Note: Transcranial CROS fittings, where a power hearing aid inserted into the poorer side ear canal stimulates the better ear via bone conduction involves a different fitting protocol than outlined below. The interested reader is referred to Valente et al[40] for more information.

7.4.10 Fitting Protocol: CROS

Goals

- Transfer sound from unaidable ear to better (normal) ear.
- Match normal ear's natural amplification (i.e., REUG).

1. Measure the response for the better ear side (▶Fig. 7.31).
   a. Conduct otoscopy.
   b. Insert probe tube into the ear canal of the better ear as you would for traditional REM testing.
   c. Turn the patient and/or position the loudspeaker so it is angled at 45* degrees to the better ear.
   d. Position (or activate) the reference microphone on the better ear (i.e., same side as loudspeaker).
   e. Measure the REUR** (Note: this response becomes your fitting "target").

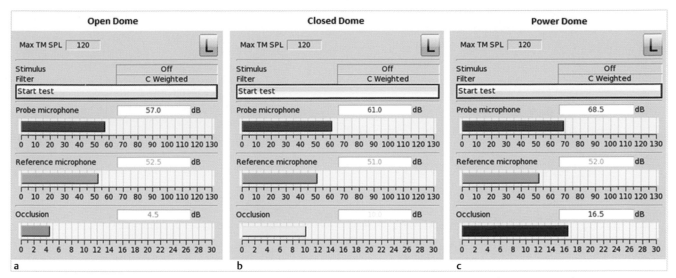

Fig. 7.30 Example of dedicated occlusion effect test from one REM system for one patient with venting conditions progressing from (**a**) open dome, (**b**) closed dome, (**c**) power dome. Note that the occlusion effect (i.e., difference in the probe microphone levels [in the ear canal] and the reference microphone levels [outside the ear canal] gradually increases as the ear canal becomes more occluded due to progressively greater signal levels being measured in the ear canal by the probe microphone).

Step 1. Measure **better side** response

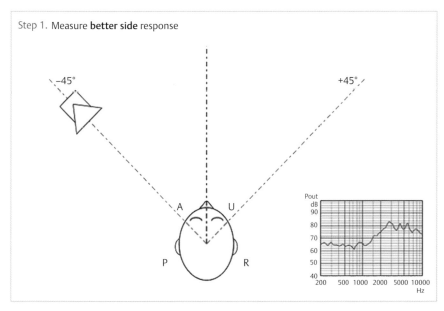

Fig. 7.31 Example of the better side measurement setup used in Step 1. The left ear is better/aidable (A), while the right ear is unaidable (U). The probe microphone (P) and the reference microphone (R) are both located at the better ear. The loudspeaker is positioned at 45 degrees azimuth relative to the better ear. Adapted from Pumford.[39]

f. Position the CROS instruments (receiver/transmitter) in the ears, turned off.

g. Measure the REOR using the same input signal and level as the REUR. The REOR should match the REUR to ensure the open coupling has not occluded the better ear. Adjust coupling as needed to match the REUR as closely as possible.

2. Measure the response for the poorer (unaidable) ear side (▶**Fig. 7.32**).

a. Turn the CROS instruments on.

b. Turn the patient and/or position the loudspeaker so it is angled at 45* degrees to the poorer ear.

c. Position (or activate) the reference microphone on the poorer ear (i.e., same side as loudspeaker).

d. Keep the probe tube in the ear canal of the better ear.

e. Measure the REAR using the same input signal and level** as used for the REUR. The REAR should match the REUR "target." Adjust device programming until the poorer side REAR matches the better side REUR as shown in ▶**Fig. 7.33**.

*Note, the desired location of the loudspeaker relative to the patient has also been reported as

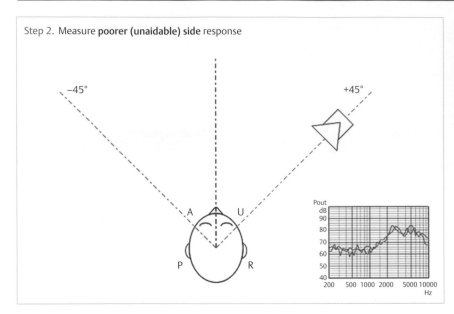

Step 2. Measure **poorer (unaidable) side** response

Fig. 7.32 Example of the poorer side measurement setup used in Step 2. The probe microphone (P) is located at the better/aidable ear (A), while the reference microphone (R) is positioned at the poorer/unaidable ear (U). The loudspeaker is positioned at 45 degrees azimuth relative to the poorer ear. Adapted from Pumford.[39]

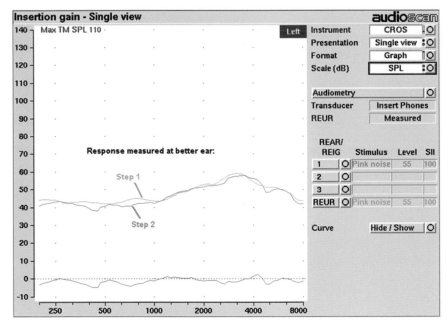

Fig. 7.33 Example of a CROS hearing aid fitting showing the REARs measured at the better (*left*) ear for Steps 1 (better ear side REUR) and 2 (transmitted signal received from poorer ear side). The lowest curve on the screen running along '0' represents the measured difference between Steps 1 and 2 showing the transmitted signal from the poorer ear side essentially matches the better ear REUR as desired based on the fitting protocol. Adapted from Pumford.[39]

90 degrees (i.e., directly to the side of the patient). Documentation of output for sound presented directly from the side (i.e., worst case scenario for head shadow) has merit, however, some data have suggested that 45 degrees azimuth may provide less test–retest variability with less sensitivity to reference microphone location than 90 degrees.[6,7] That said, the authors are not aware of any definitive study indicating the optimal position for this procedure during CROS fittings and as such a choice of either 45 or 90 degrees would appear appropriate with the key consideration being that the same position relative to either side of the patient be used for both the better ear and poorer ear side measurements.

**Various signal types and levels can be used, although typically a pink noise or standard speech signal is selected and minimally presented at a moderate level exceeding the noise floor.

7.4.11 Fitting Protocol: BiCROS

Goals

- Transfer sound from unaidable ear to better ear.
- Amplify better (hearing impaired) ear per traditional fitting formula targets.

  1. Measure the response for the better ear side.
     a. Conduct otoscopy.
     b. Insert probe tube into the ear canal of the "better ear" as you would for traditional REM testing.

c. Turn the patient and/or position the loudspeaker so it is angled at 0 to 45 degrees to the better ear.

d. Position (or activate) the reference microphone on the better ear (i.e., same side as loudspeaker).

e. Position the BiCROS instruments (receiver/transmitter) in the ears, turned on.

f. Measure the REAR and adjust programming to approximate the real-ear targets provided by the prescriptive formula you are using for the better hearing side per a traditional hearing aid.

2. Measure the response for the poorer (unaidable) ear side.

a. Turn the CROS instruments on.

b. Turn the patient and/or position the loudspeaker so it is angled at 45 degrees to the poorer ear.

c. Position (or activate) the reference microphone on the poorer ear (i.e., same side as loudspeaker).

d. Keep the probe tube in the better ear canal.

e. Measure the REARs using the same input signals and levels as used for the better ear side. Adjust device programming until the poorer side REARs match the REAR targets for the better ear.

Beyond the fitting protocol outlined above, REM can also be used to inform counseling regarding the rationale for recommending a CROS/BiCROS device by demonstrating the head shadow effect that the system is designed to overcome along with any expected benefit. Per Tecca[37] and Pumford,[39] the head-shadow effect can be documented as follows:

1. Measure the REUR for the better ear side.

a. Position the loudspeaker 45 to 90 degrees to the better ear side.

b. Position (or activate) the reference microphone on the better ear side.

c. Insert probe tube in the ear canal of the better ear.

d. Present and record an REUR.

2. Measure the REUR with sound presented to the poorer (unaidable ear) side.

a. Position speaker at 45 to 90 degrees to the poorer ear side.

b. Position the reference microphone at the poorer ear (i.e., same side as loudspeaker).

c. Keep the probe tube in the better ear canal.

d. Present and record an REUR using the same signal/input level as that is used with the better ear side.

The measured difference between the two REURs (▶**Fig. 7.34**) represents an estimate of the head-shadow effect for that client.

Special Considerations—CROS Fitting Coupling

The primary aim of conventional CROS fittings for those with normal hearing in their better ear is not to amplify sound, but to simply transfer sound from the unaidable side of the head to the better ear to minimize the head-shadow effect. As such, the primary aim is to provide acoustic transparency for sound on the better ear and match the resonance of the better ear (i.e., match the REUG) for any transmitted signal. Should the receiver provide too much gain, the user will likely complain of internal noise or tinniness and reject the fitting. Beyond programming settings, consideration should also be given to the sound delivery mechanism used on the better ear side. Specifically, with CROS devices it is important to ensure that sound originating from the better ear side can pass naturally down the ear canal and that occlusion is minimized. As such, CROS fittings typically employ "open fitting" coupling options. To document whether or not an unoccluded coupling has been provided, the clinician can either conduct a comparison between an REUG and REOG measurement on the better ear side as was previously described in the chapter or an occlusion effect test. In contrast, coupling considerations for the BiCROS patient would follow the same decision-making approach used with any traditional hearing aid for the level of hearing loss on the better ear side.

7.5 Summary

Hearing instrument technology continues to evolve, bringing with it exciting new possibilities to provide ever increasing benefit for patients with hearing loss. Beyond improvements in the basic foundational amplification components of hearing instruments, we continue to see more advanced signal processing algorithms and varied form factors designed to address various listening concerns. However, despite these ongoing advancements, the need to determine what is actually being delivered to the eardrum of the patient by the device in question remains. As research[41,42] has repeatedly shown,

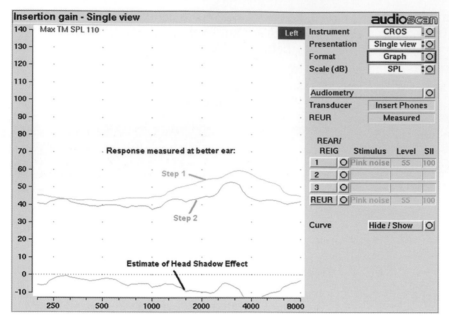

Fig. 7.34 Example of the head-shadow effect measurement showing the REUR measured at the better ear for step 1 (signal presented toward the better ear side) and the REUR measured at the better ear for step 2 (signal presented toward the poorer ear side). The lower curve represents the measured difference between the REURs for Steps 1 and 2, which provides an estimate of the head-shadow effect for this client. Adapted from Pumford.[39]

improved listening outcomes reflect not only the hearing instrument itself but also the manner in which the hearing instrument is configured. In this regard, objective verification via REMs represent a critical tool that offers clinicians valuable information to determine whether or not the device (or feature) in question is performing appropriately based on the auditory needs of the patient being fitted. By leveraging the REM tools and techniques described in this chapter, the clinician can be more confident in their decision-making when fitting hearing instruments and increase the likelihood that the benefits of amplification are maximized for every patient.

7.6 Acknowledgments

The authors would like to thank Jason Galster for his input and suggestions regarding the chapter content.

References

[1] Mueller HG, Picou E. Survey investigates popularity of real-ear probe-microphone measurements. Hear J. 2010; 63(5):27–32

[2] Northern J. Probe microphone instrumentation. In: Mueller H, Hawkins D, Northern J, eds. Probe Microphone Measurements: Hearing Aid Selection and Assessment. San Diego, CA: Singular Publishing Group Inc; 1992:21–39

[3] Bentler R, Mueller HG, Ricketts TA. Probe microphone measures: rationale and procedures. In: Bentler R, Mueller HG, Ricketts TA, eds. Modern Hearing Aids: Verification, Outcome Measures, and Follow-Up. San Diego, CA: Plural Publishing, Inc; 2016a:237–282

[4] Bentler R, Mueller HG, Ricketts TA. Probe microphone clinical uses. In: Bentler R, Mueller HG, Ricketts TA, eds. Modern Hearing Aids: Verification, Outcome Measures, and Follow-Up. San Diego, CA: Plural Publishing, Inc; 2016b:283–347

[5] ANSI. Methods of Measurement of Real-Ear Characteristics of Hearing Instruments (ANSI S3.46-R2013). New York, NY: American National Standards Institute; 2013

[6] Ickes MA, Hawkins DB, Cooper WA. Effect of reference microphone location and loudspeaker azimuth on probe tube microphone measurements. J Am Acad Audiol. 1991; 2(3):156–163

[7] Killion MC, Revit LJ. Insertion gain repeatability versus loudspeaker location: you want me to put my loudspeaker where? Ear Hear. 1987; 8 (suppl 5):68–73

[8] Mueller HG. Terminology and procedures. In: Mueller H, Hawkins D, Northern J, eds. Probe Microphone Measurements: Hearing Aid Selection and Assessment. San Diego, CA: Singular Publishing Group Inc;1992: 41–66

[9] Frye K, Martin R. Real ear measurements. In: Valente M, Hosford-Dunn H, Roeser S, eds. Audiology Treatment. 2nd ed. New York, NY: Thieme Medical; 2008

[10] Dirks DD, Kincaid GE. Basic acoustic considerations of ear canal probe measurements. Ear Hear. 1987; 8 (suppl 5) :60–67

[11] Scollie SD, Seewald RC, Cornelisse LE, Miller SM. Procedural considerations in the real-ear measurement of completely-in-the-canal instruments. J Am Acad Audiol. 1998a; 9(3):216–220

[12] Vaisberg JM, Macpherson EA, Scollie SD. Extended bandwidth real-ear measurement accuracy and repeatability to 10 kHz. Int J Audiol. 2016; 55(10):580–586

[13] Bagatto MP, Seewald RC, Scollie SD, Tharpe AM. Evaluation of a probe-tube insertion technique for measuring the real-ear-to-coupler difference (RECD) in young infants. J Am Acad Audiol. 2006; 17(8):573–581

[14] Pumford J, Sinclair S. Real-ear measurement: basic terminology and procedures. Audiology Online, Article 1229. http://www.audiologyonline.com. Accessed 24th January, 2018

[15] Bagatto M, Moodie S. (2007). Learning the art to apply the science: common questions related to pediatric hearing instrument fitting. Audiology Online, Article 1886. http://www.audiologyonline.com/articles. Accessed 24th January, 2018

[16] Folkeard P, Pumford J, Narten P, Vaisberg J, Scollie S. A comparison of wRECD and RECD values and test-retest reliability. Poster session presented at the American Academy of Audiology, Phoenix, AZ. https://www.audioscan.com/Docs/posters/2016S_poster_AudiologyNow_wRECD.pdf. Accessed 24th January, 2018

[17] Vaisberg J, Folkeard P, Pumford J, Narten P, Scollie S. Evaluation of the repeatability and accuracy of the wideband real-ear-to-coupler difference. J Am Acad Audiol. https://doi.org/10.3766/jaaa.17007

[18] Bagatto M. Optimizing your RECD measurements Hear J. 2001; 54(9):32, 34–36

[19] Bagatto M, Moodie S, Scollie S, et al. Clinical protocols for hearing instrument fitting in the desired sensation level method. Trends Amplif. 2005; 9(4):199–226

[20] Saunders GH, Morgan DE. Impact on hearing aid targets of measuring thresholds in dB HL versus dBSPL. Int J Audiol. 2003; 42(6):319–326

[21] Scollie SD, Seewald RC, Cornelisse LE, Jenstad LM. Validity and repeatability of level-independent HL to SPL transforms. Ear Hear. 1998b; 19(5):407–413

[22] Seewald RC, Moodie KS, Sinclair ST, Scollie SD. Predictive validity of a procedure for pediatric hearing instrument fitting. Am J Audiol. 1999; 8(2):143–152

[23] Cox RM, Risberg DM. Comparison of in-the-ear and over-the-ear hearing aid fittings. J Speech Hear Disord. 1986; 51(4):362–369

[24] Kuhn GF. The pressure transformation from a diffuse sound field to the external ear and to the body and head surface. J Acoust Soc Am. 1979; 65(4):991–1000

[25] Scollie SD. New RECDs and a new ANSI standard: revisiting RECD basics and applications. Audiology Online, Article 16380. http://www.audiologyonline.com. Accessed 24th January, 2018

[26] Stelmachowicz PG, Lewis DE, Seewald RC, Hawkins DB. Complex and pure-tone signals in the evaluation of hearing-aid characteristics. J Speech Hear Res. 1990; 33(2):380–385

[27] Hawkins D. Selecting SSPL90 using probe-microphone measurements. In: Mueller H, Hawkins D, Northern J, eds. Probe Microphone Measurements: Hearing Aid Selection and Assessment. San Diego, CA: Singular Publishing Group Inc; 1992:145–158

[28] Mueller HG, Alexander JM, Scollie S. 20Q: Frequency lowering—The whole shebang. Audiology Online, Article 11913. http://www.audiologyonline.com. Accessed 24th January, 2018

[29] Scollie S, Glista D, Seto J, et al. Fitting frequency lowering signal processing applying the AAA pediatric amplification guideline: updates and protocols. J Am Acad Audiol. 2016; 27(3):219–236

[30] Glista D, Hawkins M, Scollie S. An update on modified verification approaches for frequency lowering devices. Audiology Online, Article 16932. http://www.audiologyonline.com. Accessed 24th January, 2018

[31] American Academy of Audiology. American Academy of Audiology clinical practice guidelines: pediatric amplification. http://audiology-web.s3.amazonaws.com/migrated/PediatricAmplificationGuidelines.pdf_539975b3e7e9f1.74471798.pdf. Accessed 24th January, 2018

[32] Mueller HG, Ricketts TA. Open canal fittings: ten take home tips. Hear J. 2006; 59(11):24–39

[33] Smriga D. On ear verification of open fittings. Audiology Online, Article 19326. http://www.audiologyonline.com. Accessed February 2017

[34] Stach BA. Comprehensive Dictionary of Audiology, Illustrated. 2nd ed. Cengage learning; 2003

[35] Mueller HG, Bright KE, Northern JL. Studies of the hearing aid occlusion effect. Semin Hear. 1996; 17(01):21–32

[36] Dillon H. CROS, bone conduction and implanted hearing aids. In: Dillon H, ed. Hearing Aids. New York, NY: Thieme; 2001:434–450

[37] Tecca J. Use of real-ear measurements to verify hearing aid fittings. In: Valente M, ed. Strategies for Selecting and Verifying Hearing Aid Fittings. New York, NY: Thieme; 1994:88–107

[38] Mueller H, Hawkins D. Assessment of fitting arrangements, special circuitry, and features. In: Mueller H, Hawkins D, Northern J, eds. Probe Microphone Measurements: Hearing Aid Selection and Assessment. San Diego, CA: Singular Publishing Group Inc; 1992:201–225

[39] Pumford J. Benefits of probe mic measures with CROS/BiCROS fittings. Hear J. 2005; 58(10):34–40

[40] Valente M, Potts LG, Valente M, Goebel J. Wireless CROS versus transcranial CROS for unilateral hearing loss. Am J Audiol. 1995; 4(1):52–59

[41] Abrams HB, Chisolm TH, McManus M, McArdle R. Initial-fit approach versus verified prescription: comparing self-perceived hearing aid benefit. J Am Acad Audiol. 2012; 23(10):768–778

[42] Leavitt R, Flexer C. The importance of audibility in successful amplification of hearing loss. H Review. 2012; 19(13):20–238

8 Real-Ear Measurement Techniques

David Smriga, John Pumford

8.1 Interpretation of Real-Ear Measurements When Fitting to Hearing Aid Prescriptions

Real-ear measurement (REM) provides hearing care professionals with an objective and scientifically defensible method of guiding hearing aid treatment that goes beyond the simple determination of acceptable sound quality. When used in combination with a validated fitting formula, REM can help guide the clinician in their adjustment of hearing aid parameters to ensure that prescriptive targets are achieved and by association, that the underlying goals of the prescriptive approach are met.

8.2 Hearing Aid Prescriptions

Over several decades, a variety of target formulas (rules) have been developed to guide the clinician in adjusting hearing aid parameters.[1] Based on fitting goals that have been developed through research and/or consideration of hearing aid performance characteristics, these rules provide the clinician with objective targets that can be displayed on the REM screen. These targets generally specify the gain or output desirable at various audiometric frequencies. Although initially these target rules focused on a single input level and were designed primarily for use when fitting linear hearing aids, many have been updated to provide targets for different input levels across frequencies to reflect the non-linear/compression characteristics of modern hearing instruments.

Prescriptive fitting formulas are generally sorted into two main categories - generic validated fitting formulas (e.g., NAL and DSL) and manufacturer proprietary fitting formulas. These various target rules are typically available and selectable via menus that appear both in the fitting software the clinician uses to program and adjust hearing aid parameters, and in the REM system the clinician uses to verify that these targets have been delivered to the patient's tympanic membrane (eardrum). ►**Table 8.1** is a representative list of internationally recognized target rules that one might find listed in fitting software and REM system target menus.

►**Fig. 8.1** depicts an example of an insertion gain measurement as described in Chapter 7 that has been used to verify that targeted insertion gain has been delivered via the hearing aid to the patient's eardrum using the NAL-R, a linear hearing aid fitting rule. Based on the audiogram information depicted in ►**Fig. 8.1a**, the resulting fitting software screen is depicted in ►**Fig. 8.1b**. In this example, the NAL-R fitting rule has been selected, showing both the

Table 8.1 List of internationally recognized generic target rules in fitting software and REM system target menus

Fitting rule
Linear prescriptive fitting formula
Berger (1979)
Libby (1986)
NAL-R (1986)
POGO II (1988)
Nonlinear prescriptive fitting formula
Fig. 6 (1993)
IHAFF (1994)
DSL i/o (1997)
NAL-NL1 (1999)
DSL 5.0 (2005)
NAL-NL2 (2011)
CamEQ (2005)

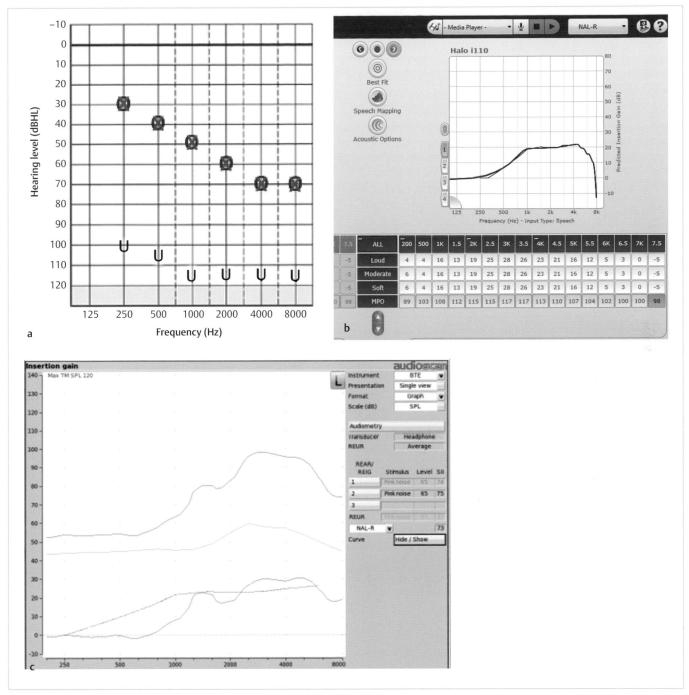

Fig. 8.1 The fitting software shown in (b) is programmed to quick-fit the hearing aid to NAL-R prescriptive targets based on the audiometric information in (a). The measured insertion gain, shown in (c), (bottom green line) indicates that the hearing aid default settings are not matching the prescribed NAL-R targets (dashed lower black line) across large portions of the frequency range, thus indicating a need for hearing aid adjustment.

insertion gain targets (thin lines) and the predicted insertion gain response (thick lines). Linear gain values are listed below the graph in the fitting software controls for input levels: soft (50 dB), moderate (65 dB), or loud (80 dB). The screen in ▶**Fig. 8.1c** is the resulting actual REM using an insertion gain approach for those same hearing aid settings. In this example, the same NAL-R fitting rule that was selected in the hearing aid fitting software has been selected in the

REM system and is shown as a dashed line near the bottom of the screen. An REAR measurement for a 65 dB input (top green line) was obtained in the patient's ear using the hearing aid programmed as indicated in the fitting software screen. The resulting REIG is shown as the bottom green line on the REM screen. With the hearing aid programmed as indicated in the fitting software, the REIG noticeably deviates from the generated REIG targets (dashed lower black line) across large portions of the frequency range. An REIG measurement such as that displayed above would indicate a need to adjust hearing instrument programming and/or ear canal coupling (or venting) for the device to deliver the targeted performance. It is this deviation from what the hearing aid fitting software predicts and what the clinician actually measures in the patient's ear canal that highlights one of the key value propositions of conducting REM.

There are several reasons why the measured real-ear response may not agree with the expected result that appears on the fitting software screen. First, the acoustic properties of the patient's outer and middle ear (e.g., resonance, volume, impedance) may differ from that of the 'average ear' data used in any software prediction. When a REM is conducted, the patient's unique ear canal properties are reflected in the result. As such, REM exposes a need for additional gain adjustments to match prescribed targets as shown in the example above. Second, certain mechanical acoustic aspects of the hearing instrument, such as the effects of venting or the depth of the earmold can affect individually measured results in ways that can only be estimated in the fitting software. For these reasons, it is not uncommon that REM findings will direct the clinician to program the hearing aid differently than the fitting software initially indicated.

In ▸ Fig. 8.2, the same hearing aid has now been adjusted via the gain controls in the fitting software so that the REIG measured in the patient's ear canal via REM matches the prescribed target response. Notice how the fitting software screen now depicts gain settings that are off target on that screen. This finding is a further indication that the clinician

should only view the fitting software depiction of aided performance as an estimate of what is happening in the patient's ear canal.

The examples described above illustrate REM with a single input, which while arguably acceptable with a linear instrument is not appropriate with today's modern compression instruments where gain (and resulting output) vary as a function of input level. As such, when conducting REM with compression devices, it is best practice to ensure that a range of inputs are delivered to the hearing instrument and that the resulting performance be assessed relative to multi-input level targets.[2]

In ▸ Fig. 8.3, the fitting rule selected in both the fitting software and the REM system is NAL-NL1. In contrast to the NAL-R fitting rule previously used, NAL-NL1 is an example of a non-linear fitting rule that provides targets for multiple input levels. For each of these input levels, differing amounts of insertion gain are calculated for each of the frequencies included in the target rule. In the software screen shown in ▸ Fig. 8.3a, the programming software has quick-fit the hearing aid to deliver the gain/output that is predicted to be required to match the prescribed fitting formula targets (in this case, REIG targets) for 50-, 65-, and 80 dB inputs based on the entered audiogram. With the hearing aid programmed in this manner, REIG measures were obtained using REM for the same three input levels depicted in the fitting software. These results are depicted in ▸ Fig. 8.3b. As was the case in the linear hearing aid example discussed earlier, this REIG result indicates that the gain and compression settings currently programmed into the hearing aid need to be adjusted to match the REIG targets across frequencies

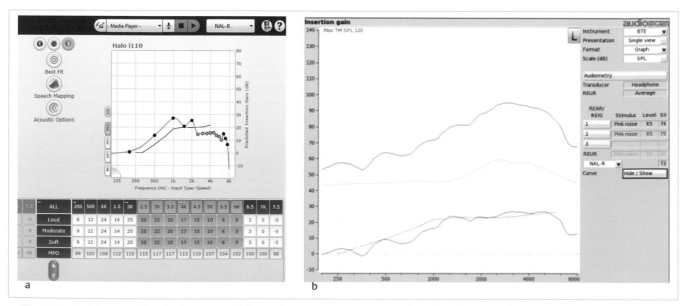

Fig. 8.2   In this example, the hearing aid device has been reprogrammed so that the REIG (lower purple curve) now more closely approximates the NAL-R target (lower black line) in (b). This improved match to REIG targets was accomplished by adjusting the fitting software controls from the original quick-fit settings as shown in (a).

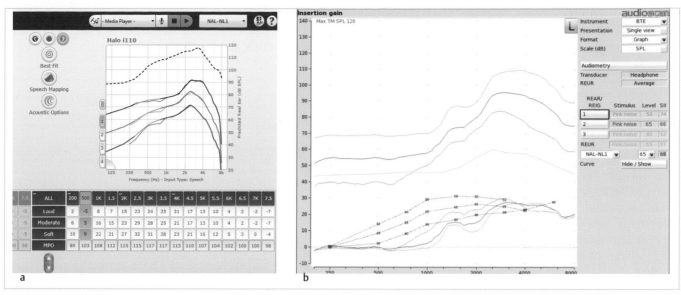

Fig. 8.3   In this example, the fitting rule selected in both the fitting software and the REM system is NAL-NL1, a nonlinear fitting rule. REIG targets now differ as a function of input level. Despite a quick-fit indicating a match to targets in **(a)**, the individually measured REIG results indicate further programming adjustments are required to match the input-level specific targets in the REM system across frequencies in **(b)**.

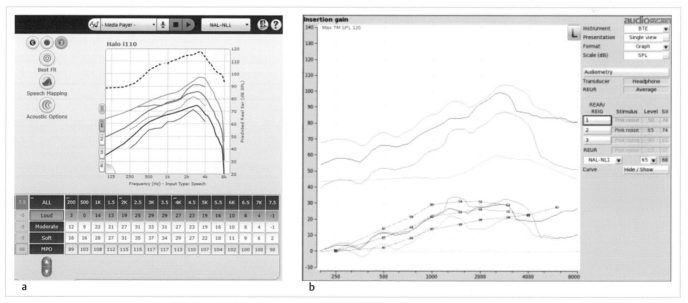

Fig. 8.4   Based on the insertion gain results obtained in ▶**Fig. 8.3**, the hearing aid was reprogrammed **(a)**, to more closely approximate the insertion gain targets at each input level across frequencies in the REM system **(b)**.

for each of the three input levels. ▶**Fig. 8.4** captures these same screens again, once the adjustments in the fitting software have been made to deliver target insertion gain to the patient's ear.

8.3 Limitations of Insertion Gain Measures

Insertion gain measurements represent a commonly used fitting approach for verifying the performance characteristics of hearing instruments. However, as

has been identified by those proponents of the more recent real-ear aided response (REAR) camp, insertion gain has a number of limitations when verifying hearing instruments.

One key drawback in the use of insertion gain measurements is the inherent assumption that the ear canal resonance properties present during the REUR measurement are also present when the audiogram is obtained.[3] This would only be the case if the audiogram is obtained in sound field. If the audiogram is obtained using circumaural headphones or insert earphones then the resonance properties of the ear present during threshold acquisition are different than the resonance properties captured in the sound field REUR.

This difference becomes particularly relevant when it is recognized that insertion gain targets are based on audiogram threshold measures. If thresholds are measured with a headphone or insert phone, but the insertion gain target is calculated based on the subtraction of the sound field REUG, then the gain targeted (and subsequently provided) may not deliver the audibility expected.

In addition, it has been noted that the REIG approach provides no frame of reference relative to the dynamic range of the patient. That is, the impact of target mismatches on audibility or loudness discomfort are not provided as there is no representation of threshold or uncomfortable loudness levels on the measurement screen. For reasons such as these, many providers now using REM to verify the function of today's multichannel wide dynamic range compression hearing aids favor measuring aided output (i.e., REAR) rather than insertion gain (i.e., REIG) and using output targets rather than insertion gain targets.

8.4 The Measurement of Aided Output

As described in Chapter 7, the REAR represents the aided output of an activated hearing aid, measured by a probe tube in the ear canal. To capture the audibility characteristics of a measured REAR, it is useful to compare that REAR to an SPL version of the patient's auditory area (i.e., the SPL-o-gram).

8.4.1 The Sound Pressure Level Audiogram

▶Fig. 8.5 depicts an HL audiogram in ▶Fig. 8.5a, and that same audiogram converted into an SPL audiogram in ▶Fig. 8.5b. Contrary to the standard HL audiogram configuration where loudness is represented as a descending scale on the y-axis, the SPL audiogram utilizes an ascending loudness representation. The dotted line at the bottom of the SPL audiogram grid represents the minimum audible pressure (MAP)[4] (i.e. 0 dB HL converted to the corresponding dB SPL values across frequencies at the eardrum).

In this example, the right ear dB HL threshold values depicted on the traditional audiogram have been converted to the right ear dB SPL threshold values on the SPL audiogram. In addition to the red threshold line, there are also a series of asterisks that represent the patient's frequency-specific UCLs. These values can either be directly measured during diagnostic testing or automatically generated by fitting rules that estimate UCLs based on threshold entries. Sounds that enter the ear canal and reach the eardrum at levels that fall between these SPL threshold and UCL indicators (i.e., fall within the dynamic range of the patient) are sounds that are both audible and tolerable. Thus,

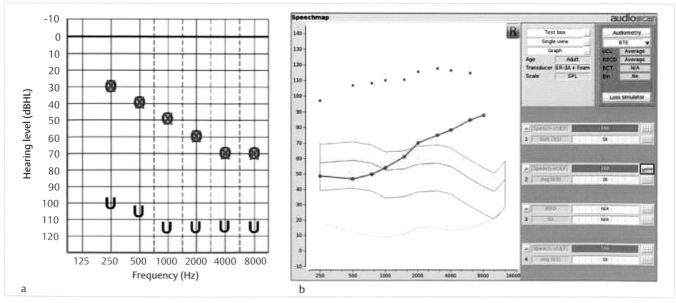

Fig. 8.5 Comparison of dB HL audiogram **(a)** (X or O = threshold; U = uncomfortable loudness level) converted to corresponding dB SPL audiogram **(b)** (O = threshold; Asterisk * = uncomfortable loudness level).

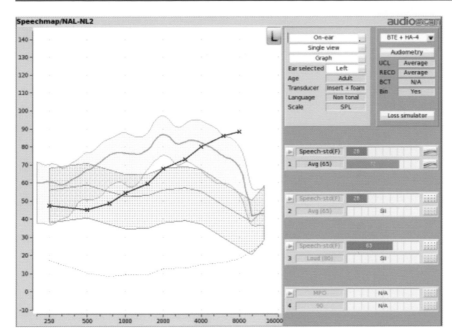

Fig. 8.6 A comparison of aided speech energy (green shaded area) to unaided speech energy (gray shaded area). Notice how much more speech energy is above threshold in the aided condition versus the unaided condition.

these two lines define the patient's residual auditory area in dB SPL at the eardrum.

In addition to the residual auditory area, there is a gray shaded region depicted on the SPL audiogram that represents average conversational speech energy in the unaided condition. This is the same "speech banana" graphic that is traditionally used on the dB HL audiogram grid, but now converted to a dB SPL form. The solid line in the middle of the gray shaded region represents the long-term averaged speech spectrum (LTASS) for average conversational speech. The top border line of the gray shaded area represents the energy level reached 1% of the time (i.e., 99th percentile) during the long-term averaging that produced the LTASS. The bottom border line of the gray shaded area represents the energy level that was reached 70% of the time (i.e., 30th percentile) during long-term averaging. These two lines define the representative dynamic range of normal conversational speech over time. By comparing the gray shaded area to the residual auditory area, a visual representation of which components of unaided average conversational speech fall into and outside of the residual auditory area is provided. Thus, this SPL-o-gram format can be a useful tool for counseling purposes.

8.4.2 Comparison of the Real-Ear–Aided Response and Sound Pressure Level Audiogram

Plotting the unaided speech spectrum on the same screen as the corresponding aided response for the same input level can offer significant fitting/counseling value. Adjusted properly, the hearing aid

should deliver an REAR with more speech energy falling within the patient's residual auditory area than in the unaided condition.

In ▶ Fig. 8.6, the green shaded area represents an REAR from a patient's ear using a 65 dB SPL overall RMS average speech input signal.

The difference between the gray shaded area and the green shaded area represents the measured change in output between the unaided and aided conditions as measured in the ear canal of the patient by the probe microphone. Using speech as the input stimuli when measuring the REAR is sometimes referred to as "speech mapping." Obtaining the aided speech banana, as indicated in the REAR in ▶ Fig. 8.6, provides the observer with an indication of changes in speech audibility associated with the fitting. If more of the green shaded area falls within the patient's residual auditory area in the aided condition than in the unaided condition, more speech energy is now audible.

8.5 Not All Speech Signals Are Alike

There are certain characteristics of speech that must be acknowledged and managed when using this signal type as an input stimulus to measure an REAR. For example, if live speech is used, it would be almost impossible to ensure consistent input signal characteristics from one measurement to the next. The intensity level, amplitude modulation patterns, and vocal effort present when one REAR is captured will not necessarily be the same upon a subsequent REAR measurement, even if the same talker and same speech material is

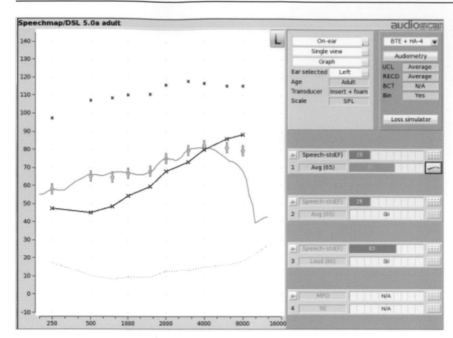

Fig. 8.7 Speechmap screen displaying the DSLv5 targets (green + signs) for one hearing loss for average speech along with the associated REAR for an average speech input (green line) after programming adjustments to match target.

used. Thus, test–retest comparisons to inform programming decisions could be compromised by the potential differences in the input condition if live speech is used. For this reason, recorded speech passages are considered preferable to live speech, particularly as it relates to target matching as the prescriptive fitting formula targets require specific input levels and spectrums.

In 1994, Dennis Byrne et al calculated an average international LTASS.[5] This internationally recognized LTASS has become one of the standards for defining the spectrum and amplitude of speech recordings that are to be used in hearing aid fitting verification.

In 2000, the engineers at Audioscan[6] introduced a recorded speech passage that has come to be known as "The Carrot Passage," which is based on the Byrne LTASS standard. "The Carrot Passage" was the first recorded speech passage provided in a clinically available REM system that produced internationally recognized average speech in both amplitude and spectrum. In 2012, the International Speech Test Signal (ISTS), which was developed by a working group of the European Hearing Instrument Manufacturers Association (EHIMA),[7] became part of the IEC and ANSI standards. These two speech recordings are so similar in average amplitude and spectrum that they can be used interchangeably. Standardized recordings like these are sometimes referred to as calibrated speech passages.

8.6 Real-Ear–Aided Response Targets

Similar to the previous discussion regarding insertion gain targets, there are also a variety of proprietary and generic fitting formula REAR target approaches. Similar to considerations regarding REIG targets for compression hearing aids, REAR targets are also generally input level and signal type specific.

Since speech is generally the most important input condition to consider when prescribing amplification, and since speech input drives the functionality of WDRC devices in a unique way when compared to swept tones or shaped noise, speech (and more specifically, calibrated speech) is generally specified as the input condition to use when programming a WDRC hearing device to an REAR target.

In ▶ Fig. 8.7, an internationally recognized REAR target rule (i.e., DSLv5) has been selected in the SPL audiogram screen of one REM system. The green target markings (+ signs) that are depicted are the REAR targets for average speech prescribed for the SPL audiogram condition represented.

Also in ▶ Fig. 8.7, an REAR result has been captured and is now displayed. The hearing aid has been adjusted in the hearing aid fitting software so that the REAR (the solid green line) is approximating the DSL target values at each frequency. Since the REAR has been measured in the patient's ear canal, any acoustic conditions present during the REAR measurement (e.g., residual ear canal resonance, pinna effects, vent effects, etc.) are contributing to the displayed REAR result.

In ▶ Fig. 8.8, the NAL-NL2 target rule has been selected for the same audiogram condition represented in the previous figure. The same procedure of gain adjustment via the fitting software was used to obtain the REAR displayed (the green line) in this figure.

In addition to using speech mapping to measure and display the REAR obtained in the presence of calibrated speech input, these systems can also be used to display the aided speech envelope (i.e., short term fluctuations in speech). ▶ Fig. 8.9 includes the same aided result screens shown in ▶ Fig. 8.7 and ▶ Fig. 8.8, but reconfigured to display the entire aided speech envelope. Using a technique known as percentile analysis,[8,9] the aided speech spectrum is analyzed over time in the presence of the calibrated speech passage for each of the one-third octave bands of the input signal. In addition to collecting the data needed to display the long term average REAR (i.e., aided LTASS), two other data sets are gathered. First, the aided output level of the band that was exceeded 1% of the time (speech peaks). Second, the aided output level of the band that was exceeded 70% of the time (speech valleys). These percentiles correspond with the peak and valley indicators defining the gray shaded area used to represent the unaided speech envelope condition. Thus, by comparing the unaided speech energy envelope (gray shaded area) to the aided speech energy envelope (the green shaded areas in ▶ Fig. 8.9), it is possible to define the overall change in speech audibility provided by the hearing aid.

The speech energy envelope is particularly valuable in calculating the Speech Intelligibility Index (SII).[10] The SII is a measure ranging from 0.0 to 1

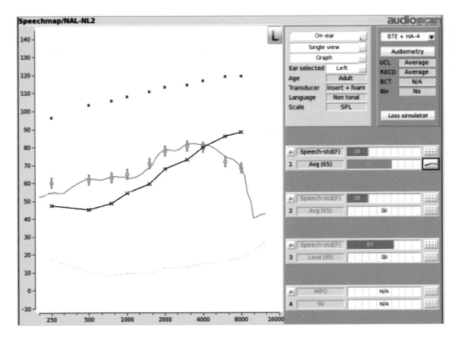

Fig. 8.8 NAL-NL2 REAR targets for average speech (green + signs) and the corresponding REAR for an average speech input (green line) positioned via programming adjustments to land on the NAL-NL2 targets.

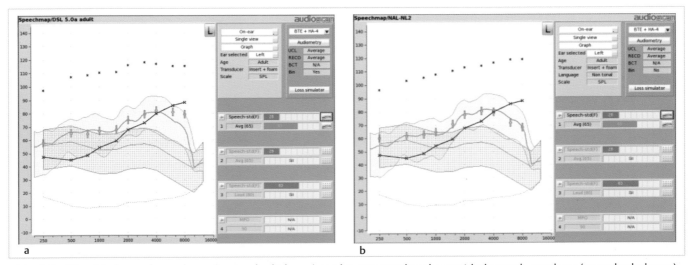

Fig. 8.9 The aided speech envelopes (green shaded area) can be compared to the unaided speech envelope (gray shaded area) for the same input condition to visualize the speech energy amplification has brought back into the patient's dynamic range. Shown is a possible measurement outcome for DSLv5 **(a)** and NAL-NL2 **(b)**.

(or 0 to 100 if multiplied by 10) that, according to ANSI S3.5-1997 is "highly correlated with the intelligibility of speech." The SII is calculated by determining the portion of speech information that is audible across a specific number of frequency bands. As the SII increases, speech understanding generally increases. Both the unaided and aided SII scores can be calculated as part of the Speechmap procedure with various REM systems by comparing the associated speech energy envelope with the dB SPL thresholds of the patient. As more of the speech energy envelope falls above threshold, the SII score increases.

In ▸**Fig. 8.10**, SII results for both the unaided average speech condition and the aided average speech condition are circled. Since a greater proportion of the aided speech energy envelope (pink shaded area) falls within the listening range than the unaided speech energy envelope (gray shaded area), the SII score is greater.

8.7 General Fitting Protocols Associated with 'Speechmap' Verification

In order to effectively utilize the objective measurement of a patient's REAR in the presence of calibrated speech input stimuli, it is necessary to coordinate the hearing aid fitting software to the extent possible with the requested prescriptive targets in the REM system. Generally, there are three main amplification characteristics that are available for adjustment: gain, compression, and maximum output. Described below are three approaches that can be

considered when deciding how to manipulate the hearing instrument to achieve the prescribed targeted performance.

1. Adjusting input-level–specific gain to match input-level–specific targets.

▸**Fig. 8.11** is an example of a manufacturer's fitting software screen. The audiogram has been entered, the hearing aids to be programmed have been selected and the fitting rule (in this case, NAL-NL2) has been chosen. Based on these three elements, the fitting software has automatically programmed channel-specific gain, compression, and output settings into the hearing aid, and has displayed a graphic representation of these settings. In this example, the display is set to 'real-ear aided response'. Note that there are three input-level–specific targets on the graph. The lower line grouping represents the NAL-NL2 target (thin line) and the hearing aid response programmed to meet that target for a 50 dB input (thick line). The middle line grouping represents the target and response programmed for a 65 dB input. The upper line grouping represents the target and response programmed for an 80 dB input. The channel-specific response values for each of these input levels are indicated in the table just below the response graphic. Since NAL-NL2 is a nonlinear target rule, the three input-level–specific targets are used to set the compression characteristics NAL-NL2 predicts are needed in each channel to accommodate the recruitment associated with the hearing loss condition entered. These initial programmed settings are often referred to as "Quick-fit" or "First-fit."

These same input-level–specific response values can be verified using real-ear measurements

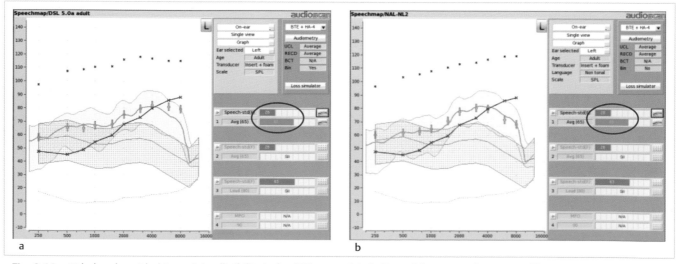

a   b

Fig. 8.10 Aided and unaided Speech Intelligibility Index (SII) scores (circled in red) for one audiogram and hearing instrument setting for average speech with (**a**) DSLv5 and (**b**) NAL-NL2. The difference between the aided and unaided SII scores quantifies the predicted improvement in overall speech intelligibility that may occur for average speech inputs as a result of this hearing instrument fitting.

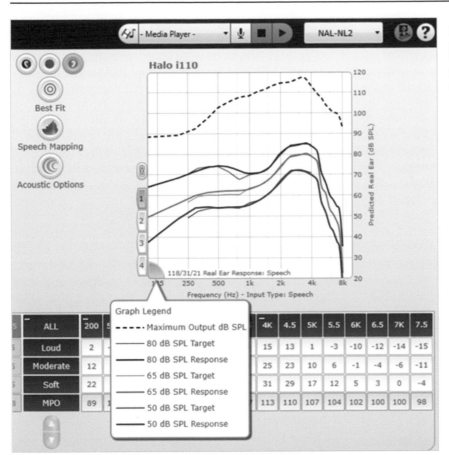

Fig. 8.11 Manufacturers fitting screen displaying "First Fit" results for NAL-NL2. On this screen, the predicted real-ear–aided response and the targeted response for each input condition appear to match.

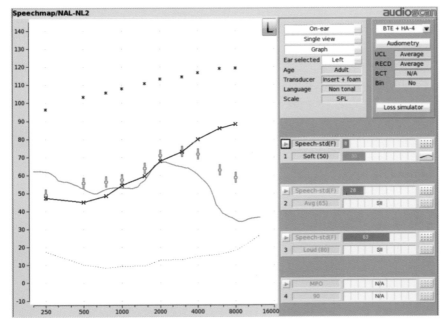

Fig. 8.12 Individually measured REAR for soft speech using the "First Fit" setting in ▶**Fig. 8.11**. While the programmed response matched REAR targets on the fitting software screen, the actual REARs obtained for this patient deviate from the REAR targets in the REM system for this particular ear.

with speech inputs. ▶**Fig. 8.12** shows a Speechmap screen where the audiogram used in the fitting software has been entered into the verification system and the same NAL-NL2 fitting formula has been selected. With a speech input level of 50 dB (soft speech) selected, the NAL-NL2 targets appear on the measurement as a set of green plus signs. Once the calibrated speech passage at this level has been averaged and recorded, a green REAR line representing the LTASS of the measured signal along with the corresponding short-term fluctuations of speech (i.e., speech envelope) is displayed. The extent to which the green-aided 50 dB LTASS line does not align with the target markings represents the deviation from prescribed target for the hearing aid as programmed.

When the clinician encounters a verification target mismatch, it will be necessary to adjust the gain settings in the fitting software for 50 dB input until the REAR more closely approximates the fitting formula targets across the widest frequency range possible. In ▶ Fig. 8.13, such adjustments were made. Note that the Speechmap screen now displays an REAR for soft speech that more closely approximates the REAR targets. However, also note that the fitting software graphic now displays a simulated measurement curve that is off-target for a 50 dB input due to differences between the predictions made by the fitting software and the actual patient and hearing aid specific variables mentioned earlier.

Once the 50 dB gain settings have been adjusted to match the associated REAR target for that input level, this same procedure can be used to adjust the hearing instrument programming to match the corresponding REAR targets for other input levels as well (e.g., 65- and 80 dB SPL). ▶ Fig. 8.14 depicts an example of a completed REAR verification process where gain settings for soft (50 dB), average (65 dB), and loud (80 dB) speech have been adjusted to match NAL-NL2 targets in the patient's ear canal.

Beyond verification of hearing aid performance for various speech input levels, it is generally recognized that the maximum output settings of the hearing instrument should be documented to ensure not only listening comfort for loud sounds (i.e., MPO not set too high relative to patient UCLs) but also

sufficient headroom for louder inputs (i.e., MPO not set too low to impact audibility and sound quality). ▶ Fig. 8.15 shows selection of the maximum power output (MPO) test signal in one REM system. With this system, an 85 dB pure tone sweep (REAR85) is presented across one-third octaves from the sound field speaker, while the output of the hearing aid is measured. The measured REAR85 curve should not exceed the predicted UCL indicators (asterisks) on the SPL audiogram or the associated REAR85/90 targets for fitting formulas that generate these values (e.g., DSLv5). Should adjustments be required, it would typically be accomplished via the MPO settings in the hearing instrument programming software. ▶ Fig. 8.16 is a summary screen of the four tests just described where the REAR targets have been approximated for soft, average and loud speech along with a MPO measurement that does not exceed the predicted UCLs of the the patient.

2. Adjusting overall gain for soft speech and verifying compression settings.

It should be noted that if the above protocol is used, the initial compression settings programmed as part of "First Fit" may change. Further, depending on the underlying signal processing architecture of the device being evaluated, the order in which the fitting handles are manipulated may result in a need to revisit previously verified input level settings. As an alternative to potentially minimize the need for additional adjustment with other input levels (or the need to revisit previously verified input levels), consider setting overall gain for soft speech as the first step in the verification protocol.

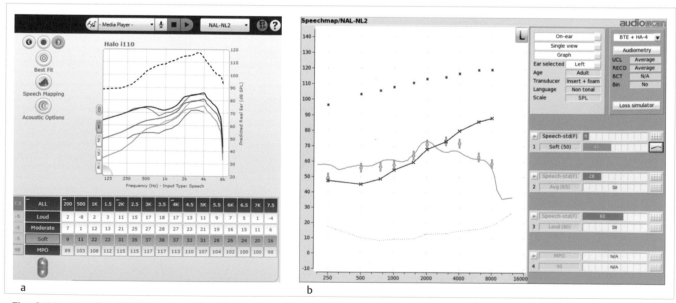

Fig. 8.13 Simulated REAR curves (a) and corresponding measured REAR curves (b) following adjustment of the hearing instrument to match targets in the REM system.

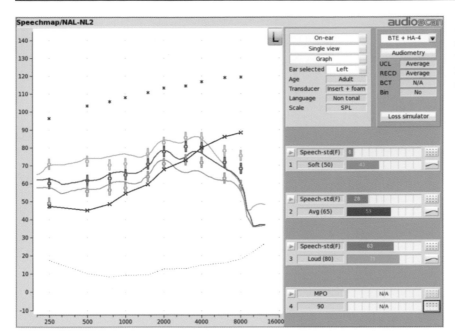

Fig. 8.14 Speechmap summary result displaying REARs and corresponding REAR targets for soft (50 dB SPL), average (65 dB SPL) and loud (80 dB SPL) speech input levels, following programming adjustments.

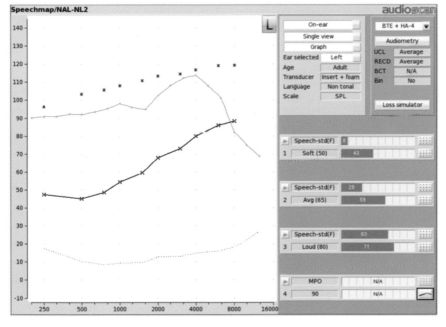

Fig. 8.15 An MPO REAR 85/90 evaluation of one hearing instrument on a representative REM system where the measured curve should not exceed the predicted UCL values (asterisks).

First obtain an REAR for 50–55 dB speech as described in the above protocol. If the aided LTASS is not on target, instead of adjusting gain values for a 50 dB input, adjust the overall gain of the device. This process will change gain for the soft (50 dB) speech input where needed while also maintaining the "First Fit" compression ratios (or input/output function).

Subsequent adjustment can then proceed as needed for the input level specific handles for 65 dB (average speech) and then 80 dB (loud speech) as needed to match their input level specific REAR targets. In some cases, this approach minimizes the need for adjustments after the initial soft speech input gain adjust-ments. Verification of maximum output (i.e., REAR 85/90) must be completed in this protocol as well, and is done in the same way that was described previously. In ▶ Fig. 8.17, this procedure was utilized to verify that soft, average, and loud speech inputs met prescribed REAR targets at each level using DSLv5 targets.

3. Using Speechmap verification as a counseling tool.

Once verification is complete, the REAR screen can be configured as an effective and compelling counseling tool. In ▶ Fig. 8.18, the result screen shown in ▶ Fig. 8.17 has been modified using the verification system display tools to show both the unaided and

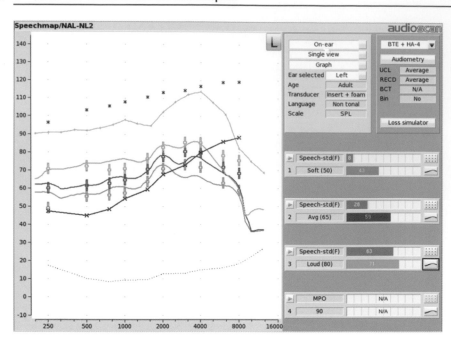

Fig. 8.16 A final REAR verification screen displaying the REARs and corresponding REAR targets for 50-, 65-, and 80 dB speech inputs along with an MPO input condition.

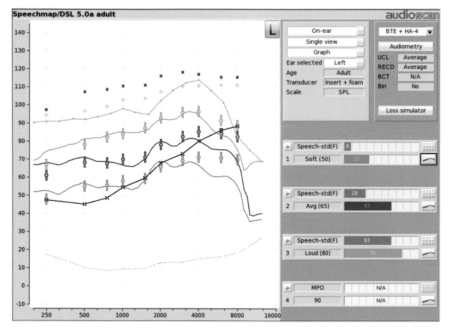

Fig. 8.17 A final REAR verification screen when setting overall gain using a 50 dB input and adjusting gain for 65- and 80 dB inputs only when needed. This programming approach may result in the need for fewer programming adjustments, as compression ratios from "First Fit" are unlikely to need modification.

aided speech energy envelopes for a 65 dB average conversational speech input. The SPL audiogram thresholds and uncomfortable loudness level (UCL) asterisks remain on the screen and when combined, they define the patient's dynamic range. Starting with the gray shaded area, the clinician can describe for the patient that portion of average conversational speech energy that is "falling outside of your listening range" without amplification. Only that portion of the gray shaded area that is above the threshold line is audible without amplification and, as a result, the associated SII score is low. The pink shaded area represents the resulting audibility of average conversational speech using hearing aid(s)

that have been programmed to the patient's hearing condition. Note that more speech energy falls inside the patient's dynamic range and the associated SII score is higher. This higher SII score indicates that a greater proportion of speech cues are audible with the hearing aid than without it, and therefore greater speech recognition is likely.

The SII value that is appropriate for a particular patient is dependent on a number of factors, not the least of which is their hearing loss.[11] The SII normative values score sheet[12] that is part of the PedAMP protocol developed by the University of Western Ontario can be a useful guide in establishing a reasonable aided SII expectation as a function of degree of hearing loss.

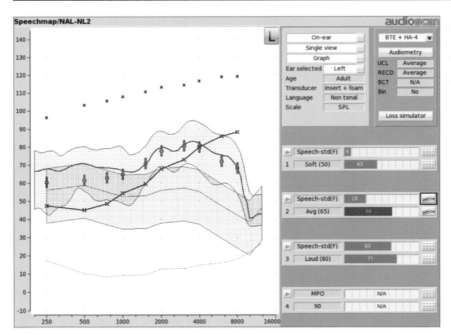

Fig. 8.18 Counseling screen showing the unaided (gray shaded area) and aided (pink shaded area) average speech curves along with the patient's 'listening range' (i.e., thresholds (X's) to UCLs (asterisks)).

8.8 Hearing Aid Function Testing

Modern hearing aids are equipped with a variety of signal processing features intended to benefit the patient with hearing loss. If these capabilities are identified by the clinician as appropriate to address communication issues impacting the patient, verifying their functionality becomes a necessary component of the treatment process.

8.8.1 Verification of Directional Microphone Performance

Directional microphone performance is often quantified in technical specifications provided by the manufacturer by including a frequency-specific polar plot diagram (▶ **Fig. 8.19**).[13] Although this technique can provide a consistent means of visually quantifying directional microphone performance, it is not a test that can readily be duplicated in a clinical setting. Therefore, clinicians often must rely on variety of techniques to assess directional microphone performance and confirm appropriate functionality including: a basic front-to-back listening check of the hearing aid, speech-in-noise testing with the directional microphone off and then on,[13,14] sequential front-to-back ratio (FBR) test of 2-cc coupler output measures,[14] or faith that the directional microphone works as specified.

Sequential FBR testing of directional microphones can be confounded by WDRC (or any compression) technology. By comparing the output levels measured in a coupler or ear canal across frequency for input stimuli coming from 0-degree azimuth, to the output levels measured across frequency for input stimuli coming from the 180-degree azimuth at the same level, one can calculate the FBR, where higher output for sounds from the front than the rear suggest directional performance and a higher FBR. However, if an FBR test is conducted on a compression hearing aid, the gain that is applied to these two separate measurements will be different, and thus, the FBR will be impacted by these gain differences.

The effects of compression on a single stimulus polar pattern measurement or a conceptually similar sequential FBR test were quantified through a FBR testing procedure utilized by Todd Ricketts in 2000.[15] In this work, data from two hearing aids were obtained, first with compression off, and then with compression on. As shown in ▶ **Table 8.2**, with the traditional sequential FBR measurement condition, where only one signal is presented sequentially during the 0- and 180-degree measures, the FBR result is less with compression on than with compression off. This is due to the fact that the directional microphone array reduces the amplitude of the signal levels from behind, relative to the amplitude of the identical signal coming from the front, which may result in more gain applied to signals from behind, as compared to those from the front.

In the modified measurement condition used in this study, two signals (one from a speaker at 0 degrees and one from a speaker at 180 degrees, each relative to the hearing aid) were presented simultaneously; the test signal was delivered from

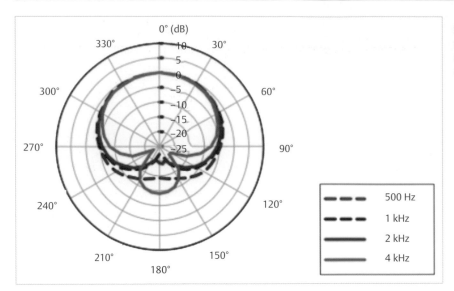

Fig. 8.19 Polar diagram showing input sensitivity at 360 degrees around a hearing aid, for frequencies of 500 Hz, 1-, 2-, and 4 kHz.

Table 8.2 Data quantifying the effects of compression on directional tests using the front-to-back ratio technique. In the modified test, where two input sources were presented simultaneously, the front-to-back ratio measurement in the presence of compression is uncompromised, which is not the case with a single-source (traditional) measurement approach.

	Traditional	Modified
Type B (compression off)	7.7 db	7.7 db
Type B (compression on)	3.9 db	7.7 db
Type C (compression off)	11.2 db	11.2 db
Type C (compression on)	3.7 db	11.1 db

the front speaker and a jamming signal presented from the rear speaker. This approach removed sequential gain as a measurement artifact during the test. In other words, to obtain a more realistic FBR when measuring compression hearing aids, the front and rear input signals should be presented at the same time.

It is possible with some REM systems to perform a simultaneous FBR test using broadband stimuli and fast Fourier transform (FFT) analysis in either test box or real-ear measurement conditions.[16] This technique allows for the output result for the 0- and 180-degree stimulus conditions to be obtained simultaneously and displayed separately, even if the aid being tested is nonlinear.

8.8.2 Simultaneous Real-Ear Front-to-Back Ratio Directional Microphone Testing

By placing a probe microphone in the patient's aided ear and delivering two input signals simultaneously from two sound field speakers located in front of and behind the patient's head, and using FFT analysis, some commercially available REM verification systems can measure the directional effect of directional hearing aids while addressing the effects of compression on sequential FBR curves as described previously. Clinicians using this type of REM directional test will see two frequency response curves representing the output produced by the directional hearing aid for signals coming from the front and back of the device at the same time.

▶ **Fig. 8.20** provides an illustration of the clinical configuration needed to conduct a simultaneous REM directional test. The patient is seated and is facing the universal sound field speaker that is used for any REM procedure. A second (auxiliary) speaker is placed behind the patient. With the probe tube and directional hearing aid placed in either ear, the reference microphone of the probe assembly will be used to regulate the level and spectrum of each speaker stimulus so that they are matched in presentation level.

8.8.3 Simultaneous Stimulus Conditions

There are various stimuli that can be employed for simultaneous front/back directional evaluation including specialized noise signals with or without the presence of speech.

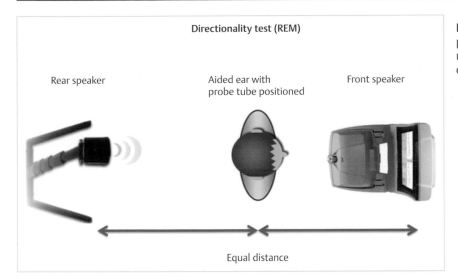

Fig. 8.20 Illustration of patient and speaker positions when measuring on-ear directional microphone performance using simultaneous measurement of the front-to-back ratio.

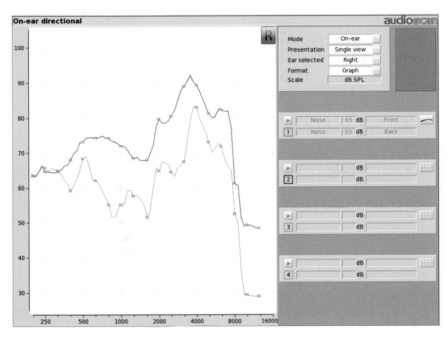

Fig. 8.21 Real-ear measurement directional test results for a simultaneous front-back noise only directional test. The upper thick line (F1) shows the output of the hearing instrument in directional mode for signals from the front, while the lower thin line (B1) shows the output of the same device for signals from behind. The separation between the 2 curves is evidence of directional performance.

▶ **Fig. 8.21** is an example of a REM directional test result from one REM system using a Noise–Noise stimulus. The upper thick curve (labeled F1) represents the output measured with a hearing instrument in a directional setting for the signal presented from the front speaker (0-degrees azimuth). The lower thin curve (labeled B1) represents the output measured for the signal presented from the rear speaker (180 degrees azimuth) for the same hearing instrument in the directional setting. Since the input level for both signals is equal, and both signals are present at the same time (i.e., under the same gain conditions) the plotted result indicates directional performance given the relatively greater output for signals from the front (F1) than behind (B1). This type of test result captures the directional effects across all frequencies being tested, a unique and valuable data set in comparison to a single-frequency polar plot. Because the compres-

sion characteristics programmed into the hearing aid device are in the "as-worn" configuration, this directional test result is a reflection of the directional performance available when the patient is using the hearing aid as programmed.

Since speech-activated directional microphone technology is available in modern hearing aids, some REM systems provide a Speech + Noise stimulus to ensure that directional devices requiring the presence of speech in noise are appropriately activated.

▶ **Fig. 8.22** shows an example of a REM directional test result using a simultaneous front/back Speech–Noise stimulus. Again, the upper thick curve (labeled F2) is the output measured for the signal presented from the front (0 degrees azimuth). The lower thin curve (labeled B2) is the output measured for the signal presented from behind (180 degrees azimuth). Curve separation

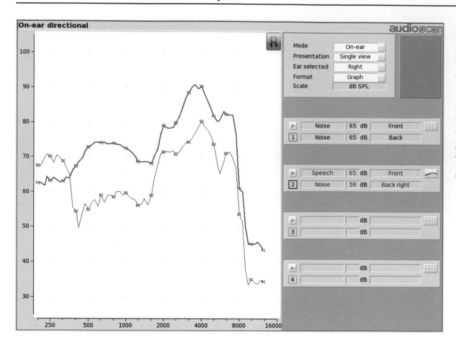

Fig. 8.22 Real-ear measurement results from a directional test. Speech and noise were presented simultaneously from the front and back, respectively, to yield these results. The upper thick line (F2) shows the output of the hearing instrument in directional mode for signals from the front, while the lower thin line (B2) shows the output of the same device for signals from behind. The separation between the 2 curves is evidence of directional performance.

indicates the directional microphone effect across all frequencies tested.

REM directional tests reflect not only the impact of the directional microphone on the FBR, but also the effects of venting and the effects of microphone port orientation relative to the horizontal plane of the input stimulus condition. As such, REM evaluation of directional microphone performance is a valuable tool when troubleshooting directional performance and can help guide decision-making and inform patient counseling.

8.9 Noise Reduction

Many modern hearing instruments are equipped with some form of digital noise reduction.[17] Generally, this feature utilizes an amplitude modulation detection algorithm in each channel or band of the hearing instrument. Since amplitude modulation patterns for speech are distinctive in comparison to other input sources, channels that do not show speech-like amplitude modulation patterns can be subject to automatic gain reduction. This gain reduction is intended to reduce the annoyance of the non-speech input signals that may dominate in any given band of frequencies.

The speed at which this gain reduction occurs and the amount of gain reduction that is applied varies among different hearing aids and their available software settings. However, REM technology can offer a way of quantifying both of these characteristics. By generating a broadband noise input signal and measuring the hearing aid's output over time, a quantification of the noise reduction feature in each band can be acquired.

▶ Fig. 8.23 shows the results of a digital noise reduction when a broadband recording of air conditioner noise is presented via the REM system's sound field speaker at a level of 80 dB SPL. After approximately the first second of stimulus measurement, an initial output curve is captured and displayed as a solid line on the output graph. Over time, the active curve should start to drop below the solid line reference curve previously captured, indicating the amount of noise reduction applied by the hearing aid. Once this active curve appears to be stable, the clinician can stop the test and capture this second curve, which is displayed as a thinner line. Because the stimulus being used contains no speech-like modulation patterns, this stimulus will typically activate the noise reduction feature in any channel where this feature is available.

The difference between the reference thick line and the noise reduction–engaged thinner line represents the magnitude of the noise reduction that has taken effect across the frequency range being measured. The stopwatch feature (available with some REM systems) allows the clinician to track the amount of time needed in order for the noise reduction to initially activate, and subsequently to fully engage. As mentioned before, the magnitude of the noise reduction can vary across different makes and models of hearing aids and can vary based on the settings programmed into the device. The attack time component is generally not a programmable feature, rather is typically defined by the algorithm's design for that particular make and model of hearing aid.

Different noise reduction algorithms can also behave differently across frequency. Some hearing aids only reduce noise in the lower frequencies. Some

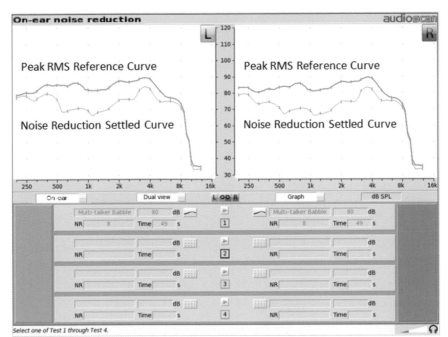

Fig. 8.23 Example of an on-ear noise reduction test from one REM system manufacturer. Shown are the peak RMS reference curve measurements for an air conditioner noise at 80 dB SPL prior to the engagement of noise reduction; and the settled noise reduction curve following continued presentation of the noise signal. The separation between the peak and settled curves represent the amount of noise reduction across frequencies.

hearing aids reduce noise in the lower frequencies first, and then in the higher frequencies at some point later in the stimulus measurement. Other systems reduce gain across all frequencies at essentially the same time and rate. These noise reduction properties, once identified, can become useful for programming decisions and to help inform counseling.

8.10 Telecoil Measurement

Many hearing aids are equipped with a small wired coil (called a telecoil) that is designed to pick up electromagnetic signals generated by either a telephone receiver or an inductive loop system sometimes installed in public locations to assist hearing aid wearers. Since the signal reaching the telecoil is electromagnetic rather than acoustic, most hearing aid verification systems include hardware designed to generate electromagnetic conditions as specified by ANSI S3.22 2009 to simulate both the telephone and loop electromagnetic input conditions. This allows the clinician to evaluate the effectiveness of the telecoil in these types of conditions and program the telecoil to ensure audibility of the inductively transmitted signal.

Although the standardized tests are designed to be conducted in a test box or coupler, some verification equipment offers a means to assess telecoil functionality on-ear as well. This is facilitated through the use of a tele-test handset (▶ Fig. 8.24) that houses the telephone magnetic field simulator (TMFS). This simulator consists of a 35.4-mm coil placed 16.5 mm below the test surface, which is identified with the "T" inside of a circle symbol. This TMFS generates the electromag-

netic input associated with the test condition that has been selected. When the handset is placed nearby the hearing aid as it is worn (▶ Fig. 8.25), the telecoil within the hearing aid then picks up this input, which is subsequently converted by the hearing aid to an amplified acoustic output that can be measured by a probe microphone. This process facilitates comparing the aided output for acoustic input conditions to the aided output for electromagnetic input conditions, thus verifying their similarities and differences.

▶ Fig. 8.26 is an example of a completed set of REAR measurements. The REAR depicted by the green curve was obtained by placing the patient in front of a sound field speaker that generated a 65 dB calibrated speech input signal. The REAR depicted by the purple curve was obtained via a tele-test handset generating a magnetic field equivalent to a 65 dB acoustic signal that was held up against the hearing aid in telecoil mode.

By comparing these two REARs, the clinician can determine if the telecoil output is equivalent to the acoustic output. As generally agreed upon in the literature (e.g., Valente, 2013), a reasonable verification goal would be to have an equivalent output for both the telecoil and acoustic modes in cases where the input level is equivalent to leave a seamless transition when switching between modes. If this is not the case, the clinician should make adjustments to the hearing aid gain associated with the telecoil memory, in an effort to match the telecoil output with the acoustic output result.

In some hearing aids, signals received by a telecoil in one hearing aid (on one ear) can also be wirelessly transmitted between ears, resulting in binaural listening for a unilateral input. In other words, a patient may hold a telephone handset to one ear, but hear

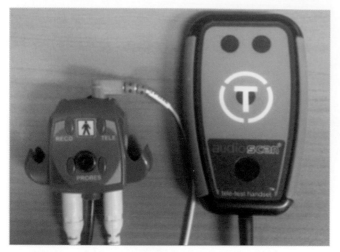

Fig. 8.24   Tele-test handset.

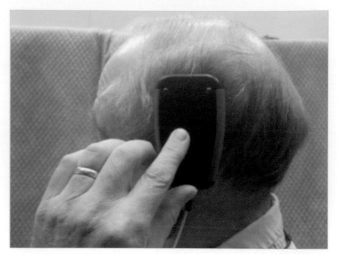

Fig. 8.25   Tele-test handset held next to patient's ear for verification procedure.

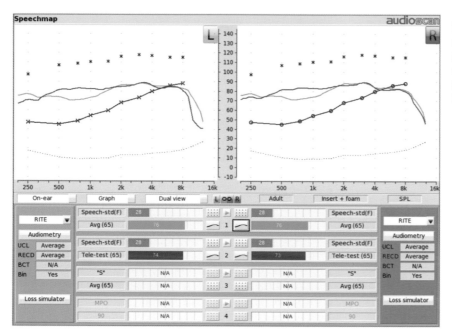

Fig. 8.26   Real-ear aided response (REAR) measurements for a 65 dB SPL (average speech) acoustic input (green curve) and an electromagnetic equivalent to 65 dB SPL speech (purple curve) using the tele-test handset while in telecoil mode.

the telephone signal in both ears. Through the use of simultaneous bilateral real-ear measurement, it is possible to measure the output produced in both ear canals at the same time, thus documenting audibility of the inductively received signal, being transmitted from one hearing instrument (phone ear) to the other (non-phone ear).

8.11 Summary

Real ear measurement can be used to directly measure insertion gain, and was originally established for this purpose. However, as hearing instrument technology has evolved, particularly in the area of nonlinear/frequency-specific compression and in the area of interactive functionality, certain limitations with insertion gain measurement became apparent. Shifting the use

of real ear measurement to the measurement of aided output overcomes many of these limitations.

A key factor in enhancing the utility of real ear measurement with today's hearing instrument technology is to use speech as the input stimulus when measuring aided output. To help insure that gain adjustments made to reach aided output goals will be appropriate for the many listening conditions a patient will likely encounter, it is important that the speech stimulus used when conducting aided output measures be a calibrated speech stimulus. This includes not only standardization of the amplitude levels presented, but also standardization of the speech spectrum being utilized. Calibrated speech signals such as "the carrot passage" or the International Speech Test Signal (ISTS) have been created for this purpose. And, when such signals are further modified at the test point via spectral analysis of a preceding calibration pulse to insure that the desired amplitude and spectrum of the speech signal is reaching that test point, then a repeatable and reliable test condition is possible.

Internationally recognized prescriptive methods such as the Desired Sensation Level (DSLv5) or the National Acoustic Laboratory (NAL-NL2) approaches provide output targets for various input levels. These targets can be used to guide the setting of gain, compression, and output of the hearing instrument. In addition, the Speech Intelligibility Index (SII) can be calculated and displayed after aided measurements have been obtained to further analyze the utility and effectiveness of aided settings. REM can also be used to troubleshoot patient concerns and identify areas of adjustment that can address these issues.

In addition to fitting hearing instruments, real ear measures can also be used to quantify and assess other hearing instrument features such as directional microphone performance, noise management technology, binaural processing, and on-ear telecoil performance. As a result, real ear measurement becomes an indispensable tool in the professional's treatment arsenal when amplification is part of the treatment strategy being utilized to address hearing loss and the communication issues associated with it.

References

[1] Mynders J. Essentials of hearing aid selection, Part 2: It's in the numbers. The Hearing Review 2003;10(12):16–20, 51

[2] Byrne D, Dillon H. The National Acoustic Laboratories' (NAL) new procedure for selecting the gain and frequency response of a hearing aid. Ear Hear 1986;7(4):257–265

[3] John AF, Santos-Sacchi J. Physiology of the Ear. New York, NY: Raven Press; 1988

[4] Olsen WO, Hawkins DB, Van Tasell DJ. Representations of the long-term spectra of speech. Ear Hear 1987;8(5, Suppl):100S–108S

[5] Taylor B. Predicting real world hearing aid benefit with speech audiometry: an evidenced-based review. 2007. Audiologyonline. Available at: https://www.audiologyonline.com/articles/predicting-real-world-hearing-aid-946

[6] Audioscan. The Audioscan Speechmap fitting system. Available at: https://www.audioscan.com/speechmap

[7] Byrne D, Dillion H, Tran K. An international comparison of long-term average speech spectra. J Acoust Soc Am 1994;96(4):2108–2120

[8] Holube I, Fredelake S, Vlaming M, Kollmeier B. Development and analysis of an international speech test signal (ISTS). Int J Audiol 2010;49(12):891–903

[9] Holube I. 20Q: Getting to know the ISTS. 2015. Audiologyonline. Available at: https://www.audiologyonline.com/articles/20q-getting-to-know-ists-13295

[10] ANSI. ANSI S3.5–1997. American National Standard Methods for the Calculation of the Speech Intelligibility Index. New York, NY: ANSI; 1997

[11] Smriga D. Speechmap as a fitting and counseling tool. May 26, 2015. Audiologyonline. Available at: https://www.audiologyonline.com/articles/speechmap-as-counseling-and-fitting-14232

[12] Aided Speech Intelligibility Index (SII) Normative Values v1.0, Revision 2. Available at: https://www.dslio.com/wp-content/uploads/2016/10/Aided-SII-Normative-Values_App-A.pdf

[13] Ricketts T, Mueller HG. Making sense of directional microphone hearing aids. Am J Audiol 1999;8(2):117–127

[14] Frye G. How to verify directional hearing aids in the office. The Hearing Review. January 6, 2006. Available at: http://www.hearingreview.com/2006/01/how-to-verify-directional-hearing-aids-in-the-office

[15] Ricketts T. Directivity quantification in hearing aids: fitting and measurement effects. Ear Hear 2000;21(1):45–58

[16] Smriga D. The Verifit directional mic test: evaluating modern directional microphone technologies. October 30, 2015. Audiologyonline. Available at: https://www.audiologyonline.com/articles/verifit-directional-mic-test-evaluating-15371

[17] Bentler R, Chiou LK. Digital noise reduction: an overview. Trends Amplif 2006;10(2):67–82

9 Hearing Aid Prescriptive Fitting Methods

Erin M. Picou

9.1 Introduction

Mr. Glenn O'Dear comes to your clinic for a hearing evaluation. He is 48 years old and reports increased difficulty understanding speech over the last 10 years, especially in noisy situations or when there are multiple people talking. In addition, his wife reports that she often has to repeat herself, especially when she is cooking in the kitchen and Mr. O'Dear is in the living room. He's been contemplating seeking help for a couple of years and is now looking for help to improve his communication. You test his hearing and find a symmetrical, moderate sensorineural hearing loss (►**Fig. 9.1**). As a result, you recommend bilateral hearing aids. The patient and his wife are ready to pursue amplification. Now what? How much gain should the hearing aids provide Mr. O'Dear? We know he wants help, so 0 dB of gain would not be enough. We also know that, although his hearing thresholds are elevated by approximately 60 dB, his loudness discomfort thresholds are not similarly elevated. Therefore, programming hearing aids with 60 dB of gain would be too much, making many sounds uncomfortably loud. So, we know he needs between 0 and 60 dB of gain, but how much?

Prescriptive fitting methods provide answers to this question, and to other related questions such as: How loud should we make whispered speech? Conversational speech? Shouted speech? What is the highest level the hearing aid should output? Generally, when we talk about a "prescriptive fitting method," it means that a clinician selects a hearing aid that is capable of providing sufficient gain based on the patient's audiometric test results. At the time of the fitting, the clinician programs or adjusts the hearing aid so that the hearing aid meets a prescriptive target. The clinician verifies that the hearing

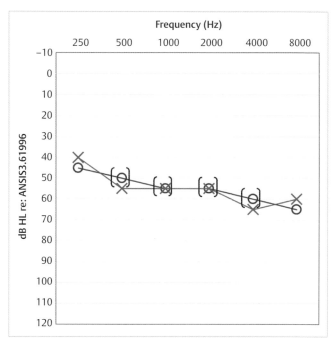

Fig. 9.1 Pure tone, air-conduction audiometric thresholds for a hypothetical patient (Mr. Glenn O'Dear) as a function of frequency for left and right ears (*blue* and *right lines*, respectively). Figure also displays bone-conduction audiometric thresholds for the patient for the left and right ears (left and right facing brackets, respectively).

aid matches the target and then the hearing aid is further adjusted for the specific patient.

This chapter discusses prescriptive fitting methods, first by focusing on how methods may vary from each other and then by reviewing some historical prescriptions. Next, the historical methods provide a context for the discussion of modern prescriptions and a review of some case studies. Finally, some of the "methods" part of prescriptive fittings are reviewed by highlighting the importance of verification and factors that may change the amount of gain a patient wears home.

9.2 Ways Prescriptions Vary

Over the years, there have been many methods of assigning hearing aid gain. These methods vary considerably not only in the amount of gain they assign, but also in their underlying rationale, the type of input, whether amplitude compression is applied, and how they handle bilateral fittings. In addition, the prescriptions vary based on the type of gain prescribed. Each of these factors will be discussed separately.

9.2.1 Underlying Rationale

Inherent to sensorineural hearing loss is disrupted loudness perception. Hearing thresholds are elevated, while thresholds of discomfort are not. As a result, the dynamic range of hearing is smaller and growth of loudness is steeper. A small change in level may result in a large change in perceived loudness. Therefore, when we fit a patient with hearing aids, we have a limited range to work with. It's why we can't give Mr. O'Dear 60 dB of gain. However, how much gain we do give him will depend on whether we try to amplify speech to his **most comfortable listening (MCL) level**, try to restore his loudness perception to normal (**loudness normalization**), or try to make all frequencies equally loud (**loudness equalization**).

One rationale underlying many prescriptive methods is the idea that we want to make speech audible and comfortable. Some prescriptions are based on the rationale that to achieve this aim, we need to amplify speech so that it is at a patient's **MCL level**. For most listeners, the MCL is actually a range of levels and is approximately halfway between their audiometric hearing threshold and their threshold of discomfort. Amplifying speech to a patient's MCL level was common for many of the historical prescriptions, although the prescriptions recommended various methods of achieving their goal, including measuring MCL levels, predicting MCL levels based on measured audiometric thresholds and loudness discomfort levels, and predicting them based only on measured audiometric thresholds.

The **loudness normalization rationale** suggests that aided loudness perception should be the same as the loudness perception of listeners with normal hearing. Without amplification, a listener with bilateral, moderate sensorineural hearing loss might rate soft sounds as inaudible, average sounds as "soft," and loud sounds as "loud." Thus, the goal of a loudness normalization prescription would be to prescribe gain such that, with hearing aids, listeners with

hearing loss would rate soft sounds as "soft," average sounds as "average," and loud sounds as "loud" and these ratings would be similar to those from listeners with normal hearing. To accomplish loudness normalization, a prescription needs to be based on loudness perception for listeners with normal hearing, which has been well documented.[1] Much like the MCL level-based prescriptions, loudness normalization prescriptions base prescriptive targets on a patient's measured loudness perception ratings across a variety of signals and levels or base the prescription on predicted loudness perception based on available scientific evidence. Most loudness normalization methods do not consider the relative importance of specific frequencies to speech recognition. As a result, loudness perception could be normal, but speech understanding is not optimized because some important speech sounds could be inaudible.

Conversely, the **loudness equalization rationale** suggests that aided loudness perception should be equal across a broad range of frequencies, even if the result is perceived loudness that is different than would be expected for someone with normal hearing. For listeners with normal hearing, loudness of low frequencies tends to dominate loudness perception of a signal. However, the middle- and high-frequencies contain important information. By making the low and the high frequencies equally loud, we can improve audibility of high-frequency sounds, while preventing a specific-frequency region from dominating loudness perception. If a particular frequency region was too loud for a patient, the patient would likely say "this is too loud," rather than "signals from 1,000 to 1,500 Hz are too loud." The result of such a complaint would likely be a reduction in overall level, either at the hands of a clinician or at the fingertips of a patient with a volume control wheel. Unfortunately, overall gain reduction in this case would have been too aggressive, since only a specific frequency region was too loud. By reducing the overall gain when only some frequencies were too loud, we could have made other frequencies inaudible, possibly negatively impacting speech intelligibility. Therefore, by equalizing loudness across frequencies, the rational suggests we may be able to maximize audibility and comfort by ensuring that all frequencies contribute equally to loudness perception, even if the resulting perception of loudness is not "normal."

9.2.2 Prescription Input

Prescriptions also vary based on whether they calculate gain based on a patient's measured hearing threshold, measured growth of loudness, or a combination. Formulae that base the prescription on hearing thresholds predict a patient's growth of loudness. Conversely, some prescriptive methods suggest measuring not only a patient's hearing threshold, but also other points on the loudness scale, such as the MCL level or the loudness discomfort level. Some prescriptions offer the option to base a prescriptive target for a patient on either the patient's threshold or a combination of hearing threshold and other loudness data. Basing targets on threshold alone is quicker clinically, because only the audiogram is used. In addition, loudness can be predicted, to some extent, based on thresholds. However, knowledge about an individual patient's actual loudness perception could lead to a better, more accurate fitting, particularly if it ensures the hearing aid stays below a patient's loudness discomfort level.

9.2.3 Linearity

Prescriptions can recommend gain that is independent of input level (**linear prescription**) or gain that varies based on input level (**nonlinear prescription**). Reflective of the technology available at the time, the early prescriptions were all linear because hearing aids were not equipped to provide level-dependent gain. In contrast, nearly all modern hearing aids are capable of providing level-dependent gain via **amplitude compression**. As a result, most modern prescriptions are nonlinear.

▶ **Fig. 9.2** illustrates hypothetical hearing aid output as a function of input (also known as an "**input/output curve**") for linear and nonlinear prescriptions in one frequency channel. In this figure, the hearing aids have similar outputs for a moderate input (65 dB SPL). Both hypothetical hearing aids are providing 20 dB of gain (85 dB SPL output for a 65 dB SPL input). Both hearing aids also include output limiting; regardless of input level, neither hearing aid allows an output response of greater than 110 dB SPL. However, the two hearing aids differ from each other for input levels above and below a moderate input level. Regardless of input level (below about 95 dB SPL where output limiting is active), the linear hearing aid always provides 20 dB of gain. A 10 dB change in input always leads to a 10 dB change in output.

Conversely, the nonlinear hearing aid provides 20 dB of gain for a 65 dB SPL input but, relative to the linear hearing aid, provides less gain for loud sounds and more gain for soft sounds. As a result, a 10 dB change in input results in only a 5 dB change in output. For example, when the input changes from 80 to 100 dB SPL, the output changes from 91 to 101 dB SPL. This is a 2:1 compression ratio. As the compression ratio increases, the difference between

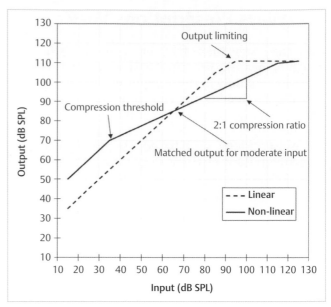

Fig. 9.2 Hearing aid output (dB SPL) as a function of input (dB SPL) for two hypothetical hearing aids, a linear one (*dashed line*) and a nonlinear one (*solid line*). Also indicated are compression thresholds, compression kneepoints, and compression ratios.

a linear and nonlinear hearing aid also increases, providing even more gain for soft sounds and even less gain for loud sounds. In ▶ **Fig. 9.2**, increases in compression ratios would lead to a flattening out of the input/output function; the input/output curve of the nonlinear hearing aid becomes increasingly more horizontal as the compression ratio increases.

▶ **Fig. 9.2** also demonstrates that the nonlinear hearing aid has a 2:1 compression ratio across a wide range of inputs, but not across all inputs. For inputs less than 35 dB SPL, or outputs less than 70 dB SPL, the hearing aid is linear. We call this threshold the **compression threshold** or the **compression kneepoint;** it is the threshold of activation for compression, below which the hearing aid is linear. Above inputs of 115 dB SPL, or outputs greater than 110 dB SPL, the compression ratio is much higher, approximately 10:1. This is called **output limiting** or **compression limiting** and it is implemented to ensure that the patient is not exposed to very loud sounds through the hearing aid. Of course venting and slit leaks will affect the extent to which the patient is actually exposed to loud sounds.

In general, we call this kind of nonlinear compression **wide dynamic range compression** or **low-threshold amplitude compression** because it is active across a broad range of levels. ▶ **Fig. 9.2** displays the input/output curve for a single-frequency channel. To fully describe the response of a nonlinear hearing aid, an input/output curve would need to be created for each frequency channel.

9.2.4 Bilateral Consideration

Prescriptive methods also vary in how they handle bilateral fittings. We know that when a signal is presented to both ears, it is perceived as louder than if the same signal is presented to only one ear, a phenomenon called **binaural loudness summation.**[2] As a result, some prescriptive methods suggest reducing hearing aid gain for bilateral fittings. The degree to which prescriptions adjust gain for bilateral fittings varies due in part to the era the method was established (many early fittings were unilateral) and also due in part to the variable estimates of binaural loudness summation. Bilateral summation for listeners with hearing loss is generally reported to be 3 to 7 dB but is influenced by a number of factors including presence of hearing loss, stimulus bandwidth, and stimulus frequency.[3,4] Many of the earliest fitting methods always assumed a unilateral fitting, while many modern prescriptions generally account for bilateral fittings with a 2 to 6 dB reduction in prescribed gain (►**Table 9.1**).

9.2.5 Type of Gain

Use gain versus full-on gain. Historically, most hearing aids had volume controls. As a result, prescriptions needed to prescribe gain for the volume control setting that was most likely to be used routinely (also known as "**use gain**") and gain for when the volume control setting was at its highest point (also known as "**full-on gain**"). The difference between use gain and full-on gain is "**reserve gain,**" or how much headroom the hearing aid has for additional gain when in a user's setting. Many methods will prescribe use or full-on gain, and corrections are necessary to convert to the other by taking into consideration reserve gain. Generally, the reserve gain is about 10 dB; in other words, a formula that provides values in use gain would have 10 dB added to achieve the prescription for full-on gain.

Insertion gain versus coupler gain. Insertion gain is the amount of gain provided by the hearing aid, as measured in the ear. It usually takes into consideration the input signal and also the natural resonances of the ear canal. **Coupler gain** is the gain measured in a coupler designed for measuring hearing aid responses (usually a 2-cc coupler) and requires a correction factor applied to estimate gain in the ear. Whether a method prescribes insertion or coupler gain would likely be related to the verification procedures recommended by the particular method. If a method focused on selecting an appropriate hearing aid and associated frequency response, the gain values might only be expressed in 2-cc coupler gain, as hearing aid selections were historically based

Table 9.1 Comparison of current prescriptive methods popular in the United States, NAL-NL2 and DSL v 5.0 on how they handle some prescriptive target parameters.

Parameter	NAL-NL2	DSL v 5.0
Experience	Level-specific adjustments for previous hearing aid experience; experienced users are prescribed 10 dB more gain for hearing thresholds greater than 65 dB HL; differences are smaller for milder losses	No adjustment
Gender	1 dB increase in gain for males; 1 dB decrease in gain for females	No adjustment
Bilateral correction	Level-specific adjustments for bilateral fittings; 2 dB for input levels up to 40 dB SPL sloping to 6 dB adjustment for levels greater than 85 dB SPL	3 dB reduction in targets for bilateral fitting (adults only)
Noise	No adjustment	3 to 5 dB reduction of less important speech frequencies for listening in noise
Conductive component	75% of conductive component is added to the prescription for the sensorineural component	25% of the conductive component is added to the upper limit of comfort, resulting in small gain corrections
Loudness discomfort measures	No adjustment	Adjusts prescription based on patient-specific loudness discomfort levels
Adult–child differences	5 dB more gain for children at moderate inputs; higher compression ratio for children than adults	More gain for children; higher compression ratio for children than adults

on the hearing aid specification sheet. A clinician would determine the prescribed gain (and possibly output) and select the hearing aid based on its matrix, which displayed the amplification characteristics in a coupler. Conversely, if a prescriptive method included verification via functional gain testing (or later probe-microphone measures) a method might prescribe insertion gain. Many prescriptions offered both (or did not specify which gain was being prescribed). Converting between coupler gain and insertion gain is relatively easy, but does require knowledge or estimation of the real-ear-to-coupler difference.

Special Considerations: Conductive Components

Generally, this chapter focuses on prescriptions for sensorineural hearing losses. However, not all patients have pure sensorineural losses. Clinicians also fit hearing aids on patients with mixed or even purely conductive hearing losses. Conductive components, quantified as the difference between air conduction and bone conduction thresholds, require special consideration because the nature of the hearing loss is different. Unlike sensorineural hearing loss, conductive hearing losses typically elevate threshold of sensitivity and also loudness discomfort levels. As a result, the residual dynamic range of hearing is relatively unchanged. For example, if Mr. O'Dear had a 20 dB conductive component in addition to his 60 dB sensorineural hearing loss at 1,000 Hz, full restoration would be to add 20 dB of gain to the 30 dB of gain you prescribed for the sensorineural component, using the half-gain rule. However, most prescriptions do not recommend that much gain, in part due to output limitations of the hearing aids.[5] For example, a prescription might suggest providing 50% of the conductive component, or 10 dB for a 20 dB conductive loss. In general, much less research attention has focused on the handling of conductive components and it remains a source of considerable variability across prescriptive methods. Future work is necessary to determine the best method of accounting for conductive components in hearing aid fittings.

9.3   History

As a profession, audiology is relatively young, with its historical roots planted in the rehabilitation for soldiers returning from the First World War. Throughout this brief history, significant attention has been focused on the testing of hearing and also on the

fitting of hearing aids. As a result, the question of identifying the "best" prescription has received considerable commentary and also scientific inquiry. Some history highlights are reviewed here in an effort to place our modern prescriptive approaches into the broader historical context and to provide evidence to support current clinical practice.

9.3.1   Prescriptions Are Born

One of the early prescriptions was from Knudsen and Jones,[6] who prescribed hearing aid gain as the degree of hearing loss minus a constant. This type of prescription has been referred to as an **audiogram mirror** because the targets look exactly like the audiogram, except they shifted by a fixed amount. Although this method might provide reasonable gain for inputs near threshold, higher-level inputs would be too loud as a result of the reduced dynamic range that accompanies sensorineural hearing loss.

Another one of the early recommendations for prescribing gain came from the Harvard Report.[7] In it, Davis and colleagues argued that the same frequency response can be used for nearly all patients and the only consideration needed to be a patient's "tolerance" test to determine maximum hearing aid output. They recommended fitting every patient with the same frequency response and suggested that this **uniform response** could yield better outcomes than individualized or "selective" amplification. The authors acknowledged at the time that the recommendations were unconventional, but maintained that the future of hearing aid prescriptions would be determined by size, weight, or instrument expense, rather than frequency response based on a patient's audiometric characteristics.

Clearly not everyone agreed with the idea that hearing aid gain could be prescribed independent of audiometric thresholds and Davis et al's[7] predictions did not come to fruition. Instead, nearly all other prescriptive methods, since the 1940s until today, have involved the prescription of gain based on an individual patient's hearing characteristics (e.g., pure tone air conduction threshold, loudness discomfort level, growth of loudness, and/or speech recognition performance). For example, Watson and Knudsen[8] recommended **selective amplification** (or gain that varies as a function of frequency based on an individual's hearing abilities) that amplified speech to a patient's MCL level, which involved measurement of both hearing thresholds and MCL level for a 1,000-Hz signal. In their paper, they presented data demonstrating the advantage of this type of amplification over uniform amplification, such as the prescription suggested by Davis et al.[7]

One of the first audiology books, Hearing Tests and Hearing Instruments,[9] included an entire chapter on hearing aid prescriptions. Watson and Tolan argued that compensating for an individual's hearing loss based on the individual's own audiometric traits was critical because an inappropriate frequency response could negatively affect speech production and because poor hearing is tied with depression and feelings of exclusion. As a result, Watson and Tolan remark that "anything less than the maximum possible utilization of an individual's residual hearing capacity is a failure of responsibility,"[9] highlighting the importance of the use of individualized prescriptions to maximize a patient's residual dynamic range and optimize hearing aid outcomes. Their chapter included recommendations for prescribing amplification based on a patient's residual range of hearing, incorporating both hearing thresholds and loudness discomfort levels. They recommended that hearing aid gain be set so that signals are presented 40 dB above threshold.

Another fitting rationale from the early years in audiology was offered by Lybarger.[10,11] At the time, Lybarger was working for a hearing aid manufacturer (RadioEar). His patent applications recommended fitting patients with one-half of their hearing loss. For example, Mr. O'Dear, with a flat 60 dB hearing loss, would have been prescribed 30 dB of gain. The **half-gain rule** was a prescription for use gain; to achieve full-on gain, 10 to 15 dB of reserve gain would be added. Lybarger's formula evolved to be a little more complicated than a straight "half-gain" rule. For frequencies above 1,000 Hz, gain was prescribed to be one-half of the patient's hearing threshold. For 500 Hz, gain was prescribed to be one-third of the patient's hearing threshold. Despite its age, the half-gain rule remains a handy way to estimate prescribed gain without assistance of powerful computers or correction factors.

Although the expressed rationales underlying Watson and Knudsen[8] and Lybarger[11] are different, amplifying speech to MCL and half-gain rule, respectively, the resultant prescriptions are relatively similar. For most patients, we would expect the MCL to be approximately half-way between the hearing thresholds and loudness discomfort levels. However, some consideration needs to be made for the long-term average frequency response of speech, which is more intense in the low frequencies than the high frequencies. As a result, prescriptions need to be modified to account for this frequency spectrum; most do it by reducing low-frequency gain.

Pitfalls: Comparing Across Prescriptions ✕

Be wary of direct comparisons between prescriptive methods, especially the early prescriptive methods, if you do not take into account the type of gain prescribed. If you find some formulae in the early manuscripts describing gain prescriptions and do not consider whether the prescription is for use gain or full gain and whether it is for insertion gain or coupler gain, you could make comparison errors as large as 30 dB! For example, if Prescription A provides a formula for use, insertion gain and Prescription B provides a formula for full-on, coupler gain, the formula may start off being 30 dB different even before you consider how much gain is prescribed (10 dB of reserve gain and 20 dB real-ear-to-coupler difference at some frequencies).

9.3.2 Comparative Testing

The preceding review of prescriptive methods in the early years of audiology is not comprehensive, but does highlight some of the issues relevant to clinicians at the time. Should gain be personalized or uniform across all patients? Should gain be prescribed based on audiometric threshold or should we try to amplify speech so that it reaches a patient's MCL level? Around the same time, Captain Raymond Carhart introduced a fitting method that, at first glance, appeared to be quite different from the other prescriptive fitting methods. Carhart[12] outlined the extensive 12-step program for the selection and provision of hearing aids. Instead of explicitly prescribing gain, Carhart's program advocated for his comprehensive testing program that has been called "**comparative testing**." The general idea behind comparative testing is to select some hearing aids (or hearing aid frequency responses) that are potentially appropriate for a patient and then test the patient with each response, ultimately prescribing the hearing aid that resulted in the best performance or had the highest user preference.

Carhart's comprehensive procedure included 12 steps divided into four phases. The first phase (steps 1 through 5) included an exploration of the patient's needs with diagnostics, an interview, and earmold impressions. In the second phase, unsuitable hearing aids were eliminated through interviews between the patient and clinician; typically 7 to 10 hearing aids were identified for further testing. In the third phase, a patient would wear one of the hearing aids for 24 hours, testing the hearing aid in typical listening situations. At the end of the use trial, the patient wore the hearing aid in the clinic while listening to a range of environmental sounds and also speech. During the fourth, and final, stage, three hearing aids were selected and a patient's performance in each was evaluated on tasks of speech recognition and listening comfort. After all the testing with each hearing aid has been accomplished, a hearing aid was selected based on all of the test results.

9.3.3 Resurgence of Prescriptions

Carhart's comparative testing protocol dominated hearing aid selection for several decades. However, around the mid-1970s to early 1980s, several factors converged to reshape the hearing aid prescriptive method landscape. First, the implementation of the Carhart method evolved away from weeklong comprehensive testing over the course of weeks to only 1 or 2 hours of comparative testing. To achieve shorter testing times, procedures often included comparative testing with only a single word list of speech in quiet instead of the recommended comprehensive 12-step program. These shortened versions of testing were minimally effective.[13]

In addition, around this time audiologists' roles were changing. Before 1971, the American Speech-Language Hearing Association (ASHA) deemed that it was unethical for audiologists to sell hearing aids. By 1979, ASHA's scope of practice and ethical guidelines had changed to include hearing aid dispensing and sales.[14] As a result, audiologists sought ways to expedite hearing aid fittings, leaning toward prescriptive approaches and away from the lengthy, comprehensive comparative testing procedures.

Finally, around this time, custom hearing aids were becoming popular, taking market share away from behind-the-ear instruments.[14] When you have access to a hearing aid library of 200 stock hearing aids, as Carhart did,[12] comparative testing is time consuming but feasible. When you need to make 7 to 10 custom hearing aids (or sets of hearing aids in a bilateral fitting), comparative testing might be prohibitively expensive for clinicians and manufacturers.

As a result of this convergence of factors, the late 1970s and early 1980s saw a resurgence of prescriptions. Below is a list of just some of the influential prescriptions of the time.

- **Pascoe's method**: Pascoe[15] aimed to amplify average speech to the MCL level. For his dissertation, he tested eight participants with mild-to-moderate sensorineural hearing loss with six different hearing aid responses and found the one whose gain amplified average speech to a patient's MCL level provided the best word discrimination performance (18.4% better than the second best frequency response). Although, the data

set was limited to a few participants with a relatively homogenous hearing loss, many later prescriptions were based on Pascoe's loudness data.

- **Berger's method**: Berger[16,17] recommended prescription of frequency-specific gain and also hearing aid maximum output for hearing aids. Relative to a half-gain rule, the Berger method prescribes more hearing aid gain, especially for 1,500 and 2,000 Hz (▶Fig. 9.3). The Berger method includes corrections for bilateral fittings (3 dB correction), hearing aid style, and conductive hearing loss (one-fifth of conductive component). In addition, Berger recommended verification with functional gain testing.

- **Prescription of gain and output (POGO)**[18]: POGO provided prescriptive insertion gain targets and these values were quite similar to the Lybarger half-gain rule. Specifically, prescribed insertion gain was one-half of the hearing loss at a given frequency, with a 10 and 5 dB subtraction for 250 and 500 Hz, respectively. The low cut was introduced to limit the effects of low-frequency ambient noise, but it also is consistent with altering gain based on the long-term average spectrum of average speech. In addition, POGO provided specific recommendations for maximum output, which should never exceed a patient's uncomfortable listening level. POGO became popular clinically because it was easy to implement.

- **POGO II**[19]: POGO was revised in 1988 to include prescriptions for patients with severe hearing loss. For hearing losses greater than

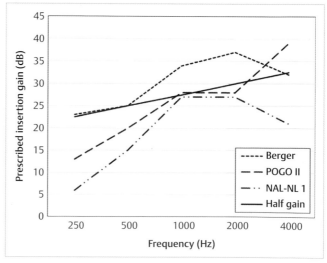

Fig. 9.3 Calculated insertion gain for Berger, POGO II, NAL-NL1, and half-gain rule as a function of frequency for Mr. O'Dear's audiometric thresholds (relatively flat loss). Prescription assumes a moderate, speech-shaped input signal.

65 dB, POGO II prescribed an additional half gain of the difference between the threshold and 65 dB HL. For example, at 1,000 Hz, for a patient with a threshold of 80 dB HL, the POGO II prescribed gain would be 47.5 dB (½ of 80 dB + ½ of 15 dB). The modifications were necessary because, in cases of severe and profound losses, the MCL level increases and this additional gain is necessary to amplify speech to the elevated MCL level.

- **Libby**[20]: The Libby **insertion gain prescription** was similar to the Lybarger half-gain rule, except it was modified based on a patient's degree of hearing loss. Patients with mild-to-moderate loss were prescribed a one-third gain, whereas patients with moderate-to-severe hearing loss were prescribed a one-half gain. Patients with severe hearing loss were prescribed a two-thirds gain. These recommendations were based on Libby's beliefs that listeners with less hearing loss preferred less gain, whereas patients with more hearing loss needed more gain. Libby's prescription included a correction for bilateral fittings (3 dB) and conductive components (one-fourth of the conductive component).

- **Cambridge formula**[21]: The Cambridge formula was developed to equalize loudness of a moderate input across 500 to 4,000 Hz. The Cambridge formula is approximately similar to half gain, with a low-cut modification. For listeners with mild-to-moderate losses, the Cambridge frequency response has been shown to be effective.[22]

9.3.4 Early Nonlinear Years

The advancement of digital technologies propelled the proliferation of prescriptive fitting methods. The effects of digitalization and miniaturization influenced prescriptive fittings on two fronts, verification systems and hearing aids. First, probe microphone verification systems became readily available. These systems are capable of calculating prescriptive targets, displaying the targets on a screen, and displaying the level of sound in a patient's ear canal (or calculating insertion gain) using probe tubes combined with small microphones. The advancement of these systems made it possible to precisely measure a hearing aid's performance and accurately adjust its response to match the prescribed target.

Second, hearing aids themselves became far more flexible with the introduction of digitally programmable hearing aids in the late 1990s. With

nonprogrammable hearing aids, clinicians had a limited range of possible frequency responses and gain levels they could achieve. Their options for changing the frequency response were limited to plumbing modifications (e.g., vents, dampers, and horns) or to analog potentiometers. Fine-tuning instruments to meet precise prescriptive targets was not always possible. However, by 2001, more than half of instruments dispensed were digitally programmable.[23] Today, it would be rare to find a hearing aid that was not programmable, with many channels, and seemingly infinite flexibility to shape the frequency response for multiple input levels. As a result, prescriptive targets can be more individualized and more refined. This is reflected in the increased complexity of the formulae for modern prescriptive fitting methods.

Also around this time, gain targets could vary as a function of input level. The preceding discussion included only prescriptive methods that were linear. However, in the 1990s with programmable instruments and advances in hearing aid technologies, nonlinear fittings were possible and increasingly common. Many of the early nonlinear prescriptions were based on the principle of loudness normalization. For example, one of the first nonlinear prescriptions was the **loudness growth in half-octave bands (LGOB) procedure**.[24] The LGOB procedure required patients to categorize narrow-band noise using a seven-category loudness scale, ranging from 1 (not audible) to 7 (too loud). Gain was prescribed so that the patient with hearing loss achieved similar loudness perception as a listener with normal hearing. Other examples of early nonlinear prescriptions include the **Ricketts and Bentler (RAB) method**[25] and the **FIG 6 strategy**.[26] The RAB method started with the NAL-R prescription for average inputs and then modified the prescription to be nonlinear based on a patient's measured growth of loudness. In contrast, the FIG 6 strategy prescribed hearing aid gain that would restore loudness perception based on average loudness growth data, rather than requiring measurement of loudness growth from a patient.

The Cambridge formula has also been modified to accommodate nonlinear hearing aids. The current version of the Cambridge formula, whose aim is still loudness equalization for 500 to 4,000 Hz, is known as **Cambridge loudness equalization with high frequencies (CAMEQ2-HF)**.[27] CAMEQ2-HF, sometimes called CAM2, also includes recommendations for gain for 6,000 to 10,000 Hz. Specifically, CAM2 recommends these high-frequency signals be amplified to a patient's thresholds at these frequencies, unless the result is greater than normal loudness perception.

9.4 Modern Prescriptions

Now let's turn our attention to current prescriptive methods. In the United States, probably the two most commonly implemented prescriptions come from the National Acoustics Laboratory (NAL) and the University of Western Ontario (UWO). Each of these organizations has a long history of publishing and validating prescriptive methods. Perhaps because of the large body of evidence supporting the prescriptions from both organizations, they have been some of the only survivors in the modern era of prescriptive fitting methods. Prescriptions from each of the organizations will be discussed in turn, rather than chronologically, since each iteration from an organization is founded largely on a similar set of guiding principles.

9.4.1 National Acoustics Laboratory

The researchers from the Australian NAL have guided and influenced hearing aid selection and fittings for decades. Although the prescriptions have evolved over the years based on empirical evidence, they have not wavered in their fundamental philosophy, which is of loudness equalization. The goal of the NAL prescriptions continues to be to maximize speech intelligibility, while maintaining loudness comfort. The original NAL method prescribed 4.6 dB of gain for every 10 dB of hearing loss, but with corrections for the spectral shape of speech and for 2-cc coupler gain.[28]

The revised version of the NAL method, called **NAL-R**,[29] modified the original NAL procedure by accounting for audiogram slope. Steeper slopes necessitated steeper hearing aid frequency responses. Byrne and Cotton[30] provided validation for the NAL-R prescription by comparing the NAL-R prescription to responses with various low- and high-frequency slopes. The authors evaluated participants' preferred gain, judgements of speech intelligibility in quiet, and pleasantness of speech in noise. On average, the results suggested that the NAL-R prescription was better than the alternatives. The NAL method was again revised to incorporate considerations for listeners with severe-to-profound hearing losses; the result was **NAL-Revised Profound (NAL-RP)**.[31] In NAL-RP, additional gain was prescribed if the hearing threshold was greater than 60 dB. In addition, a correction was applied for hearing losses greater than 90 dB HL at 2,000 Hz.

The next modification of the NAL formula incorporated level-dependent gain prescriptions and was called **National Acoustics Laboratories–nonlinear 1 (NAL-NL1)**.[32] Like its predecessors, the goal of NAL-NL1 was to maintain comfort by not exceeding normal loudness perception and to maximize speech intelligibility. For moderate input levels, NAL-RP and NAL-NL1

are very similar; the differences emerge in prescription for soft and loud inputs, where NAL-NL1 prescribes more and less gain, respectively. NAL-NL1 was incorporated into most hearing aid software and probe-microphone equipment, which made it easily accessible and consequently very popular for clinic and research.

The current NAL prescription is **NAL-nonlinear 2 (NAL-NL2)**.[33] Consistent with its predecessors, NAL-NL2 focuses on optimizing speech intelligibility and loudness comfort through loudness equalization. However, the prescription was modified based on data suggesting that the NAL-NL1 prescription was too loud for some patients. Harvey Dillon, a leading researcher at NAL, analyzed the results from several studies and found that NAL-NL1 was "just right" for about 49% of patients and "too loud" for 46% of them.[34] Therefore, NAL-NL2 targets were reduced overall. Other adjustments included in NAL-NL2 were less gain for new users, higher compression ratios, less gain for bilateral fittings, and still higher compression ratios for children.

9.4.2 University of Western Ontario

The researchers from the University of Western Ontario have also been guiding and influencing hearing aid selection and fittings for decades. The first prescription from this organization was called the **desired sensation level (DSL)**.[35] DSL was founded on the principles that infants and young children require specialized amplification considerations. Most notably, speech needs to be amplified to a certain sensation level to maximize intelligibility.[36] As a result, the guiding principle of DSL is to maximize the audibility of speech cues, while maintaining comfort. In general, DSL has traditionally been referred to as a loudness normalization procedure. Although the formulae have evolved over the decades since the first version, the foundations of the DSL prescriptions have been consistent. In addition, throughout the evolution, DSL has been consistent in its emphasis on consideration of infants and young children by providing corrections for individual real-ear-to-coupler differences, diagnostic transducers, diagnostic testing methods (auditory brainstem responses vs. behavioral testing), and maximum hearing aid outputs.

The first nonlinear version of DSL was called the **DSL input/output formula (DSL [i/o])**[37] and has been implemented since DSL v4.0.[36] The nonlinear version of DSL shared many similarities with the previous version of DSL, but included prescriptions for nonlinear parameters (compression threshold, compression ratio). The DSL (i/o) procedure was validated by several studies that indicate that patients prefer the DSL targets to other prescriptive alternatives.[38]

The current version of DSL, the **DSL multistage input/output (DSL m[i/])**[39] is implemented in DSL v5.0. This version includes a family of targets that vary as a function of age. That is, targets for children and adults are different, in part because children prefer higher gain than adults and also because higher sensation levels are important for language development.[39] Relative to the previous versions of DSL, there were several important changes implemented in DSL v5.0, as summarized by Scollie.[40] First, DSL v 5.0 prescribes lower targets than previous versions, especially for high-level inputs or severe losses. The purpose of this change was to ensure that the peaks of speech stay below a patient's upper limit of comfort. Second, DSL v 5.0 provides specific targets for noisy situations based on evidence that the frequency-importance function of speech changes in noise. Third, DSL v 5.0 includes a bilateral correction that lowers targets by 3 dB. Fourth, gain for low-input sounds has been reduced.

Finally, the current DSL prescription includes age and etiology corrections, rather than only the birth date. There are separate prescriptions for children with presumed congenital hearing losses, for adults with presumed acquired hearing losses, and for adults with presumed congenital hearing loss. As a result, an adult with congenital hearing loss would be fit with DSL targets that are more similar to those of children, whereas an adult with acquired hearing loss would be prescribed lower targets, as language acquisition is not a consideration for this type of hearing loss. This distinction is outlined further below in the Case Studies section of this chapter.

Special Consideration: The Cambridge Formulae

Although this chapter has largely focused on the prescriptions from the National Acoustics Laboratory and the University of Western Ontario, the work of Brian Moore and his colleagues at Cambridge University warrants further consideration. Much like the histories of both NAL and DSL, Moore and his colleagues established a linear Cambridge formula and later published several modifications, including nonlinear versions which seek to equalize loudness (CamEQ)[41] or to normalize loudness (CamREST).[42] CamEQ and CamREST are based on similar principles as NAL and DSL, respectively. Although there is considerable research and validation into the Cambridge formulae, they have not reached the clinical popularity of those proffered by NAL and UWO. However, there is some evidence to suggest that CamEQ may be preferred by patients relative to other modern popular prescriptive methods, at least in laboratory settings.[43,44]

9.4.3 Comparison of Current Procedures

Now that we have reviewed some generalities of each of the modern prescriptions, let's compare the two side-by-side. As is evident in ►**Table 9.1**, the prescriptions are more similar than they are different. Few studies have directly compared the latest versions of NAL and DSL, but there are some published model-based comparisons for adults and children. Each will be considered separately.

Adults: In a recent paper, Johnson and Dillon[45] calculated prescribed gain for a variety of example audiograms, capturing a range of hearing loss configurations, which were sensorineural, conductive, or mixed in origin. In addition to calculated gain, Johnson and Dillon modeled perceived loudness and predicted speech recognition with each prescription by using existing models of loudness perception and speech intelligibility. Although they did not include participants, they completed comprehensive predictions of performance based on well-established models. For sensorineural hearing losses, their results suggested that, despite differences across prescriptive targets, NAL-NL2 and DSL v5.0 resulted in similar predicted loudness perception but less overall perceived loudness than NAL-NL1 and CAM2, and also less than "normal" for the same signals. The differences between the most recent versions of NAL and DSL also did not affect predicted speech intelligibility in quiet or in noise. The results of this study suggest that if the models used are an accurate reflection of patient performance, NAL-NL2 and DSL v5.0 would result in similar perceived loudness and speech intelligibility for moderate-level speech for most patients with sensorineural hearing loss.

For predominately conductive losses, the differences between NAL-NL2 and DSL v 5.0 become more apparent. DSL prescribes significantly less gain to compensate for conductive components (►**Table 9.1**). Thus, it is not surprising that Johnson and Dillon found lower predicted overall loudness for conductive losses using DSL v 5.0 than either NAL-NL1 or NAL-NL2. All three of those prescriptions resulted in less predicted overall loudness than "normal." Despite large differences in prescriptive targets and predicted loudness for these three methods, Johnson and Dillon found no differences in predicted speech intelligibility for moderate-level speech, either in quiet or in noise, for the conductive or mixed losses.

Children: Because of the historical focus on children, we might expect differences between NAL and DSL to be larger when we consider the pediatric population. Indeed, Teresa Ching and her colleagues (who included Johnson and Dillon) also modeled predicted loudness and speech intelligibility, this time for a pediatric population.[46] Based on 200 pediatric patients, Ching et al made model-based predictions of loudness and speech intelligibility based on real audiograms and real-ear–aided responses. Their results suggest that the comparison between predicted perception with NAL and DSL are level dependent. For moderate-level inputs (e.g., average speech), Ching et al found that NAL and DSL resulted in similar speech intelligibility, but fittings with DSL were expected to be perceived as twice as loud as fittings with NAL. For high-level inputs (e.g., shouted speech), DSL fittings resulted in higher predicted loudness and poorer predicted speech intelligibility. For low-level inputs (e.g., whispered speech), DSL fittings resulted in better predicted speech intelligibility than NAL.

In addition to predicted loudness and speech intelligibility, Ching and her colleagues also studied the effect of the choice of prescriptive method on pediatric outcomes at 3 years of age. They randomly assigned infants and small children to be fit with either NAL-NL1 or DSL v4.0 and evaluated their language, speech production, and functional performance, in addition to parental reports of hearing aid use and loudness discomfort. The results revealed no effect of hearing aid prescription on any of the outcomes. Instead, factors such as additional disability and maternal education level were more likely to affect outcomes than choice of prescriptive targets. It is unclear how these results would be different with the latest version of NAL (NAL-NL2) or with older children whose auditory demands might be quite different from those of infants.

9.5 Case Studies

To put these differences into practice, let's take a look at some case studies. These cases are not actual patients; any resemblance to a real patient is coincidence.

9.5.1 Case Study 1: Glenn O'Dear

We briefly met Mr. O'Dear at the beginning of this chapter. He has bilateral, flat, moderate sensorineural hearing loss (▶Fig. 9.1). The hearing loss etiology is unknown, although he has a maternal family history of acquired hearing loss. ▶Fig. 9.3 displays calculated prescriptive insertion gain for Mr. O'Dear for several of the prescriptive targets mentioned in this chapter. As you can see, the prescriptions vary dramatically. The Berger method prescribes the most gain, whereas NAL-NL1 provides the least. Most of the prescriptions provide similar gain values for the middle frequencies (1,000–2,000 Hz). All prescriptions are frequency dependent, with the least gain in the low frequencies. This is the result of a combination of the patient's (very) gently sloping hearing loss and the low-frequency emphasis of natural speech.

Now imagine that you are actually fitting Mr. O'Dear. You enter his thresholds into the probe-microphone verification system available to you in your clinic. In this case, let's assume that is an AudioScan Verifit. You record Mr. O'Dear's hearing aid response in his ear canal and match the response to NAL-NL2 prescriptive targets (for an adult with a bilateral fitting). The results look something like the top left panel of ▶Fig. 9.4, which displays Mr. O'Dear's thresholds (in blue), predicted loudness discomfort levels (black asterisks), and prescriptive targets (green crosses). The hearing aid response (green line) runs through the prescriptive targets 250 to 6,000 Hz, although the hearing aid response is about 2 dB lower than the target at 3,000 Hz and about 5 dB lower than target at 6,000 Hz.

Now imagine using the exact same hearing aid in Mr. O'Dear's left ear and changing the prescriptive targets. The top right panel of ▶Fig. 9.4 demonstrates the effect in the real ear of changing from NAL-NL2 bilateral fitting to a NAL-NL2 unilateral fitting. If Mr. O'Dear was only going to pursue a single hearing aid, NAL-NL2 prescribes slightly more gain. As a result, the hearing aid we fit assuming a bilateral fitting is now 2 to 6 dB lower than targets.

The bottom left panel of ▶Fig. 9.4 displays the same hearing aid response in Mr. O'Dear's ear, but with the DSL v 5.0 instead of the NAL-NL2 targets (both for an adult with bilateral fitting). You can see that the hearing aid matches targets pretty well 2,000 to 4,000 Hz, but is below prescriptive targets slightly at 1,000 Hz and significantly at 250, 500, and 6,000 Hz. Although there are some significant differences displayed in the top left panel of ▶Fig. 9.4, the fitting could be considered a fair approximation to prescriptive target. The choice of adult DSL v 5.0 or NAL-NL2 targets for Glenn would have a relatively small clinical impact during the selection or fitting processes.

9.5.2 Case Study 2: Dahlia O'Dear

Mr. O'Dear returns to your clinic with his 24-month-old daughter, Dahlia. Dahlia has an identical hearing loss to her dad, but her hearing loss is congenital. She has been wearing hearing aids since she was 9 months old. ▶Fig. 9.5 displays Mr. O'Dear's hearing aid response and the NAL-NL2 prescriptive output targets for a bilateral, behind-the-ear fitting for a 24-month-old, as would be appropriate for Dahlia. Mr. Glenn O'Dear's hearing aid response is displayed in ▶Fig. 9.5 to demonstrate the difference between NAL-NL2 prescriptions for adults and children. Recall that the hearing aid approximated bilateral, adult NAL-NL2 prescriptive targets well. However, as you can see in ▶Fig. 9.5, the same hearing aid response

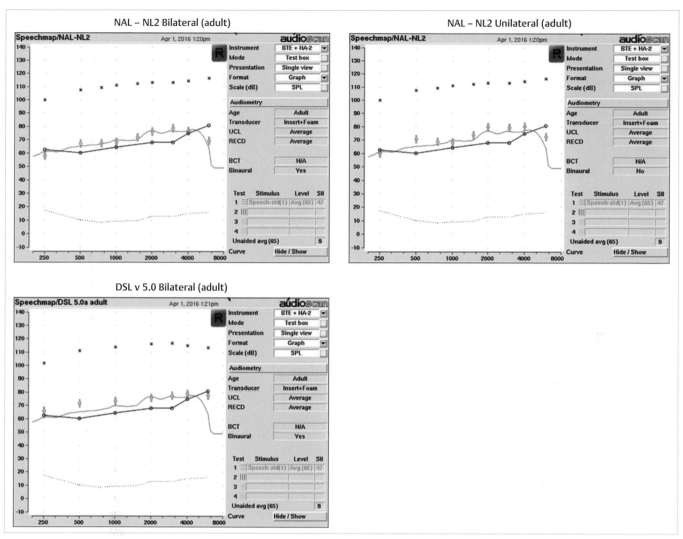

Fig. 9.4 Screen capture images from the AudioScan Verifit displaying match to target when the prescriptive targets are based on the prescriptions from NAL-NL2 (bilateral), NAL-NL2 (unilateral), and DSL v 5.0 (bilateral) in the top left, top right, and bottom left panels, respectively. The hearing aid response is unchanged in all three panels. Prescriptive targets are based on Mr. Glenn O'Dear (48-year-old man).

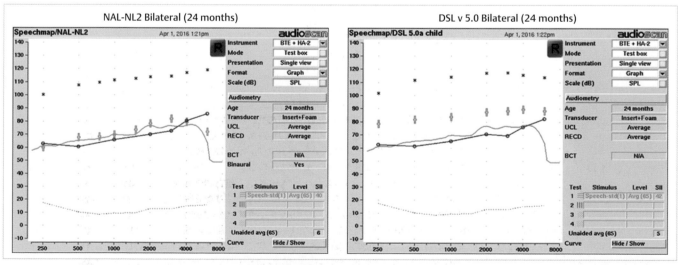

Fig. 9.5 Screen capture images from the AudioScan Verifit displaying match to target when the prescriptive targets are based on the prescriptions from NAL-NL2 (bilateral) and DSL v 5.0 (bilateral) in the left and right panels, respectively. The hearing aid response is unchanged in both panels. Prescriptive targets are based on Dahlia O'Dear (24-month-old girl).

that matches adult targets well, is under the pediatric prescriptive target for many frequencies, especially 3,000 to 6,000 Hz.

However, the largest differences between the adult and child targets are evident in the right panel of ►**Fig. 9.5**. This figure displays the same hearing aid response, but with DSL v 5.0 prescriptive targets for a 24-month-old with a bilateral fitting. If you decided to fit with this version of DSL, the hearing aid would not be appropriate for Dahlia. The hearing aid is 10 to 30 dB under prescriptive targets from 250 to 6,000 Hz. This striking difference in the match to target in the left and right panels underscores the underlying difference in prescriptive rationales. Recall DSL was specifically developed for children with the intent of maximizing audibility in order to optimize language development. Conversely, NAL was developed to maximize speech intelligibility while maintaining comfort.

9.5.3 Case Study 3: Gavin O'Dear

Mr. O'Dear also brought his 48-month-old son, Gavin, to your clinic. Gavin also has congenital hearing loss and has been wearing hearing aids since he was 12 months old. However, Gavin's hearing loss looks different than that of his father and sister. Gavin has a bilateral, mild sloping to severe sensorineural

hearing loss (►**Fig. 9.6**). ►**Fig. 9.7** displays calculated insertion gain values for several of the historical prescriptions described, as well as NAL-NL1. Much like the flat loss (►**Fig. 9.3**), the insertion gains for the various prescriptions are similar to each other for the middle frequencies (1,000–2,000 Hz), except for the Berger procedure, which prescribes significantly more gain than the other prescriptions. Also note the steep slope of prescribed insertion gain. Although Berger and a pure half-gain rule prescribe 10 dB of gain for 250 to 500 Hz, the others prescribe very little low-frequency gain.

►**Fig. 9.8** displays images of the AudioScan Verifit with the same hearing aid response relative to NAL-NL2 or DSL v 5.0 prescriptive targets in the left and right panels, respectively. In the left panel, you can see that the hearing aid matches prescriptive targets relatively well. It is a few decibels over target 750 to 2,000 Hz and 20 dB under target at 6,000 Hz, but otherwise close to the NAL-NL2 prescription. Conversely, the right panel displays that this hearing aid would be 15 to 20 dB under target if DSL prescriptions were used. Similar to the findings for those reported for Dahlia O'Dear (►**Fig. 9.5**), these results likely reflect the difference in prescriptive rationale. Clinically, for children, the decision to use DSL or NAL prescriptions will likely have a big impact on hearing aid selection and on how much gain you program into the hearing aid(s).

9.5.4 Case Study 4: Eugene O'Dear

Finally, during Mr. O'Dear's initial appointment, he mentioned his father, Eugene (76 years old), has hearing loss. Glenn O'Dear was so impressed with

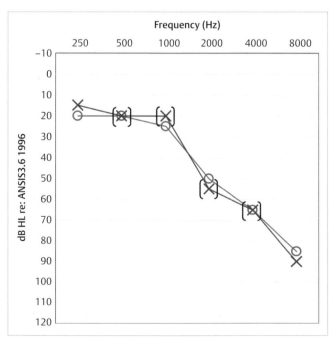

Fig. 9.6 Pure tone, air-conduction audiometric thresholds for a hypothetical patient (Gavin O'Dear) as a function of frequency for left and right ears (*blue* and *right lines*, respectively). Figure also displays bone-conduction audiometric thresholds for the patient for the left and right ears (*left* and *right facing brackets*, respectively).

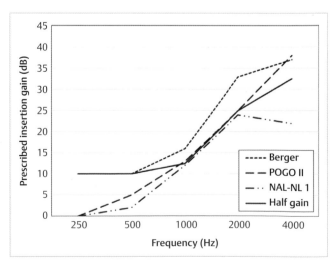

Fig. 9.7 Calculated insertion gain for Berger, POGO II, NAL-NL1, and half-gain rule as a function of frequency for Dahlia O'Dear's audiometric thresholds (sloping loss). Prescription assumes a moderate, speech-shaped input signal.

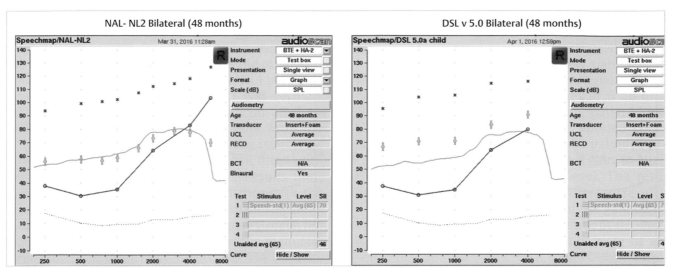

Fig. 9.8   Screen capture images from the AudioScan Verifit displaying match to target when the prescriptive targets are based on the prescriptions from NAL-NL2 (bilateral) and DSL v 5.0 (bilateral) in the left and right panels, respectively. The hearing aid response is unchanged in both panels. Prescriptive targets are based on Gavin O'Dear (48-month-old boy).

your clinical service, including your knowledge of prescriptive methods, that he convinces his father to become your patient as well. The elder O'Dear has acquired hearing loss, consistent with his history of noise exposure in the military. His hearing loss, despite the etiology, manifests itself as the same audiogram as his grandson (▶ **Fig. 9.6**). You proceed with a selection and decide to fit him with behind-the-ear hearing aids. ▶ **Fig. 9.9** displays the match to target with the same hearing aid response for NAL-NL2 (aged adult), DSL v 5.0 (adult, aged adult), and DSL v 5.0 (child, aged adult). First, let's focus on the top panels. In both cases, the hearing aid matches targets relatively well, although the hearing aid is a little over target 750 to 2,000 Hz and under target at 6,000 Hz (and under at 4,000 Hz for DSL). These top panels reflect patients whose hearing loss is assumed to be acquired. NAL doesn't differentiate between acquired and congenital losses, but by selecting DSL adult and inputting the age as "adult," DSL's targets, as implemented by the AudioScan Verifit, are appropriate for acquired hearing losses. In this case, the targets are quite similar between NAL and DSL. Conversely, if the "child" option is selected for DSL, but the age "adult" is selected, the targets are adjusted to reflect a presumed congenital, or perhaps prelingual, hearing loss. ▶ **Fig. 9.9** demonstrates that the hearing aid response that was appropriate for an acquired hearing loss would be undertarget for a congenital loss, according to the DSL prescriptions. For Eugene, a clinician would likely select NAL-NL2 or DSL adult, since his hearing loss was

acquired. However, significantly more gain would be prescribed if his loss was congenital.

> ### Pearl: How Much Gain Does My Patient Need?   ✔
>
> At the beginning of the chapter, we asked: "How much gain should we prescribe?" Although the precise answer to this question is complicated and depends on a variety of factors, it can be useful to be able to estimate required gain without the help of sophisticated computers or verification systems. For most adults with sensorineural hearing loss in the United States, the quick answer to the question is probably somewhere between one-third and one-half the patient's threshold at 2,000 Hz. This estimate will likely capture the highest amount of gain necessary for the patient across frequencies (▶ **Fig. 9.3** and ▶ **Fig. 9.7**).

9.6 The Methods of Prescriptive Fitting

The preceding discussion focused almost exclusively on prescribing hearing aid gain. However, the prescriptive targets are only a component of a prescriptive fitting method. These gain values need to be selected and programmed into the hearing aid, and the actual hearing aid response needs to be verified. In addition, the prescribed values reflect an appropriate starting place for selecting gain. There are many factors that influence the amount of gain a patient ultimately uses.

Special Consideration: Testing Dead Regions

Identifying dead regions based on audiometric information alone can be problematic. You might expect that a patient with a dead region at a particular frequency would have no response at the limits of the audiometer for that particular frequency. However, we know that at high presentation levels, the cochlea loses its fine tuning and more frequency regions start to respond. As a result, clinically a patient with a dead region at a particular frequency region may have measurable hearing at that frequency because the neighboring inner hair cells are responding. Thus, patients with measurable hearing on an audiogram may still have a dead region. To measure the presence of dead regions clinically, Brian Moore and his colleagues introduced the **threshold-equalizing noise (TEN) test**.[60] Although the original TEN test required threshold measurement twice, the more recent version, the TEN(HL) test[61] has simplified the process. Using the TEN(HL) test, the measurement of potential dead regions can be accomplished relatively quick and easy within a clinic appointment (typically during the diagnostic or prefitting stages).

audibility through 285 Hz (0.57 × 500 = 285). For high-frequency dead regions, the recommendation for hearing aid gain is improve audibility up to 1.7 times the beginning edge of the dead region.[62] Consider Eugene O'Dear (▶ **Fig. 9.6**). If you tested him and found a dead region at 4,000 Hz, you would only provide hearing aid gain through 6,800 Hz (1.7 × 4000 = 6800). Considering the limitations of current hearing aids, that is likely as high (or higher) in frequency than you would consider amplifying anyway. However, consider a different patient who has a steeply sloping, sensorineural hearing loss. He has thresholds of 30 and 80 dB HL at 500 and 2,000 Hz, respectively. If you identified dead regions at 2,000 and 4,000 Hz, you would probably not need to amplify above 3,400 Hz (1.7 × 2000 = 3400). The presence of this dead region could cause you to alter your prescription by limiting hearing aid gain above 3,400 Hz. Consistent with this, Vinay and Moore[63] recommend only testing for the presence of dead regions above 3,000 Hz, since the presence of dead regions below 3,000 Hz will not change your hearing aid fitting.

For typical patients, the presence of dead regions might not significantly affect your prescription. Cox et al[64] tested patients with and without dead regions and fit members of each group with hearing aids matched to NAL-NL1 and to NAL-NL1 with a

high-frequency roll-off. The authors investigated differences between hearing aid settings in each group for a variety of outcomes, including laboratory measures (speech recognition in quiet, speech recognition in noise) and field measures (ratings of speech understanding, preference). Results revealed that performance was better, or at least no worse, with NAL-NL1 prescriptions than with the fittings with less high-frequency amplification. This was the same for both groups, suggesting that the high-frequency amplification was not contraindicated for patients with dead regions. However, Preminger et al[65] did find a relationship between the presence of dead regions and hearing aid satisfaction, suggesting that although the presence of dead regions may not affect the prescribed hearing aid gain, dead regions may affect expectations for hearing aid outcomes.

Special signals: The quest for the "best" frequency response, as outlined above, has generally focused on speech signals. However, we know that the optimum frequency response for other types of signals is likely very different, in part because the spectral content of signals other than speech might be very different, and also because a listener's needs might be different. For example, in acoustically poor listening situations, such as those with poor signal-to-noise ratios (SNRs), digital noise reduction algorithms decrease gain for channels dominated by steady-state noise, often the lowest-frequency channels. As a result, many patients report improved sound quality in these listening situations.[66] Therefore, the ideal frequency response for comfort in noise is likely different than one prescribed by one of the aforementioned prescriptions. Similarly, DSL prescribes different targets for listening in noise than for listening in quiet, acknowledging that the frequency-importance function changes in noise and thus gain can be reduced for those frequencies.

Music is another case where prescriptions are sometimes modified for patients from the original prescription. In general, music has a wider bandwidth, a larger dynamic range, and a more tonal quality than speech.[67] As a result, a smooth frequency response and perhaps uniform gain may be important for listening to music. In addition, Moore[68] evaluated preferences for NAL-NL2 or CAM while listening to music (jazz or classical). Patients indicated a consistent preference for CAM over NAL-NL2, likely because CAM prescribes a broader bandwidth, which listeners tend to prefer for music. Based on patient reports, investigators have also advocated for extending the low-frequency hearing aid response for music.[69] Furthermore, patients may prefer music signals while listening to hearing aid with limited compression.[70]

Signals from the telephone are another type of specific signal that require modification from prescribed targets. Telephone signals are bandlimited from approximately 300 to 3,000 Hz. As a result, there is no need to provide gain above 3,000 Hz and doing so with an acoustic telephone program increases the risk of feedback unnecessarily. Even with a telecoil or other wireless streaming telephone options where acoustic feedback is not a risk, providing gain above 3,000 Hz would be unnecessary.

Streamed signals may also require special consideration. Streamed signals are those which are transmitted wirelessly directly from technologies, like a cellular telephones or portable music devices. Streaming is accomplished via Bluetooth or other proprietary streaming algorithm and sometimes requires an intermediary device. Because these signals originate from the technology directly, only those frequencies which have programmed gain will be transmitted. For a patient with normal low-frequency hearing, the modern prescriptive methods would provide minimal low-frequency gain. Patients may not be satisfied with these settings; more low-frequency gain might be added to the streamed signals in order to compensate for the lack of natural sound entering the ear canal from the streaming device.

Sometimes these special signals are handled separately by programming multiple programs in a multi-memory hearing aid. Other times, special signals are handled automatically by the hearing aid classifier, which will adjust gain settings based on a classifier's determination. Regardless of how these special signals are handled, it is valuable to understand how and why the gain settings differ from prescriptions. However, in many cases, the answer to the "best" prescription for special signals is still unknown as signals other than speech receive comparatively little research attention.

9.7 Summary

The purpose of this chapter is to describe prescriptive fitting methods for hearing aids. Prescriptive fitting methods have evolved since the early days of audiology. Many differences between methods can be attributed to differences in underlying rationale. Some prescriptions prioritize maximizing audibility or restoring loudness perception to normal, whereas others prioritize maximizing speech intelligibility or equalizing loudness perception across frequencies. Case studies are included to highlight the similarities and differences between two currently popular prescriptive methods for adults and children. For all prescriptions, the targets provided are generally considered a good starting place for hearing aid gain. There are several factors, in addition to patient variability in preferences, which may influence the hearing aid settings ultimately fit to a patient. Among these are adaptation to gain, choice of initial prescription, the presence of dead regions, and special signals. Finally, to actually use a prescriptive method for fitting hearing aids, it is critical to verify that the hearing aid is providing the prescribed amplification.

References

[1] Moore BC. Cochlear Hearing Loss: Physiological, Psychological, and Technical Issues. 2nd ed. West Sussex, Englad: John Wiley & Sons, Ltd; 2007

[2] Marks LE. Binaural summation of loudness: noise and two-tone complexes. Percept Psychophys. 1980; 27(6):489–498

[3] Moore BC, Glasberg BR. Loudness summation across ears for hearing-impaired listeners. J Acoust Soc Am. 2014; 135(4):2348

[4] Oetting D, Hohmann V, Appell J-E, Kollmeier B, Ewert SD. Spectral and binaural loudness summation for hearing-impaired listeners. Hear Res. 2016; 335:179–192

[5] Walker G. The required frequency responses of hearing aids for people with conductive hearing losses. Aust J Audiol. 1999; 21:39–43

[6] Knudsen VO, Jones IH. Symposium on the viiith nerve. III.—Artificial aids to hearing. Laryngoscope. 1935; 45(1):48–69

[7] Davis H, Hudgins CV, Marquis R, et al. The selection of hearing aids. Laryngoscope. 1946; 56(4): 135–163

[8] Watson N, Knudsen V. Selective amplification in hearing aids. J Acoust Soc Am. 1940; 11(4):406–419

[9] Watson L, Tolan T. Hearing Tests and Hearing Instruments. Baltimore, MD: Williams and Wilkins; 1949

[10] Lybarger SF. Wearable hearing aid with inductive pickup for telephone reception. Google Patents; 1953

[11] Lybarger S. Development of a new hearing aid with magnetic microphone. Electrical Manufacturing. 1947; 1947:11

[12] Carhart R. Selection of hearing aids. Arch Otolaryngol. 1946; 44(1):1–18

[13] Walden BE, Schwartz DM, Williams DL, Holum-Hardegen LL, Crowley JM. Test of the assumptions underlying comparative hearing aid evaluations. J Speech Hear Disord. 1983; 48(3):264–273

[14] Goldstein BA. Factors contributing to the changing hearing aid scene. Ear Hear. 1981; 2(6):260–266

[15] Pascoe DP. Frequency responses of hearing aids and their effects on the speech perception of hearing-impaired subjects. Ann Otol Rhinol Laryngol. 1975; 84(5 pt 2, suppl 23):1–40

[16] Berger KW. Prescription of hearing aids: a rationale. J Am Audiol Soc. 1976; 2(3):71–78

[17] Berger KW, Hagberg EN, Rane RL. Prescription of Hearing Aids: Rationale, Procedure, and Results. Kent, OH: Herald Press; 1984

10 Outcome Measures in the Prescription of Hearing Aids for Adults

Harvey B. Abrams

"If you don't know where you are going, you'll end up someplace else."

— Yogi Berra

10.1 Introduction

In addition to being a hall-of-fame catcher, a manager of several world series champion teams and an oft-quoted "peoples' philosopher", Yogi seemed to know something about the importance of measuring outcomes. The primary reason we measure outcomes as part of the hearing aid selection and fitting process is to provide objective information to patients concerning the extent to which their goals have been achieved and to promote data-driven decision made by health care policy makers and other stakeholders. In the context of this chapter, the term "outcome measures" refers to those methods and tools that can be used to evaluate a patient's status as a result of audiological intervention. While the use of outcome measures is critical for all audiological services, the focus of this chapter will be on hearing aid selection and fitting. It is the hearing aid and its associated services that currently define the profession and discipline of audiology. Turner[1] argues that by virtue of their education, research productivity, knowledge transfer, and clinical services, audiologists should be the recognized hearing aid expert. In order to truly claim the right to declare themselves as the hearing aid providers of choice, however, it is imperative that audiologists objectively document the benefits achieved as a result of their expertise.[a]

---

[a] The interested reader is referred to the 1993 Carhart Memorial Lecture delivered by Dr. Earl Harford[2] to the annual meeting of the American Auditory Society. Dr. Harford delivered an eloquent and convincing case for the indispensable role of the hearing aid in the past, present, and future of Audiology.

These collective measures of treatment effectiveness coupled with carefully conducted clinical trials create a foundation of evidence upon which the clinician can draw to maximize the opportunity for positive patient outcome—a process known as evidence-based practice (EBP). EBP is defined as the "conscientious, explicit, and judicious use of current best evidence in making decisions about the care of individual patients. The practice.... means integrating individual clinical expertise with the best available external clinical evidence from systematic research.[3]"

> **Pearl**
>
> Use outcome measures to modify the fitting as well as to determine the success of the fitting.

The move to EBP requires data-driven decision making and underscores the need for performance measures that provide quantitative information on the outcomes of care. As the evidence base grows, the profession of audiology will be in a position to develop clinical practice guidelines (CPGs) which will lead to the following:

- Reduced variability.
- Increased reproducibility.
- Consistent outcomes.
- High-quality patient care.
- Minimized risks.
- An increased relationship between knowledge and clinical practice.

10.2 Rationale for Hearing Aid Outcomes Assessment

We are firmly entrenched in an era characterized by an everchanging health care environment and increasing requirements for accountability. As a result, administrators, third-party payers, health care policy makers, and our patients are seeking evidence that our treatments make meaningful differences in our patients' lives. An impressive array of outcome measures is available to the practicing audiologist for documenting the effectiveness of intervention with hearing aids. In addition to the obvious benefits to the clinician and patient of demonstrating improvement as a result of intervention, another, less obvious, application of outcome measures is the performance of an economic analysis of hearing aid options. For example, in order to economically justify the selection of a "premium" technology instrument compared to a less expensive "basic" technology alternative, the measured benefits with the more expensive option would need to increase in proportion to the additional costs in order to demonstrate cost-effectiveness. Beck[4] posited that while cost will always remain a concern in health care decision making, the question will be reframed to determine if the most expensive treatment necessarily leads to the best outcome. In fact, recent studies have called into question the superiority of high-end devices.[5] In addition to their use in measuring treatment effectiveness and in conducting economic evaluations of treatment options, outcome measures can be used for purposes, such as (1) adjusting the hearing aid parameters; (2) counseling patients regarding expectations of benefit; and (3) documenting patient satisfaction.

Special Consideration

Outcomes are for all of your stakeholders—patients, employer, families, insurers, coworkers, and accrediting organizations.

10.3 A Conceptual Framework for Hearing Aid Intervention

The choice of an appropriate outcome measures is dependent on the establishment of clear goals for hearing aid intervention. This process can be facilitated by application of the World Health Organization (WHO) classification scheme for describing the consequences of health conditions (i.e., disorders and diseases). Initially, the WHO[6] used the terms "impairment," "disability," and "handicap" to describe the multidimensional impact of a health condition. More recently, however, as a result of changes in health care practices and a new social understanding of disability, the classification system was revised and is now referred to as the International Classification of Functioning, Disability, and Health (ICF; WHO).[7] The WHO-ICF is a biopsychosocial model of functioning and disability that provides a framework for evaluating success in all areas of intervention and treatment,

including hearing aid rehabilitation.[8,9] The WHO-ICF systematically organizes and codifies the consequences of an individual's health condition such as a hearing loss, into the broad dimensions of body structure and function, activity, and participation.

Special Consideration

The World Health Organization deleted the domains "disability" and "handicap" from its revised classification document due to negative connotations associated with this terminology.

As illustrated in ▶Fig. 10.1, these three dimensions interact and are influenced by contextual factors related to the environment and the person. Environmental factors include social attitudes, architectural characteristics, legal and social structures, etc., while personal factors allow for consideration of a person's gender, age, coping style, socioeconomic background, education, and other demographic variables. The WHO-ICF can be accessed at http://www3.who.int/icf/.

Special Consideration

A major change from the 1980 to the 2001 WHO classifications is the inclusion of "contextual" factors (environment, law, accessibility, social attitudes, etc.) that impact on the patient's activity and participation.

The WHO-ICF is important, not only because it provides a conceptual framework, but also because it allows for a detailed classification of human functioning. In theory, any function or disability can be assigned an ICF alpha-numeric code that identifies a functional category and a level of functioning. To clarify the classification principles, consider the code for "hearing functions" which is b230. This code refers to "sensory functions relating to sensing the presence of sounds and discriminating the location, pitch, loudness, and quality of sounds" (WHO-ICF,).[7] The "b" refers to body functioning. The "2" refers to Chapter 2 in the ICF, titled "Sensory Functions and Pain." The "30" refers to the section of that chapter on hearing functions. Most domain codes at this level have statements about "inclusions" and sometimes "exclusions" that help coders to avoid some common errors. In the case of b230 inclusions are specified as "functions of hearing, auditory discrimination, localization of sound source, lateralization of sound, speech discrimination," and "impairments such as deafness, hearing impairment, and hearing loss" (WHO-ICF).[7]

ICF coding for body structures and function, activity, and participation are applicable

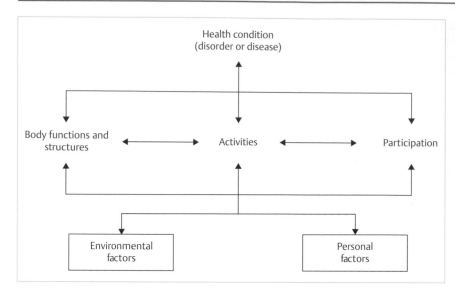

Fig. 10.1 Interactions between the components of WHO-ICF.

to all aspects of audiology. For example, body structures are the anatomical parts of the body including the external (s240; WHO-ICF[7]), middle (s250; WHO-ICF[7]), and inner (s260; WHO-ICF[7]) parts of the ear. Body functions are the physiological and psychological functions of body systems and include the aforementioned hearing functions (b230; WHO-ICF[7]). An anatomical deviation, such as occurs in otosclerosis results in an *impairment* in body structure. A deviation in function that occurs when middle ear pathology or cochlear damage results in elevated auditory thresholds causes a person to exhibit an *impairment* in body function. Surgical treatment for otosclerosis would be aimed at alleviating an impairment of body *structure* and the use of a hearing aid by an individual with elevated auditory thresholds would be aimed at alleviating an impairment of body *function*.

The full range of life areas are encompassed in the dimensions of *activity* and *participation*. The broad domains assessed under activity and participation include learning and applying knowledge; general tasks and demands; communication; mobility; self-care; domestic life; interpersonal interactions and relationships; major life areas (e.g., employment, education, economic life); and, community, social and civic life. *Activity* is defined as a person's ability to perform or execute an action or task in a uniform environment—or more simply, what a person "can do." *Participation* is what a person "does do" in his or her everyday environment. For example, "can" a person with sensorineural hearing loss, who has difficulty with sound detection, "communicate with—receive—spoken messages" (d310; WHO-ICF[7]) or engage effectively in a "conversation" (d350; WHO-ICF[7]). Even if a person "can" do these activities, he or she may not participate in communication and conversational activities for a variety of reasons, such as

the effort involved, embarrassment from potentially misunderstanding a message, lack of readily available communication partners, etc. The process of audiological rehabilitation, the cornerstone of which is the use of hearing aids, is aimed not only in assuring that a person "can" engage in activities dependent on hearing, but also to help a person to participate fully in hearing-related communication and conversational activities. Indeed, addressing the whole of a person's functioning through audiological rehabilitation is necessary in order to minimize the potential impact of a hearing impairment on an individual's *health-related quality of life* (HRQoL). While "health-related quality of life"[b] is not a specific dimension within the WHO-ICF classification system, it is understood that HRQoL represents the sum of the effects of each of the dimensions shown in ▶ **Fig. 10.1**.

It is generally accepted that activity limitations, participation restrictions, and consequent reductions in HRQoL are related to the magnitude and type of hearing loss. However, there is widespread clinical recognition that it is not possible to accurately predict the nature and extent of an individual's limitations and restrictions solely on the basis of audiometric data alone. Two persons with the same degree of impairment may have very different perceptions regarding their health-related quality of life. Similarly, we cannot measure the effects of audiological intervention solely in terms of a reduction of impairment. If this were the case, the provision of reasonably good audibility across a broad frequency range, without making average and loud speech uncomfortable, would be the

---

[b] The term health-related quality of life is used here, but in the health care literature this term is often used interchangeably with health status, functional status, and quality of life to refer to the same concept of "health."

only determinant of a successful hearing aid fitting. Since activity limitations and participation restrictions are significantly influenced by the individual's personality, communication needs, and the environment, as well as the degree of impairment, assurance of audibility at comfortable listening levels, unfortunately, does not guarantee an improvement in HRQoL.

> ### Pitfall ✕
>
> Assuring audibility at comfortable listening levels does not guarantee an improvement in quality of life.

10.3.1 Goals of Hearing Aid Intervention

Impairment

Based on the WHO-ICF, hearing aid intervention can be conceived of as having several general goals. The first general goal is to alleviate, as much as possible, the *impairment* resulting from health conditions affecting the auditory system's structure and/or function. As is well known, the primary impairment resulting from a conductive disorder is a decrease in the ability to detect sounds. When there is damage to the sensorineural mechanism, however, impairments in loudness perception, temporal resolution, and frequency resolution often accompany the impairment in detection. While future technology may allow us to address frequency and temporal resolution impairments, current hearing aid technology provides the audiologist with the ability to address impairments of detection and loudness perception through the preselection of electroacoustic characteristics, while also considering the style of the instrument (e.g., behind-the-ear [BTE],in-the-ear [ITE], in-the-canal [ITC], completely in-the-canal [CIC], receiver-in-canal [RIC]), the hearing aid arrangement (e.g., unilateral, bilateral, CROS), circuitry options (e.g., linear, output compression, wide dynamic range compression), special features (e.g., frequency lowering, adaptive directionality, wireless streaming), and user options (e.g., T-coil, directional/omnidirectional switching, multiple programs).

In current practice, the selection of hearing aid parameters begins with obtaining data from a complete audiological evaluation. Standard audiometric data are often supplemented with information from additional perceptual measures, such as speech recognition performance in quiet and in noise, and loudness comfort and growth. In addition, relevant information may be obtained through informal discussions or formal assessment of an individual's self-perceived listening difficulties, needs, concerns,

and cognitive status. To select an initial set of electroacoustic characteristics, these data are often applied to one of several available prescriptive approaches. The prescription defines several parameters including the frequency/gain response at one or more input levels, the OSPL90, and additional characteristics such as cross-over frequency between channels and dynamic/static characteristics of compression circuitry.[c]

Electroacoustic and other hearing aid parameters are typically selected to meet three specific goals: (1) make soft sounds audible; (2) make normal conversational speech comfortably loud and understandable; and (3) make loud sounds loud but tolerable. Outcome measures selected to demonstrate that these specific goals are achieved involve *verifying* that the electroacoustic and other hearing aid characteristics meet the objective criteria used in their preselection. Once it is determined that the electroacoustic and other characteristics of the hearing aid(s) are optimal for meeting the impairment-level goals, we need to determine that general and specific goals set at the levels of activity and participation are also met. At these levels, the outcome measures selected will be used to *validate* that the use of hearing aid(s) makes meaningful differences; that is, that the treatment is efficacious and the goals, as defined by the patient, have been achieved.

> ### Pearl
>
> Use outcome measures to modify the fitting as well as to determine the success of the fitting.

Activity Limitations

The general goal of hearing aid fitting in the *activity* domain is to improve a person's ability to understand speech, thus leading to improvement in communication functioning. Currently, outcome measures used to validate the effectiveness of hearing aid intervention in this domain include objective, performance measures and subjective, self-report measures of speech understanding, and communication performance. It is important to keep in mind that as more sophisticated signal processing technologies are introduced, other types of outcome measures aimed at validating the effectiveness of hearing aid intervention at the activity level may be seen in the audiology clinic. For example, it would not be unreasonable

---

[c] Although not common in current clinical practice, technological advances may result in the incorporation of techniques such as paired-comparisons of sound quality and/or perceived intelligibility for selection and/or adjustment of electroacoustic characteristics.

to include a measure of sound localization ability when evaluating multiple-microphone and ear-to-ear wireless technologies. Indeed, techniques for addressing localization performance in the clinic are currently available.[10,11] In addition, questionnaires such as The Speech, Hearing, Spatial Hearing and Qualities of Hearing Questionnaire (SSQ)[12,13] and the Spatial Hearing Questionnaire (SHQ)[14] include several questions designed to access the patient's perceptions of distance and movement and sound source segregation. Another example is the need to verify high-frequency audibility, as frequency-lowering technology becomes a more commonly selected feature among clinicians, using outcome measures specifically designed for this purpose.[15]

Participation Restrictions

The measurement of *restrictions in participation* resulting from a hearing impairment, as a consequence of activity limitations, is not a common focus in standard audiological testing protocols. We often infer this data, however, through the case histories we obtain from our patients. For example, patients may report seeking our services because they can no longer enjoy attending social gatherings or are having difficulty with communication at work. As part of post–hearing aid fitting services, we may informally ask our patients if they experience less difficulty in these or similar situations. While this informal approach may satisfy us that we have accomplished our goals, more formal assessments allow for the quantification of successful outcomes at the level of *participation*. There are a variety of self-report measures that can be used for this purpose which will be detailed further in this chapter. Since the level of participation is highly influenced by the environmental factors described earlier, the audiologist may need to take a more active role in evaluating the social, occupational, and living environments in which the patient exists. As a result, the audiologist may become involved in the development of hearing accessibility programs for communities or groups of listeners with hearing impairments.[16,17] Such programs are designed to address the needs, wishes, and abilities of the listener within specific communication situations with specific communication partners in specific communication environments.

Health-Related Quality of Life

We are also concerned that meeting our clinical objectives in terms of reductions of *impairment, activity limitations*, and *participation restrictions* will result in measurable changes in self-perceived *health-related quality of life (HRQoL)*. Although HRQoL measurement has received little clinical application among audiologists, it is a construct that is receiving increasing attention in the health care research literature, including those studies aimed at demonstrating the efficacy of hearing aid intervention.[18,19,20] A review of this literature provides information regarding available tools and approaches that can be adopted for use in our clinical protocols.

Satisfaction

Finally, no hearing aid fitting could be considered fully successful without demonstrating that the patient was *satisfied* with the device and services received. *Satisfaction* does not always correspond to significant or quantifiable reductions in *impairment, activity limitations, participation*, or *HRQoL*. In addition to improvements in communication and real-world functioning, the domain of *satisfaction* involves the patient's relationship with service providers, the ease of access to services, as well as the influence of factors such as cosmetics, comfort, expectations and perceived value. It is a construct that needs independent assessment.

10.3.2 Clinically Useful Outcome Measures

The remainder of this chapter provides detailed discussion of clinically useful outcome measures which provide a means for demonstrating that in the clinical processes of selection, fitting, and counseling in the appropriate use of hearing aid(s) we have met the goals selected at the levels of *impairment, activity limitation, participation restriction, HRQoL*, and *satisfaction*. These data can be used to demonstrate treatment effectiveness for individual patients and/or as part of program evaluation. The discussion focuses on measures appropriate for use in the adult population. It is important to note that outcome assessment for children requires age-appropriate tests, tasks, and approaches.

Measuring Outcomes for Impairment-level Goals: The Verification Process

As discussed, the general goal at the level of impairment is to improve audibility of speech, while maintaining listening comfort. This goal is accomplished through the selection of appropriate electroacoustic parameters and other hearing aid characteristics (i.e., style, arrangement, circuitry). While 2-cm^3 coupler measurements may be used to ensure that the hearing aid satisfies manufacturer quality control standards and to make initial adjustments on the hearing aid, it is now standard practice to use real-ear measurements (probe microphone measurements of real-ear insertion gain [REIG] and real-ear–aided response [REAR], or functional gain for severe to profound losses) in order to individually adjust the parameters of the hearing aid and verify results. The primary goals of this verification process are to ensure that the measured electroacoustic characteristics are as close as possible to those prescribed for the patient, and that the hearing aid provides adequate audibility of the important speech energy without feedback or loudness discomfort. Several commercially available probe microphone systems incorporate "live speech mapping" capabilities. While using actual speech (recorded or live) may intuitively seem preferable to speech-shaped stimuli (e.g., composite noise), there is no evidence that patient outcome is any better with live speech mapping. This should come as no surprise as composite or speech-like noise used in most systems closely resembles the long-term average speech spectrum (LTASS). There are those who argue that "mapping" the response to a particular voice (e.g., spouse) will lead to better hearing and understanding of that person. Unfortunately, the acoustic properties of the spouse's voice in the real world will vary as a function of distance, reverberation, direction, and presence of background noise and will likely bear very little resemblance to those properties in the clinic environment.

RMS difference: Documentation that the impairment-related goals have been met can be accomplished in several ways. For example, one approach would be to determine the extent to which the measured aided response deviates from the prescribed target by calculating the root mean square (RMS) difference between the probe microphone-measured REAR from the prescribed target REAR. Byrne[21] described such a procedure using the following formula:

$$\text{RMS difference} = \sqrt{\frac{d_1^2 + d_2^2 + d_3^2 + d_4^2}{4}} \quad (1)$$

Where $d_1^2 \ldots d_4^2$ equals the difference between the target-aided response and measured-aided response at 500, 1,000, 2,000, and 4,000 Hz. Byrne discovered that his subjects were able to detect a difference in the sound quality of the hearing aid with an RMS difference of as little as 3 dB.

Articulation (speech intelligibility) index: Another approach to verifying audibility as part of the hearing aid fitting process is calculating the Articulation Indices (AIs), sometimes referred to as the Speech Intelligibility Index (SII). The AI provides a numerical value between 0.0 and 1.0. Higher AI scores are achieved by placing more of the acoustic speech signal in the audible range. Theoretically, the higher the AI score, the greater the ability to understand speech at comfortable levels. Several calculation methods are available, each with benefits and limitations.[22,23] The ANSI[22] and Fletcher[24] methods require complex calculations and are not appropriate for routine clinical use. The Pavlovic[23] methods involve simpler calculations and are easy to use but lack precision. Unfortunately, existing AI approaches which best predict performance are not presently available for clinical implementation.[25] That said, commercial probe microphone systems are available that automatically calculate a version of the SII which can be informative when comparing unaided to aided predicted audibility.

Patient acceptability factors: In addition to documenting improvements in speech audibility, it is also important to achieve a good physical fit, acceptable cosmetics, adequate volume wheel range, and satisfactory sound quality. The assessment of these important outcomes is typically determined at follow-up visits, through telephone interviews, or by mailed questionnaires.

Pitfall	
"Hitting the REAR target" is of little value if the patient won't wear the hearing aids due to dissatisfaction with cosmetics or comfort.	

Acclimatization: Following the hearing aid fitting process and a complete orientation to their use and care, patients will wear their instruments in their real-world environment for a period of time (at least a few weeks) prior to obtaining measures which provide *validation* of the efficacy of hearing aid selection and fitting as part of their follow-up appointment. During the period between fitting and follow-up, it is expected that the patient will have experienced a variety of listening environments and that "acclimatization" to amplification may occur, at least for some new hearing aid users.[26] Acclimatization may result in improved speech recognition ability over time, particularly for those patients who have more severe losses, but may merely be reflected in the fact that the patient has become accustomed to wearing the hearing aids at a higher gain setting (as modified by the patient, clinician, or as part of an automated adaptation feature) or has become less bothered by such side effects of amplification as the occlusion effect, common background sounds, and the physical presence of the instruments in the ear.

> **Controversial Point**
>
> Some acclimatization studies suggest that speech recognition outcome measures may change over time. Other investigations failed to demonstrate any significant changes in performance.

Measuring Outcomes for Activity Limitation and Participation Restriction Goals: The Validation Process

Outcome measures used to *validate* the efficacy of hearing aid intervention at the activity and participation levels include objective, performance measures of speech recognition, and self-report measures assessing activity limitations and/or participation restrictions. Each of these categories is discussed.

Objective, performance measures of speech recognition: The use of speech recognition testing as an outcome assessment tool in hearing aid fitting is controversial. Such testing has generally fallen out of favor since the Carhart comparative speech approach to hearing aid fitting[27] was determined to be too time consuming and the PB-word lists were found to be insensitive to small differences among hearing aids.[28] In addition, it has not been adequately demonstrated that performance on these clinical tests accurately predicts performance in everyday listening environments. There are those who argue, however, that the use of phoneme scoring, rather than whole-word scoring of PB words, allows for an increase in the reliability of test scores without increasing test time, such that their use as a hearing aid outcome measure warrants further consideration.[29] However, the use of phoneme scoring does not appear to be gaining widespread acceptance among clinicians.

New speech-in-noise testing materials continue to be developed, ranging from phoneme-level identification tasks to whole-sentence recognition. In the last few decades multiple-target words concatenated into syntactically correct sentences or whole-sentence recognition tests, both administered in noise, have begun to gain popularity among clinicians, on the assumption that speech that includes contextual cues and is presented in a background of noise will have greater predictive validity as an outcome measure for amplification. Two tests that have seen increasing use both clinically and in hearing aid research are the Hearing-In-Noise test (HINT; Nilsson[30]) and the QuickSIN.[31] In the HINT, the speech spectrum noise level is fixed at a moderate-intensity level. The signal-to-noise ratio is varied adaptively to determine the signal-to-noise ratio at which a 50% correct sentence performance is obtained. The patient is required to repeat the entire sentence correctly.

The QuickSIN uses a descending paradigm with administration of one sentence, composed of five target words, at each of six signal-to-noise ratios that start at 25 dB S/N and decrease in 5 dB decrements. The level of the sentences is fixed and the level of the multitalker babble, which is continuous throughout the list of sentences, is varied in 5 dB increments from 25- to 0 dB S/N. The QuickSIN is scored by quantifying the 50% point in terms of dB S/N and subtracting 2 dB, which is the mean score for young normal hearing listeners, to identify the signal-to-noise ratio loss of an individual. The QuickSIN manual[32] provides the number of pairs of sentences required for comparison between two conditions such as two different hearing aids, or two different hearing aid adjustments.

A similar approach to measuring signal-to-noise ratio as described above was created using NU No. 6 words in multitalker babble. The Words-In-Noise protocol (WIN)[33] consists of (1) 35 monosyllabic words from NU No. 6 spoken by the female speaker on the VA compact disc, which enabled the evaluation of recognition performance in quiet and in babble with the same materials spoken by the same speaker, (2) 5 unique words presented at each of 7 signal-to-babble ratios from 24 dB S/B to 0 dB S/B in 4 dB decrements, (3) the level of the babble, which is presented continuously, is fixed and the level of the words vary, and (4) the 50% point was quantifiable with the Spearman-Kärber equation.[34] Both the QuickSIN and the WIN provide an approximate 8 dB separation in terms of signal-to-noise ratio between performance by listeners with normal hearing and performance by listeners with hearing loss.

Two benefits of signal-to-noise ratio testing that quantifies the 50% point are that for the majority of patients, there is no ceiling or floor effect and the test can be administered quickly. In addition, a speech-in-noise task can be administered in the sound field such that the signal and the noise are both presented from the same speaker, thereby estimating the patient's performance in the most challenging of listening situations. Caution is advised when using speech-in-noise testing procedures to compare performance between hearing aids that have nonlinear signal processing functions, since the presentation level of the test materials may result in different amounts of gain with each hearing aid and differentially affect performance as a function of level more so than as a function of signal-to-noise ratio.

There remain a number of outstanding issues in speech recognition testing. Some of the speech materials available do not have normative data, are not available in languages other than English, or the recordings are not standardized. One issue that has been noted by some is that the recording or playback process may seriously limit the dynamic range (DR) of the test materials relative to everyday listening environments, which may be an issue in predictive validity, particularly with nonlinear signal processing hearing aids. Another issue is that most of the speech materials use a male voice, which may not tap into the perception of important high-frequency phonemes that are so difficult for many patients who have sloping hearing losses. Finally, there are still questions about what levels the speech and noise should be set at to represent the "real world," what type of noise should be used, and what loudspeaker array should be used to simulate everyday environments.

Pitfall	

Most of the recorded speech materials use a male voice, which may not tap into the perception of important high-frequency phonemes that are so difficult for many patients who have sloping hearing losses.

Subjective, self-report measures examining activity limitations and/or participation restrictions. In real world, rather than clinical or laboratory conditions, the activity of speech understanding and the participation in events that require speech understanding are heavily influenced by contextual factors related to both the environment and the individual. As a result, many inventories have been developed to assess the impact of a hearing impairment on the individual in the areas of communication functioning, activity limitation, and participation restrictions. ▶Table 10.1 provides references to some of the more commonly used self-report hearing aid outcome measures for use in the general adult population. This list is by no means exhaustive. Numerous additional inventories are available for use in assessing the outcomes of hearing aids' intervention in other populations (e.g., children, communication partners, prelingual deafened adults, etc.; see Chapter 11) and for assessing outcomes in other areas of audiological intervention (e.g., tinnitus management, dizziness, etc.; see Chapter 17)

The inventories reviewed in detail here are those reported to be most commonly used by audiologists who dispense hearing aids and other instruments, less commonly used, but which meet criteria that are considered important for clinical utility: (1) they are valid—that is, the inventories measure what they claim to measure; (2) they are easy to administer in a short period of time—that is, they are practical; (3) they are sensitive—that is, the measure is able to detect change if change occurs; (4) they have test–retest reliability and/or critical difference data available; and, (5) they are comprehensible—that is, they are understandable

to the end users of the information.[35] The exclusion of any instrument here is not intended as a commentary on its psychometric properties or utility in research endeavors. Rather, we have chosen to focus our discussion on inventories that we believe are likely to be the most useful in clinical practice.

Pearl	

A clinically practical outcome measure should be easy to administer in a short period of time, provide easily quantifiable scores, and have established test–retest reliability data.

Three well-documented questionnaires warrant special mention although they are not discussed in detail. The first is the Communication Profile for the Hearing Impaired (CPHI),[36] which is an excellent research tool and useful for in-depth clinical assessment. With 145 items, however, the CPHI is time consuming to administer. Another useful instrument is the Hearing Aid Performance Inventory (HAPI),[37] which at 64 items is also quite long to administer. Although shortened versions of the HAPI (SHAPI/SHAPI-E) have been introduced, these inventories provide aided scores only. As they do not allow for difference scores, their value, for individual patients, is likely to be most applicable to examining differences between hearing aids. The final measure of note is the Speech, Spatial Hearing and Qualities of Hearing Questionnaire (SSQ).[12] This instrument assesses auditory attention, perceptions of distance and movement, sound-source segregation, listening effort, prosody, and sound quality. While the SSQ takes a more ecological approach to examining self-perceived hearing difficulties than does any other available self-report instrument, with 80 questions, the SSQ like the CPHI and the HAPI is a time-consuming instrument to administer. A shortened version (12 items), however, of the SSQ[13] is available as is the 24-item SHQ which also assesses spatial abilities.[11]

Abbreviated Profile of Hearing Aid Benefit (APHAB). A commonly used tool for quantifying the changes in the WHO-ICF *activity* dimension as a result of hearing aid use is the APHAB, developed by Cox and Alexander.[38] The APHAB, a 24-item questionnaire, is composed of situational-specific questions which assess speech understanding and hearing in a variety of situations (▶Fig. 10.2). Scores are provided for four categories: (1) ease of communication (EC), which examines the communication effort under favorable conditions; (2) reverberation (RV), which examines communication in reverberant environments such as classrooms; (3) background noise (BN), which examines communication in high

Table 10.1 Comparison of self-report outcome measures

Instrument/authors	Purpose	Domain	Number of items	Scoring and interpretation
Abbreviated Profile of Hearing Aid Benefit (APHAB) Cox and Alexander[38]	Quantify hearing loss disability and reduction of disability after using a hearing aid	Activity	24	Four subscale scores provided: ease of communication (EC); background noise (BN); reverberation (RV); aversiveness (AV). EC, BN, and RV combine to provide global score. Equal percentile profiles determined for aided, unaided, benefit scores. Lower scores are indicative of fewer problems for EC, BN, and RV, while higher scores indicate fewer problems for AV.
Client Oriented Scale of Improvement (COSI) Dillon et al[39]	Subjective identification of situations of listening difficulty and benefit from hearing aid intervention	Activity Participation	1–5	Patient judges degree of change attributable to intervention and final ability as a result of intervention. Higher scores indicate better outcomes. Proportion of patients obtaining degree of change and final ability scores is available.
Communication Profile Hearing Inventory (CPHI) Demorest and Erdman[36]	Provides systematic and comprehensive assessment of a wide range of communication difficulties and reactions to those difficulties	Activity Participation	145	Results plotted as a profile of three importance ratings and 22 scale scores grouped into four categories: communication performance, communication environment, communication strategies, and personal adjustment. Higher scores indicate lesser difficulty or involvement. Data can also be examined as z-scores for five factors: communication importance, communication performance, adjustment, reaction, and interaction.
Glasgow Hearing Aid Benefit Profile (GHABP) Gatehouse[40]	Assess hearing aid benefit and satisfaction over time	Activity Participation HRQoL	Four to eight items; up to seven questions per item	5-point scale; can convert to 100-point scale; higher score indicates greater problems.
Hearing Aid Users Questionnaire (HAUQ) Dillon et al[41]	Quantify hearing aid use, difficulty, and benefit	Satisfaction	11	Different scale for each question. In all cases, a higher score indicates greater hearing aid satisfaction.
Health Utilities Index (HUI) Furlong et al[42]	Measure comprehensive health status and HRQoL for a broad range of subjects	HRQoL	15	Scoring algorithm based on eight attributes: vision, hearing, speech, ambulation, dexterity, emotion, cognition (including memory and thinking ability), and pain or discomfort, with five or six levels each, ranging from severely impaired to normal, describing 972,000 unique health states. The single-attribute utility functions provide utility scores for each level with scores ranging between 0, dead, and 1, full health. Scores provide a measure of attribute-specific morbidity and a single summary measure of HRQoL.
Hearing Aid Performance Inventory (HAPI) Walden et al[37]	Assesses effectiveness of hearing aids in a variety of listening situations	Activity	64	5-point scale where 1 is very helpful and 5 hinders performance, based on four listening situations: noisy, quiet, reduced signal, and nonspeech stimuli. Numbers are added for individual items and the sum divided by total number items answered. The closer the score is to 1, the greater the hearing aid benefit.
Hearing Handicap Inventory for Adults (HHIA)/the Elderly (HHIE) Ventry and Weinstein[43]	Measure perceived handicap from hearing loss	Participation	25	Three scores can be generated: 0–52 for emotional score; 0–48 for social/situational score; 0–100 for total score. Higher scores indicate greater difficulty.

Table 10.1   *(Continued)* Comparison of self-report outcome measures

Instrument/authors	Purpose	Domain	Number of items	Scoring and interpretation
International Outcome Inventory for Hearing Aids (IOI-HA) Cox et al[44]	Assess a broad range of outcome domains in a short, practical mini-profile	Use Benefit Activity Participation Satisfaction HRQoL	7	5-point scale, where 1 is most negative and 5 is most positive. Norms for each item are available.
Medical Outcomes Study-Short Form 36 (MOS-SF 36) Ware and Sherbourne[45]	Assess limitations in daily life and general health	HRQoL	36	Eight subscale scores, 2 to 10 items each: physical function, role-physical, bodily pain, general health, vitality, social function, role-emotional, and mental health. Subscale aggregate scores: physical component summary (PCS) and mental component summary (MCS), reported as standardized scores with mean of 50 (SD = 10) in general healthy U.S. population.
Satisfaction with Amplification in Daily Life (SADL) Cox and Alexander[46]	Quantify satisfaction in social daily life from hearing aid intervention	Satisfaction	15	Four subscale scores provided: positive effects, service and costs, negative features, and personal image, and a global score. Higher scores indicate greater satisfaction.
Sickness Impact Profile (SIP) Bergner et al[47]	Measure changes in behavior based on the impact of sickness	Participation	136	Overall score, 2 domain scores, and 12 category scores; items are weighted according to a standardized weighting scheme. Subscales: ambulation, mobility, body/care movement, social interaction, communication, alertness, emotional, sleep/rest, eating, work, home management, and recreation/pastimes. A high score suggests greater functional difficulty. Based on three scales of health (physical, psychosocial, and overall function).
Speech Hearing, Spatial Hearing and Qualities of Hearing Questionnaire (SSQ) Gatehouse and Noble[12]	Measures disability and handicap in a realistic range of contexts	Activity	80	0–10 scale, where 0 is not at all and 10 is perfectly. Higher score indicates greater ability. In addition to traditional speech intelligibility items, addresses issues of sustaining and switching attention, monitoring multiple input streams, analysis of spatial hearing (location, distance, and movement), and qualities of hearing such as listening effort, sound segregation, and prosody.
World Health Organization Disability Assessment Schedule 2.0 (WHO-DAS 2.0) WHO[48]	Examine consequences of a disease or disorder in three dimensions: body function and structure, activities, and participation.	HRQoL	36	5-point scale: 1 (none) to 5 (extreme/cannot do). Six domain scores: communication, mobility, self-care, interpersonal, life activities at home and work, and participation. Can convert to a 100-point scale; lower score indicates greater difficulty.

Abbreviations: HRQoL, health related quality of life; SD, standard deviation.

levels of background noise; and, (4) Aversiveness of sound (AV), which examines the unpleasantness of environmental sounds.

Cox[49] describes the administration and application of APHAB. Patients are asked to indicate the percentage of time they experience problems hearing under these situations. There are seven response alternatives ranging from always to half the time to never. The patient uses these response alternatives to indicate answers to the 24 situational-specific items both "without my hearing aid" and "with my hearing aid." Responses can be recorded in a paper-and-pencil format or keyed directly onto a computer keyboard. A software program available from Cox is used for scoring. The scores generated are displayed graphically and numerically. A subscale score can

ABBREVIATED PROFILE OF HEARING AID BENEFIT

A

NAME: _____   ☐ Male   ☐ Female   TODAY'S DATE: ___/___/___
Last   First

INSTRUCTIONS: Please circle the answers that come closest to your everyday experience. Notice that each choice includes a percentage. You can use this to help you decide on your answer. For example, if a statement is true about 75% of the time, circle "C" for that item. If you have not experienced the situation we describe, try to think of a similar situation that you have been in and respond for that situation. If you have no idea, leave that item blank.

A   Always (99%)
B   Almost Always (87%)
C   Generally (75%)
D   Half-the-time (50%)
E   Occasionally (25%)
F   Seldom (12%)
G   Never (1%)

	Without Hearing Aid	With Hearing Aid
1. When I am in a crowded grocery store, talking with the cashier, I can follow the conversation.	A B C D E F G	A B C D E F G
2. I miss a lot of information when I'm listening to a lecture.	A B C D E F G	A B C D E F G
3. Unexpected sounds, like a smoke detector or alarm bell are uncomfortable.	A B C D E F G	A B C D E F G
4. I have difficulty hearing a conversation when I'm with one of my family at home.	A B C D E F G	A B C D E F G
5. I have trouble understanding the dialogue in a movie or at the theater.	A B C D E F G	A B C D E F G
6. When I am listening to the news on the car radio, and family members are talking, I have trouble hearing the news.	A B C D E F G	A B C D E F G
7. When I'm at the dinner table with several people, and am trying to have a conversation with one person, understanding speech is difficult.	A B C D E F G	A B C D E F G
8. Traffic noises are too loud.	A B C D E F G	A B C D E F G
9. When I am talking with someone across a large empty room, I understand the words.	A B C D E F G	A B C D E F G
10. When I am in a small office, interviewing or answering questions, I have difficulty following the conversation.	A B C D E F G	A B C D E F G
11. When I am in a theater watching a movie or play, and the people around me are whispering and rustling paper wrappers, I can still make out the dialogue.	A B C D E F G	A B C D E F G
12. When I am having a quiet conversation with a friend, I have difficulty understanding.	A B C D E F G	A B C D E F G

Fig. 10.2   Abbreviated Profile of Hearing Aid Benefit (APHAB). First 12 items of Form A.

then be produced for unaided and aided listening. Benefit is defined as the difference between the aided and unaided scores. For individual subscale scores for "EC," "RV," or "BN" a difference of 22 percentage points is needed between aided and unaided scores for the clinician to be reasonably certain that the scores represent a real difference between conditions. When pattern performance across these three subscales is examined, the clinician can be confident that real benefit has been achieved (at least for linear hearing aids) when the aided scores exceed the unaided ones by at least 10 percentage points. A downloadable version of APHAB as well as normative data and other information can be found at http://harlmemphis.org/index.php/clinical-applications/.

Clinical experience with APHAB suggests several factors to consider in its use. One of these is the administration format. In one approach, the unaided responses are provided prior to hearing aid fitting, and aided responses are obtained following an appropriate (~ 30 days) period of hearing aid use. During the second administration, Cox[49] suggests that reliability and validity are increased if the patients are allowed to see their unaided responses. If they no longer agree with their assessment of their unaided difficulties, they are permitted to change the response. While this is acceptable, this format differs from the one used when the APHAB was normed, where subjects were asked to provide unaided and aided responses in the same sitting. In addition, research conducted by Joore and colleagues[50] demonstrated "response shift" through administration of a retrospective pretest completed at the time of posttest on hearing-specific measures in adults being fitted with hearing aids for the first time. A response shift may occur for a variety of reasons including the individual undergoing changes in (1) internal standards of measurement; (2) values; or (3) conceptualization of a target construct (Schwartz and Sprangers).[51]

Another problem associated with the APHAB is that not all of the situational-specific items are relevant to individual patients. Because patients are discouraged from leaving items blank, they need instruction about how to respond to situations that they do not or are not likely to experience. Finally, there is some concern regarding the reading level associated with the scale. It is recommended that questionnaires and other documents designed for patient use and education (e.g., informed consents, drug information pamphlets) be written at the seventh to eighth grade reading level. The readability level of the APHAB exceeds the eleventh grade level according to the Flesch–Kincaid grade level score.

> **Pitfall** ✕
>
> The validity of some self-report questionnaires is limited because they require the patient to respond to situations that the patient does not, and never will, encounter.

Hearing Handicap Inventory for the Elderly (HHIE). One of the most commonly used, and studied, outcome measures for audiological intervention is the HHIE[42] (▶**Fig. 10.3**). This measure focuses on how a hearing loss might impact on *participation*. The original version, with 25 questions, contains 13 items that are classified as eliciting information from an "emotional" domain and 12 from a "social" domain. The inventory is scored on the basis of the total number of "yes" (4 points), "sometimes" (2 points), and "no" (0 points) responses. The total score (range 0–100) provided the clinician with a relative indication of how handicapping the patient perceives the hearing impairment to be. That is, the higher the value, the greater the self-perception of hearing handicap. The questionnaire is repeated after audiological intervention, which may include hearing aids and/or aural rehabilitation. The change in the HHIE score provides the outcome measure. When administered in a face-to-face format, a reduction in score of 18.7 point is needed for the clinician to conclude that real benefit has been attained. If a paper-and-pencil format is used, however, test–retest reliability diminishes and the 95% confidence interval for a true change in score becomes 36 points.[52] An example of an emotional-domain item from the HHIE is "Does a hearing problem cause you to feel embarrassed when meeting new people"; whereas" Does a hearing problem cause you difficulty when listening to radio or TV?" would fall into the "social domain" group of questions.

Variations of the HHIE include the HHIE-S, a 10-item short-form version[53]; the HHIA, which is a 25-item version including occupationally related questions (and its shortened version, HHIA-S)[53]; and a full length Spanish version[54] as well as a shortened one.[55] Clinical experience suggests that the HHIE is most effective with inexperienced hearing aid users as experienced users may not accurately recall their "prehearing aid" self-perception of hearing handicap after a significant period of hearing aid use.

Client-Oriented Scale of Improvement (COSI). As noted, one of the concerns associated with inventories such as APHAB and the HHIE is that some items may not be relevant to some individuals. In contrast to scales that list specific questions or situations, the COSI[39] requires the patient, with guidance from the clinician, identify up to five situations that cause

HEARING HANDICAP INVENTORY

Please answer "yes" or "no" or "sometimes" to each of the following items. Do not skip a question if you avoid a situation because of a hearing problem.

		(4) YES	(2) SOME-TIMES	(0) NO
S-1.	Does a hearing problem cause you to use the phone less often than you would like?	____	____	____
E-2.	Does a hearing problem cause you to feel embarrassed when meeting new people?	____	____	____
S-3.	Does a hearing problem cause you to avoid groups of people?	____	____	____
E-4.	Does a hearing problem make you irritable?	____	____	____
E-5.	Does a hearing problem cause you to feel frustrated when talking to members of your family?	____	____	____
S-6.	Does a hearing problem cause you difficulty when attending a party?	____	____	____
E-7.	Does a hearing problem cause you to feel "stupid" or "dumb"?	____	____	____
S-8.	Do you have difficulty hearing when someone speaks in a whisper?	____	____	____
E-9.	Do you feel handicapped by a hearing problem?	____	____	____
S-10.	Does a hearing problem cause you difficulty when visiting friends, relatives, or neighbors?	____	____	____
S-11.	Does a hearing problem cause you to attend religious services less often than you would like?	____	____	____

Fig. 10.3 Hearing Handicap Inventory for the Elderly (HHIE). First 11 items.

the most communication difficulties (▶ Fig. 10.4). At the completion of treatment, the patient assesses the degree to which the identified problems have resolved. Degree of change is ranked on a five-point scale from worse to slightly better to much better or from hardly ever to occasionally to almost always. A score of 5 corresponds to much better and a score of 1 corresponds to worse. Patients also rate their final ability on a five-point scale, with 1 corresponding to hardly ever and 5 indicating almost always. Test–retest correlation coefficients for COSI degree of change ($r = 0.73$) and COSI final ability ($r = 0.84$) were found to be higher than that obtained for the HHIE total score ($r = 0.54$) in 98 adults fitted with hearing aids for the first time, leading Dillon et al[39] to conclude that COSI was particularly suitable for clinical use. An individual patient's score can be compared to the proportion of patients with

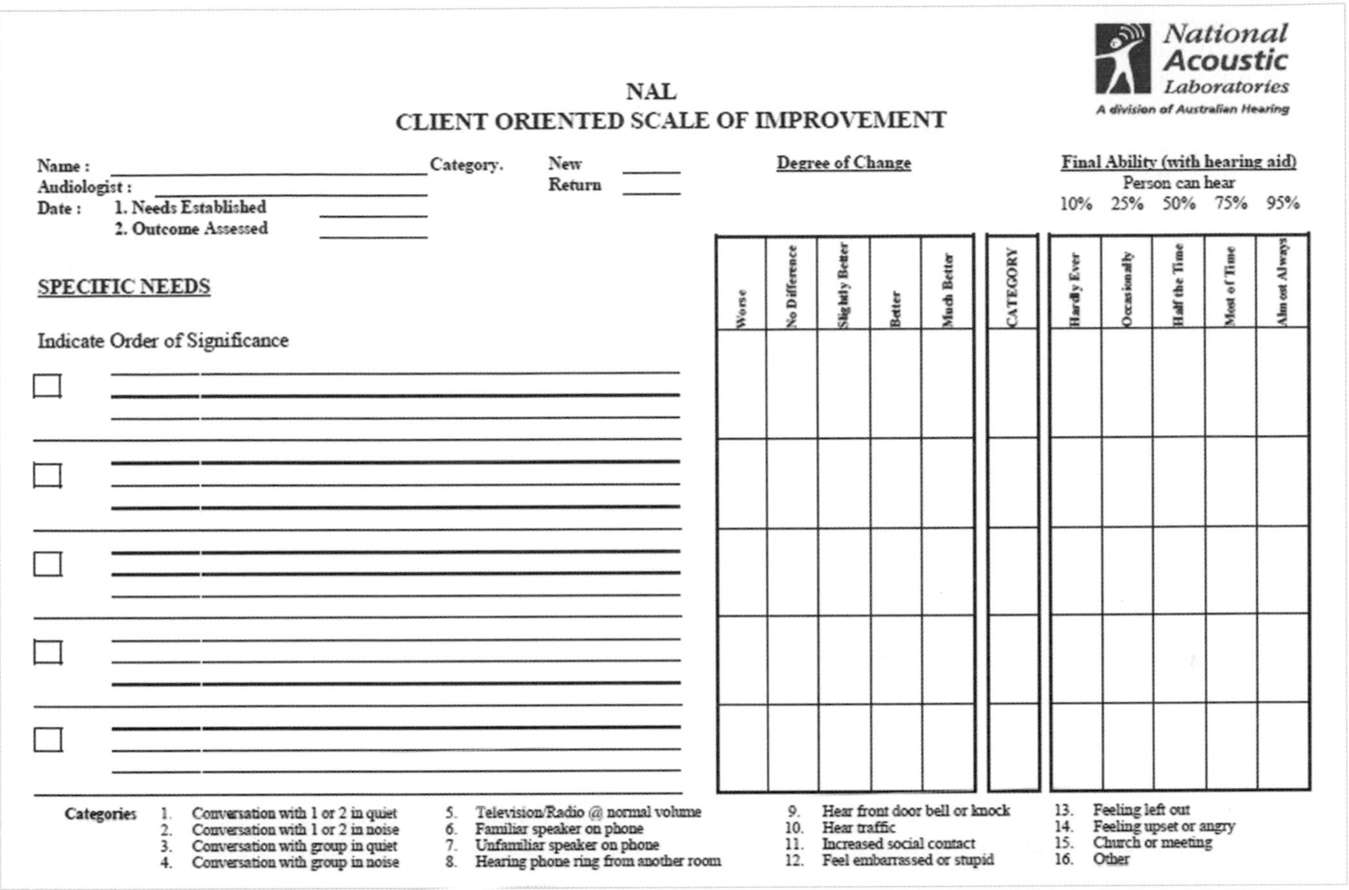

National Acoustic Laboratories
A division of Australian Hearing

NAL
CLIENT ORIENTED SCALE OF IMPROVEMENT

Name : _____   Category. _____   New _____   Degree of Change   Final Ability (with hearing aid)
Audiologist : _____   Return _____   Person can hear
Date :   1. Needs Established   _____   10%   25%   50%   75%   95%
           2. Outcome Assessed   _____

SPECIFIC NEEDS

Indicate Order of Significance

(Degree of Change columns: Worse, No Difference, Slightly Better, Better, Much Better, CATEGORY, Final Ability columns: Hardly Ever, Occasionally, Half the Time, Most of Time, Almost Always)

Categories			
1. Conversation with 1 or 2 in quiet	5. Television/Radio @ normal volume	9. Hear front door bell or knock	13. Feeling left out
2. Conversation with 1 or 2 in noise	6. Familiar speaker on phone	10. Hear traffic	14. Feeling upset or angry
3. Conversation with group in quiet	7. Unfamiliar speaker on phone	11. Increased social contact	15. Church or meeting
4. Conversation with group in noise	8. Hearing phone ring from another room	12. Feel embarrassed or stupid	16. Other

Fig. 10.4 Client-Oriented Scale of Improvement (COSI).

mild-to-moderate hearing loss who obtained different COSI change and final ability scores.[56] The COSI goals can be focused on WHO-ICF dimensions of *activity* and/or *participation*, depending on the specific situations identified. In one reported survey, the COSI was used by more respondents than any other standardized outcome measure.[57] One reason for COSI's popularity may be the assumption that by focusing on and measuring the treatment effect of problems that are most relevant to the patient, the outcomes measured will most accurately reflect the true functional impact of intervention as perceived by the patient.

The COSI is not without critics. One concern is that the COSI's application to program evaluation may be limited because each patient identifies problem situations that are unique to him or her. It may be problematic, then, to compare the relative performance among clinicians in the same clinic or across clinics in a multioffice practice for program evaluation purposes. Dillon et al,[41] however, reported on their use of COSI and the Hearing Aid Users Questionnaire (HAUQ) as outcome measures for monitoring the National Australian Hearing Services Program. The authors determined that many individual needs identified by the participants could

be classified into 16 categories that can be analyzed for program effectiveness. For example, communication needs associated with hearing or understanding speech in restaurants, parties, or unique social situations can be categorized as "conversation with one or two in noise" or "conversation with group in noise." Approximately, 75% of the subjects reported wanting to be able to hear television or radio at normal levels. The question remains, however, the extent to which different clinicians would be in agreement in terms of which of the 16 categories to place a patient's stated problem. To this point, Zelski[58] found interrater agreement for assignment of specific needs into the 16 COSI categories was quite high, that is, 0.887.

Controversial Point

While the COSI may be an effective outcome measure for individual patients, there is concern that it may be inappropriate for analyzing programs. Research[41,58] suggests otherwise.

Glasgow Hearing Aid Benefit Profile (GHABP). Another instrument that allows for the assessment changes in both *activity limitations* and *participation restrictions* as a function of hearing aid use through identification of individualized listening needs is the GHABP.[40] In addition to allowing for the identification of four patient-specific goals, the GHABP includes four prespecified questions: listening to television with other people; conversing with one another in quiet; conversing in a busy street or shop; and, conversing with several people in a group. For the preset items, patients are first asked whether the situation occurs in their lives. If it does, they are then asked how much difficulty they have in the situation and how much any difficulty in the situation caused them to feel worried, annoyed, or upset. For each question, patients can report that the item is not applicable or select on a scale of 1 to 4, the amount of difficulty and degree of emotional response, with 1 equivalent to no difficulty/not at all and 4 indicating great difficulty/quite a lot. Patients are also asked to answer the same two questions for individually identified situations. Gatehouse[59] refers to the first of these questions as assessing *initial disability*, which in current WHO-ICF (2001) terminology would be equivalent to initial activity limitations; and, the second as assessing *hearing handicap*, or in current WHO-ICF[7] terminology, initial participation restrictions. After a period of hearing aid use, patients are asked, for each situation, how often they use their hearing aids, how much the hearing aid helps (i.e., hearing aid *benefit*), how much difficulty they still have (i.e., residual *disability* or activity limitations), and how satisfied they are with their hearing aids (i.e., *satisfaction*). Response scales for each question range from 1 to 4, with 1 indicating the least favorable response and 4 the most favorable. Test–retest correlations are reported to be a minimum of 0.86, indicated excellent stability across time.[40] Gatehouse[59] reports that each of these scales can be manipulated on a scale varying from 0 to 100 with higher scores indicating more positive responses. Although quite comprehensive, the fact that up to six questions can be addressed for up to eight items (four preset and four individualized), the GHABP can become time consuming in a clinical situation.

> ### Pearl ✔
>
> A comprehensive outcome assessment is best achieved by using a combination of instruments or a single instrument which is designed to measure the treatment effect on impairment, activity, participation, satisfaction, and health-related quality of life.

International Outcomes Inventory for Hearing Aids (IOI-HA). In 1999, an international workshop "Measuring Outcomes in Audiological Rehabilitation Using Hearing Aids" took place in Eriksholm, Denmark. The workshop was focused on issues related to the use and promotion of outcome measures, as well

as the design and selection of appropriate tools.[44] As a result of the workshop, a new instrument, the IOI-HA was developed. The instrument, which contains seven questions, was designed to be practically oriented and was viewed as more of a mini-profile than a scale. The IOI-HA was not intended to be used as a substitute outcome measure rather as a supplement. If used as a supplement in research studies, the IOI-HA has the potential to generate a core set of data that can be compared across the investigations,[60] and thus increase the evidence to direct practitioners in the use of the most efficacious approaches to hearing aid intervention. Each of the IOI-HA items is designed to target a different outcome domain: number of hours per day of hearing aid use; benefit in terms of improvement in hearing-related activities; residual activity limitations; satisfaction; residual participation restrictions; impact on others; and, quality of life. Each item has five response choices and is scored on a scale of 1 to 5, with 1 indicating the most negative response and 5 the most positive. Psychometric data for the IOI-HA have been developed.[60] Initially designed to be appended to research protocols without significant cost in time or other resources, the brevity and inclusiveness of the IOI-HA has made it attractive to practitioners as well as researchers.[61] Thus, Cox and colleagues[61] provided normative data which can be used by clinicians to determine the relative success of a hearing aid fitting for an individual patient. Information about the IOI-HA is available at http://harlmemphis.org/index.php/clinical-applications/.

The outcome measures reviewed here as well as others that assess activity limitations and/or participation restrictions are useful for documenting hearing aid treatment efficacy (e.g., Cox et al).[44] Currently, however, less than half of individuals (46%) dispensing hearing aids report using a standardized self-report outcome measure in the hearing aid fitting process.[57] As we move forward in this era of evidence-based practice, it will be increasingly more important that the routine use of clinically applied standardized outcome measures becomes usual and ordinary practice for all practitioners. Only by routinely obtaining outcome measures can audiologists be assured that their interventions make a difference and that their patients have benefited from their care.

Measuring Outcomes for Health-Related Quality of Life: An Important Outcome Measures

There is increased interest in examining the impact of hearing impairment in terms of HRQoL. An assessment of an individual's HRQoL involves more global considerations than those normally associated with impairment, activity limitations, or participation restrictions although each of these necessarily impacts on an individual's perceived HRQoL. A HRQoL assessment commonly involves consideration of four separate factors, or domains: (1) *physical* and *occupational* function, (2) *psychological* function, (3) *social* interaction, and (4) *somatic* sensation. HRQoL assessments are *multifactorial,* that is, they encompass more than one domain of human experience; they are *self-administered*; they are *time-variable,* that is, one's HRQoL may change from day to day depending on changes to any one of the four domains; and they are *subjective.* While specific clinical disciplines such as psychiatry, rehabilitation, cardiology, and oncology use HRQoL measurements to assess outcome, less is known about how audiological disorders and interventions affect HRQoL, particularly when compared to other health-related disorders and treatments.

HRQoL measures can be categorized as *disease specific* or *generic.* Disease-specific measures are useful for comparing different treatment options for the same health condition. Generic HRQoL measures, on the other hand, are designed for use across health conditions. For example, a generic HRQoL measures have been used to demonstrate the cost-effectiveness of cochlear implantation relative to other health disorders.[62] In choosing to a specific or a generic instrument, the benefits and limitations of both approaches should be considered. Disease-specific instruments are clinically sensible; that is, the questions are similar to those used when talking to a patient anyway. As a result, these instruments tend to be sensitive to the effects of treatments that are directed toward alleviating the specific problems identified. Using disease-specific instruments creates problems, however, when comparing treatment benefits across populations or conditions. Conversely, generic instruments allow comparisons across populations or conditions, but may be insensitive to a particular condition and treatment. As a result of these benefits and limitations, the National Institutes of Health consensus statement on HRQoL[63] currently recommends both types of measures.

Pearl ✔

The National Institutes of Health consensus statement on HRQoL currently recommends the use of both disease-specific and generic measures when assessing patient outcome.

Disease-Specific HRQoL Measures: The HRQoL disease-specific instruments were created to measure a specific portion of an individual's health. The questions associated with this type of measure are customized to the HRQoL burden of a specific disorder and its treatment options. The IOI-HA, GHABP, and other measures summarized in ▶ **Table 10.1** may be considered as disease-specific HRQoL measures. For example, Mulrow and colleagues[64] used the HHIE, a disease-specific measure of hearing aid benefit, in a randomized trial of the effect of hearing aid use on HRQoL.

Generic HRQoL Measures: There are two styles of generic measures: health profiles and utilities. Health profiles are self-report instruments that attempt to measure all important aspects of HRQoL. These aspects often include mobility, self-care, depression, anxiety, well-being, etc. Utility measures are derived from economic and decision theory. They represent the preferences of patients for treatment process and outcomes. With utilities, HRQoL is summarized as a single number on a continuum from 0.0 (usually representing death) to 1.0 (usually representing full health) (although there can be scores less than 0.0 which represent states worse than death). Thus, with utilities, an individual can express positive and negative effects of a health disorder or treatment protocol within one score. One utility measuring device utilizes a scale, also known as a *"feeling thermometer"* (▶ **Fig. 10.5**). A patient may be asked to rank her present health state on this thermometer before and after audiological intervention to determine the extent to which our treatment has improved the patient's perceived quality of life.

Standard Gamble. Another utility measure technique is known as the "Standard Gamble" (▶ **Fig. 10.6**). In this approach, the patient is offered a choice between two alternatives: living with health state "B" with certainty (which is presumably their present health state) or gambling on treatment "A." Treatment "A" can lead to either perfect health or immediate death. The interviewer manipulates the probabilities of perfect health and death in choice "A" until the patient is indifferent between his present health state ("B") and choice "A." Obviously, the higher the probability of death the patient is willing to consider, the lower is the health state (or quality of life) inherent in remaining with choice "B."

While the Standard Gamble is most commonly used for theoretical purposes to elicit "utility values" associated with serious life-threatening diseases such as cancer and heart disease, this technique may be useful in determining the impact of an individual's hearing impairment on his/her overall perceived quality of life. It might be useful, for example, to apply the Standard Gamble approach to potential cochlear implant recipients, particularly if candidacy continues to become less stringent. Instead of choosing between "perfect health" and "immediate death," the choice for the cochlear implant candidate might be "normal hearing" and "total deafness." If the patient is reluctant to gamble on a small risk of total deafness, the clinician may assume that the patient perceives his quality of life to be relatively good and not likely to significantly improve with an implant, even if hearing is substantially improved.

Time Trade-Off. An alternative approach to the Standard Gamble is Time Trade-Off (▶ **Fig. 10.7**). In this technique, the patient is offered a choice between living a normal life span in his or her present health state or a shortened life span in perfect health. The interviewer reduces the life span spent in perfect health until the patient is indifferent between the shorter period of perfect health and the longer

period in the less desirable state. An individual who is willing to "trade off" a significant part of his or her life for a shorter life in perfect health is revealing a great deal about his or her perceived quality of life.

Several computer-assisted programs have been developed to measure utilities including the U-titer[65] and the Utility Measures for Audiology Application (UMAA) software.[66] The U-titer was used by Yueh and colleagues[67] in a comparative evaluation of the effect of different amplification strategies on HRQoL and by Abrams et al[68] who demonstrated the sensitivity of utilities to hearing aid intervention.

Profiles. As noted earlier, health profiles are designed in the form of a questionnaire and provide individual scores for each category of health separate from a general health score. Examples of generic profiles referenced in the audiological literature are (1) Sickness Impact Profile (SIP)[47]; (2) MOS SF-36 Health Survey[45]; (3) Health Utilities Index[42]; and (4) World Health Organization's Disability Assessment Schedule 2.0 (WHO-DAS 2.0; WHO).[48] Information about these measures is included in ▶ **Table 10.2**. The SIP measures sickness-related behavior by either direct report from the individual or from observations by another respondent referring to the individual. The MOS SF-36 measures eight subscales of general health that can be categorized into physical and mental components of health status. The Health Utilities Index (HUI) is a generic, preference-scored, comprehensive system for measuring health status, health-related quality of life, and producing utility scores. Individuals are required to select their level of functioning for several attributes. For example, in the Health Utilities Index Mark 3 (HUI3), a person is asked to select one of six descriptors that best represents his/her hearing. Each descriptor (1–6) is associated with a different utility value such that 1 = 1.0, 2 = 0.95, 3 = 0.89, 4 = 0.80, 5 = 0.74, and 6 = 0.61. In the HUI3, utilities are measured for the multiple domains of vision, hearing, speech, dexterity, ambulation, emotion, cognition, and pain and a summary measure is calculated to provide an overall utility value. There have been several studies that

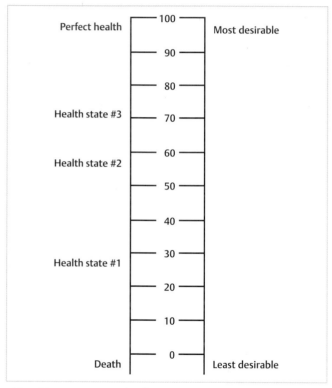

Fig. 10.5 An example of a generic, utility measure known as a "feeling thermometer." The patient is asked to rate their overall quality of life on the thermometer before and after treatment. The difference may indicate the degree to which intervention has improved the patient's overall quality of life.

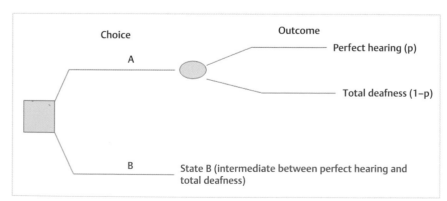

Fig. 10.6 Standard gamble technique to determine the degree to which a patient's hearing impairment impacts on their perceived quality of life. (p), the probability of perfect hearing; (1–p), the probability of total deafness. (p) and (1–p) are manipulated until the patient is indifferent between choice A with its associated risk and choice B, their present health state.

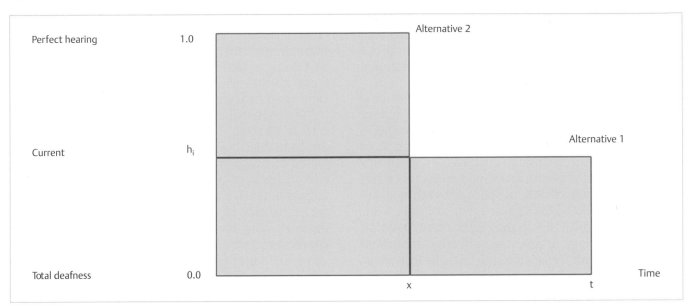

Fig. 10.7 Time trade-off technique to determine perceived quality of life associated with hearing loss. h_i, perceived quality of life; x, total time with perfect hearing. x and t are manipulated until the patient is indifferent between a normal life span with existing hearing and shorter life expectancy with "perfect" hearing.

Table 10.2 Comparison of cost analysis procedures

This economic measure	Answers this question	As measured by
Cost analysis	How much does it cost me to deliver my service?	Dollars
Cost-benefit analysis	Will the generated revenue or cost avoidance associated with delivering my service exceed my expenditures?	Dollars vs. dollars
Cost-effectiveness analysis	Which service option, among several, offers the best clinical results for each dollar spent?	Clinical improvement (%, dB, etc.) per dollars spent
Cost-utility analysis	Which service option, among several, offers the largest improvement in quality life, as determined by the patient, for each dollar spent?	Dollars per quality-adjusted life-years

utilized the HUI3 to determine the effect of hearing aids on self-perceived HRQoL.[69,70] The WHO-DAS 2.0 consists of 36 items organized into six domains: communication, mobility, self-care, interpersonal, life activities, and participation in society. The WHO-DAS 2.0 assesses difficulties with functioning and disability in each of these six domains over the past 30 days. For each question an individual is asked "In the last 30 days how much difficulty did you have in....," responses are given on a five-point Likert-type scale from 1 (none) to 5 (extreme/cannot do). Six domain scores are generated along with a total score. Raw scores are transformed into standardized scores that range from 0 indicating the highest level of functioning to 100 indicating the lowest level of functioning. The domains of communication, mobility, and self-care reflect the WHO-ICF dimension of activity and the interpersonal, life activities, and participation domains reflect the WHO-ICF dimension of participation.

The SIP and the SF-36 were designed to measure the impact of illness and disease on an individual's HRQoL. The SIP is devised of multiple subscales with a grand total of 136 items. It is time consuming and not easy to administer, which limits its clinical utility. The SF-36 is much shorter, easy to administer, and is commonly used among quality-of-life researchers. Unfortunately, in reviewing the use of the SIP and the SF-36 as outcome measures for hearing aid intervention, Bess[71] concluded that while currently available generic health status instruments were successful in determining the impact of hearing loss on functional status and health-related quality of life, the instruments were not particularly responsive to hearing aid intervention. Since Bess's review, the responsiveness of the WHO-DAS 2.0 to hearing aid intervention was demonstrated in a large clinical trial.[19] A systematic review and meta-analysis of the impact of hearing aids on HRQoL among adults was conducted by Chisolm and her colleagues[18] which concluded that the provision of hearing aids does, indeed, improve HRQoL by reducing the psychosocial and emotional consequences of sensorineural hearing loss.

One reason that HRQoL assessment is receiving increased attention throughout health care is that the outcomes data obtained can be combined with economic data to examine the cost-effectiveness of particular treatments. In one approach, the relationships among cost, benefit, and time are examined and reported in terms of dollars spent for each quality-adjusted life-year (QALY) gained. For example, Mulrow and colleagues[64] using the HHIE determined that hearing aids were a very cost-effective treatment for veterans with sensorineural hearing loss, costing only $200 per hearing QALY gained. In a study comparing hearing aid use alone with hearing aid use in conjunction with short-term group postfitting audiological rehabilitation (AR), Abrams et al[72] determined that hearing aid alone treatment cost $60.00 per QALY gained, while hearing aids plus AR cost only $31.91 per QALY gained, making hearing aids plus AR the more cost-effective treatment. The concept of QALY and other economic assessments of outcome will be discussed in greater detail later in this chapter.

Pearl

Quality-adjusted life-year analyses demonstrate that maximum benefit is achieved per dollar spent when intervention is begun as early as possible.

Measuring Outcomes for Satisfaction

The measurement of *satisfaction* as a clinical outcome presents unique problems. Whereas measures of impairment, activity, participation, and HRQoL can be referenced to a specific treatment intervention, a patient's perception (judgment) of satisfaction involves a constellation of factors, many of which are peripheral to the treatment. These may include, but are not limited to, expectations of success, perceived value, cosmetic appeal, comfort, ease of use, and competent, efficient service delivery.

The concept of value warrants elaboration. For paying patients, the issue is fairly clear—they can return the hearing aid if they don't feel they are getting their money's worth. For Veterans Affairs (VA) patients, on the other hand, the issue of determining the influence of value on satisfaction is problematic. Individuals might keep the instruments even if they are dissatisfied, as there is no economic incentive to return the aids. For these individuals, however, the

concept of value is often related to such noneconomic factors as their perception of service-related entitlement. Interestingly, an investigation of the impact of cost on perceived benefit[73] revealed that HHIE scores were no different between groups of insured and uninsured hearing aid recipients.

The most common way of documenting satisfaction is through questionnaires. Numerous surveys are available; however, only a few have been subjected to psychometric evaluation. The most extensive instrument assessing satisfaction with hearing aids and service delivery is the MarkeTrak Survey series developed by Kochkin[74] for the hearing aid industry. The MarkeTrak survey has been administered every few years with the last (the ninth) in 2014.[75] Other questionnaires include the Hearing Aid Users Questionnaire,[76] an 11-item clinical instrument developed and evaluated on an Australian adult population that assesses both device and service delivery satisfaction; and, the Satisfaction with Amplification in Daily Life (SADL),[46] which is a 15-item instrument that assesses the patient's level of satisfaction among several hearing aid–related dimensions including perceived positive and negative effects of amplification, service and cost, and perceived effect on personal image. The Device-Oriented Subjective Outcome Scale (DOSO; Cox et al[77]) is not specifically purported to be a satisfaction measure; however, many of the 40 items in the full form (and 25 items in the short version) query the patient regarding "how good" the hearing aids are at, for example, making music pleasant, providing a pleasing sound quality, not whistling during use, and making the batteries easy to change. Finally, many clinics have developed their own measures to assess patient satisfaction.

10.4 The Economics of Outcomes

The emphasis on the "bottom line" in health care has refocused discussion of outcomes to the costs as well as the results of treatment. It is no longer sufficient to demonstrate that an intervention has made a difference in the impairment, participation, activity, satisfaction, or quality-of-life domains. Sufficiency now demands that the outcome has been achieved at "reasonable costs." The definition of "reasonable" is often left up to the entity paying the bills—the insurer, HMO, government agency, or patient. It is becoming increasingly important for audiologists to understand the concepts of health care economics in order to analyze their costs, compare the costs of different treatment options, operate efficient and competitive practices, and determine costs as a function of benefit achieved for audiological intervention. An understanding of health care economics is essential for analyzing costs and benefits of present services as well as for planning future programs. The discussion below is designed to introduce the reader to the basic concepts of health care economics. ▶ Table 10.3 illustrates the differences among several commonly used health economic measures. For a comprehensive treatment of the subject, the interested reader is referred to Drummond et al.[78]

> **Pitfall**   ✕
>
> Just whose outcomes are you measuring, the patient's or yours?

10.4.1 Cost Analysis

Cost analysis is the simplest and most straightforward of health care economic analyses. It answers the question, "what does it cost to deliver my service?" To answer this question, the clinician needs to identify the resources required to deliver the service. These resources can be separated into direct and indirect costs. ▶ Fig. 10.8 illustrates how a spreadsheet can be used to calculate the cost of an audiological assessment. Labor costs include not only the time spent by the audiologist, with the patient, but also the time spent by the receptionist who checks the patient in and schedules the patient for a return appointment, and the file clerk who is responsible for locating the file, transporting it to the clinic, and reshelving the records (assuming the clinic has not converted to electronic health records). Fringe benefits must also be included in the calculation of labor costs. These include vacation and sick time, employer-paid health and disability insurance, employer contributions to retirement and social security programs, employer-paid continuing education and professional licensing, worker's compensation, etc. Fringe benefits can add 25 to 30% to the labor costs. Supplies and materials used for the procedure are also considered as direct costs. The indirect costs are primarily associated with equipment and space. If these are leased, the costs can be easily calculated. If the equipment and space (building) are owned, the costs

are depreciated over the life expectancy of the equipment and building.

A spreadsheet can be a very powerful tool for cost analysis purposes. The clinician can easily manipulate components of the analysis (salary, equipment, time) to examine various alternatives and the resultant costs. For example, the clinician or manager can answer the following questions: "How will my audiological evaluation costs change if I buy a new audiometer?" "What will happen if I reduce my evaluation time by 10 minutes?" "How will my costs be affected by the 10% increase in the lease for my office space?"

While a cost analysis is critical for determining the dollars spent to deliver services, it reveals nothing about the value of those services; that is, what are the benefits achieved for the dollars spent? As part of an economic evaluation of health care services, the costs of treatment, both direct and indirect, can be compared to the measured outcomes resulting from the treatment. Three methods are used to evaluate the relationship between costs and outcomes. *Cost-benefit analyses* (CBAs) measure outcome by assigning monetary values to morbidity and suffering incurred from treatment. *Cost-effectiveness* evaluations measure outcomes as specific increments of clinical effects such as percent correct for word recognition tasks when comparing various hearing aids, for example. Finally, *cost-utility analyses* (CUAs) measure outcomes in terms of quality of life produced by the clinical effects. CUAs are widely used in the medical field since this type of analysis allows for comparison of the cost-effectiveness between different treatment interventions.

10.4.2 Cost-Benefit Analysis

A CBA answers the question, "If I apply this intervention strategy, will the dollars earned or saved exceed the dollars spent?" A CBA requires assigning monetary units to both the costs of treatment and the benefits achieved. For example, the costs of a balance rehabilitation program, including evaluation and therapy (as calculated through a cost-analysis process), are compared against the dollars saved by

Table 10.3 Example of hearing aid cost-effectiveness analysis

Hearing aid (RIC 312)	Cost (retail)	Outcome score (% correct on speech-in-noise test)	Cost per % increase (cost-effectiveness)
A. Nonwireless, fixed directional, 8 channels	$1,104.42	24%	$46.02
B. Nonwireless, adaptive directional, 16 channels	$1,357.74	16%	$84.86
C. Wireless, adaptive directional, 24 channels	$2,472.64	18%	$137.37

Procedure: audiological assessment (AA)
Number of procedures: [ ]

I. Direct costs:

A. Labor costs:

Position	Salary/hour[1]	Procedure time (MIN)	Cost/procedure
Audiologist			$ -
Receptionist			$ -
Audiology assistant			$ -
			$ -
			$ -

[1] Divide yearly salary by 2080 to determine salary/hour and multiply this value by .26 (or other %) to account for fringe benefits.

Total labor costs per procedure $ -

B. Supplies & materials:

Item	Cost per item	No. per procedure	Cost/procedure
Specula			$ -
Impression material			$ -
Earphone covers			$ -
Impedance tips			$ -
Insert phones			$ -
Miscellaneous			$ -

Total supplies & materials costs per procedure: $ -
Total direct costs per procedure: $ -

Figure 4 (continued)

II. Indirect costs:
A. Equipment costs:

Item	Purchase cost	Life expectancy	Depreciated value	Cost/procedure
Computer				
Audiometer				
Immittance				
Otoscope				
Otoacoustic system				
Sound booth				
Probe mic system				
	Actual cost	Contract	Ttl m&r	

Total equipment costs per procedure: $ -

B. Building depreciation

Bldg cost/yr	# Sq ft	Cost/sq ft	Audio sq ft	Total cost	Cost/proc
[ ]	[ ]				

Bldg cost/yr is calculated by dividing the cost of the building by 40 (life expectancy)

Total building depreciation costs per procedure: $ -

C. administrative support:

Ttl direct costs/proc	% Admin support(default is 15%)
$ -	0.15

Total administrative support costs per procedure: $ -
Total indirect costs per procedure: $ -
Total cost per audiological assessment: $ -

Fig. 10.8   An example of a spreadsheet for analyzing costs associated with a comprehensive audiological assessment.

reducing the need for office visits and medication or the dollars gained by allowing the individual to return to work. If the money gained and/or avoided exceeds the money spent, the service can be considered as "cost-beneficial"—an outcome dearly appreciated by CEOs. However, health care is not a manufacturing business where the price of a widget must exceed the cost of manufacturing the widget for the outcome to be considered successful. As a society, we do not treat cancer or kidney disease with the expectation that the monetary benefits associated with treatment will exceed the costs spent on that treatment. There is an expectation that properly delivered health care will improve outcomes in domains that are not necessarily economic. Nonetheless, a CBA may be a useful exercise when comparing treatment alternatives that have the potential to reduce personal or societal costs.

Willingness-to-Pay (WTP) Concept. A special subset of cost-benefit analysis is the WTP concept; that is, how much is the individual willing to pay for the increased benefits associated with the intervention? There are several examples in the audiological literature that have examined this issue. Palmer, et al[79] asked subjects to make sound quality judgments while listening to Classes A and D amplifiers. The subjects were then asked how much they would pay for a hearing aid with the associated sound quality. The results indicated that the subjects would be willing to pay up to $200 more for a hearing aid with better sound quality. Newman and Sandridge[80] compared objective and subjective outcome measures among subjects who were fitted with three levels of hearing aid technology. While more than 75% of the subjects preferred the fully digital technology, one-third of those switched their preference to a lower level of technology after being informed of the cost. Chisolm and Abrams[81] used a willingness-to-pay approach to examine the value associated with self-perceived hearing aid benefit as measured by the APHAB global score. Results suggested that the participants were willing to pay $22.06 more for a hearing aid for each 1-point increase in APHAB global benefit. In a study of how much individuals were willing to pay above the base price of a hearing aid for specific signal processing features, Abrams et al[82] asked 100 participants to view several video vignettes that simulated advanced signal processing features. Experienced hearing aid users were willing to pay the most for feedback cancellation, followed by directional technology, expansion, and noise management, in that order.

There are some problems associated with WTP assumptions. The same amount of money may be perceived as having inherently greater or lesser *value* depending on one's income. An individual who earns minimum wage, for example, is likely to assign a much greater value to hearing aids for which he or she is willing to pay $500,00 than an individual with a six-figure income.

10.4.3 Cost-Effectiveness Analysis

A cost-effectiveness analysis (CEA) compares the costs of treatment alternatives against a specific outcome measure that is a result of that treatment. For exam-

ple, we accept the fact that improved intelligibility in noise is a highly desirable outcome of hearing aids. We may want to examine the cost-effectiveness of several hearing aid alternatives—a nonwireless, fixed directional microphone instrument with eight channels; a nonwireless, adaptive directional microphone instrument with 16 channels; and a wireless, adaptive directional microphone instrument with 24 channels—by determining the relative cost per intelligibility point gained (▶Table 10.3). There has been little research examining relative cost-effectiveness of hearing aid technologies. Newman and Sandridge,[80] however, conducted a comprehensive benefit, satisfaction, and cost-effectiveness analysis comparing three hearing aids representing different levels of technology: a one-channel linear hearing aid, a two-channel, nonlinear hearing aid, and a multichannel, multiband, digital signal processing (DSP) hearing aid. The investigators found that the subjects scored higher on a speech recognition test with the DSP instrument, but no significant differences were found among the instruments on the self-report measure of benefit or satisfaction survey. The cost-effectiveness analysis revealed that it cost $49.67 for each percentage point improvement achieved with the single-channel linear hearing aid compared to $51.88 with the two-channel, nonlinear instrument and $109.76 with the hearing aid incorporating DSP technology.

> ### Controversial Point
>
> A cost-effectiveness analysis reported in the literature revealed that it cost $49.67 for each percentage point improvement achieved with a single-channel linear hearing aid compared to $109.76 with a fully digital signal processing instrument.

A third-party payer may use the results of the cost-effective analysis in ▶Table 10.4 to determine which hearing aid technology it will cover, or the maximum hearing aid allowance permitted under their policy. However, these choices may not coincide with patient satisfaction. The outcome measure used in the CEA may not be the one of primary interest to the patient. The patient may place a premium on cosmetics, the ability to change programs, or simply possessing the latest technology. As discussed earlier in this chapter, there is a large number of outcome measures from which to choose (objective, performance measures of speech recognition; and, self-report measures assessing activity limitations and/or participation restrictions) any one of which may represent a better measure of outcome than percentage correct, for example. Another limitation of CEA is that it cannot be used to make comparisons across different disorders. For example, while we may know that it costs $46.02 for each 1% improvement

Table 10.4 Four examples of quality-adjusted life-year calculations

QALY example #1	QALY example #2	QALY example #3	QALY example #4
Age of patient—70	Age of patient—70	Age of patient—5	Age of patient—65
Cost of hearing aids —$2,000/pair	Cost of hearing aids —$4,000/pair	Cost of implant—$50,000	Cost of implant—$50,000
Benefit obtained—25% (APHAB)	Benefit obtained—60% (APHAB)	Benefit obtained—30% (open set monosyllables)	Benefit obtained—70% (open set monosyllables)
Life expectancy—5 y	Life expectancy—5 y	Life expectancy—70 y	Life expectancy—10 y
Cost per QALY = $\dfrac{\$2,000}{0.25 \times 5}$ = $1600.00	Cost per QALY = $\dfrac{\$4,000}{0.60 \times 5}$ = $1,333.33	Cost per QALY = $\dfrac{\$50,000}{0.30 \times 70}$ = $2,380.95	Cost per QALY = $\dfrac{\$50,000}{0.70 \times 10}$ = $7,142.86

in intelligibility with hearing aid A, and $46.02 for each 1-mm reduction in blood pressure with medicine C, we know nothing about how improved hearing compares to reduced blood pressure in improving that individual's quality of life. Nor are we able to determine which $46.02 expenditure represents the better utilization of limited health care dollars. Cost analyses which measure the association between cost and quality of life are best examined using cost utility analyses (CUAs).

Controversial Point

Can the sale of a "premium-featured" hearing aid costing over twice as much as a "basic-featured" hearing aid be justified if there is no significant difference in measured outcomes between the two levels of technology?

10.4.4 Cost-Utility Analysis

A CUA focuses on the quality of health outcome achieved by a particular intervention. The analysis typically involves determining (1) the costs of treatment, both direct and indirect, for each intervention approach; (2) the change in scores as a function of treatment on a HRQoL measure; and (3) the estimated quantity of years of life remaining that any treatment effects may influence HRQoL (usually the life expectancy of the individual as indicated by an actuarial table). These data are then used to calculate the cost of treatment for different diseases or disorders per QALY. QALYs are used in a cost-utility analysis to place a monetary value on specified treatment protocols. While CEAs and CUAs are similar from the cost perspective, they differ from the outcome perspective. CEAs examine the cost per unit of some specific outcome achieved; CUAs examine the cost per quality of life years gained.

▶ **Table 10.5** illustrates how CUAs may be used to examine the effects of various hearing aid intervention options on costs per QALYs. Examples 1 and 2 demonstrate that the cost per QALY for more expensive instruments may be *lower* if the improvement in outcome is high enough. On the other hand, examples 3 and 4 illustrate that even a very large difference in outcome cannot overcome the effects of longevity when

Table 10.5 Cost per QALY provided by cochlear implants as compared with other medical devices and services

Technology	cost/QALY
Neonatal intensive care	$7,968
Cochlear implant	$9,325
Coronary artery bypass	$11,255
Coronary angioplasty	$11,485

Abbreviation: QALY, quality-adjusted life year.
Source: With permission from Wyatt et al.[83]

intervention is begun early enough (assuming the device does not need to be replaced). Such an analysis may be very useful for insurers and health care planners when determining what services to offer as part of a comprehensive health care plan. Wyatt et al[83] conducted a CUA on cochlear implants and compared the implant costs with those associated with other common medical interventions. The results of this analysis are summarized in ▶ **Table 10.6**. Cochlear implants compare very favorably with other high-cost medical interventions due to the age at which the patients received their implants and the benefits achieved from using the device. The power of early intervention is nicely illustrated with the neonatal intensive care example. This resource-intensive intervention can cost hundreds of thousands of dollars, but may be a "bargain" when the costs and benefits are spread out over an individual's lifetime. CUAs have been used in several hearing aid–related studies. As previously noted, Abrams et al[62] examined the cost utility of postfitting group AR treatment and found it more cost-effective than fitting hearing aids alone. Joore and colleagues[84] calculated the cost per QALY among hearing aid recipients in the Netherlands and found the fitting of hearing aids to be a cost-effective health care intervention.

10.5 Counseling Patients on the Outcomes of Care

The primary objective of measuring outcomes of care is to determine the extent to which the patient-identified treatment goals have been achieved. Measuring the real-ear–aided response

Table 10.6 Clinically useful measures to assess outcomes in the WHO, generic, and audiology domains

WHO domains	Generic domains	Audiology domains	Outcome measure
Impairment		Verification	a. 2 cc/REM b. Functional gain
Activity limitations and/or participation restrictions		Validation	a. QuickSIN (objective) b. WIN (objective) c. HHIE (subjective—new users) d. APHAB (subjective—experienced users) e. COSI (subjective—new and experienced users) f. IOI-HA (subjective)
	HRQoL	Validation	a. HHIE (disease-specific) b. IOI-HA (disease-specific) c. WHO-DAS 2.0 (generic)
	Satisfaction	Validation	a. selected items from MarkeTraK b. SADL c. HAUQ

Abbreviations: COSI, Client-Oriented Scale of Improvement; HAUQ, Hearing Aid Users Questionnaire; HHIE, Hearing Handicap Inventory for the Elderly; HRQoL, health-related quality of life; IOI-HA, International Outcomes Inventory for Hearing Aids; QuickSIN, Quick Speech-in-Noise Test; SADL, Satisfaction with Amplification in Daily Life; WHO-DAS 2.0, World Health Organization's Disability Assessment Schedule 2.0; WIN, Words-in-Noise Test.

of a hearing aid or administering a standardized questionnaire is of no value unless the information helps in determining whether the patient's stated communication problems have been resolved. It is assumed that the patient and, if appropriate, the patient's significant communication partners have been involved in all aspects of the treatment planning including the establishment of goals—a process known as shared decision making. If so, the patient will want to be informed and counseled concerning the results of each measure along the way from the initial examination through postfitting validation. This is why the establishment of specific and measurable treatment goals at the initial visit is critical to optimizing the outcome of care.

Just as the selection of hearing aid style and feature decisions need to be based on the patient's needs, so do the selection of outcome measures. For example, recall that the electroacoustic and other hearing aid parameters are typically selected to meet three specific goals: (1) make soft sounds audible; (2) make normal conversational speech comfortably loud and understandable; and (3) make loud sounds loud but tolerable. These three goals are verified through the measurement of the output of the hearing aid response at the tympanic membrane. Counseling the patient as to why you are performing real-ear measures and what is happening during the measurement (i.e., what the lines on the graph represent and why you are adjusting those lines)

informs the patient regarding the extent to which the audibility and comfort goals have been achieved.

More importantly, however, are the benefits associated with counseling the patient on the results of your validation measures. After all, these measures inform the clinician, patient, and family members whether the treatment objectives have been achieved. While comparing unaided to aided speech recognition scores may yield some measure of benefit, those results don't provide much of an opportunity for counseling other than to communicate the scores (which are not particularly representative of the patient's real-world experiences). By contrast, self-reported benefit questionnaires like the APHAB and HHIE also provide pre- and postfitting scores, but the counseling opportunity does not lie in the numbers but, rather, in the individual questionnaire items. For example, if the patient still answers "Yes" to the question, "Does a hearing problem cause you difficulty in the movies or theater?" this is an outstanding opportunity to counsel and educate the patient about hearing assistive technology options for the theater. Similarly, if one of the patient's treatment priorities, as identified on the COSI, was to be able to understand conversations with her husband at her favorite restaurant and posttreatment results indicate persistent problems in this situation, this offers an excellent opportunity to counsel the patient and communication partner concerning the benefits of employing remote microphone technology, completing a computerized auditory training program to improve speech-in-noise understanding, and/or participating in your practice's group AR program where communication strategy skills will be taught and practiced.

A comprehensive discussion of effective counseling techniques for audiologists is beyond the scope of this chapter but specific behaviors that have been identified by Terrie[85] as being particularly important include the ability to do the following:

- Establish trust.
- Communicate verbally.
- Communicate nonverbally.
- Listen.
- Ask questions.
- Remain clinically objective.
- Show empathy and encouragement.
- Provide privacy and confidentiality.
- Tailor counseling to meet patient needs.
- Motivate patients.

10.6 Outcomes and Evidence-Based Practice

In examining the available evidence for hearing aid outcomes, Maki-Torkko and colleagues[86] noted a paucity of studies that provide high-quality evidence to guide the practitioner in determining candidacy, amplification characteristics, and rehabilitation plans for individuals with hearing loss. Rather, as Van Vliet[87] points out, practitioners have tended to depend on clinical experience. The recent emphasis on EBP makes the measurement of hearing aid treatment outcomes of great importance on the national health care stage. By routinely measuring clinical outcomes and engaging in carefully controlled clinical trials, audiologists can build a foundation for evidence-based CPGs. To examine the current state of evidence for practices related to hearing aid rehabilitation in adults, the interested reader is referred to the American Academy of Audiology's *Proposed Guideline for the Audiological Management of Adult Hearing Impairment.* CPGs help to minimize variability in outcome, maximize treatment effectiveness, reduce risks, decrease waste, and improve patient satisfaction. The development and implementation of EBP clinical practice guidelines have the potential to elevate the profession of Audiology among third-party payers, other health care providers, and, most importantly, current and future patients.

A key player in EBP clinical practice guideline development is the Agency for Health Care Research and Quality (AHRQ; www.ahrq.gov). The AHRQ is the health services research arm of the U.S. Department of Health and Human Services (HHS). One of its missions, through the National Guideline Clearing House (NGC), is to provide physicians, health professionals, health care providers, health plans, integrated delivery systems, purchasers, and others objective and detailed information on clinical practice guidelines and to further their dissemination, implementation, and use. In addition, the AHRQ reviews and synthesizes scientific evidence for conditions or technologies that are costly, common, or important to the Medicare or Medicaid programs. To accomplish this goal, the AHRQ supports 13 EBP centers throughout the United States and Canada. There are several reviews and clinical practice guidelines that would be of interest to audiologists including a review of the evidence on the effectiveness of universal hearing screening among newborns and EBP guidelines for the medical management of otitis media. While there are EBP guidelines for contact lens care, there are no evidence reports related to hearing aids or the nonmedical management of hearing loss.

AHRQ evaluates the evidence for a specific condition or technology assigning a recommendation across three major categories: the *level* of evidence, the *grade* of the evidence, and the *strength of recommendations* that can be made based on the evidence review and which often forms the foundation for a CPG. Each of these categories is briefly described below.

Levels of evidence:

- Level 1 evidence results from large randomized trials with clear-cut results where there is low risk of error.
- Level 2 evidence results from small, randomized trials with uncertain results (moderate to high risk of error).
- Level 3 evidence is collected from nonrandomized, contemporaneous controls.
- Level 4 evidence is from nonrandomized, historical controls and expert opinion.
- Level 5 evidence is the result of uncontrolled studies, case series, and expert opinion.

Grades of evidence:

- Grade A study requires level 1 evidence—randomized clinical trials.
- Grade B studies involve level 2 evidence (well-designed clinical trials that may not be randomized).
- Grade C studies involve levels 3, 4, or 5 evidence.

Strength of recommendations: As a result of the review and grading of the evidence by AHRQ, recommendations are made for a particular intervention. Such recommendations become the basis of a CPG.

- Level I recommendations are usually indicated, always acceptable, and considered useful and effective (requires grade A evidence).
- Level IIa recommendations are considered acceptable, of uncertain efficacy, and may be controversial. The weight of evidence is in favor of usefulness/efficacy (requires grade B evidence).
- Level IIb recommendations are acceptable, of uncertain efficacy, and may be controversial. Level IIb recommendations may be helpful, and are not likely harmful (requires grade C evidence).
- Level III recommendations are not acceptable, of uncertain efficacy, and may be harmful.

Sources of evidence: While there are no audiological specific evidence reviews conducted by the AHRQ, there are numerous available sources of evidence to assist the audiologist with an EBP approach and Cox[88] presents a detailed outline of how to engage in an EBP-based review of a clinical question. These sources of evidence available to the audiologist include books, nonpeer-reviewed journals (e.g., The Hearing Review, The Hearing Journal), peer-reviewed journals (e.g., The International Journal of Audiology, Ear & Hearing, American Journal of Audiology, Journal of the American Academy of Audiology), electronic bibliographic databases (e.g., Google Scholar, PubMed http://www.ncbi.nlm.nih.gov/pubmed; CINAHL: https://health.ebsco.com/products/the-cinahl-database and EBP websites (e.g., Center for Evidence-Based Medicine: http://www.cebm.net/; ASHA: http://www.asha.org/Research/EBP/EBSRs/; the Cochrane Collaboration: http://www.cochrane.org/; and AHRQ).

Critical review of the evidence: Even without a systematic review of the audiological evidence, research concerning the clinical efficacy of audiological intervention is continually being conducted and reported. Not every article published necessarily represents good science or research. As a matter of fact, the AHRQ often rejects many articles as part of its evidence reviews due to poor quality research. Abrams et al[89] and Cox[88] delineate the criteria with which clinicians need to become familiar so that they can learn to distinguish higher quality from poorer quality research. These criteria include (1) knowledge of participant selection procedures; (2) whether participants were truly randomized into treatment arms; (3) the importance of "blinding" both participants and examiners to treatment arms; (4) the importance of having an adequate sample size to detect clinically meaningful effects;

(5) a clear description of the therapeutic regimen, including descriptions of how the hearing instruments were selected and fit; (6) use of well-selected outcome measures with known psychometric properties; (7) detailed information about study procedures; (8) discussion of withdrawals and study dropouts; (9) consideration of confounds and biases and if discovered how they were resolved; and, finally (10) justification of statistical analyses with results properly reported and interpreted.

10.7 Conclusion

As the demand for EBP increases in health care, audiologists need to incorporate outcome measures such as those reviewed in this chapter as part of their standard clinical protocol. It is not enough for patients to simply express satisfaction with the services or devices they receive. Audiologists must be able to document the impact of those services through the use of standardized measures of objective and/or subjective benefit and satisfaction.

Measuring outcomes is nothing more than applying the scientific method to a clinical application. We develop a hypothesis that a particular hearing aid with specific features (independent variables) will have a certain effect in the activity and participation domains, as well as the quality of life of our patient (dependent variables). We apply the chosen treatment to our patient, measure and analyze the results and determine whether or not we have proven our hypothesis. In a sense, every clinical intervention is a scientific experiment.

Clinicians are probably familiar with many of the measures presented in this chapter and have likely used the data they provide to adjust hearing aid parameters, counsel patients, or assess satisfaction. ▶Table 10.6 illustrates how some of these measures can be applied to the WHO-ICF domains, the domains of HRQoL and satisfaction, as well as the common Audiology terminology applied to these outcome measures. The measures selected for this table were chosen for their clinical practicability. They are easy to use, quickly administered and scored, and empirically tested. It is important for us to realize that these as well as many of the other outcome measures available to us can be used to demonstrate to administrators, insurers, referral sources, other health care providers, our patients and their families that hearing aids are an effective and economical treatment for hearing impairment.

Audiologists, particularly those whose practice primarily depends on the provision of hearing aids, are facing unprecedented pressure from competing market forces including big-box retailers,

[64] Mulrow C, Aguilar C, Endicott J, et al. Quality of life changes and hearing impairment. Ann Intern Med. 1990; 113:188–194

[65] Sumner W, Nease R, Littenberg B. U-titer: a utility assessment tool. In: Clayton PD, ed. Proceedings of the Fifteenth Annual Symposium on Computer Applications in Medical Care. Washington, New York: McGraw-Hill; 1991:701–705

[66] Roberts R, Lister J. Utility Measures for Audiology Application (UMAA) [Computer software]. Bay Pines, FL: VA Medical Center Bay Pines; 2005

[67] Yueh B, Souza PE, McDowell JA, et al. Randomized trial of amplification strategies. Arch Otolaryngol Head Neck Surg. 2001; 127(10):1197–1204

[68] Abrams H, Hnath Chisolm T, Kenworthy M. Utility approach to measuring hearing aid outcomes. Presented at the International Hearing Aid Research Conference Lake Tahoe; August 23, 2002

[69] Barton GR, Bankart J, Davis AC, Summerfield QA. Comparing utility scores before and after hearing-aid provision : results according to the EQ-5D, HUI3 and SF-6D. Appl Health Econ Health Policy. 2004; 3(2):103–105

[70] Grutters JPC, Joore MA, van der Horst F, Verschuure H, Dreschler WA, Anteunis LJC. Choosing between measures: comparison of EQ-5D, HUI2 and HUI3 in persons with hearing complaints. Qual Life Res. 2007; 16(8):1439–1449

[71] Bess FH. The role of generic health-related quality of life measures in establishing audiological rehabilitation outcomes. Ear Hear. 2000; 21(suppl 4):74–79

[72] Abrams H, Chisolm TH, McArdle R. A cost-utility analysis of adult group audiologic rehabilitation: are the benefits worth the cost? J Rehabil Res Dev. 2002; 39(5):549–558

[73] Newman CW, Hug GA, Wharton JA, Jacobson GP. The influence of hearing aid cost on perceived benefit in older adults. Ear Hear. 1993; 14(4):285–289

[74] Kochkin S. Introducing MarkeTrak: a consumer tracking survey of the hearing instrument market. Hear J. 1990; 43(5):17–27

[75] Abrams H, Kihm J. An introduction to MareTrak IX: a new baseline for the hearing aid market. Hear Rev. 2015; 22(6):16–21

[76] Forster S, Tomlin A. Hearing aid usage in Queensland. Paper presented at: the Audiological Society of Australia Conference; May 1988; Perth

[77] Cox RM, Alexander GC, Xu J. Development of the Device-Oriented Subjective Outcome (DOSO) scale. J Am Acad Audiol. 2014; 25(8):727–736

[78] Drummond M, O'Brien B, Stoddart G, Torrance G. Methods for the Economic Evaluation of Health Care Programmes. 2nd ed. New York, NY: Oxford University Press; 1997

[79] Palmer CV, Killion MC, Wilber LA, Ballad WJ. Comparison of two hearing aid receiver-amplifier combinations using sound quality judgments. Ear Hear. 1995; 16(6):587–598

[80] Newman CW, Sandridge SA. Benefit from, satisfaction with, and cost-effectiveness of three different hearing aid technologies. Am J Audiol. 1998; 7(2):115–128

[81] Chisolm TH, Abrams HB. Measuring hearing aid benefit using a willingness-to-pay approach. J Am Acad Audiol. 2001; 12(8):383–389, quiz 434

[82] Abrams H, Block M, Chisolm TH. The effects of signal processing and style on perceived value of hearing aids. Hear Rev. 2004; 11:16

[83] Wyat J, Niparko J, Rothman M, deLissovoy G. Cost effectiveness of the multichannel cochlear implant. Am J Ontol. 1995; 16(1):52–62

[84] Joore MA, Van Der Stel H, Peters HJ, Boas GM, Anteunis LJ. The cost-effectiveness of hearing-aid fitting in the Netherlands. Arch Otolaryngol Head Neck Surg. 2003; 129(3):297–304

[85] Terrie Y. 10 behaviors of effective counselors. Pharmacy Times. http://www.pharmacytimes.com/publications/issue/2008/2008-05/2008-05-8527. Accessed March 1, 2008

[86] Mäki-Torkko EM, Brorsson B, Davis A, et al; Mair LWS. Hearing impairment among adults—extent of the problem and scientific evidence on the outcome of hearing aid rehabilitation. Scand Audiol Suppl. 2001; 54(54):8–15

[87] Van Vliet D. The current status of hearing care: can we change the status quo? J Am Acad Audiol. 2005; 16(7):410–418

[88] Cox RM. Evidence-based practice in provision of amplification. J Am Acad Audiol. 2005; 16(7):419–438

[89] Abrams H, McArdle R, Chisolm TH. From outcomes to evidence: best practices for audiologists. Semin Hear. 2005; 26(3):157–169

Suggested Reading

Bentler RA, Kramer SE. Guidelines for choosing a self-report outcome measure. Ear Hear. 2000; 21(suppl 4):37–49

Johnson CE, Danhauer JL. Handbook of Outcomes Measurement in Audiology. Clifton Park, NY: Thomson Delmar Learning; 2002

11 Hearing Aid Selection and Prescription for Children

Ryan W. McCreery

11.1 Introduction

Hearing aids are an essential intervention for most infants and children who have permanent hearing loss. Recent policy changes related to universal newborn hearing screening and early detection and intervention programs around the world have enabled professionals to diagnose hearing loss and provide early intervention at an early age. The age of identification of hearing loss and subsequent hearing aid fitting has been lowered from an average of two and a half years around the turn of the century[1] to more than half of children receiving amplification by 7 months of age in recent years.[2] Despite this rapid progress, the quality of hearing aid fitting in infants and children remains unacceptably low. Recent evidence suggests that over half of infants and children with hearing loss are provided with less gain than pediatric prescriptions and up to one-third may not receive adequate access to speech for their degree of hearing loss.[3] The good news is that these inadequacies are largely preventable through appropriate selection and verification of amplification using child-specific approaches. The purpose of this chapter and following two chapters will be to describe an evidence-based process for optimizing hearing aids for children and monitoring outcomes.

The first stage of the amplification process is to determine when amplification is warranted for children. The issue of hearing aid candidacy for children is constantly evolving as we learn more about the effects of hearing loss on auditory and communication development. Once the decision to initiate amplification for children is made, professionals must decide which types of signal processing features may help to benefit the child. The hearing aid selection process for children must not only take into account the child's current needs, but also the child's future growth and development. The specific prescriptive method should also be decided to ensure that each child has consistent access to speech for their degree of hearing loss. These introductory steps to the pediatric amplification process provide a solid foundation for minimizing the potential for developmental delays in children with permanent hearing loss.

11.2 Hearing Aid Candidacy for Children

For adults who have hearing loss, the hearing aid candidacy process is based on multiple factors beyond the degree of hearing loss, including the patient's perception of their hearing problem, the patient's motivation, and the listening demands of their daily communication environments. Adults have developed a full complement of cognitive abilities and semantic and episodic memory to allow them to understand when the speech signal is less audible due to hearing loss. The impact of hearing loss on children's communication is more fundamental than in adults, since hearing loss can inhibit development. Not only does hearing loss reduce the child's access to the acoustic signal, but children are in the process of developing the knowledge and skills that are needed to understand speech in degraded listening conditions well into adolescence.[4] In general, children require more of the speech signal to be audible to reach the same level of speech recognition than adults.[5,6]

> **Pearl** ✔
>
> Audiologists are likely to fit children with milder degrees of hearing loss than would be considered for adults. Even mild hearing loss can disrupt a child's communication development.

Additionally, hearing loss during infancy and early childhood can negatively affect cognitive[7,8] and linguistic[9] abilities that are crucial scaffolds for listening and learning. Therefore, a main criterion of hearing aid candidacy in children is based on the extent to which hearing loss disrupts their access to speech.

The primary method of quantifying the effects of hearing loss on a child's access to speech is by estimating audibility for speech. A standardized method of estimating audibility is the Speech Intelligibility Index (SII).[10] The SII is a number between 0 and 1 (or a percentage between 0 and 100) that estimates the weighted proportion of the speech spectrum that is audible to the listener. A value of 0 indicates that none of the long-term average speech spectrum (LTASS) is audible to the listener, whereas a value of 1 indicates that the entire LTASS is audible. Most often, the SII is estimated for average speech using an LTASS with an input level of 60- or 65 dB sound pressure level (SPL), though audibility at higher or lower speech input levels also may be of interest. The SII may be calculated without amplification (unaided SII), where the unamplified LTASS is compared to the listener's audiometric thresholds. The SII can also be expressed as an aided estimate of audibility, where the amplified LTASS measured during hearing aid verification is compared to the listener's thresholds. A comparison of the unaided and aided audibility provided by a hearing aid can be used to estimate the increase in auditory access that a listener would receive with amplification.

Controversial Point

How much of a reduction in audibility compared to normal hearing should be considered sufficient to warrant a hearing aid? There is limited direct evidence available to guide clinical practice in this area. Walker et al[11] found that children with pure tone averages around 23.5 dB had disruptions in speech and language abilities compared to peers with normal hearing. Many of these children had SII values around 0.80. This suggests indirectly that hearing losses that reduce the audibility of speech to around 0.80 may impact speech and language development and should warrant a discussion about hearing aid candidacy. However, more direct evidence is needed to answer this question.

Another factor that influences hearing aid candidacy in children is the consideration of individual differences in ear canal acoustics, which can influence the measurement of thresholds for transducers like insert earphones that couple with the child's ear canal. A more extensive discussion of the influence of ear canal acoustics on audiometric thresholds and amplification will be highlighted in Chapter 12, but a brief discussion of key issues is essential for discussion of hearing aid candidacy for children. The volume of the ear canal not only varies widely across children of the same age, but also increases for any given child as they grow and develop. For a given SPL, the level in the ear canal increases as the volume of the ear canal decreases. This means that the sound level in the ear canal during hearing assessment or from a hearing aid can be higher or lower than calibrated values. Insert earphones often used to measure thresholds in children are calibrated using a 2-cm^3 coupler designed to approximate the ear canal volume of an average adult. The calibrated dB HL level from the audiometer or auditory brainstem response (ABR) equipment used to measure thresholds may be considerably higher in an infant's or child's ear canal that is smaller than the 2-cm^3 coupler used for calibration. The higher dB SPL level in the smaller ear canal can lead to an underestimation of threshold levels, if individual ear canal acoustics are not taken into consideration. Determinations of hearing aid candidacy in children should not be based solely on dB HL threshold levels from the audiogram or estimated threshold levels from ABR systems due to the risk of underestimation of thresholds for children with small ear canal volume, particularly infants. Ear canal acoustics also affect the output of the hearing aid in the ear canal. Children with smaller ear canal volumes may have significantly higher hearing aid output in their ear canal. The amount of amplification required to make speech audible will increase over time as the child's ear canal increases in size and the effective output level of the hearing aid decreases.

The individual variability related to differences in ear canal acoustics across children and increase in ear canal volume over time as children grow mean the same audiometric thresholds may have vastly different implications for audibility across children or over time. As a result, standard audiometric thresholds in dB HL are not always an effective indicator of hearing aid candidacy in children. For example, the same audiogram in ▶Fig. 11.1a has very different effects on audibility for two children with different ear canal acoustics.

Child 1 (▶Fig. 11.1b) has a much greater reduction in unaided audibility because the level of the signal during the audiometric testing was significantly higher than it was for Child 2 (▶Fig. 11.1c) for the same dB HL dial setting on the audiometer. In order to avoid this conundrum, the impact of the thresholds on unaided audibility can be estimated as an objective way to assess amplification

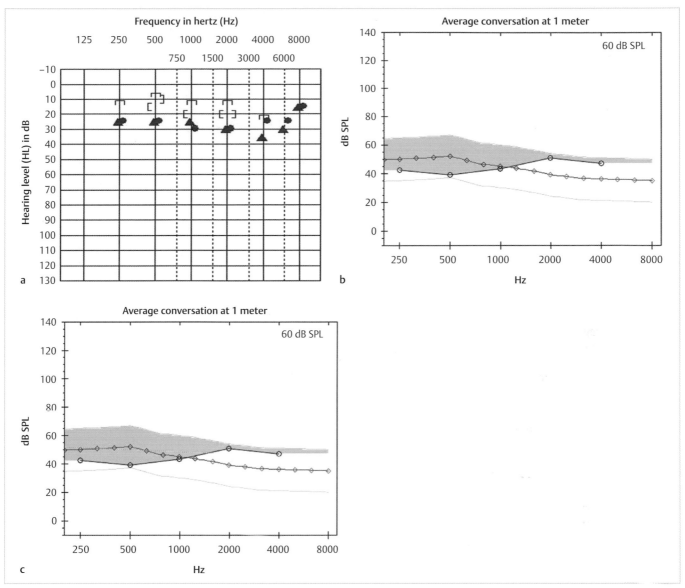

Fig. 11.1 **(a)** Audiogram for a child with mild-to-moderate hearing loss. Circles are the thresholds in the right ear, and triangles are thresholds in the left ear. **(b)** Displays the unaided SPL-o-gram (dB SPL by frequency in Hz) for the audiogram in **(a)** based on the real-ear-to-coupler difference (RECD) for a 2-month-old infant. **(c)** Displays the unaided SPL-o-gram for the same audiogram with an RECD for a 9-year-old child. Note that the same dB HL audiogram can result in different amount of unaided audibility depending on the ear canal acoustics of the child.

candidacy. The unaided SII requires that the child's thresholds be converted to dB SPL at the eardrum by incorporating the child's individual ear canal acoustics. The frequency-specific measure used to quantify the difference in dB between the child's ear canal acoustics with an insert earphone or an earmold and the 2-cm³ coupler is known as the real-ear-to-coupler difference (RECD). The RECD is applied to the dB HL threshold, along with a transducer-specific reference equivalent threshold for sound pressure level (RETSPL) to convert the audiometric thresholds to dB SPL in the ear canal. The unaided audibility of the LTASS can be estimated using the SII by evaluating the proportion of the

unamplified LTASS that is above the child's threshold. The unaided SII allows for an individualized estimate of how the hearing loss affects access to speech and how much access can be restored once amplification is provided. Using unaided audibility as one criterion for hearing aid candidacy in children reveals that nearly any amount of threshold elevation outside of the normal range (20 dB HL) can reduce audibility for the average LTASS. Therefore, children with bilateral hearing loss of any degree should be considered candidates for hearing aids due to the potential for reduced access to the acoustic cues that are needed to develop speech and language.

11.3 Diagnostic Assessment for Hearing Aid Candidacy

Estimation of the degree and configuration of hearing loss is essential for determining whether a child is a candidate for amplification. Audiometric thresholds also will be used to prescribe frequency- and ear-specific gain values that will be needed to make speech audible and maximize auditory function. The availability of universal newborn hearing screening in many countries around the world has led to the need to determine candidacy and fit hearing aids on infants at an earlier age than the behavioral audiogram can be measured. Most infants with hearing loss at birth are fit with hearing aids based on estimates of the behavioral audiogram from ABR or auditory steady-state response (ASSR). Rudimentary behavioral responses to sound can be observed in unconditioned paradigms prior to 6 months of age,[12] using behavioral markers such as cessation of sucking, eye-widening, head turns, and preferential looking. Unconditioned behavioral responses for infants younger than 6 months can be observed at levels that may be 20 to 30 dB higher than electrophysiological estimates from ABR or ASSR. The presence or absence of unconditioned responses may be valuable in assessing general auditory development and responsiveness to sound, but present data suggest that such measures are not accurate enough to be used for determination of hearing aid candidacy or prescription of amplification.

Pearl ✔

The presence or absence of unconditioned responses may be valuable in assessing general auditory development and responsiveness to sound, but present data suggest that such measures are not accurate enough to be used for determination of hearing aid candidacy or prescription of amplification.

Other physiological assessments of auditory function can be used to rule out the presence of middle ear dysfunction and to confirm the site of lesion. Tympanometry provides valuable information about the status of the middle ear and potential presence or absence of middle ear dysfunction. For infants younger than 6 months, 1,000-Hz probe tone should be used with tympanometry to minimize the potential for false-negative results. The absorbance of the infant ear canal for low-frequency sound energy can lead to tympanometric results consistent that appear to show normal middle ear pressure and tympanic membrane mobility with a 226-Hz probe tone.[13]

Special Consideration

Classification of 1,000-Hz tympanograms in infants can be more challenging than those obtained with 226-Hz probe tones, which has led to the development of separate classification schemes (Baldwin et al[14]). The clinician draws a horizontal line from the negative tail to the positive tail. If the tympanometric peak is above the horizontal line, the tympanogram is considered normal. If the tympanometric peak is below the line or crosses the line multiple times, the interpretation is abnormal.

In cases where tympanometry confirms the presence of middle ear dysfunction, immediate referral for medical management by an otolaryngologist or primary care provider prior to the initiation of amplification for children is preferable. Resolution of middle ear dysfunction may not always be possible prior to initiation of amplification for children with hearing loss who also have persistent middle ear problems. The contributions of middle ear dysfunction to elevation in thresholds should be evaluated using bone conduction, if possible. Clinicians should attempt to minimize the likelihood for delays in the fitting of amplification related to persistent middle ear dysfunction by making timely referrals for medical evaluation, scheduling follow-up assessments to monitor thresholds and middle ear status, and communication with parents and families about the implications of middle ear dysfunction for amplification in children.

Otoacoustic emissions can also provide valuable supplemental information about the site of lesion in children with hearing loss, though not about the specific degree of hearing loss. Otoacoustic emissions are acoustic responses that can be measured from the outer hair cells in the cochlea. Once the degree of sensorineural hearing loss is greater than mild, otoacoustic emissions are frequently absent or reduced in level. If otoacoustic emissions are absent and middle ear function is normal, there is a high likelihood that there is a hearing loss in that ear that is mild or greater in degree. Otoacoustic emissions are also frequently absent in even mild conductive hearing losses because the presence of hearing loss in the outer or middle ear disrupts the forward transmission of the stimulus used to evoke the otoacoustic emission and the reverse transmission of the emission from the cochlear back to the ear canal where it is measured. In cases where middle ear function is abnormal, otoacoustic emissions are expected to be absent and statements about the status of the cochlea cannot be reliably made. If otoacoustic emissions are present in an ear with hearing loss that is greater than mild in degree, there can be several potential reasons.

First, the reliability of the behavioral or electrophysiological thresholds should be verified to determine if the degree of hearing loss is accurate. The presence of otoacoustic emissions in an ear with significant hearing loss also may indicate that a child could have auditory neuropathy spectrum disorder. Auditory neuropathy spectrum disorder is a type of hearing loss that occurs at a level beyond the outer hair cells in the cochlea, where otoacoustic emissions are generated. In auditory neuropathy spectrum disorder, otoacoustic emissions can be present along with significant elevations in thresholds. Though auditory neuropathy spectrum disorder is rare, children with present otoacoustic emissions and thresholds which are moderate or greater should receive a specialized diagnostic evaluation to rule out the presence of this disorder. As noted in the next section, hearing aid candidacy may be different in children with auditory neuropathy spectrum disorder than in children who have other types of permanent hearing loss.

11.4 Special Cases of Hearing Aid Candidacy

11.4.1 Mild Hearing Loss

Children with mild degrees of hearing loss often experience delays in communication, academic, and psychosocial outcomes compared to peers with normal hearing,[15,16] but deficits are not uniform or routinely observed.[17,18] The mixed developmental outcomes reported in the literature for children with mild hearing loss have led to an inconsistent approach in determining hearing aid candidacy for children. For example, in a recent study of developmental outcomes in children with hearing loss, many children with similar mild degrees of hearing loss received interventions that varied from hearing aids plus regular early intervention to no intervention at all.[11] Objective methods of determining hearing aid candidacy prior to the point where developmental delays are evident are clearly needed.

A comparison of the unaided and aided SII can offer one such objective approach to determining hearing aid candidacy for children with mild hearing loss. Although the SII offers an objective method of quantifying the effects of hearing loss on the child's access to speech, the degree of reduction in audibility that warrants hearing aids has not been definitively established. Some children with mild hearing losses who have unaided audibility of approximately 0.85 experience disruptions in acquisition of speech and language, but others with similar unaided audibility do not.[11,18] Some clinical protocols suggest

ongoing monitoring of communication development milestones in children with mild hearing loss, but this approach requires that children experience disruptions in development before intervention is provided, which is not effective in preventing developmental delays related to mild hearing loss. Emerging evidence suggests that children with mild hearing losses who receive early intervention services and use amplification have improved speech and language outcomes compared to peers with mild hearing loss who do not receive intervention or amplification.[11] Based on emerging evidence and the importance of providing intervention to minimize developmental delays, the American Academy of Audiology Pediatric Amplification guidelines suggest that children with any degree of hearing loss be considered for amplification.

11.4.2 Unilateral Hearing Loss

Hearing loss that occurs only in one ear can also create substantial difficulties in development and communication, despite the presence of normal hearing in the other ear.[19,20,21] Like children with mild bilateral hearing loss, however, the outcomes of unilateral hearing loss have been inconsistent across individuals and studies. Some children with unilateral hearing loss experience few difficulties even without amplification, whereas others seem to experience auditory and communication deficits in line with peers who have bilateral hearing loss. Predicting which children with unilateral hearing loss will experience problems with development and targeting those children for intervention has not been possible up to this point. The number of children with unilateral hearing loss who have been fit with amplification in previous studies varies from 9[22] to 49%,[23] which reflects the lack of consensus about whether or not and how to intervene in children with unilateral hearing loss. Clinicians must weigh several factors when deciding whether to provide amplification for children with mild hearing loss. One major consideration is the degree of hearing loss in the impaired ear. As with bilateral hearing loss, the degree of unilateral hearing loss can range from mild to profound. For children with hearing loss that ranges from mild to moderate, many guidelines recommend a trial with a hearing aid in the impaired ear. In cases where children have aidable hearing in the impaired ear, there is potential to provide binaural stimulation with amplification.

For children with severe or profound degrees of hearing loss in the impaired ear, the impaired ear is unlikely to benefit from direct stimulation. There also is limited evidence that stimulation of the impaired ear with hearing aids can reduce performance overall, a phenomenon known as binaural interference.[24] There is less consensus about the best approach for management in children with severe or profound unilateral hearing loss, but the approaches fall into the following three categories:

1. Routing of sound from the side of the impaired ear to the normal-hearing ear.
2. Provision of hearing assistance technologies in noise or for specific listening situations.
3. Cochlear implantation.

The first approach to amplification in children with severe or profound unilateral hearing loss will involve routing the signal to the opposite ear, known as contralateral routing of sound (CROS). There are several approach to CROS for children with severe or profound bilateral hearing loss, including placing a receiver on the impaired ear that wirelessly transmits sound from that side to a transducer on the normal hearing or using a bone conduction device to route the sound from the impaired ear to the normal ear. The decision about whether to use a wireless CROS or bone conduction CROS approach for a given child may depend on the degree of occlusion that occurs with the transducer on the normal-hearing ear. In infants and young children, the placement of a receiver in the normal-hearing ear for CROS devices can create some occlusion that reduces audibility. The degree of occlusion that occurs with any CROS receiver placed in the ear canal should be individually measured using probe microphone measures of the real-ear–unaided response (open ear canal) to the real-ear–occluded response (CROS receiver in the normal-hearing ear). CROS devices that reduce access in the normal-hearing ear based on comparison of the unaided and occluded response are not recommended for the obvious reason that the child's increased access to sound from the impaired ear may occur at the expense of reduced access in the ear with normal hearing.

Special Consideration

CROS devices do not restore binaural hearing, as the signal is still being routed to a single cochlea. This means that while CROS devices can improve access to sounds on the side of the impaired ear in cases of unilateral hearing loss, the devices may not necessarily result in benefits that would be achieved with the restoration of input to both ears.

Bone-conduction CROS devices use mechanical vibration through the bones of the skull to route the sound to the ear with normal hearing. Bone-conduction CROS devices have the relative advantage over air-conduction CROS devices that they do not occlude the normal-hearing ear. However, bone-conduction CROS devices must be word on a headband for infants and young children. In older children, bone-conduction CROS devices can be surgically implanted. The evidence supporting the use of CROS devices in infants and children with severe-to-profound unilateral hearing loss is limited and shows mixed outcomes. In a study with three teenagers with profound hearing loss, improvements were reported for speech-in-noise in conditions where the speech and noise were spatially separated, as well as parent- and child-reported benefit, were reported.[25] Pennings and colleagues,[26] however, reported that only 50% of older children and adults who received a 2-week in-home trial with a bone-conduction CROS on a soft band elected to pursue surgical implantation of device based on that experience. This research suggests that the perceived benefit of bone-conduction CROS devices may be limited, and extended trials with the device on a soft band with outcome measures may be needed to support candidacy for surgery.

In the past, cochlear implants were not considered an option for individuals with profound unilateral hearing loss due to the presence of a normal-hearing ear. However, emerging research suggests that cochlear implants may be an option for individuals with severe or profound unilateral hearing loss, though the current evidence is limited, particularly for children.[27,28] Even as evidence regarding the benefits of cochlear implantation for unilateral severe or profound hearing loss increases, many children with unilateral hearing loss may not meet candidacy requirements. Some children with profound unilateral hearing loss have anatomical abnormalities to the cochlea or eighth nerve that are contraindications to cochlear implantation.[29] Therefore, professionals should approach cochlear implant candidacy discussions for children with unilateral hearing loss cautiously until the status of the cochlear and auditory nerve can be assessed through imaging.

The negative effects of unilateral hearing loss are sufficient to warrant consideration of amplification, hearing assistance technology, or cochlear implantation. However, the evidence to guide clinical decision making around which options are preferable for a specific child are extremely limited at the present time. Cincinnati Children's Hospital and Medical Center published a comprehensive evidence statement on the treatment of unilateral hearing loss that provides recommendations for outcome measures and further evidence on the topics related to CROS devices. Amplification should be considered as an option for children with unilateral hearing loss to help minimize the potential for problems in development and communication. Further research is clearly needed to better guide candidacy decision related to unilateral hearing loss in children.

11.4.3 Auditory Neuropathy Spectrum Disorder

As noted in the previous section about diagnostic considerations for pediatric amplification, auditory neuropathy spectrum disorder (ANSD) is a specific type of neural hearing loss. In sensorineural hearing loss, the damage to the auditory system occurs at the level of the cochlea and/or the auditory nerve. ANSD is a unique subtype of sensorineural hearing loss where part of the cochlear appears to function normally, while the interface between the cochlea and auditory nerve or auditory nerve are specifically impaired. Diagnostically, ANSD is characterized by normal cochlear outer hair cell function, evident from present otoacoustic emissions or observable cochlear microphonic response from the ABR, combined with severely abnormal neural function, such that ABR waveforms are absent or grossly abnormal. The clinical management of ANSD is complicated by the fact that numerous auditory problems originating from different sites of lesion all have the same clinical presentation. Many different auditory problems within the auditory system are grouped together under the diagnostic umbrella of ANSD. Individuals with an absent auditory nerve can produce the same diagnostic profile as another patient with an intact auditory nerve, but limited neural synchrony of the auditory pathways. The lack of diagnostic specificity has led to criticism of the auditory tests and the use of the diagnostic term as a whole.[30] Perhaps not surprisingly, the variance in etiology for ANSD and lack of diagnostic specificity leads individuals with widely varying auditory skills being labelled as having ANSD. Behavioral audiograms from individuals with ANSD have been noted to vary across individuals from normal hearing to profound degrees of hearing loss with a wide range of audiometric configurations.[31] Conflicting evidence and numerous anecdotal reports have led to conflicting recommendations about whether hearing aids should be recommended for children who have been diagnosed with ANSD.[32,33] (see Roush et al[34] for a review). Children with ANSD who have behavioral thresholds in the profound hearing loss range are most often referred for cochlear implantation, due to limitations in the ability to make speech audible, just as in cases of sensorineural hearing loss.[35] Amplification benefit in children with ANSD who have behavioral thresholds in the mild-to-severe range is considerably more variable than in age-matched peers with sensorineural hearing loss.

Whether or not children with ANSD will accept and benefit from hearing aids is generally not predictable based on the audiogram. Instead, success with hearing aids may be related to suprathreshold deficits in temporal resolution.[36] Preliminary evidence suggests that cortical auditory-evoked potentials may offer some additional diagnostic specificity as to which patients have intact auditory pathways,[37] but so far have not proven to differentiate definitively which patients with ANSD will be successful hearing aid candidates.

Our limited understanding of the factors that influence hearing aid benefit in children with ANSD has led to the development of the stepwise management protocol for ANSD by researchers from the University of North Carolina, Chapel Hill.[35] In the stepwise management protocol, every child who is diagnosed with ANSD is provided with a trial with amplification based on their degree of hearing loss from the behavioral audiogram. Children with ANSD are fitted and verified using pediatric prescriptive approaches based on their degree of hearing loss, using the same procedures as children with sensorineural loss. Because the ABR is absent or grossly abnormal in ANSD, behavioral thresholds must be obtained prior to initiating amplification, which often leads to delays in hearing aid fitting. Because conditioned behavioral audiometric techniques cannot be reliably completed until after 6 months of age or later, this can lead to considerably delays in the initiation of amplification for children with ANSD. Once fit with amplification, communication and auditory development milestones must be closely monitored. Children who demonstrate acquisition of speech and language with amplification continue to use hearing aids, and children who show limited auditory responsiveness or development are referred for a cochlear implant evaluation. Recent evidence suggests that infants with ANSD who are fit with amplification using the stepwise approach can achieve speech and language outcomes that are similar to children with sensorineural hearing loss.[33] Children with ANSD who have thresholds in the mild-to-severe hearing loss range should be provided with a hearing aid trial as early as behavioral threshold can be obtained to avoid long delays in the provision of hearing aids or cochlear implant candidacy.

11.5 Prescription of Amplification for Children

Once an infant or child has been identified as having permanent hearing loss, a hearing aid is selected that will provide the child with a sufficient amount of amplification to make speech audible. The determination of what constitutes a sufficient amount of amplification for a given degree of hearing loss is usually determined from validated, evidence-based prescriptive approaches. The audiometric thresholds for the individual child are used to generate the prescription for each ear. Modern prescriptive approaches have been developed based on the assumption that the input–output function of hearing aids has multiple stages of gain and that the input–output functions are typically nonlinear. Thus, the amount of gain prescribed is dependent on their degree of hearing loss and the input level of the signal. The two most widely studied and used prescriptive approaches for prescribing amplification for children are the Desired Sensation Level multistage prescriptive approach (DSL v5.0a),[38] and the second generation of the National Acoustics Laboratory nonlinear prescriptive approach (NAL-NL2).[39] Both prescriptions have pediatric versions that provide greater gain and audibility than the adult prescriptions. The rationale for increasing the gain prescription for children compared to adults is that children require more audibility than adults[5] and that greater audibility has been shown to enhance language development[9] and speech recognition in children who wear hearing aids.[3] Children with hearing loss also show higher preferred listening levels compared to adults with the same degree of hearing loss.[40] However, there are differences between the pediatric versions of NAL and DSL prescriptive approaches in how much gain and audibility are prescribed. ▶ **Fig. 11.2** shows the

differences in prescription between DSL and NAL for three different audiograms.

In general, DSL provides more gain and greater audibility for the same audiogram than DSL, but the differences are minimal in some cases. In a study by Ching and colleagues[41] that compared aided audibility and loudness ratings for DSL and NAL prescriptions for the same audiograms, the results showed that DSL provided slightly greater audibility than NAL-NL2, but that loudness ratings were significantly higher for DSL than for NAL. The authors suggested that the prescriptions provide comparable audibility for most hearing losses, but that NAL-NL2 might be preferred due to lower loudness ratings.

Despite the apparent differences in audibility between DSL and NAL pediatric prescriptions for the same audiogram, research comparing the two prescriptions has indicated roughly equivalent outcomes for children across a wide range of measures. Using a randomized, controlled trial, Ching and colleagues[42] demonstrated no differences in an aggregate measure of language outcomes for children fit with NAL compared to children fit with DSL. However, a modelling study by Ching and colleagues[41] suggested that the higher output levels prescribed by DSL could lead to the potential for amplification-related hearing loss, particularly in listeners with severe or profound hearing loss. The paper defined safety limits for amplification and suggested that children with more than 70 dB thresholds might be at risk for progression of hearing loss if fit with the DSL prescription.

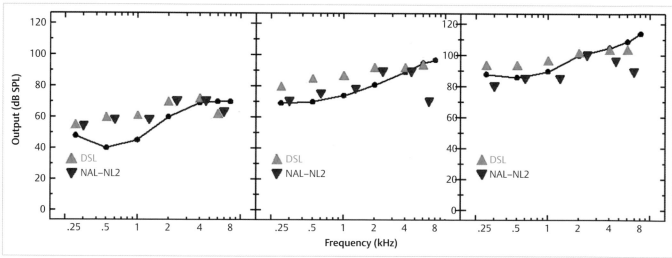

Fig. 11.2 A comparison of aided audibility for a 60dB SPL input between NAL-NL2 and DSL m i/o prescriptions for three different audiograms: mild-to-moderate (left panel), moderate-to-severe (middle panel), and severe-to-profound (right panel). The black dots connected by the black line represents the audiometric thresholds in dB SPL for each audiogram. The green symbols represent DSL targets and blue symbols represent NAL targets for each audiogram based on the real-ear-to-coupler difference of a 3-year-old child. The difference in audibility between DSL and NAL prescriptions increases as the degree of hearing loss increases.

A follow-up study by McCreery et al[43] evaluated whether or not children who wore hearing aids fit to the DSL prescription who were over the safety limits proposed in the model by Ching et al.[41] Children who had hearing aid outputs above the amplification safety limit and wore their hearing aids for at least 10 hours per day were compared to a group of children who had hearing aids below the safety limit over a period of 4 years. The results indicated that children over the safety limit did not experience significant degradation in hearing thresholds over the course of the study. Children with mild-to-severe hearing loss who are fit to DSL m i/o do not appear to be at risk for amplification-related progression of hearing loss, as long as the output of their hearing aids is verified using appropriate clinical techniques. Verification methods will be discussed in greater detail in the next two chapters.

Controversial Point

Some researchers have argued that if comparable outcomes can be obtained with the lower output associated with the NAL-NL2 prescriptive approach, NAL-NL2 should be preferred to DSL as it lowers the risk of loudness discomfort and overamplification. Other researchers believe that the greater audibility that results from the higher output from DSL may help children in specific listening situations. Further research may help to resolve this important issue.

In summary, both the NAL-NL2 and DSL m i/o prescriptive approaches are validated prescriptive approaches that are appropriate for children who wear hearing aids. In most cases, comparable audibility can be achieved for the same audiogram using either prescriptive approach. Prescriptions provide a standardized approach to determining the amount of amplification that is needed for a specific hearing loss, but as children get older and are able to express their preferences about amplification, adjustments of the frequency response of the hearing aid away from prescriptive targets may be needed based on personal preferences. Failure to take individual listening preferences into account can result in the child being unwilling to wear the hearing aids. However, reduction in the gain of hearing aids should occur with the corresponding reduction in audibility in mind. Prior to reducing the output of the hearing aid to address complaints about loudness or sound quality, discussion about alternative strategies that might improve listening comfort in particularly problematic listening situations should occur. An alternative program or frequency response for noisy

situation may be advisable, such as the DSL-noise prescription which reduces audibility for noisy situation in a way that optimally maintains audibility for speech.[44] Noise management strategies are another option that can be used to improve listening comfort in noise[45] without negatively impacting speech understanding.[46] Prescriptive methods for fitting children's hearing aids can be a helpful starting point for any fitting, particularly for infants and young children who cannot describe how well they hear with their hearing aids. As children get older and can express their personal preferences, prescriptions should still be used, and any adjustments away from target based on listening preferences should be documented in terms of the impact on audibility for speech.

11.6 Essential Hearing Aid Features

In addition to selecting a hearing aid that is capable of providing sufficient audibility, there are numerous considerations for hearing aid selection that are specific to infants and children. As noted in the previous section about prescription, the hearing aid must be able to provide adequate gain to match prescription for the child's degree of hearing loss, but infants and children with hearing loss have other unique needs that will influence decisions about the style of the hearing aid, how the hearing aid will be coupled to their ear, and what advanced signal processing features might be beneficial. Each of these issues requires careful evaluation of the listening needs of children, not only at the time of the fitting, but as they grow and develop.

11.6.1 Hearing Aid Style

Behind-the-ear (BTE) hearing aids are generally the most common hearing aid style selected for children who have hearing loss. The durability and reliability of BTE hearing aids typically is much higher compared to custom, in-the-ear devices. As the child's ear canal grows, the earmold that is used to couple the hearing aid to the child's ear can be replaced periodically, unlike custom in-the-ear devices, where the entire device must be returned to the manufacturer for a new shell. In general, the fitting range of BTE hearing aids can accommodate a wider range of hearing losses than in-the-ear devices. This allows the device to be reprogrammed to meet the child's needs for audibility, even if their hearing thresholds change over time. In fact, many models of BTE hearing aids can accommodate degrees of hearing loss from mild to severe. Most BTE hearing aids offer compatibility with a wide range of devices that promote connectivity, such as frequency- or digital-modulation (FM or DM) systems that can be used in the classroom or wireless connections to computers and phones. Because of space constraints related to having to put all of the hearing aid components into the ear, in-the-ear hearing aids may not offer the same level of connectivity as BTE devices. Overall, BTE hearing aids offer the flexibility, connectivity, and durability that children need in hearing aids.

In recent years, the size of BTE devices has been reduced, and new options for coupling the device to the ear have become popular solutions for adults with hearing loss. Receiver-in-the-ear (RITE), also known as receiver-in-canal (RIC), devices are BTE devices where the receiver of the device is placed in the ear canal, rather than being in the case of the hearing aid like traditional BTE devices. (see ▶Fig. 11.3 for illustration.)

Hearing aids with RITE have grown in popularity with adults who wear hearing aids because of their small size and the fact that their appearance is often more discrete than a BTE hearing aid coupled to an earmold. Improvements in the ability to suppress acoustic feedback, often noticed as whistling or buzzing from the hearing aid, have also led to the development of a wide range of BTE devices that can be fit with minimal occlusion of the ear canal, often known as open-fit hearing aids. Some open-fit devices are also RITE, but others are traditional BTE devices with a special tone hook that allows coupling to an open dome. Both open-fit and RITE devices offer adults with hearing loss significant advantages related to occlusion and cosmetics, compared to traditional BTE hearing aids coupled to an earmold. This recent development in the hearing aid market has led some audiologists to question whether or not children may be able to realize some of the same benefits that adults have achieved with RITE and open-fit devices.

Like other decisions related to amplification for children, there are additional considerations when RITE or open-fit devices might be selected for children. One significant consideration is the ability of the RITE or open-fit device to accommodate the child's current audibility needs and also potential increases in gain should the child's hearing loss progress. Most RITE and open-fit devices are designed for adults with mild-to-moderate high-frequency hearing loss related to aging or noise exposure. Children are considerably more likely than adults to have audiometric configurations that include low-frequency sensorineural hearing loss than their adult counterparts.[47] The higher prevalence of audiometric configurations with low-frequency hearing loss in children means that in some cases, RITE and open-fit devices may not provide sufficient gain to improve audibility. Also, the overall fitting ranges for many RITE and open-fit devices are limited and could not be adjusted to provide audibility if the child's hearing loss progresses. The fitting range of RITE and open-fit hearing aids should be verified to determine whether the device can meet the child's current and future audibility needs.

There are other limitations related to RITE and open-fit devices for children. Hearing aids with RITE or that are open-fit may present challenges related to retention of the device on the child's ear. The minimal occlusion of the ear canal with open-fit devices in particular might result in limited retention, particularly on the ear of a physically active young child. Additionally, RITE receivers must often be replaced one to two times per year due to their placement in the ear canal, which can create an added expense for parents and caregivers. As will be discussed in the next chapter, RITE and open-fit devices have limited options for coupler verification, in that these devices must be verified in the ear using probe microphone measures. These verification methods may not be practice or possible for infants or young children. The smaller size of many RITE and open-fit devices also may limit the options for connectivity for FM or DM systems or telecoils. For these reasons, RITE

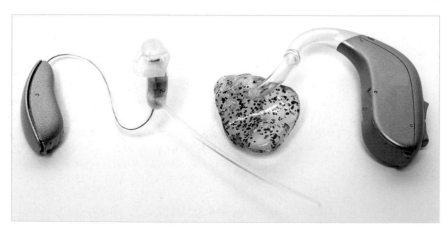

Fig. 11.3 A comparison of a receiver-in-the-ear (RITE) and behind-the-ear (BTE) hearing aids. Note the location of the receiver for each device.

and open-fit devices may not be appropriate until children have reached adolescence.

11.6.2 Hearing Aid Coupling

Because BTE hearing aids are the preferred style of hearing aid for infants and children, most hearing aids for children will be coupled to an earmold. Earmold selection for children has some important facets beyond what would be considered for adults. The preferred earmold material for children is often a softer material than for adults. Vinyl or silicone earmold materials are often recommended for children, as acrylic may be more difficult to modify and may cause skin irritation with soft, flexible pinnae of infants and young children. Once children reach older school age or adolescence, the earmold material may change to acrylic for specific patients to aid with retention or based on the child's preference for a firmer material. Earmolds of all materials are available in a wide range of colors, which not only can be fun for parents and child to choose, but can also be helpful in finding hearing aids that have fallen out of the ear or that are lost.

Earmold venting is also different for children than for adults, related to both acoustic and physical factors. For infants, venting may not be possible due to the very small size of the ear canal. Even in toddlers and preschool-aged children, the ear canal size may not be sufficient to permit a vent or may require a vent that intersects the sound bore due to ear canal size constraints. Intersecting vents in children should be avoided, as the intersecting vent can reduce the high-frequency response of the hearing aid. Once a child's ear canal is large enough to accommodate a sound bore and a vent, venting may be helpful, particularly for children with regions of normal hearing below 1,000 Hz who may experience occlusion with an unvented earmold. Venting can reduce the output of the hearing aid in the low frequencies, which may limit the amount of audibility in the low frequencies that can be provided by a hearing aid.

Whereas adults often can use the same earmolds for a period of several years, earmolds must be replaced much more frequently in children, particularly during the first year of life. Ear canal growth during the first year of life often necessitates replacement earmolds every 3 months. After the first year, earmolds must often be replaced every 6 to 12 months depending on the material and the child's individual rate of ear canal growth. In years past, the need for earmold replacement could be judged based on problems with retention of the earmold in the ear and the occurrence of acoustic feedback. An unfortunate side effect of effective feedback suppression signal processing algorithms in hearing aids is that the fit of earmolds can be very poor before problems with feedback occur. Problems with the effectiveness of the transmission of amplified sound through the earmold or the loss of sound due to gaps in the earmold that function like unintended vents can reduce the output of the hearing aid in the child's ear and audibility. These acoustic changes can occur long before problems with retention are apparent. Therefore, earmold replacement should occur for infants and young children when problems with feedback or retention occur, but also when the output of the hearing aid is reduced to a point where effective audibility can no longer be provided.

Parents should be oriented to watch for problems with acoustic feedback and retention that might occur between regular hearing aid evaluations. In cases where problems with retention or feedback are occurring and the earmold cannot be immediately replaced, slightly lubricating the earmold can improve the fit temporarily until the earmold can be remade.

11.6.3 Tamper-Resistant Features

Most adults who wear hearing aids can manage changing their batteries and adjusting the volume control on their hearing aids as needed. Not only can infants and young children not manage these aspects of their hearing aids, but in some cases there may be a risk of battery ingestion by children who wear hearing aids or inadvertent changes to the hearing aid output if a volume control is moved. Hearing aids that are selected for children must have the option to lock the battery compartment and disable the volume control as needed. Tamper-resistant battery compartments on hearing aids are often special battery doors with a locking mechanism that require either special tools or manipulation of the hearing aid to open. Parents should be oriented to how to access the battery compartment in order to change the batteries as needed. Deactivation of the volume control can be achieved in most cases using the hearing aid programming software. In some cases with older hearing aids, the volume control must be manually blocked using a plastic cover. The use of tamper-resistant features should also be continuously evaluated as children get older and take on the care and maintenance of their hearing aids. Once children are older enough to change and understand how to properly dispose of their hearing aid batteries, tamper-resistant battery compartment

can be replaced with a standard model in most cases. In the case of the volume control, the audiologist may select a hearing aid for a child that has the capability of a volume control, knowing that the child may eventually need access to a volume control as they get older.

11.6.4 Hearing Aid Retention

Keeping hearing aids on children's ears can be a challenging proposition. The challenge can be minimized through the use of a wide range of retention devices that keep the hearing aids in place or at least keep the hearing aid attached to the child when it is removed to avoid losing the earmold or device. Anderson and Madell[48] provided an overview of the most popular retention options for families of children who wear hearing aids, including advantages and disadvantages for each type. Retention devices can broadly be categorized into three groups: (1) corded devices, (2) caps or hats, and (3) adhesives. Examples of all three devices are provided in ►Fig. 11.4.

Corded devices are popular retention strategies that have a sleeve or loop that goes around the device that is attached to a cord that is connected to the child's clothing via a clip. The best corded devices have cords that are stretchable and sleeves that cover the hearing aid and can also reduce the device's exposure to perspiration. Caps and hats have more limited use as retention devices, but can be effective for infants who are occasionally prone to reach up and remove their hearing aids. Because the caps or hats cover the hearing aids, the caps should be verified to ensure that sound input to the hearing aid is not reduced with the cap in place. A cap or hat that does not reduce the output of the hearing aid is said

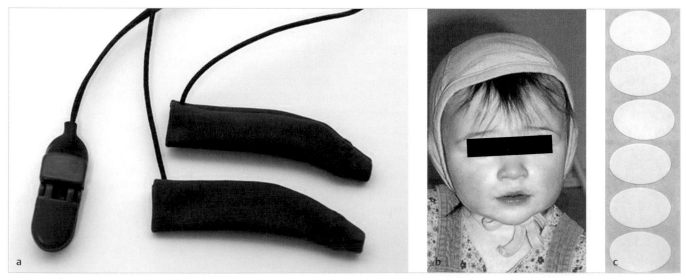

Fig. 11.4 Retention devices for hearing aids for children from left to right: (**a**) corded device, (**b**) cotton pilot cap, (**c**) biocompatible adhesive tape.

to be acoustically transparent, which can be verified using the techniques described in the following chapter. Caps and hats may also be uncomfortable to wear in the summer or in hot climates. Adhesives are biocompatible tape or glue that can be used to affix the child's hearing aid directly to their skin. Wig or toupee tape can be placed on the side of the BTE hearing aid that is adjacent to the child's head for adhesive. Some hearing aid manufacturers also sell biocompatible tape that is already the same size as the hearing aid. A wide range of retention strategies are available and can help provide peace of mind for families who may be concerned about losing the child's hearing aids and earmolds if the child removes them.

Pearl

All retention strategies are not equally effective for every family. Each family should be provided with multiple retention options to choose from for their child. Anecdotally, our experience in our clinic suggests that some families may use multiple retention strategies at the same time to minimize the likelihood that the device will be removed or lost.

11.7 Selection of Advanced Hearing Aid Features

Hearing aids increasingly have a wide range of advanced signal processing features that are designed to process the input to the hearing aid in ways that are beneficial to the user. However, much of the research with current hearing aid signal processing strategies has been completed with adults. Even when research can be completed with children who have hearing loss, it may take many years before the research gets published, leading to gaps in our knowledge about how current hearing aid signal processing strategies may affect perception in children. This section will describe the unique considerations related to the selection of advanced hearing aid features and signal processing strategies for children. In some cases, the recommendations and decision-making process are nearly identical to the process of fitting an adult. In other cases, features may be recommended at a specific age or developmental stage. Hearing aids for children often come with many advanced features and signal processing included, but the audiologist must determine if and when these features should be made available to the child. Five different hearing aid signal processing strategies or features will be discussed:

1. Amplitude compression.
2. Digital noise reduction.
3. Directional microphones.
4. Feedback suppression.
5. Frequency lowering.

A brief description of each feature will be provided, along with a pediatric-specific rationale for activation or delaying activation.

11.7.1 Amplitude Compression

Amplitude compression refers to the fact that most hearing aids reduce the amount of gain provided to a signal as the input level increases. Amplitude compression is so widely available in hearing aids that it is often not considered to be an advanced feature. The alternative to amplitude compression would be to provide linear amplification, which does not match with the specifications of modern hearing aid prescriptions for children. Thus, the decision with amplitude compression is not whether a hearing aid should be selected to have amplitude compression, rather making sure that the amplitude compression in a specific hearing aid allows for the output of the device to match prescriptive targets across a wide range of speech input levels. Whether or not a specific amplitude compression algorithm provides adequate audibility across a range of input levels can be confirmed using the verification techniques described in the next chapter.

The evidence to support the use of amplitude compression in children, beyond the need to use amplitude compression to satisfy the recommendations of nonlinear pediatric hearing aid prescriptions, was summarized in a systematic review.[49] Most of the research with amplitude compression that is specific to children was primarily completed in the early 2000s. Though significant changes in amplitude compression systems have occurred since that time, many of the findings still apply. Studies that have evaluated amplitude compression in children have generally evaluated three types of outcomes: audibility, speech recognition, and listener preference.

Amplitude compression improves audibility overall[50] and for soft sounds,[50,51] compared the linear processing. The improvements in audibility with amplitude compression compared with linear amplification occur because a larger proportion of the speech spectrum can be placed within the listener's dynamic range. The dynamic range can be generally defined as the difference between a listener's thresholds and the level where loudness discomfort occurs. Linear amplification provides the same amount of gain regardless of the input level, which means that when average speech input levels are audible, soft input levels may be inaudible and loud input levels may be uncomfortable. By gradually reducing the amount of amplification as the input level increases, soft sounds can be made audible, while loud sounds can receive less amplification to better avoid discomfort. The relationship between audibility across a wide range of inputs for linear amplification and amplitude compression is illustrated in ▶ **Fig. 11.5**.

The improvements in audibility that occur with amplitude compression might be predicted to also result in improvements in speech recognition. Children, in particular, might be expected to be more likely than adults to benefit from improvements in audibility, as has been the case across several studies.[5,6] For conversational levels, amplitude compression does not appear to enhance speech recognition compared to linear amplification.[52,53] This is not surprising, however, since improvements in audibility with amplitude compression are most pronounced for soft input levels. For soft speech input levels, the findings have been either that amplitude compression improves speech recognition compared to linear amplification[50,51,54] or that performance for linear amplification or amplitude compression conditions are not different.[53,55] In summary, the audibility improvements with amplitude compression for soft input levels may result in improvements in speech recognition under some specific conditions.

Controversial Point

There is some evidence to suggest that the improvements in audibility that occur with amplitude compression come at a cost of increased distortion for specific speech sounds (e.g., Bor et al[56]). Most of this research has been conducted with adult listeners, but raises an obvious potential concern for fitting children with amplitude compression. Few studies of this kind have been done in children, but the general pattern of speech recognition across studies with amplitude compression is either null or positive, suggesting that degradation in speech recognition may be limited to adults or specific listening conditions that have not been explored in children.

Another key outcome with amplitude compression was whether children preferred amplification with amplitude compression over linear amplification. Improvements in audibility for soft sounds combined with greater comfort for louder sounds with amplitude compression were expected to lead to greater listening satisfaction compared to linear amplification. Overall, a greater number of children preferred amplitude compression compared to linear amplification for real-world listening in two studies.[52,53] However, in

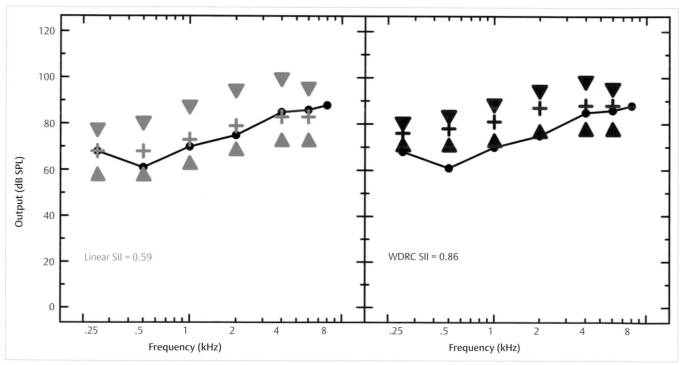

Fig. 11.5 A comparison of linear and nonlinear amplification for the same audiogram. The black dots connected by the black line represents the audiometric thresholds in dB SPL for a child with moderate-to-severe hearing loss. The left panel (green symbols) shows the soft (upward triangles), average (plus), and loud (downward triangles) for a linear prescription. The right panel (blue symbols) shows the soft (upward triangles), average (plus), and loud (downward triangles) for a nonlinear prescription with amplitude compression. Note the higher audibility for a 60dB SPL speech input for the nonlinear prescription, as well as the greater audibility for soft speech.

each study, there were a small number of children who preferred linear amplification over amplitude compression. The preference for linear amplification may have been related to the fact that many participants in these studies had been previously fit with linear amplification prior to the study, and preferred to listen to something that was similar to their own hearing aids. Alternatively, there may be some group of listeners who prefers linear amplification over amplitude compression. The number of participants in these studies is small, so specific indicators that might be used to predict individual preferences for linear amplification or amplitude compression are not available. The decision to use linear amplification for children based on individual sound quality preferences should be weighed against the reduction in audibility that would be anticipated to occur when switching from amplitude compression to linear processing.

Overall, amplitude compression has been shown to enhance audibility and speech recognition for soft speech input levels. Additionally, most children with hearing loss prefer listening to amplification processed with amplitude compression compared to linear amplification. Additionally, both NAL-NL2 and DSL prescriptive approaches assume that amplitude compression will be used to maximize audibility for soft sounds, while maintaining comfort for louder

sounds. As a result, amplitude compression is widely accepted as being appropriate for children for these reasons. The process of verifying amplitude compression to ensure audibility across a wide range of input levels will be discussed in the next chapter.

11.7.2 Digital Noise Reduction

Digital noise reduction refers to a group of signal processing strategies that are generally designed to reduce the perception of background noise. Digital noise reduction typically works by reducing gain when the hearing aid detects that the input is primarily noise. Gain reduction with most digital noise reduction algorithms either can occur across a wide range of frequencies or may be limited to the frequencies where noise is detected. Clinicians must decide whether to activate digital noise reduction, and also may need to determine the amount of gain reduction that occurs when the feature is activated. Because digital noise reduction reduces gain, there is a high likelihood that audibility will be reduced when this feature is activated. Several examples of digital noise reduction are displayed in ▶ Fig. 11.6.

If speech and noise are both present in the input to the hearing aid, the gain reduction will reduce audibility for the speech and the noise. This has

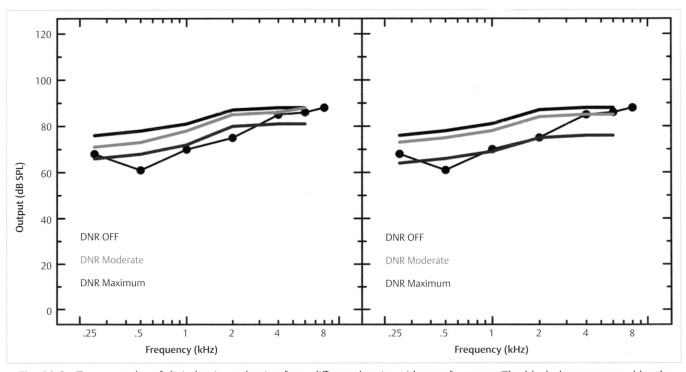

Fig. 11.6 Two examples of digital noise reduction from different hearing aid manufacturers. The black dots connected by the black line represents the audiometric thresholds in dB SPL for a child with moderate-to-severe hearing loss. In each panel, the black line represents the response of the hearing aid for a 60 dB SPL speech noise signal with digital noise reduction off. The green and red lines in each panel represent the respond of the hearing aid to speech noise for moderate and maximum digital noise reduction settings, respectively. The digital noise reduction in the left panel has greater gain reduction in the low frequencies. The digital noise reduction in the right panel reduces gain across all frequencies, particularly for the maximum setting.

led to questions about whether or not digital noise reduction algorithms are appropriate for children, since audibility is an important predictor of their outcomes with hearing aids.

> ## Controversial Point
>
> Reviews of the research literature for adults (Bentler[57]) and children (McCreery et al[58]) indicate that digital noise reduction does not enhance or degrade speech recognition in children or adults with hearing loss. The lack of measurable effects in the research has not changed the perception among consumers that digital noise reduction can improve speech recognition in noise. Patients and their families may need to be counselled about appropriate expectations for noise reduction.

The decision about whether or not to activate digital noise reduction in hearing aids worn by children can be informed by several factors. First, several recent studies indicate that speech recognition is neither improved nor degraded when digital noise reduction is activated for children with normal hearing[59] or children who wear hearing aids.[46,60] This suggests that gain reduction associated with some digital noise reduction systems are unlikely to have a positive or negative impact on speech recognition. Few studies have examined preference for digital noise reduction in children who wear hearing aids, but the study by Gustafson and colleagues[59] found that children with normal-hearing–rated speech processed with digital noise reduction higher on a visual scale of clarity than speech processed without digital noise reduction. However, the magnitude of this effect varied across children, suggesting that not all children rated the digital noise reduction as the preferable condition. Scollie et al[45] recently compared children's preference ratings of noise reduction processing for multiple different digital noise reduction algorithms and found that the effect on preference was either equivalent to amplification without digital noise reduction or enhanced for digital noise reduction. These results suggest that children may not perceive a difference between hearing aid settings with digital noise reduction activated or may prefer it in some cases.

In summary, the effects of digital noise reduction on speech recognition in children is minimal. However, digital noise reduction has the potential to improve listener comfort in background noise for school-aged children. Importantly, the effects of digital noise reduction on perception and sound quality have not been evaluated in children with hearing loss who are younger than 5 years. Given the lack of evidence in this age range, clinicians may choose to approach the decision to activate digital noise reduction in infants and young children on an individual

basis. The amount of gain reduction that occurs with the activation of digital noise reduction should also be verified to ensure that changes in audibility are acceptable for a child's degree of hearing loss.

11.7.3 Directional Microphones

Like digital noise reduction, directional microphones are activated in hearing aids to minimize the perceptual consequences of background noise. Directional microphones process sounds differently depending on the location of the sounds relative to the listener. In most directional microphone systems, sounds arriving from the front of the listener on the azimuthal place are maintained, while amplification for sounds arriving from the sides or behind the listener is reduced. Directional microphones assume that the listener is oriented toward the signal of interest in their environment. If signal of interest is in front of the listener and the background noise primarily originates from the sides or behind the listener, directional microphones have the potential to improve the signal-to-noise ratio through spatialized processing of the noise. In practice, the degree to which the signal-to-noise ratio is enhanced in real-world environments is often limited by the fact that noise sources may be diffuse and reverberation may result in reflections of noise energy from the sides or behind the listener being reflected into the frontal plane.[61]

The question about whether or not children can benefit from directional microphones has been studied in groups of children during early childhood[62] and school age.[63,64] For example, Ching and colleagues[62] examined looking behavior in a group of infants and preschoolers to attempt to simulate the potential directional benefit that they might receive from hearing aids based on their real-world listening situations. Parents of children with hearing loss kept diaries of the types of listening situations that their children encountered. In general, speech was the primary signal of interest in the frontal plane less than 50% of the time, and parents reported that their children spent a limited amount of time in one-on-one situations with a talker in front of them, where directional microphones might be predicted to be most helpful. However, they also found that the decrements that occurred with the directional microphone were small, even when the talker of interest was at the child's side or behind them. This led them to conclude that while the benefits of directional microphones for infants and young children were likely to be limited, the potential negative effects were also small. Importantly, none of the children in the study were wearing directional microphones, which limited the ability to measure the effects of this feature on the child's looking behavior or other outcomes. Ricketts and colleagues[63] also evaluated directional microphone benefit in the classroom for older school-age children. Similar to the results from Ching and colleagues,[62] directional benefit was highest when the talker of interest was in front of the child and the noise was either behind or to the sides and lowest when the talker of interest was to the side or behind the child or the noise was diffuse. In a follow-up study, Ricketts and Galster[64] demonstrated that children who wear hearing aids can effectively orient toward the talker of interest when the talker is to the side or behind, although the children in the study did not have directional microphones activated in their hearing aids.

Controversial Point

The potential benefits of directional microphones have led to the recommendation that they can be activated for school-age children in specific situations, but questions about how the microphone mode should switch and who should switch the mode remain unresolved. One option would be to have the child switch the hearing aid from omnidirectional to directional when they encounter a noisy environment (and back to omnidirectional when the listening situation dictates), but studies have not been reported to determine whether or not school-age children can make this switch reliably for directionality. Another option would be to allow the hearing aid to switch the directionality based on the noise characteristics of the environment. Automatic switching algorithms have also not been evaluated as a strategy in children who wear hearing aids. Clinicians who elect to activate directional microphones in children's hearing aids must have a clear plan for how the microphones will be switched between modes, but have little evidence to inform these choices.

Directional microphones have the potential to provide benefit for speech recognition in noise in specific listening situations for school-age children. However, even when the talker of interest is not in front of the listener, school-age children are likely to be able to orient toward the talker of interest consistently. Limited research with infants and preschoolers suggests that the potential benefits are likely to be similar, but there is limited evidence to suggest whether or not infants and young children can reliably orient toward talkers of interest. If clinicians determine that directional microphones should be activated for a specific child, a switching strategy should be developed so that parents or caregivers or the child can manage this aspect of the signal processing or the microphone switching can occur automatically.

11.7.4 Feedback Suppression

Recent advances in hearing aid signal processing have led to the development of novel approaches to minimizing acoustic feedback. Acoustic feedback can occur any time that amplified sound is received by the hearing aid microphone, creating a feedback loop of amplified sound that often results in a whistling or buzzing sound. An example of acoustic feedback is shown in ▶ **Fig. 11.7**.

Feedback suppression algorithms often use multiple approaches to minimizing feedback including setting gain limits, frequency shifting, and phase cancellation. Some devices may use multiple strategies to minimize the likelihood for feedback. Children may be at particular risk for acoustic feedback because of the ear canal growth that they experience over time, which may result in decreasing occlusion of the ear canal over time. To date, feedback suppression research with

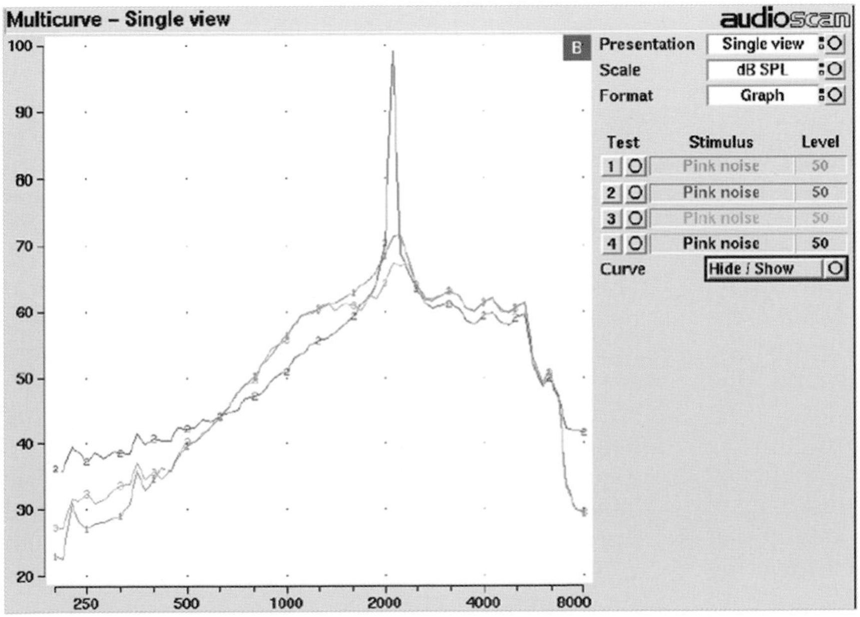

Fig. 11.7 The output of a hearing aid in dB SPL as a function of frequency in Hz. The green line represents the output of the hearing aid in a 2-cc coupler with no acoustic feedback. The pink line represents the response of the hearing aid with a feedback loop introduced to the test box via a speaker that is placed in the test box. The blue line represents the output of the hearing aid with feedback suppression activated in the hearing aid. The response of the hearing aid is only slightly reduced at the frequency where feedback is present, but the feedback peak has been eliminated.

adults has indicated that the amount of gain that can be achieved when feedback suppression is activated is higher,[65] which means that more audibility can be provided prior to the occurrence of feedback. Feedback suppression can also help to extend the amount of time that earmolds can be used as a child grows, since the likelihood of feedback is reduced. In general, feedback suppression is recommended for use with children as a way to maximize audibility and extend the length of time that earmolds can be used.

> ### Pearl ✔
>
> The effectiveness of feedback suppression should have led to the potential for a poorly fitting earmold to be used longer than it should be. When an earmold no longer fits adequately to provide retention or the amount of amplification that can be provided is limited, the earmold should be replaced, even if feedback is not a problem.

11.7.5 Frequency Lowering

The maximum upper-frequency limit of hearing aids is often less than the frequency range of speech. For adults with hearing loss acquired later in life, the limited bandwidth of hearing aids does not have a significant impact on their ability to understand speech under most conditions,[6] although adults may rate the sound quality of speech to be higher with access to high-frequency cues.[65] Children, on the other hand, need to hear high-frequency sounds in order to learn those sounds and understand the linguistic functions that are associated with those sounds. Research from Moeller and colleagues[66] highlights the speech and language problems that can be associated with limited high-frequency audibility. When Moeller et al[66] surveyed the speech sound inventories of children who were fit and identified with hearing loss prior to 6 months of age, they found that these children were developing speech sounds at a similar rate as their normal hearing peers, with the exception of two categories of sounds: affricates and fricatives. They hypothesized that this lack of development for fricative sounds was related to the limited audibility for these sounds through conventional amplification.

Around the same time, several hearing aid manufacturers were developing solutions to improve the high-frequency audibility of amplified sound. One of these strategies was a group of signal processing strategies known collectively as frequency lowering. Early attempts to extend the upper-frequency limit of hearing aids resulted in only modest gains,[67] particularly for listeners with greater degrees of high-frequency hearing loss. Frequency-lowering algorithms were designed as an alternative to extending the high-frequency response of the hearing aid. Most frequency-lowering algorithms alter the frequency of high-frequency sounds so that they occur at lower frequencies in the hearing aid output. Though a number of different frequency-lowering strategies are available (see Alexander[68] for a review), two approaches or a combination of approaches have been most extensively researched with children: frequency compression and frequency transposition. Frequency compression condenses high-frequency sounds into a smaller range of frequencies in the output, much in the same way that amplitude compression condenses a range of different input levels into the dynamic range of the listener. Frequency transposition moves a band of high-frequency energy to a lower frequency, typically without compressing the band.

Both approaches to frequency lowering have shown mixed results for speech recognition in children. In an evidence-based systematic review, McCreery and colleagues[58] concluded that both types of signal processing could be used to improve audibility of high-frequency sounds, but that the improvements in audibility did not always translate to measureable improvements in speech recognition. Many studies of frequency lowering with children are characterized by significant individual variability in benefit across subjects.[69,70] In research with adults, some researchers have concluded that improvements in audibility with frequency lowering may be offset in some cases by distortion that comes from modifying frequency relationships that are important for understanding speech. However, it is important to note that very few studies of frequency lowering in children have indicated poorer performance with frequency lowering than with conventional amplification.

The mixed results from the literature do not provide a clear picture for clinicians about whether or not frequency lowering should be activated for children, and if so, how much frequency lowering should be used. In one experiment by McCreery et al,[70] children and adults with hearing loss had their best performance when frequency lowering was optimized to limit the lowering to highest frequencies, so that only speech energy that was above the highest frequency that the child could hear would be lowered. This approach has been adopted in a recent clinical recommendation for prescribing frequency lowering for children.[45] In general, frequency lowering should not be activated by default. Rather, frequency lowering strategies should only be activated when the bandwidth in the high frequencies is limited above 4 kHz due to the child's degree of hearing loss, the bandwidth of the hearing aid, or a combination of these factors. Examples of variation in maximum audible frequency with the same hearing aid are shown in ▶ Fig. 11.8.

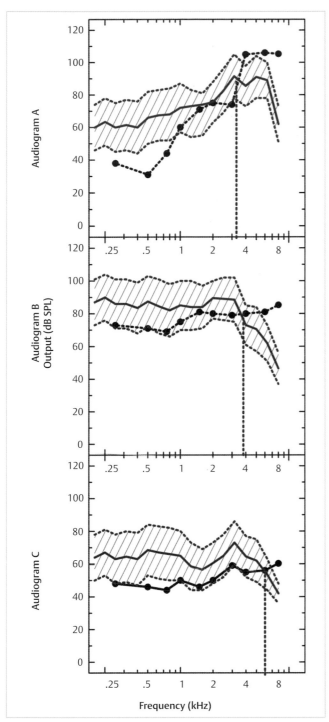

Fig. 11.8 The maximum audible frequency for three different audiograms with the same hearing aid. Hearing aid output in dB SPL as a function of frequency in kHz. The black dots connected by the black line represents the audiometric thresholds in dB SPL for a child with mild-to-profound (Audiogram A), moderate-to-severe (Audiogram B), and mild (Audiogram C) hearing loss. The amplified long-term average speech spectrum (LTASS) is displayed as the red cross-hatched area in each graph. The maximum audible frequency for each audiogram is designated by the vertical red line from where the average of the LTASS intersects the audiogram. The maximum audible frequency for the same hearing aid decreases as the degree of high-frequency hearing loss increases.

In terms of the strength of frequency lowering, the weakest setting that can restore audibility for the inaudible high-frequency information should be utilized in order to minimize the potential negative effects related to lowering information that is already audible. Appropriately prescribed frequency lowering may not have large impacts on the child's perception, simply because the processor should be used ideally to move the smallest amount of speech energy that it possibly can into the range of audibility.

In general, frequency lowering can be used to increase children's access to high-frequency speech cues, but the impact on speech recognition remains mixed in the previous literature. Despite the fact that improving the development of high-frequency speech sounds is a major justification for the development and implementation of frequency-lowering strategies, surprisingly few studies have been conducted to evaluate whether or not children fit with frequency lowering have better speech sound development than peers without frequency lowering. In a randomized controlled trial, Ching and colleagues[42] reported no differences in speech and language outcomes at age 3 for children who were randomly assigned to either receive frequency-lowering or conventional amplification. However, the study provided limited information about the method used to fit frequency lowering, so it is unclear whether or not access to high-frequency sounds was increased for the children fit with frequency lowering. Similarly, Bentler and colleagues[71] conducted a nonrandomized comparison of children in a longitudinal study who were fit with conventional amplification and children in the same study who were fit with frequency lowering. In this study, the audibility provided to the frequency-lowering group was equivalent to the group without frequency lowering, and the language and speech outcomes were equivalent between the two groups. This suggests that similar outcomes can be provided for language development when audibility is equated between conventional processing and frequency lowering, but does not address the primary question of interest for children, which is whether or not the development of speech and language could be better than conventional amplification with frequency lowering.

In summary, children with limited high-frequency audibility should be considered to be candidates for frequency-lowering signal processing. The weakest setting that can restore the frequency regions that are inaudible should be used to minimize distortion. Children who have audible bandwidth up to 6 to 8 kHz with conventional amplification are unlikely based on the current research to experience improvements in speech recognition or development of speech and language with frequency lowering. In the future, improvements in hearing aid technology may help to improve the bandwidth that can be provided by hearing aids, which could minimize the need for frequency lowering for some individuals. However, frequency lowering is likely to continue to remain a viable option for individuals with limited high-frequency residual hearing, but who are not candidates for cochlear implantation.

11.8 Conclusions

Hearing aid candidacy and the selection of features for children is a fundamentally different process for children than it is for adults. Hearing aid characteristics that promote access to the acoustic cues needed to develop speech and language are the foremost concern when selecting hearing aid technology for children. Devices that have the flexibility to change as the child grows and develops are crucial. The selection of hearing aid features for children has grown increasingly complex, as hearing aid signal processing has led to the implementation of hearing aids that analyze the sound environment and adapt the processing. The pace of research into the unique effects of these advanced hearing aid signal processing features on perception and development in children has not kept up with innovation in this area, which leaves clinicians with the task of evaluating the effectiveness of many of these features. Fortunately, verification methods discussed in the next chapter can help clinicians to make more objective determinations of the effects of different features on audibility, and to ensure that children have adequate auditory access over time.

11.9 Summary

The process of determining hearing aid candidacy for children with hearing loss is fundamentally different than for adults. Hearing in children is a pathway for development, and hearing aids must provide access to the acoustic cues needed for communication, socialization, and learning for children with mild-to-severe hearing losses. The process of determining hearing aid candidacy in children is reviewed, including hearing disorders that warrant particularly consideration such as mild hearing loss, unilateral hearing loss, and auditory neuropathy spectrum disorder. Considerations such as the style of hearing aid, how the hearing aid is coupled to the ear, and retention of the device are discussed. Different prescriptive approaches for providing amplification to children are reviewed. The rationale for the selection and activation of advanced hearing aid features such as digital noise reduction, directional microphones, feedback suppression,

and frequency lowering are also highlighted. Audiologists and other professionals will improve their understanding of the process of selection and prescription of amplification for infants and children.

References

[1] Moeller MP. Early intervention and language development in children who are deaf and hard of hearing. Pediatrics. 2000; 106(3):E43

[2] Holte L, Walker E, Oleson J, et al. Factors influencing follow-up to newborn hearing screening for infants who are hard of hearing. Am J Audiol. 2012; 21(2):163–174

[3] McCreery RW, Walker EA, Spratford M, et al. Speech recognition and parent ratings from auditory development questionnaires in children who are hard of hearing. Ear Hear. 2015; 36(suppl 1):60–75

[4] Corbin NE, Bonino AY, Buss E, Leibold LJ. Development of open-set word recognition in children: speech-shaped noise and two-talker speech maskers. Ear Hear. 2016; 37(1):55–63

[5] Stelmachowicz PG, Pittman AL, Hoover BM, Lewis DE. Effect of stimulus bandwidth on the perception of /s/ in normal- and hearing-impaired children and adults. J Acoust Soc Am. 2001; 110(4):2183–2190

[6] McCreery RW, Stelmachowicz PG. Audibility-based predictions of speech recognition for children and adults with normal hearing. J Acoust Soc Am. 2011; 130(6):4070–4081

[7] Pisoni DB, Cleary M. Measures of working memory span and verbal rehearsal speed in deaf children after cochlear implantation. Ear Hear. 2003; 24(suppl 1):106–120

[8] Willis S, Goldbart J, Stansfield J. The strengths and weaknesses in verbal short-term memory and visual working memory in children with hearing impairment and additional language learning difficulties. Int J Pediatr Otorhinolaryngol. 2014; 78(7):1107–1114

[9] Tomblin JB, Harrison M, Ambrose SE, Walker EA, Oleson JJ, Moeller MP. Language outcomes in young children with mild to severe hearing loss. Ear Hear. 2015; 36(suppl 1):76–91

[10] American National Standards Institute (ANSI). American National Standards methods for calculation of the speech intelligibility index. ANSI/ASA S3.5–1997 (R2007). Washington, DC: ANSI; 1997

[11] Walker EA, Holte L, McCreery RW, Spratford M, Page T, Moeller MP. The influence of hearing aid use on outcomes of children with mild hearing loss. J Speech Lang Hear Res. 2015; 58(5):1611–1625

[12] Tharpe AM, Ashmead DH. A longitudinal investigation of infant auditory sensitivity. Am J Audiol. 2001; 10(2):104–112

[13] Sanford CA, Keefe DH, Liu YW, et al. Sound-conduction effects on distortion-product otoacoustic emission screening outcomes in newborn infants: test performance of wideband acoustic transfer functions and 1-kHz tympanometry. Ear Hear. 2009; 30(6):635–652

[14] Baldwin M, Choice of probe tone and classification of trace patterns in tympanometry undertaken in early infancy. Int J Audiol. 2006; 45(7):417–427

[15] Bess FH, Dodd-Murphy J, Parker RA. Children with minimal sensorineural hearing loss: prevalence, educational performance, and functional status. Ear Hear. 1998; 19(5):339–354

[16] Porter H, Sladen DP, Ampah SB, Rothpletz A, Bess FH. Developmental outcomes in early school-age children with minimal hearing loss. Am J Audiol. 2013; 22(2):263–270

[17] Ching TY, Dillon H, Marnane V, et al. Outcomes of early- and late-identified children at 3 years of age: findings from a prospective population-based study. Ear Hear. 2013; 34(5):535–552

[18] Wake M, Tobin S, Cone-Wesson B, et al. Slight/mild sensorineural hearing loss in children. Pediatrics. 2006; 118(5):1842–1851

[19] Lieu JEC. Speech-language and educational consequences of unilateral hearing loss in children. Arch Otolaryngol Head Neck Surg. 2004; 130(5):524–530

[20] Lieu JE, Tye-Murray N, Karzon RK, Piccirillo JF. Unilateral hearing loss is associated with worse speech-language scores in children. Pediatrics. 2010; 125(6):e1348–e1355

[21] McKay S, Gravel G, Tharpe AM. Amplification considerations for children with minimal or mild bilateral hearing loss and unilateral hearing loss. Trends Amplif. 2008; 12(1):43–54

[22] English K, Church G. Unilateral hearing loss in children: an update for the 1990s. Lang Speech Hear Serv Sch 1999;30(1):26–31

[23] Davis A, Reeve K, Hind S, Bamford J, Seewald R, Gravel J. Children with mild and unilateral hearing impairment. In: Seewald R, Gravel J, eds. A Sound Foundation through Early Amplification 2001 - Proceedings of the Second International Conference. Chicago, IL;2001:179–186

[24] Jerger J, Silman S, Lew HL, Chmiel R. Case studies in binaural interference: converging evidence from behavioral and electrophysiologic measures. J Am Acad Audiol 1993; 4(2):122–131

[25] Christensen L, Dornhoffer JL. Bone-anchored hearing aids for unilateral hearing loss in teenagers. Otol Neurotol. 2008; 29(8):1120–1122

[26] Pennings RJE, Gulliver M, Morris DP. The importance of an extended preoperative trial of BAHA in unilateral sensorineural hearing loss: a prospective cohort study. Clin Otolaryngol. 2011; 36(5):442–449

[27] Arndt S, Aschendorff A, Laszig R, et al. Comparison of pseudobinaural hearing to real binaural hearing rehabilitation after cochlear implantation in patients with unilateral deafness and tinnitus. Otol Neurotol. 2011; 32(1):39–47

[28] Vermeire K, Van de Heyning P. Binaural hearing after cochlear implantation in subjects with unilateral sensorineural deafness and tinnitus. Audiol Neurotol. 2009; 14(3):163–171

[29] Vlastarakos PV, Nazos K, Tavoulari EF, Nikolopoulos TP. Cochlear implantation for single-sided deafness: the outcomes. An evidence-based approach. Eur Arch Otorhinolaryngol. 2014; 271(8):2119–2126

[30] Rapin I, Gravel J. "Auditory neuropathy": physiologic and pathologic evidence calls for more diagnostic specificity. Int J Pediatr Otorhinolaryngol. 2003; 67(7):707–728

[31] Zeng FG, Kong YY, Michalewski HJ, Starr A. Perceptual consequences of disrupted auditory nerve activity. J Neurophysiol. 2005; 93(6):3050–3063

[32] Berlin CI, Hood LJ, Morlet T, et al. Multi-site diagnosis and management of 260 patients with auditory neuropathy/dys-synchrony (auditory neuropathy spectrum disorder). Int J Audiol. 2010; 49(1):30–43

[33] Walker EA, McCreery RW, Spratford M, Roush PA. Children with ANSD fitted with hearing aids applying the AAA Pediatric Amplification Guideline: current practice and outcomes. J Am Acad Audiol. 2016; 27(3):204–218

[34] Roush P, Frymark T, Venediktov R, Wang B. Audiologic management of auditory neuropathy spectrum disorder in children: a systematic review of the literature. Am J Audiol. 2011; 20(2):159–170

[35] Teagle HF, Roush PA, Woodard JS, et al. Cochlear implantation in children with auditory neuropathy spectrum disorder. Ear Hear. 2010; 31(3):325–335

[36] Rance G, Cone-Wesson B, Wunderlich J, Dowell R. Speech perception and cortical event related potentials in children with auditory neuropathy. Ear Hear. 2002; 23(3):239–253

[37] He S, Grose JH, Teagle HF, et al. Gap detection measured with electrically evoked auditory event-related potentials and speech-perception abilities in children with auditory neuropathy spectrum disorder. Ear Hear. 2013; 34(6):733–744

[38] Scollie S, Seewald R, Cornelisse L, et al. The Desired Sensation Level multistage input/output algorithm. Trends Amplif 2005; 9(4):159–197

[39] Keidser G, Dillon H, Flax M, Ching T, Brewer S. The NAL-NL2 prescription procedure. Audiology Res 2011; 1(1):e24

[40] Scollie SD, Ching TY, Seewald RC, et al. Children's speech perception and loudness ratings when fitted with hearing aids using the DSL v.4.1 and the NAL-NL1 prescriptions. Int J Audiol 2010; 49(1, suppl 1): S26–S34

[41] Ching TY, Johnson EE, Seeto M, Macrae JH. Hearing-aid safety: a comparison of estimated threshold shifts for gains recommended by NAL-NL2 and DSL m[i/o] prescriptions for children. Int J Audiol 2013; 52(2, Suppl 2):S39–S45

[42] Ching TY, Dillon H, Hou S, et al. A randomized controlled comparison of NAL and DSL prescriptions for young children: hearing-aid characteristics and performance outcomes at three years of age. Int J Audiol. 2013; 52(suppl 2):S17–S28

[43] McCreery R, Walker E, Spratford M, Kirby B, Oleson J, Brennan M. Stability of audiometric thresholds for children with hearing aids applying the American Academy of Audiology Pediatric Amplification Guideline: implications for safety. J Am Acad Audiol. 2016; 27(3):252–263

[44]   Crukley J, Scollie SD. Children's speech recognition and loudness perception with the Desired Sensation Level v5 Quiet and Noise prescriptions. Am J Audiol 2012; 21(2):149–162

[45]   Scollie S, Levy C, Pourmand N, et al. Fitting noise management signal processing applying the American Academy of Audiology Pediatric Amplification Guideline: Verification protocols. J Am Acad Audiol 2016; 27(3):237–251

[46]   Stelmachowicz P, Lewis D, Hoover B, Nishi K, McCreery R, Woods W. Effects of digital noise reduction on speech perception for children with hearing loss. Ear Hear 2010; 31(3):345–355

[47]   Pittman AL, Stelmachowicz PG. Hearing loss in children and adults: audiometric configuration, asymmetry, and progression. Ear Hear 2003; 24(3):198–205

[48]   Anderson KL, Madell JR. Improving hearing and hearing aid retention for infants and young children: A practical survey and study of hearing aid retention productions. Hear Rev 2014; 21(2):16–20

[49]   McCreery RW, Venediktov RA, Coleman JJ, Leech HM. An evidence-based systematic review of amplitude compression in hearing aids for school-age children with hearing loss. Am J Audiol. 2012; 21(2):269–294

[50]   Jenstad LM, Seewald RC, Cornelisse LE, Shantz J. Comparison of linear gain and wide dynamic range compression hearing aid circuits: aided speech perception measures. Ear Hear 1999; 20(2):117–126

[51]   Gou J, Valero J, Marcoux A. The effect of non-linear amplification and low compression threshold on receptive and expressive speech ability in children with severe to profound hearing loss. J Educ Audiol 2002; 10:1–14

[52]   Marriage JE, Moore BCJ, Stone MA, Baer T. Effects of three amplification strategies on speech perception by children with severe and profound hearing loss. Ear Hear 2005; 26(1):35–47

[53]   Christensen LA. A comparison of three hearing aid sound-processing strategies in a multi-memory hearing aid for adolescents. Semin Hear 1999; 20:183–195

[54]   Marriage JE, Moore BCJ. New speech tests reveal benefit of wide-dynamic-range, fast-acting compression for consonant discrimination in children with moderate-to-profound hearing loss. Int J Audiol 2003; 42(7):418–425

[55]   Stelmachowicz PG, Kopun J, Mace A, Lewis DE, Nittrouer S. The perception of amplified speech by listeners with hearing loss: acoustic correlates. J Acoust Soc Am 1995; 98(3):1388–1399

[56]   Bor S, Souza P, Wright R. Multichannel compression: effects of reduced spectral contrast on vowel identification. J Speech Lang Hear Res. 2008; 51(5):1315–1327

[57]   Bentler R, Chiou L-K. Digital noise reduction: an overview. Trends Amplif. 2006; 10(2):67–82

[58]   McCreery RW, Venediktov RA, Coleman JJ, Leech HM. An evidence-based systematic review of frequency lowering in hearing aids for school-age children with hearing loss. Am J Audiol. 2012; 21(2):313–328

[59]   Gustafson S, McCreery R, Hoover B, Kopun JG, Stelmachowicz P. Listening effort and perceived clarity for normal-hearing children with the use of digital noise reduction. Ear Hear 2014; 35(2):183–194

[60]   Pittman A. Children's performance in complex listening conditions: effects of hearing loss and digital noise reduction. J Speech Lang Hear Res 2011; 54(4):1224–1239

[61]   Amlani AM. Efficacy of directional microphone hearing aids: a meta-analytic perspective. J Am Acad Audiol 2001; 12(4):202–214

[62]   Ching TY, O'Brien A, Dillon H, et al. Directional effects on infants and young children in real life: implications for amplification. J Speech Lang Hear Res 2009; 52(5):1241–1254

[63]   Ricketts T, Galster J, Tharpe AM. Directional benefit in simulated classroom environments. Am J Audiol 2007; 16(2):130–144

[64]   Ricketts TA, Galster J. Head angle and elevation in classroom environments: implications for amplification. J Speech Lang Hear Res 2008; 51(2):516–525

[65]   Moore BC, Tan CT. Perceived naturalness of spectrally distorted speech and music. J Acoust Soc Am 2003; 114(1):408–41

[66]   Moeller MP, Hoover B, Putman C, et al. Vocalizations of infants with hearing loss compared with infants with normal hearing: Part I–phonetic development. Ear Hear 2007; 28(5):605–627

[67]   Kimlinger C, McCreery R, Lewis D. High-frequency audibility: the effects of audiometric configuration, stimulus type, and device. J Am Acad Audiol 2015; 26(2):128–137

[68]   Alexander JM. Individual variability in recognition of frequency-lowered speech. Semin Hear 2013; 34(2):86–109

[69]   Glista D, Scollie S, Bagatto M, Seewald R, Parsa V, Johnson A. Evaluation of nonlinear frequency compression: clinical outcomes. Int J Audiol; 2009; 48(9):632–644

[70]   McCreery RW, Alexander J, Brennan MA, Hoover B, Kopun J, Stelmachowicz PG. The influence of audibility on speech recognition with nonlinear frequency compression for children and adults with hearing loss. Ear Hear. 2014; 35(4):440–447

[71]   Bentler R, Walker E, McCreery R, Arenas RM, Roush P. Nonlinear frequency compression in hearing aids: impact on speech and language development. Ear Hear. 2014; 35(4):e143–e152

Suggested Reading

Gustafson SJ, Pittman AL. Sentence perception in listening conditions having similar speech intelligibility indices. Int J Audiol. 2011; 50(1):34–40

Hoetink AE, Körössy L, Dreschler WA. Classification of steady state gain reduction produced by amplitude modulation based noise reduction in digital hearing aids. Int J Audiol. 2009; 48(7):444–455

McCreery RW, Venediktov RA, Coleman JJ, Leech HM. An evidence-based systematic review of directional microphones and digital noise reduction hearing aids in school-age children with hearing loss. Am J Audiol. 2012; 21(2):295–312

12 Cochlear Implants in Adults

Sarah A. Sydlowski

12.1 Introduction

The first device to replace one of the five senses, cochlear implants (CIs) have been successfully utilized in nearly half a million recipients worldwide. A cochlear implant system consists of both internal and external components (▶Fig. 12.1). The internal equipment consists of an implanted electrode array and a receiver/stimulator and the external equipment consists of a microphone, speech processor, transmitting coil, and battery (it may optionally include an acoustic component when residual hearing is preserved; ▶Fig. 12.1). The microphone converts the incoming acoustic signal into electrical signals that are shaped and amplified by the sound processor. The signal is then transmitted to the receiver/stimulator via transcutaneous communication between transmitting coils. Depending on the sound coding strategy utilized, the signal is then converted into a series of biphasic electrical pulses which directly stimulate the auditory neurons. Whereas hearing aids simply amplify incoming sounds and rely on the partially intact peripheral auditory system to further process the amplified signal, a cochlear implant essentially bypasses the peripheral auditory system and replaces the function of the nonfunctioning sensory hair cells in the cochlea. In this way, cochlear implant recipients have the potential for significantly improved speech recognition ability.

While the basic design of the multichannel cochlear implant system has remained relatively unchanged since its U.S. Food and Drug Administration (FDA) approval and release to the market in the mid-1980s, recent advances in cochlear implant system design have improved battery life and usability, have increased the potential for the preservation of residual acoustic hearing in an implanted ear, and have excellent outcomes even in complex listening environments such as background noise. As a result,

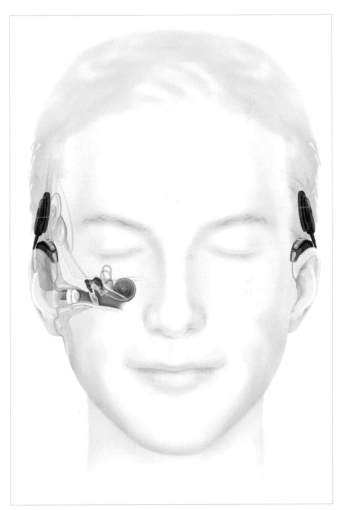

Fig. 12.1 Cochlear implant system. Image courtesy of Cochlear Americas, © 2017.

cochlear implant candidacy criteria have rapidly expanded. Initially reserved for adult patients with bilateral profound sensorineural hearing loss (SNHL) and no benefit from hearing aids, FDA indications now include children as young as 12 months of age and adult patients with moderate-to-profound (standard arrays) and normal-to-profound (short arrays) SNHL.

> ### Pearl
>
> The youngest cochlear implant recipient to date was 2 months old and the oldest was 102 years old.

The expansion of cochlear implant candidacy criteria has allowed this technology to be made available to more patients who receive only limited benefit from hearing aids. Clinicians understand that a variety of factors influence the benefit appreciated by cochlear implant recipients, including duration of hearing loss, consistency of use of appropriate amplification, etiology of hearing loss, and postoperative auditory rehabilitation and this information can be utilized to appropriately counsel patients regarding expected prognosis. As a result of increased understanding regarding the benefits of cochlear implantation sooner and with more residual hearing, outcomes have also improved such that many recipients have excellent speech recognition ability, even in challenging listening environments like background noise or when talking on the phone. New potential clinical applications for cochlear implantation are beginning to emerge, including use in special populations such as those patients suffering from intractable tinnitus and patients with severe-to-profound unilateral SNHL, or single-sided deafness (SSD). The purpose of this chapter is to provide an introduction to the design and function of available devices, the candidacy process, the impact of cochlear implantation on speech recognition, and the influence of various factors (both patient and implant related) on cochlear implant outcomes in adults.

12.2 Cochlear Implant Design

12.2.1 History and Development

Modern cochlear implant design is the result of hundreds of years of study and development. Although multichannel cochlear implants have only been approved by the FDA for clinical use for less than 40 years, early investigation into the ability to stimulate the auditory system electrically began as early as the late 18th century when Alessandro Volta, an Italian physicist inserted two metal rods attached to a battery into his ears, producing a sound mimicking the hissing of boiling soup. Perhaps it was this initially negative experience that

dissuaded research in the area for nearly 150 years until 1957 when Andre Djourno and Charles Eyries, a French scientist and surgeon, directly stimulated the auditory nerve of a patient with bilateral profound hearing loss after the resection of cholesteatomas. Unfortunately, the implant they developed failed in only a few weeks, but during that time, the patient reported some auditory perception, although there was no speech discrimination.[1] Eventually, an otologist in California, William House, heard about the work of Djourno and Eyries. At the time, he was working with John Doyle, an electrical engineer, to discover a way to stimulate the auditory nerve and restore hearing. They first implanted a patient in January 1961 and although the recipient did have some auditory perception, the device had to be explanted because he couldn't tolerate the perception. A second device had to be explanted from another patient due to concern for infection. Around the same time, F. Blair Simmons, an otolaryngologist at Stanford University, began experimenting with a six-channel percutaneous device. Unlike House and Doyle's device, a five-wire design where the same signal was delivered across the length of the cochlea, Simmons' design was able to stimulate each of the six channels separately, resulting in distinct pitch perceptions. These results were encouraging, and suggested to researchers that creating useable auditory perception may eventually be possible.[2]

As other implantable technologies (such as pacemakers) advanced, auditory implant researchers borrowed knowledge regarding biocompatibility to make advancements of their own. By the early 1970s, William House and Jack Urban, an engineer, developed the House/3M single-channel device that was eventually approved for commercial use by the FDA in 1984. Nearly concurrently, a team of researchers at the University of California San Francisco compiled by Francis Sooy worked to prove that auditory input from implants could send meaningful signals to the brains of recipients. They filmed their experiments, and in one such episode, recorded a patient humming the melody of a song that was being played, while tapping out the rhythm.[2] This video garnered the attention of the National Institutes of Health (NIH) and finally convinced many in the field that cochlear implants held potential. However, at the time, they were highly experimental and their use was unstandardized. In 1975, the NIH contracted Robert Bilger to head a team who would evaluate the 13 currently implanted recipients and determine whether the progress thus far warranted further support in the form of funding. The outcomes of this investigation, known as the Bilger Report, ultimately concluded that cochlear implants offered benefit to deaf patients by supporting lipreading skills, improving quality of life, and improving their speech production skills, all with minimal risk to their safety.[3] The Bilger Report stimulated increased funding and attention for cochlear implants and progress in the introduction and development of multichannel cochlear implants rapidly followed. By the late 1970s, four primary teams emerged: the UCSF group led by Francis Sooy that included Michael Merzenich, Robert Schindler, and Robin Michelson; a group in Melbourne led by otolaryngologist Graeme Clark; a group in Vienna, Austria using an implant designed by Ingeborg and Erwin Hochmair; and a group in France that included Claude-Henri Chouard. The separate works of these teams eventually resulted in the development of the electrode arrays used by the current four cochlear implant manufacturers worldwide: Advanced Bionics, Cochlear, MED-EL, and Oticon Medical (respectively). Beginning in the mid-1980s, the multichannel devices developed by these groups surpassed the House/3M single-channel implant (the first FDA-approved cochlear implant), earning FDA approvals of their own. Following their continued success, FDA labeling continued to expand to include children, pre- and postlingually deafened adults, and eventually, individuals with residual hearing.

12.2.2 Currently Available Devices and Outcomes

Modern day cochlear implants have undergone remarkable developments since the earliest designs (▶Fig. 12.2 and ▶Fig. 12.3). With advancements in electrode array designs, surgical techniques, and signal processing, increases in speech understanding have come as well. Whereas the earliest cochlear implants offered a supplement to lipreading and basic sound awareness, today's cochlear implant recipients talk on the telephone, have high levels of speech understanding in background noise, and even enjoy music in many cases.

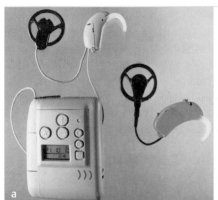
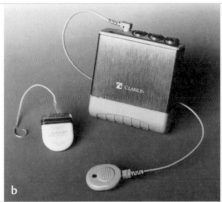
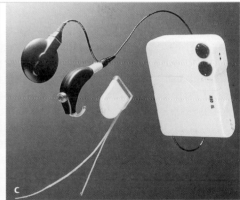

Fig. 12.2 (a–c) Legacy cochlear implant sound processors.

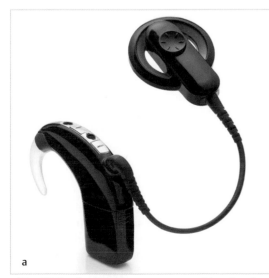
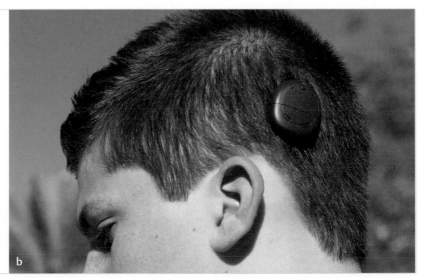

Fig. 12.3 (a, b) Contemporary cochlear implant sound processors. Image courtesy of Cochlear Americas, © 2017.

> **Pearl** ✔
>
> Today's cochlear implant recipients talk on the telephone, have high levels of speech understanding in background noise, and even enjoy music in some cases.

Electrode array portfolios are comprehensive and offer options for surgeons for a variety of frequently encountered scenarios that span the spectrum from ossified or malformed cochleae to cochleae with significant functional residual capability in the apex. Furthermore, modern devices incorporate acoustic advantages for patients with residual hearing in the implanted or contralateral ear in the form of integrated acoustic components and bimodal or bilateral streaming capabilities, which will be discussed shortly.

12.2.3 Cochlear Anatomy and Electrical Stimulation of the Auditory Nerve

Unlike normal hearing which involves the transition of an incoming acoustic signal into mechanical energy in the middle ear and hydraulic energy at the level of the cochlea before an electrical signal is generated at the level of the auditory nerve, a cochlear implant bypasses the outer and middle ear and is directly inserted into the inner ear. The primary cause of SNHL is nonfunctioning inner and outer hair cells; a cochlear implant is designed to essentially replace the function of those sensory cells by directly stimulating the neural fibers of the auditory nerve. While modern cochlear implant designs allow for the preservation of any intact cochlear structures and continued acoustic benefit in those circumstances, the cochlear implant itself does not rely on any functioning components within the cochlea. Rather, from its position within the scala tympani, the cochlear implant electrode array delivers a series of biphasic electrical pulses to the surviving auditory neurons. Over time, or with certain etiologies of hearing loss, the peripheral auditory neurons may suffer retrograde degeneration.[4,5] However, the cell bodies, called spiral ganglion cells, are more proximally located and are often more robust. These structures are hypothesized to be the site most responsive to stimulation from a cochlear implant.

The cochlear implant electrode array may be inserted into the cochlea by drilling a small opening called a cochleostomy, just anterior–inferior to the round window. The round window itself has also been shown to be an optimal point of entrance, and is often preferred by surgeons using a soft surgical technique to preserve residual cochlear structures, although similar outcomes have been observed with both round window and cochleostomy insertions.[6] The cochlea is tonotopically organized, with corresponding neural populations traversing the modiolus and forming the afferent components of the auditory nerve. Cochlear implant systems attempt to capitalize on this frequency-ordered system and electrode contacts are ordered in a corresponding manner. However, due to power and space limitations, a relatively small number of electrodes (generally no more than 22, depending on the implant manufacturer) are tasked with replacing the function of thousands of sensory cells. Because of the limited number of physical electrode contacts, each electrode stimulates a relatively broad population of neurons. Further, each electrode corresponds to a particular channel, which delivers current that corresponds to the presence of a range of frequencies within an incoming signal. A critical goal when designing cochlear implants is to maximize the number of mostly nonoverlapping populations of neurons, thus minimizing the opportunity for loss of spatial specificity.[7] An exception is the use of "virtual channels" or "current steering" which are available in a number of contemporary coding strategies and will be discussed shortly.

The ability of the cochlear implant to effectively stimulate auditory neurons depends on a number of key factors including the proximity of the electrode array to the modiolus, the anatomy of the cochlea, including the presence of fibrosis or ossification, the integrity of the neural structures of interest, and the signal processing and delivery mechanism.

12.2.4 Basics of Implant Function

In the United States, there are three cochlear implant manufacturers with devices approved by the FDA: Advanced Bionics, Cochlear Corporation, and MED-EL Corporation. At the time of this writing, Oticon Medical has not received FDA approval in the United States. Regardless of manufacturer, the basic design of a cochlear implant system is the same. As previously described, the cochlear implant system consists of internal (magnet, telemetry coil, receiver/stimulator, and electrode array) and external (microphone, processor, transmitting coil, battery) components. The processing of the incoming signal begins with the external equipment. The microphone detects the incoming acoustic signal and converts that energy into an electrical signal. Typically, that signal passes through a preamplifier in order to improve the signal-to-noise ratio (SNR) before passing to a digital signal processor (DSP) which classifies the input according to intensity, frequency, and timing information. The incoming sound signal is a complex sound which must be broken down into its more basic components.

The signal is divided into channels, or specific frequency bands. Contemporary systems then use digital bandpass filtering, fast Fourier transformation, or Hilbert's transformation[8] to extract the envelope of the signal, preserving information regarding amplitude. The electrical signal is then sent via a transmitting cable to the radio frequency (RF) coil which is held in position over the internal receiving coil using a magnet. The electrical signal is converted into an electromagnetic signal which is transmitted to the receiving coil. The receiving coil is attached to the internal stimulator which converts the electrical signal back into digital code. A coding strategy, which will be discussed shortly, is applied, and determines the rules that should be applied to generate electrical pulses that will accurately represent the incoming acoustic signal. These pulses are sent from the pulse generator along the electrode lead to the intracochlear electrode array. The number of physical electrode contacts varies among manufacturers, but each electrode is associated with a particular frequency band. Each physical electrode contact delivers electrical stimulation to the auditory fibers to which it lies in close proximity. Low-frequency information is delivered to more apical electrodes, while more high-frequency information is delivered to more basally situated electrodes. Electrical stimulation of the auditory system is successfully produced as a result of a complete electrical circuit between an active electrode a reference electrode which delivers the necessary current to the nearby neural elements.[9]

Cochlear implant coding strategies are algorithms used to transfer critical aspects of the incoming system into electrical code that the implant can utilize. Coding strategies vary among manufacturers and utilize different philosophies in the extraction of relevant aspects of the incoming sound signal. A sound signal can be considered in terms of its two principal components, the envelope and the fine structure.

> **Pearl** ✔
>
> Cochlear implant systems primarily encode the envelope cues of the incoming signal.

The majority of cochlear implant systems utilize the envelope of the signal primarily or exclusively to generate relevant pulse trains; however, Advanced Bionics and MED-EL Corporation have both introduced clinically available fine structure coding strategies. ▶Table 12.1 summarizes the processing strategies offered in each current cochlear implant system available in the United States. A thorough discussion of the details of signal coding is beyond the scope of this chapter; however, these coding strategies can be generally summarized into three main categories: spectral peak picking (n-of-m), CIS-type, and fine structure processing. Research has not suggested superiority among various strategies and comparable performance can be achieved with any current strategy.

CIS-type: Continuous interleaved sampling (CIS) strategy forms the foundation of most contemporary cochlear implant coding strategies. In this strategy, an incoming acoustic signal is divided into *m* number of bandpass filter banks, where *m* equals the number of electrode contacts. High-frequency information is delivered to corresponding basally situated electrode contacts, while low-frequency information is delivered to corresponding apically situated electrode contacts. Importantly, using a CIS strategy, (1) biphasic pulses are delivered sequentially, not simultaneously, and (2) every electrode fires in every cycle, regardless of whether the incoming signal contribute high- or low-amplitude input (or even no input) to its associated filter bank.

Spectral Peak Picking (n-of-m): While *n-of-m* strategies are fundamentally similar to the CIS strategy, the major difference is that the acoustic

Table 12.1 Cochlear implant coding strategies

Cochlear implant manufacturer	CIS-type	Spectral peak picking (n-of-m)	Fine structure
Advanced Bionics[a]	HiRes-S HiRes-P CIS[b] MPS[b]		HiRes-S Fidelity 120 HiRes-P Fidelity 120 Optima-S Optima-P
Cochlear		ACE or ACE(RE) SPEAK	
MED-EL	HDCIS		FSP FS4 FS4p

[a]Advanced Bionics C1 internal devices may utilize Simultaneous Analog Stimulation (SAS) which delivers a continuous electrical waveform, not a biphasic pulse.
[b]Legacy processors only.

energy present in each channel is determined and only those electrodes whose channels have the highest amplitude inputs deliver stimulation. In n-of-m strategies, n is usually defined by maxima, or the number of electrodes that will deliver stimulation in any given cycle. The m is the total number of channels. The n-of-m strategies are designed to deliver the most inputs that are most significant, while eliminating those that are less pronounced (and therefore hopeful, less critical, and more likely to be noise). Because fewer electrodes are delivering stimulation in any given cycle, there may be less channel interaction, the opportunity for faster stimulation rates, and better battery life.[8]

Fine Structure Processing: Fine structure processing also has CIS as its foundation, but where CIS strategies deliver stimulation sequentially, or in sequential pairs in the case of HiRes-P and MPS, fine structure processing strategies intentionally overlap either the input filter bank upper and lower limits (in the case of FSP, FS4, and FS4p) or the firing of neighboring electrodes (in the case of Fidelity 120, Optima, and FS4p) to provide better spectral resolution by current steering. MED-EL's fine structure strategies go one step further and modulate the timing of the pulse train in the most apical electrodes to try to mimic the natural time-locked firing pattern of the auditory nerve.

12.3 Implant Process

The process to cochlear implant candidacy can be long and involves a multidisciplinary team consisting of experts in a variety of subject matter areas. Typically, the team minimally consists of an otologist or otolaryngologist who ensures the patient is a medically and surgically appropriate candidate and an audiologist who evaluates the need for a cochlear implant based on the individual's hearing history and ability. Hearing implant teams may also include a speech language pathologist or auditory verbal therapist, a social worker, or a psychologist. These other specialists contribute valuable perspectives regarding the candidate's ability to regain and utilize auditory reception and their ability to handle the challenges of a rehabilitative process, as well as the presence of adequate postoperative support.

Pearl ✔
Multidisciplinary teams are essential to successful determination of cochlear implant candidacy.

12.3.1 Candidacy

One of the most critical aspects of the cochlear implant process is identifying appropriate candidates to utilize the technology, and then, among those candidates, selecting the appropriate cochlear implant system to maximize their benefit. The preoperative assessment determines whether the patient is medically and audiologically appropriate for implantation and, if so, assists in the choice of ear to be implanted. Recent research has suggested less than 9% market penetration of cochlear implants[10,11]; in other words, more than 90% of individuals who could likely benefit from a cochlear implant *don't have one*. While there are a variety of factors that may contribute to this disheartening figure, one likely reason is the misperception of who is a candidate for cochlear implantation. The criteria for cochlear implantation have changed substantially since adults began receiving cochlear implants for the treatment of deafness in the late 1970s. At that time, adult candidates had to demonstrate profound, bilateral, SNHL and no benefit from hearing aids. "No benefit" was often defined as a score of 0% on open-set speech materials in the best-aided condition. At that time, a more conservative approach was considered reasonable due to the novelty of the technology and the uncertainty about the potential for benefit. Over time, improvements in technology and remarkable outcomes for recipients have paved the way for expansion of cochlear implant candidacy criteria. Contemporary cochlear implant criteria are much less restrictive today than in the early years of cochlear implantation. However, it is important to realize that each individual device has been independently labeled by the FDA based on submissions from each cochlear implant manufacturer and, as a result, there is significant variability in across the approved labels. For all devices, there are two primary aspects to approved labeling: audiometric thresholds and aided speech recognition performance. The indications for each manufacturer's devices are summarized in ▶ Table 12.2.

Clinically, it is generally accepted that if patients meet the least stringent criteria, they are deemed candidates for cochlear implantation and are free to select the cochlear implant that best suits their needs. However, in some circumstances, the cochlear implant center may recommend a cochlear implant "off-label," or outside of the guidelines approved by the FDA. Although manufacturers are prohibited from promoting any off-label use of its devices, individual clinicians may make recommendations for the device's use provided they are using their best clinical judgment which is well-supported by scientific evidence. One exception to this rule is for those

Table 12.2   Primary aspects to FDA-approved labeling

		Unaided aud thresholds iometric	Aided speech recognition ability
Advanced Bionics HiRes90K HiRes90K Ultra		Severe-to-profound bilateral SNHL (> 70 dB HL)	50% or less on a test of open-set sentence recognition (HINT sentences)
Cochlear Corporation CI24RE CI512 CI522 CI532		Moderate-to-profound hearing loss in the low frequencies and profound (≥ 90 dB HL) hearing loss in the mid-to-high speech frequencies	50% correct or less in the ear to be implanted (60% or less in the best-aided listening condition) on recorded tests of open-set sentence recognition
Cochlear Corporation Hybrid L24 (unilateral use only)	Synchrony EAS	Severe-to-profound high frequency SNHL in both ears; better ear PTA (2,3,4 kHz) ≥ 60 dB HL	10–60% correct on CNC words in ear to be implanted; better ear ≤80% on CNC words
MED-EL PulsarCI100 Sonata 100 TI Concert Synchrony	Standard	Bilateral severe-to- profound SNHL determined by a pure tone average of 70 dB HL or greater at 500, 1,000, and 2,000 Hz	40% correct or less in best-aided listening condition on recorded tests of open-set sentence recognition tests (HINT sentences)
		Normal hearing to moderate sensorineural hearing loss in the low frequencies (thresholds ≤ 65 dB HL up to and including 500 Hz) with severe-to-profound mid-to high-frequency hearing loss (≤ 70 dB HL at 2,000 Hz and above) in the ear to be implanted. Nonimplanted ear may be worse than the implanted ear, but may not be better.	Monosyllable word score ≤ 60% at 65 dB SPL in both the ear to be implanted and the contralateral ear
		Centers for Bilateral moderate sloping to **Medicare/Medicaid** profound sensorineural **services (CMS)** hearing loss **National Coverage Determination (for all cochlear implants)**	< 40% in best-aided listening condition on recorded tests of open-set sentence recognition

Abbreviations: CNC, consonant-nucleus-consonant; HINT, Hearing in Noise Test; PTA, pure tone average; SNHL, sensorineural hearing loss.

Source: Adapted with permission from Cochlear Implant Patient Assessment: Evaluation of Candidacy, Performance, and Outcomes by René H. Gifford, © 2013 Plural Publishing, Inc. All rights reserved.

patients on Medicare which has much more stringent criteria (▶**Table 12.2**). In general, cochlear implantation in adults tends to be reserved for those patients who demonstrate limited benefit from hearing aids as measured on aided tests of speech recognition ability. The limitation of current evaluation methods is that most clinicians interpret "best-aided" condition to mean bilaterally aided.

Particularly for patients with asymmetric hearing loss, determining cochlear implant candidacy by evaluating performance with two hearing aids may mask the difficulty encountered by the poorer hearing ear. Furthermore, candidacy for standard length cochlear implants is determined using sentence materials which are highly contextual and may allow candidates to achieve higher scores because they can extrapolate the overall meaning of the sentence and fill in the gaps of the words they may have missed. The most recently labeled devices, Cochlear's Hybrid

cochlear implant (2014) and MED-EL's Synchrony EAS system (2016), represent a significant advancement in the determination of cochlear implant candidacy as they are the first device to utilize expanded criteria that allow clinicians to base candidacy on the performance of each individual ear (as opposed to the best-aided condition) using word recognition (instead of more highly contextual sentence recognition). Clinical trials investigating these expanded candidacy criteria in standard cochlear implant recipients are ongoing. Unlike audiometric and speech recognition abilities, FDA labeling of contraindications to cochlear implantation is consistent across manufacturers. Cochlear implantation is contraindicated for those individuals with hearing loss originating in auditory nerve or central auditory pathway; active external or middle ear infections; cochlear ossification preventing electrode insertion; cochlear nerve deficiency; tympanic membrane

limited by the presence of the cochlear implant magnet. Historically, cochlear implant recipients could not undergo MRI over 0.2 Tesla without having the magnet removed. At the time of this writing, all three manufacturers have received FDA approval for recipients of contemporary receiver/stimulator platforms to undergo MRI up to 1.5 Tesla *with the magnet in place* so long as a special splinting system is utilized. Advanced Bionics and Cochlear are labeled for MRI up to 3.0 Tesla with the magnet removed, and recipients of the most current MED-EL Synchrony implant may undergo MRI up to 3.0 Tesla with the magnet in place. It should be noted that the magnet does create artifact on the image up to approximately 4 in, so for those scans where good visibility of structures of the head are desired, magnet removal is still preferred. Please refer to manufacturer package inserts for specifics of MRI compatibility with each implant system.

Cochlear implant recipients have higher risk than the general population for contracting bacterial meningitis from the bacteria *Streptococcus pneumoniae* (pneumococcus). For this reason, reviewing immunization records and recommending appropriate pneumococcal immunizations and boosters is an important component of the cochlear implant candidacy process. The Centers for Disease Control and Prevention (CDC) recommends that all persons with cochlear implants receive age-appropriate pneumococcal vaccination with 7-valent pneumococcal conjugate vaccine (PCV7) (Prevnar), 23-valent pneumococcal polysaccharide vaccine (PPV23) (Pneumovax), or both. The CDC offer updated information and vaccination schedules on their website, www.cdc.gov.

Another important aspect in the cochlear implant candidacy process is vestibular assessment. It is not uncommon for individuals with certain types of hearing loss to exhibit reduced or absent vestibular function. Furthermore, Buchman et al[23] reported a 38% chance of vestibular damage and 10% of severe or profound vestibular loss as measured by caloric tests subsequent to cochlear implantation, even in patients with normal vestibular function preoperatively. Thus, the primary goal of preoperative vestibular assessment is to identify whether there is a side with reduced labyrinthine function such that it would be inadvisable to implant the better functioning side as it would present great risk to the patient's overall vestibular function. While preoperative vestibular assessment may be considered routinely, it is arguably most critical when considering a sequential bilateral cochlear implant. In these cases, it is important to assess whether there was any vestibular insult during the first cochlear implantation for which the patient has compensated and perhaps does not exhibit functional limitations. The potential for subsequent bilateral vestibular weakness should be considered in the implant evaluation as the presence of bilateral vestibular hypofunction can be debilitating and may perhaps outweigh the auditory benefits of a second cochlear implant.

Typically, caloric nystagmography is used to quantify existing vestibular function. An asymmetry of greater than 20% in the sum of responses to 30 and 44°C irrigations suggests hypofunction on the weaker side, while the absence of a caloric response to ice water irrigation suggests profound vestibular loss. The cochlear implant team may utilize this information to select the most appropriate ear to implant or even to counsel the patient regarding the advisability of undergoing implantation at all.

In recent years, substantial progress has been made in the atraumaticity of electrode array design and insertion technique which may influence both the likelihood of vestibular insult and the loss of residual hearing in an implanted ear. While the potential of these developments to positively influence vestibular outcomes are in the early stages of investigation,[24] the ability to preserve residual acoustic hearing in cochlear implant recipients has been well documented.[6,25,26] For decades, cochlear implant candidates were informed that losing any remaining hearing they had in the ear to be implanted was a certainty. Because of advances in electrode array design as well as refinement of "soft" surgical technique, loss of residual hearing is no longer a certainty. In fact, many reports suggest the possibility of routine preservation of some or even all of the residual preoperative acoustic thresholds. On average, reports in the literature (as summarized by Gifford and Dorman[27]) suggest that mean postoperative threshold elevation ranges from 10 to 20 dB depending on a number of factors, including the electrode array, surgical technique, and surgeon experience. The benefits of hearing preservation will be discussed later; at this point the focus will remain on the factors that make hearing preservation possible. First, electrode array design has developed with a focus on atraumaticity. Electrode arrays are thinner, more flexible, and have softer tips such that their insertion into the cochlear can be as smooth as possible.

Recent designs have focused on lateral wall placement where the electrode array hugs the lateral wall and avoids contacting more medial structures like the organ of Corti. Cochlear and advanced Bionics have developed a mid-scala electrode array that floats away from either the medial or lateral walls in order to minimize trauma within the cochlea. Shorter electrode arrays designed to stimulate only the basal portion of the cochlea (Cochlear Hybrid, MED-EL Flex 20 and Flex 24) and slim variable insertion depth arrays (Cochlear CI522) are specifically designed to minimize damage to delicate cochlear structures. Furthermore, research has suggested that a primary traumatic result of cochlear implantation can be translocation of the electrode array from the scala tympani through the basilar membrane into the scala vestibuli. Aside from causing destruction to the delicate structures of the cochlea, translocation results in the mixing of endolymphatic and perilymphatic fluids and the subsequent loss of the endocochlear potential necessary for acoustic hearing. Insertion techniques that minimize the potential for translocation have therefore come into favor for surgeons practicing hearing preservation surgery. While insertion through a cochleostomy (a small hole typically drilled anterior and inferior to the round window) was traditionally the insertion technique of choice for precurved, perimodiolar electrode arrays, the slimmer, straighter lateral wall electrode arrays are designed to be inserted through either a cochleostomy or directly through the round window itself. Other soft surgical techniques include very slow insertion of the electrode array over minutes, avoidance of drilling, excursion of bone dust into the cochlea, excessive irrigation or suction, use of lubricants, and the administration of preoperative, perioperative, and postoperative steroids.[28] ▶ Fig. 12.4 shows the position of a cochlear implant at the conclusion of surgery.

At the time of device selection in the preoperative period, selection of an appropriate electrode array is of utmost importance. Factors that should be considered by the cochlear implant team when selecting a device should include the potential for residual postoperative hearing that is sufficient to utilize acoustic amplification, contralateral residual hearing that may benefit from bimodal (cochlear implant on one side, hearing aid on the other) stimulation, cochlear structure including anatomical malformations or ossification, configuration of the hearing loss, electrode array length, whether the procedure is for an initial implant or a revision, and probable spiral ganglia survival.

12.3.3 Programming and Postoperative Follow-Up

Successful adoption of the cochlear implant system requires periodic programming, aural rehabilitation, and time to adapt to the new sound quality provided by a cochlear implant.

> **Pearl** ✔
>
> Successful outcomes following cochlear implantation require frequent programming, auditory practice (training), and patience while acclimatization occurs.

The process begins by setting realistic expectations prior to activation. As will be discussed, a variety of factors influence the prognosis for individual patients. It is important for patients to realize that cochlear implants offer a very different auditory experience than normal hearing and even hearing aids. Whereas hearing aids amplify incoming acoustic signals, the cochlear implant is converting incoming acoustic information into electrical signals. Although contemporary coding strategies are very advanced in their abilities to accurately replicate auditory information, it is completely different signal processing than that typically conducted by the peripheral auditory system. To put this difference in patient-friendly terms, nearly 18,000 highly specialized sensory cells have been replaced with 12 to 22 physical electrode contacts. Thus, information is conveyed to the auditory system via a very different mechanism than that to which the individual has been accustomed. Furthermore, the physical electrode contacts to which certain frequency bandwidths are assigned may not be situated exactly in line with the natural tonotopicity of the cochlea. Thus, the recipient's auditory system must undergo some degree of neural reorganization in order to interpret the resulting signal. Most patients initially report the sound quality of their cochlear implant to be "squeaky" or "tinny" due to the primary location of the cochlear implant within the basal and middle turns of the cochlea. Some patients are unable to initially

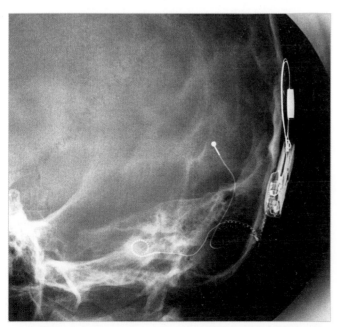

Fig. 12.4 Stenvers' view of Nucleus 24 taken at time of surgery.

decipher speech and may report the sensation of hearing to more closely approximate a sound of "ringing bells" or "chimes." The more recently that the recipient has had appropriately aided residual hearing, the more quickly he or she will typically develop open-set speech understanding, but achieving this goal is usually a process. Stable programming is typically accomplished within the first 3 months, but it can take up to 1 to 2 years for recipients to reach their full potential from their cochlear implant systems.[29,30] It is important to convey that cochlear implants are not a direct replacement of normal hearing, rather a remarkable way to improve speech understanding ability when hearing aids cannot do so effectively enough.

The postoperative cochlear implant process may vary among cochlear implant centers, but typically consists of a series of cochlear implant programming or "MAPping" sessions scheduled at increasing intervals. The process of mapping a cochlear implant is complex and beyond the scope of this chapter; however, it is important to understand that programming a cochlear implant is a process and development of open-set speech perception may take several days, weeks, or months postactivation. The programming process begins with initial activation, which may occur over one or two appointments. During these initial visits, initial programming adjustments are made and equipment is reviewed. Subsequent programming appointments may be scheduled in 1 week, 1 month, 3 months, 6 months, and annually, at a minimum.

Again, while this specific schedule may vary among centers, the general premise will remain consistent. Routine programming and adjustment is necessary with the fastest adaptation to the changing signal presented to the auditory system perceived in the earlier appointments, eventually reaching a plateau and needing more infrequent visits and more minimal adjustments. While the time frame to a stable MAP varies due to a variety of factors, many patients begin achieving open-set speech understanding by 1 month postactivation and often have a relatively stable MAP by 3 to 6 months post-activation.

12.4 Special Factors

12.4.1 Bilateral Cochlear Implantation

There are a number of known advantages to binaural hearing, including head shadow effect, binaural squelch, and binaural summation. The term "head shadow effect" describes the acoustic imbalance between the SNR of the poor ear and the better ear in the unaided condition; that is to say, the head and torso shield the better hearing ear from the deleterious effects of noise from the contralateral side. This phenomenon is most effective in the important speech frequencies of 2,000 Hz and above.[31] Binaural squelch describes the ability of binaural listeners to attenuate competing background noise and reverberation to improve speech understanding in noise. Finally, binaural summation is an advantageous result of binaural hearing that creates a system of redundancy and maximizes the incoming speech signal for optimal understanding. Auditory localization also requires intact bilateral hearing. There are three primary cues responsible for auditory localization and all rely on bilateral hearing: interaural timing difference (ITD), interaural level difference (ILD), and the head-related transfer function. As a result, in the absence of bilateral hearing, an individual would experience significant difficulty knowing the direction from which sound is traveling and understanding speech in background noise and other challenging listening environments.

In the early days of cochlear implantation, adult patients with bilateral profound SNHL received one cochlear implant, improving their potential for sound awareness and even open-set speech understanding, but limiting their abilities in more complex auditory environments. By the late 1990s, the significant advantages of binaural hearing became a focus of cochlear implant researchers and today bilateral cochlear implantation is considered to be standard of care for adults with severe-to-profound SNHL.[12] Along with consideration of bilateral cochlear implantation came associated questions and concerns: longer time under anesthesia, particularly in the case of simultaneous bilateral implants, potentially increased risk for vestibular trauma; cost-effectiveness; bilateral loss of residual hearing; and achieving bilateral balance. Despite these initial concerns, the benefits of bilateral hearing were soon demonstrated to outweigh the potential risks and bilateral implantation has become common practice.

Specifically, research has consistently demonstrated that bilateral cochlear implant recipients demonstrate improved localization ability, speech in noise capability, and bilateral sound awareness which is particularly critical in situations where the speaker is necessarily lateral to the recipient, such as restaurant booths and driving a car.[32,33,34,35] Most bilateral cochlear implant recipients experience bilateral summation, or an overall increase in perceived loudness by receiving stimulation in two ears. Importantly, these benefits are in no way restricted by recipient's age.[36] For these reasons, in adult cochlear implant candidates with severe-to-profound SNHL, often the biggest obstacle to bilateral implantation is insurance coverage, at least in the case of Medicare, whose criteria are vague on the matter of coverage of more than one implant. With increasing experience with bilateral cochlear implants, opportunities to optimize the bilateral cochlear implant experience have gained attention. For example, not surprisingly, no two cochlear implants are placed identically within different cochleae and even in the same recipient, symmetrical anatomy and associated physiological responsiveness is unlikely.

> **Pearl**   ✔
>
> Recent advancements with cochlear implantation in individuals with SSD may allow us to better understand what a cochlear implant sounds like to a recipient.

Thus, recent research has focused on optimizing programming by focusing on loudness balancing pitch-matching, and electrode deactivation using high-resolution imaging to achieve better overall sound quality.[37] Finally, while bilateral cochlear implantation may be an obvious recommendation for patients with bilateral severe-to-profound SNHL who attain limited-to-no benefit from acoustic stimulation, a particularly relevant question is for what degree of hearing loss and at what interval bilateral implantation should be considered for adult patients. Most commonly, in adult patients, bilateral implantation is conducted in a sequential manner, unless there is substantial risk for ossification of the cochleae. For patients with residual hearing in the nonimplanted ear, it is increasingly common for patients to continue to utilize a hearing aid in addition to their cochlear implant in a configuration called bimodal stimulation (▶ Fig. 12.5).

12.4.2 Bimodal Stimulation

The term bimodal describes the combination of electric hearing through a cochlear implant on one side and acoustic hearing through a hearing aid on the nonimplanted side. Schafer et al[38] reported that both bilateral and bimodal stimulation was found to provide listeners with an overall average improvement ranging from 15.3 to 30.7 percentage points across the combined effects of binaural summation, binaural squelch, and the head shadow effects compared to a monaural CI or hearing aid. While there are substantial advantages to hearing in complex environments offered by bilateral cochlear implantation, the addition of residual acoustic hearing to electric hearing, even in the contralateral ear, can offer measurable benefit to recipients for speech perception in quiet, in noise, and for localization compared with monaural conditions.[39,40] In particular, the addition of residual hearing in the contralateral ear provides improved spectral resolution and temporal fine structure cues in the low to mid frequency region.[12] Thus, before proceeding to bilateral implantation, most centers closely evaluate the clinical benefit of adding a hearing aid for a unilateral CI recipient and will typically only advanced to a second implant when limited benefit from the hearing aid is demonstrated. Adding to the diagnostic challenge is the limitation that binaural advantages are often observed only in more complex listening environments

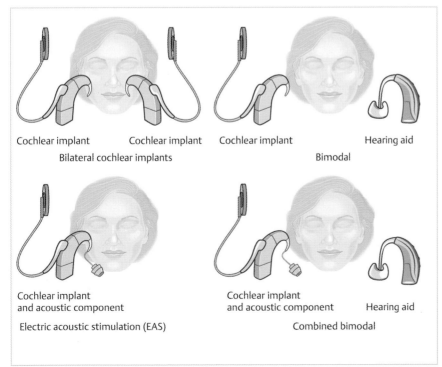

Cochlear implant   Cochlear implant

Bilateral cochlear implants

Cochlear implant   Hearing aid

Bimodal

Cochlear implant
and acoustic component

Electric acoustic stimulation (EAS)

Cochlear implant
and acoustic component   Hearing aid

Combined bimodal

Fig. 12.5 Hearing configurations. Reprinted with permission, Cleveland Clinic Center for Medical Art & Photography © 2017. All Rights Reserved.

that are not always clinically accessible. Fortunately, Gifford et al[12] identified AzBio Sentences in +5 SNR as a reliable tool for identification of sequential bilateral candidates; the authors proposed recommending a second cochlear implant for those patients not exhibited a clinically significant improvement in the bimodal condition as compared to unilateral CI.

Bimodal listeners anecdotally tend to report that the addition of a contralateral hearing aid provides a sensation of balance and "roundedness" that improves the overall sound quality. While bilateral CI recipients tend to demonstrate superior performance on localization tasks and perception of semantically unpredictable sentences with spatially separated noise, bimodal recipients tend to perform better than bilateral CI recipients on perception of natural prosody of speech and are better able to utilize acoustic cues for benefits in background noise.[41] These clear differences in auditory strengths are likely due to the bimodal recipient's ability to take advantage of ITD, a low-frequency phenomenon that is largely inaccessible to bilateral CI recipients without residual acoustic hearing. Thus, the determination of when to move from bimodal to bilateral electric stimulation is variable and patient-specific.

Importantly, bimodal stimulation ensures that the nonimplanted ear is also adequately stimulated to minimize the risk of auditory deprivation. Once an ear cannot be adequately stimulated, bilateral implantation should be considered in order to capture the maximal potential benefit of electrical stimulation in an ear that has been recently acoustically stimulated. Bimodal stimulation is most appropriate when the nonimplanted ear retains thresholds that can be consistently and appropriately amplified. This configuration is increasingly common as centers are becoming ever more considerate of CI candidacy for patients with more residual hearing in the contralateral ear. Specifically, patients with asymmetric hearing loss, where one ear is a candidate for cochlear implantation while the other ear is outside of FDA labeling criteria, are more commonly receiving an implant off-label, when insurance coverage can be obtained. Thus, in addition to those traditional cochlear implant recipients with bilateral moderate-to-profound SNHL, patients with normal-to-moderate SNHL in the unimplanted ear not only exist, but are also fairly common. They are even more likely to demonstrate significant benefit from bimodal stimulation than more traditional cochlear implant candidates due to the presence of more aidable residual hearing.

12.4.3 Electric Acoustic Stimulation and Combined Bimodal Stimulation

As previously discussed, the development of less traumatic electrode arrays has successfully introduced the possibility of preserving residual acoustic hearing, presumably by protecting the delicate structures of the cochlea. As a result, it is not uncommon to observe measurable and even useable residual acoustic hearing postoperatively. Perhaps surprisingly, hearing preservation has been shown to be achievable not only with short arrays designed to stimulate only the basal section of the cochlea, but also with full-length electrode arrays.[26] As a result, patients with variable degrees of residual preoperative hearing have the potential to preserve some or all of that ability postoperatively. Even more importantly, recent advances in external processor design allows clinicians to amplify residual acoustic hearing using a single, integrated device (▶ **Fig. 12.6**). At the time of this writing, there is considerable debate in terms of how to define "hearing preservation" and subsequently integrate acoustic hearing with electric stimulation. More specifically, it is heavily debated whether the evaluation of residual acoustic hearing should focus on the presence of measurable thresholds (audibility) or take a more functional approach aidability. While this debate rages on, clinicians are currently struggling to identify the most appropriate approach to identify appropriate candidates for potential hearing preservation arrays and postoperative use of acoustic amplification in an implanted ear as well as identifying efficacious clinical batteries for monitoring postoperative performance. Regardless of these logistical challenges, the benefits of hearing preservation are well documented and extensive. Similar to bimodal stimulation, the presence of residual acoustic hearing, particularly in the low frequencies, offers significant advantages in challenging listening environments.

Pearl	✔
Residual hearing enhances speech recognition in noise, appreciation of music, and sound quality.

Cochlear implants are known to have limited spectral resolution that curtails recipients' ability to understand speech in background noise; however, the presence of residual acoustic hearing, even if it is only the low frequencies, may offer access to some spectral cues that allow these listeners more opportunities for release from masking.[27] Interestingly, the degree of both pre- and postoperative residual acoustic hearing seems to be unrelated to the degree of successful postoperative speech recognition ability.[27]

Furthermore, it does not appear that the residual hearing needs to extend across a wide frequency

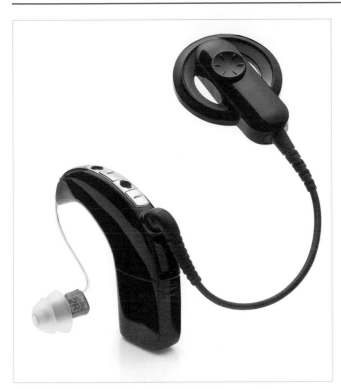

Fig. 12.6 Electric-acoustic sound processor. Image courtesy of Cochlear Americas, © 2017.

range in order to be useful; rather the information contained in the region of the fundamental frequency (< 200 Hz) is most impactful on electric acoustic stimulation (EAS) benefit.[27,42,43]

In light of the numerous advantages observed in groups with bilateral CI, bimodal stimulation, and EAS, there has been considerable attention given to quantifying and ranking the advantages of each aspect of hearing: monaural versus binaural, acoustic versus electric, residual acoustic hearing in contralateral or ipsilateral ear. Using a within-subjects repeated measures design, Gifford et al[12] demonstrated that bilateral CI recipients performed significantly better than they had in the bimodal condition, even when their speech recognition scores approach the performance ceiling. Further, those bilateral CI recipients with bilateral residual acoustic hearing (BiBi) exhibited significant benefit over patients using bilateral CI. The benefits of bilateral preservation of low-frequency acoustic hearing were further supported by Loiselle et al[44] who reported the advantages demonstrated by patients with symmetric residual hearing compared to those with asymmetric residual hearing. To summarize, it is critical to restore binaural audibility whenever possible. Importantly, the ability to incorporate residual acoustic hearing from one or both ears with electric stimulation is always advantageous although the degree of benefit may vary.

12.4.4 Single-Sided Deafness

The degree of residual acoustic hearing in the contralateral ear is taken to the extreme in cases of unaidable unilateral SNHL, more commonly referred to as SSD. SSD is a potentially disabling condition that may be the result of a variety of etiologies including acoustic neuroma resection, viral or autoimmune involvement, or idiopathic causes. SSD typically describes hearing loss that is isolated to one ear with normal hearing retained in the other ear. The hearing loss is generally profound, although in some situations there is residual ability to detect sound at better than profound levels, but residual speech recognition is so poor that the individual cannot benefit from traditional amplification. If medical intervention is unsuccessful in restoring serviceable hearing, then the individual is left with several communication challenges resulting from the loss of binaural benefits. Specifically, individuals with SSD typically have difficulty determining the direction from which sound arises (localization), hearing sounds arising from the deafened side, and understanding speech in background noise.

Although patients with SSD retain normal hearing in the contralateral ear, there are myriad negative consequences of unilateral hearing loss (UHL). These consequences are perhaps intensified by the fact the UHL is a nearly invisible disorder[45] and many communication partners may be unaware of the disability. Individuals with SSD commonly report perceived hearing handicap at levels that often approach severe levels.[46] This perceived handicap is most often related to the characteristic triad of SSD impairment.[47] Consequently, individuals with SSD commonly report difficulty participating in group environments, inability to converse in lateralized communication settings such as when riding in the car, and general fatigue from increased listening effort, particularly when in challenging hearing environments. Many patients report social consequences that include feelings of embarrassment and isolation resulting from the inability to accurately follow conversations in a noisy environment or unawareness of a speaker on their deaf side. Wie et al[47] reported 93% of patients with permanent unilateral deafness claimed the condition was a communication handicap that had a negative effect on their interactions with other people. This communication handicap was most pronounced in a background of noise where only 13% of participants reported they are able to hear "most" words. Douglas et al[48] reported individuals with profound unilateral SNHL had significant difficulties with speech in the presence of noise, situations of multiple stimuli (such as listening to the television and someone speaking at the same time), determining the location of unseen objects, and resultant increased listening effort. Without adequate intervention, individuals with SSD rely on coping mechanisms that may include strategic positioning in group situations (83%), reliance on visual inputs including speechreading (97%), or avoidance strategies, such as opting out of challenging communication situations like noisy environments (40%).[47]

There are currently a variety of management options for this population, all of which attempt to deliver stimuli from the poorer hearing side to the normally functioning contralateral cochlea in order to improve sound awareness and speech understanding in noise. Management options include a contralateral routing of signal (CROS) hearing aid, bone-anchored auditory implant, transcranial CROS, or TransEar®. All of these devices function to alleviate the head shadow effect, but do not restore any of the binaural benefits related to binaural squelch or summation, nor do they improve the recipient's ability to localize sound.

Recently, several clinical trials have investigated the safety and efficacy of cochlear implantation in patients with SSD and particularly with intractable tinnitus, which will be discussed shortly. Positive outcomes increased interest in expanding the candidacy for cochlear implantation to include more ear-specific measures without restrictions due to a better, or even normal, hearing contralateral ear. Specifically, studies have suggested that for adult patients with acquired SSD, cochlear implantation offers improved spatial release from masking, improved speech understanding, and improved localization ability.[49,50,51] As a result of improved speech awareness, understanding, and overall functionality, SSD CI recipients tend to also demonstrate associated improvement in health-related quality of life (HRQoL).[52] Despite these positive reports, a recent systematic review of the literature suggested that larger studies are necessary to better define the tangible outcomes for the SSD population.[53] At the time of this writing, although several devices have been CE Marked for SSD outside of the United States (indicating European Conformity, a term used for devices marketed in Europe), FDA approval for the SSD population has not been achieved and therefore, insurance coverage remains challenging.

12.4.5 Tinnitus

Tinnitus is a phenomenon that is not entirely understood; however, a primary hypothesis is that tinnitus arises from changes in neural activity caused by reduction in or loss of auditory inputs, for example, as results from hearing loss. Because of the close association with hearing loss, it is not surprising that as many as 66 to 86% of cochlear implant candidates report the presence of tinnitus with variable severity preoperatively.[54] Postoperatively, tinnitus has the potential to worsen, or to partially or even completely resolve. Tinnitus has been reported as a frequent complication post-cochlear implantation. Tinnitus that develops or worsens after cochlear implantation can be transient or permanent. One hypothesis for the potential for observed changes in tinnitus postimplantation is that intracochlear trauma occurs with electrode array placement that may damage the delicate structures of the inner ear.

Although candidacy criteria have expanded to include patients with substantial residual hearing, where there may be concern that the risk of trauma-induced tinnitus may be worse, Arts et al[55] reported that of 197 CI recipients, only 39 (19.8%) who suffered from a newly developed (25) or worsened (14) tinnitus following CI surgery were identified. No statistically significant association between perioperative deterioration of hearing thresholds measured by pure tone audiometry and the development or worsening of tinnitus was found.

Recently, cochlear implantation and the associated electrical stimulation has become a focus of researchers aiming to investigate possible interventions that can directly modulate individuals' perception of tinnitus. The approach of direct electrical stimulation is particularly relevant for those patients who have severe-to-profound hearing loss who may not be able to benefit from acoustic amplification or tinnitus maskers that aim to provide sound enrichment and subsequently minimize the impact of tinnitus on the listener. Because tinnitus has been postulated to arise, at least in part, as a direct result of the auditory system's attempt to create auditory stimulation in the absence of environmental stimulation, direct stimulation of the auditory nerve with electrical stimulation from a cochlear implant is an attractive opportunity to both restore hearing and minimize the impact of tinnitus. The SSD population has been a particularly attractive group for this investigation as the presence of tinnitus is often as bothersome, if not more bothersome, than the hearing loss in the presence of a contralateral normal hearing ear. Van de Heyning et al[56] first reported a significant and consistent reduction in tinnitus loudness and therefore suggested CI as a new treatment for tinnitus in patients with SSD. Mertens et al[57] reported that in a group of 23 CI recipients suffering from UHL and accompanied incapacitating tinnitus who had been implanted for 3 to 10 years, 100% of the subjects wears their CI 7 days a week. Their reported tinnitus significantly reduced up to 3 months after activation of the CI and tinnitus reduction persisted over the long term. Their study sample consisted of both true SSD patients, as well as individuals with asymmetric hearing loss. The SSD group reported tinnitus reduction as the primary benefit, whereas the majority of the asymmetric hearing loss (AHL) group reported improved hearing as the primary benefit, although tinnitus reduction was also noted. The period of tinnitus reduction once the cochlear implant was switched off at night is short, on the order of minutes; thus, cochlear implantation does not appear to have residual tinnitus suppressive effects in the absence of ongoing stimulation. A systematic review conducted by Arts et al[58] found cochlear implantation to be an appropriate treatment for tinnitus in SSD, although the underlying mechanism for the successful attenuation of tinnitus is unclear. Early reports suggest that tinnitus can be suppressed with intracochlear electrical stimulation independent of environmental sounds,[59] however, further investigation is necessary to identify the impact of electrical stimulation on an auditory system that is not impacted by the confounding effect of hearing loss.

12.5 Cochlear Implant Outcomes

Outcomes with cochlear implants in adults are most frequently reported in terms of improvement in postoperative speech perception. Speech perception, while critically important, is only one outcome measure that can be considered for cochlear implant recipients. Quality of life, self-perceived benefit, localization, and music enjoyment, are all important considerations when evaluating the success of cochlear implantation. Since the early days of cochlear implants, expected (and achieved) outcomes have continued to improve. Advances in the auditory abilities of contemporary cochlear implant recipients have been dependent on a variety of factors including technological improvements, better and earlier candidate selection, and enhanced surgical techniques, to name a few. In this section, outcome assessment and factors contributing to expected outcomes will be reviewed.

12.5.1 Individual Factors Influencing Outcomes

A variety of individual factors can influence outcomes with cochlear implants (▶Table 12.4).

Many of these factors are related to anatomical and/or physiological limitations of an individual's auditory system and include variables such as cochlear malformations, spiral ganglia survival and central auditory pathway integrity, and preserva-

tion of useable residual acoustic hearing, which can all contribute to the degree of successful auditory improvements achieved by the recipient. Arguably, duration of deafness and auditory deprivation are the single most influential factors related to the ability to perceive open-set speech using a cochlear implant. Successful cochlear implantation relies on the intact survival and functional integrity of the spiral ganglion cells (SGCs), the cell bodies of auditory neurons, and higher-level auditory pathways. It is believed that SGCs represent the primary site of stimulation for the electrical stimulation generated by a cochlear implant. Therefore, it is important that SGCs are both present and functionally intact in order to successfully respond to stimulation and propagate the electrical signal to the level of the brainstem and beyond. In the same vein, the more central auditory system must also be intact in order to receive and process incoming auditory information.

Research has shown that loss of inner hair cells tends to prompt retrograde neural degeneration[4,5] and degeneration tends to be more severe with longer durations of auditory deprivation, although this is not always the case. There is an abundance of research relating better speech recognition outcomes with shorter durations of deafness due to the reorganization of auditory pathways that occurs in response to lack of reliable stimulation.[60] Animal models have demonstrated that long duration of deafness, or perhaps more accurately, lack of auditory stimulation, results in degradation of more peripheral neural structures including the SGCs and cochlear nucleus.[61] The effects of this phenomenon are particularly obvious in congenitally deafened adults who receive cochlear implants compared to postlingually deafened adults who receive a cochlear implant following progressive hearing loss and amplification; however, similar effects of auditory deprivation can be observed

Table 12.4 Factors affecting cochlear implant outcomes

Appropriate device selection and programming
Anatomical malformations
Surgical technique/electrode placement
Neural survival and integrity
Preservation of cochlear structures and function
Duration of deafness
Amplification history
Etiology of hearing loss
Medical health
Electrode array placement
Aural rehabilitation
Motivation and expectations
Binaural hearing
Preoperative function (hearing levels/speech performance)

for ears that are postlingually deafened, but inadequately aided.

The postimplant expectation for an individual who has been bilaterally, prelingually sound- deprived is the ability to detect and perhaps identify environmental sounds, or "sound awareness." For postlingually deafened adults, anticipated results are much more favorable and include very good open-set speech recognition, although there are reports that an ear with more than 10 years of auditory deprivation is a poorer cochlear implant candidate than an ear that has remained adequately aided.[62] This distinction becomes particularly relevant for individuals who have asymmetric hearing and are pursuing a single cochlear implant, as frequently is the case, particularly with Medicare beneficiaries. In circumstances where a candidate has a poorer ear that has been sound deprived for many years, clinicians may prefer to implant an ear that has been more consistently stimulated. However, it can be a difficult decision for an individual to risk losing the residual hearing in an aided ear, as well as the potential benefits of bimodal hearing. In a counterpoint to the accepted clinical consensus, Boisvert et al[60] proposed that outcomes of cochlear implantation are more closely related to the period of time for which the brain is deprived of auditory stimulation from both ears, not only one and suggested that postlingually deafened adults can do equally well no matter which ear is implanted.

Pitfall ✕

Long duration of unamplified or underamplified severe-to-profound hearing loss can negatively impact outcomes with a cochlear implant and setting realistic expectations for patients should be an important aspect of the candidacy evaluation process.

While duration of deafness is a primary factor in developing a prognosis for cochlear implant candidates, age itself appears to have variable bearing on outcomes. Certainly, medical health, which may decline with increasing age, is an important consideration when identifying appropriate cochlear implant candidates to undergo implantation under general anesthesia.

Carlson et al[63] reported that patients 80 years or older were more likely to have anesthetic complications and require hospital admission than their younger counterparts. However, speech recognition outcomes may be comparable to those implanted at younger ages. Other studies have found a relationship between age and speech recognition outcomes,

but there may also be a cognitive component to consider. Although outcomes are likely more related to duration of deafness relative to age (the percentage of the patient's life lived with significant hearing loss) rather than absolute age, the effects of aging and cognitive decline can impact outcomes. It is not uncommon for older adults (> 70 years) to have more difficulty understanding speech in noise than their younger counterparts, perhaps due to age-related central auditory system degradation that is independent of age at the time of the cochlear implant.[64]

Contemporary reports agree that age should not be a limiting factor in consideration of cochlear implantation,[63,65,66] other than to say that implantation as early as hearing aids no longer provide adequate benefit is advisable over waiting until amplification provides little to no benefit. This clinical approach could result in individuals generally being implanted at younger ages.

Aside from duration of deafness, there are a variety of etiologies of acquired SNHL that result in poor spiral ganglia survival and potential atrophy of auditory neurons. These include pathologies that are prone to the development of fibrosis and ossification, such as meningitis, autoimmune disease, and otosclerosis. In addition to increasing the potential for neural atrophy, these pathologies also make optimal electrode insertion into the cochlea more challenging.

Suboptimal electrode array placement has been shown to result in poorer outcomes postimplant. As previously discussed, electrode design and insertion techniques are critical factors for hearing preservation. Insertion of the electrode array to an appropriate depth, in close proximity to the modiolus, and without translocation across the cochlear membranes is equally critical, even in patients with little to no hearing preservation. In addition to the soft surgical techniques previously discussed, research has shown that having more electrodes in the scala vestibuli instead of the scala tympani is correlated with lower open-set speech recognition.[67,68] This relationship may be due to greater distance of the electrode array from the stimulable neural elements in the modiolus, but is more likely due to the trauma to the delicate structures of the cochlea caused by rupturing the cochlear membranes and mixing the perilymphatic and endolymphatic fluids. O'Connell et al[68] reported that lateral wall electrode arrays, which are located furthest from the modiolus, had higher rates of scala tympani insertion than perimodiolar or mid-scala arrays, particularly when they were inserted through the round window or extended round window instead of a cochleostomy. Even though the electrode array may have been further from the modiolus, recipients with a lateral wall array and scala tympani insertion had higher word recognition scores. Other suboptimal electrode array placement may include bending, kinking, or folding of the electrode array, or even partial insertion. These risks are particularly high in patients with anatomical malformations of the cochlea such as Mondini malformations, common cavity, hypoplastic cochleae, or enlarged vestibular aqueducts. Use of fully banded, straight, or double electrode arrays and in some challenging cases, insertion under fluoroscopy may be necessary to ensure as complete of an insertion as possible in this challenging population. Postoperative imaging and/or intraoperative evoked compound action potentials (ECAP) testing can be extremely valuable for confirming appropriate placement and device function. It is not uncommon, even with appropriate device placement, that individuals with anatomical cochlear malformations and/or cochlear ossification will have poorer outcomes than recipients with anatomically typical cochleae. Frequently, higher current levels are necessary to overcome the anatomical challenges, which can introduce the potential for facial stimulation and poorer frequency specificity.

Along with the discussion of electrode array placement belongs the discussion of cochlear coverage. There is certainly the expectation that there will be some frequency-to-place mismatch between the physical location of the electrode contacts relative to the frequencies that the stimulated neurons are coded to transmit. It is unclear to what degree the tonotopic arrangement of the electrode array must coincide with the tonotopic arrangement of the cochlea itself. There is some plasticity to the system which can compensate for minimal frequency-to-place mismatch,[69,70] but this ability may be limited to only a few millimeters of shift from the natural tonotopic arrangement of the cochlea. There is currently interest among implant researchers regarding how to optimize programming of a cochlear implant recognizing that there are anatomical and surgical variations that result in differences in electrode array placement among implant recipients and may impact outcomes.[37,71] In addition to developments in programming approaches, there are also variations in electrode design philosophies among manufacturers in terms of how to address the anatomical and physiological limitations of a frequency-mapped cochlea where the number of possible physical electrode contacts is limited by the small size of the cochlea and the realities of current spread within it.

12.5.2 Auditory Rehabilitation/Training Post-Cochlear Implantation

Postlingually deafened cochlear implant recipients typically develop open-set speech recognition rapidly in the first months after cochlear implant activation. However, results are variable, even for recipients with similar histories, and benefit from the cochlear implant may be somewhat decreased in more challenging listening environments (e.g., speech in noise, telephone, music). Recall that a cochlear implant delivers a substantially altered signal that primarily emphasizes the envelope, but not fine structure, of the acoustic inputs. Recall further that the electrode array assigned to a particular bandpass filter may not be located in closest proximity to those neural fibers that are tonotopically arranged to be most sensitive to those frequencies.[72,73] When combined with individual patient factors (e.g., duration of hearing loss, cognitive capacity, mapping), it is clear that expectations for individual outcomes must be somewhat malleable and may be largely based on the ability of the recipient to learn the new speech patterns produced by the cochlear implant.[73]

Several studies have reported on the critical inclusion of moderate (e.g., 1–2 h/d, 5 d/wk) auditory training for achievement of optimal outcomes following cochlear implantation in adult recipients.[73,74,75,76,77] While this auditory training is most valuable immediately following implant activation, benefits have been observed years after activation.[76] Types of training include bottom-up (analytic) and top-down (synthetic) approaches. There may be benefit from both focusing on gaining meaning in context (synthetic) and focusing on phonemic discrimination (analytic) training methods.[76] Both one-on-one and computer-based strategies have been shown to be effective when the recipient is appropriately motivated.[74,75,76,77] This is not to say that cochlear implants alone do not produce remarkable improvements in speech recognition ability; rather, it is important to realize that auditory training may be a necessary complement to achieve maximal outcomes, particularly in challenging listening environments.[75]

12.5.3 Music and Cochlear Implantation

Generally speaking, cochlear implant recipients as a group tend to perform poorly on spectrally complex aspects of speech perception and these spectral components are also associated with music understanding and appreciation.[78] Recalling the earlier discussion of coding strategies in cochlear implants, cochlear implant recipients are often unable to achieve good frequency resolution because the primary coding method is envelope extraction. In such methods, primarily temporal information is preserved and is delivered in a tonotopically organized manner using a series of bandpass filters with fixed center frequencies. While this arrangement is often adequate for speech perception, even in more challenging listening environments, the perception and enjoyment of music is often limited as the listener is often unable to appreciate subtleties of pitch and timbre.[78,79]

Modern day cochlear implant coding strategies that introduce some fine structure signal processing attempt to improve on this circumstance. There is also evolving interest in postoperative music rehabilitation, particularly for postlingually deafened adults who, some reports suggest, may have more decreased satisfaction with music using cochlear implant(s) than their prelingually deafened counterparts.[80]

12.5.4 Importance of Longitudinal Postoperative Assessment

As previously mentioned, longitudinal postoperative assessment is of critical importance for cochlear implant recipients. Longitudinal assessment should include evaluation of residual hearing (in both implanted and unimplanted ears), subjective evaluation of performance, and assessment of detection thresholds in the soundfield when using the cochlear implant. Finally, speech perception testing in a variety of conditions (implant only and bilateral or bimodal) should be conducted routinely. Methodology for speech perception testing has been previously described in the "Candidacy" section of this chapter. However, beyond determining appropriate candidacy, longitudinal testing using the same measures allows the clinician to accurately assess the benefit obtained from the cochlear implant system and to quickly identify any changes in performance that need attention.

Impedance measurements should also be routinely conducted at follow-up appointments. The term impedance refers to the opposition to the flow of current from the electrode array when a certain voltage is applied and can be determined using Ohm's law: $V = IR$ or $I = V/R$, where V = voltage, I = current, and R = resistance. Recall that the cochlear implant electrode array is bathed in the highly conductive perilymph of the scala tympani. Current, therefore, should be easily conducted and impedance should be relatively low. Impedances usually stabilize within the first 1 to 2 months of device use,[81] and subsequent changes may have clinical implications that require management. Factors that may influence electrode impedances include device-related issues such as short- or open circuits which can result from damage to or malfunction of the device and physiological issues such as ossification, fibrous encapsulation of the electrode array which occurs as an autoimmune response to the presence of a foreign object, inflammatory or infectious processes, or nonuse of the device.

12.6 Device Failure and Postoperative Complications

Cochlear implant device failure is an infrequent but not uncommon occurrence.[82] The International Consensus Group for Cochlear Implant Reliability Reporting created a consensus statement[83] and standardized reporting that classifies failures as follows:

- Device failure (often called "hard failure")—all explanted devices falling outside of manufacturer specifications.
- Device failure (often called "soft failure")—all explanted devices where patient demonstrated performance decrement that improved with replacement device but explanted device was found to be in specifications.
- Medical failure—those failures due to patient factors, including CI exposure or infection, receiver/stimulator migration, or electrode array migration.

In terms of surgical complications, cochlear implantation is a safe surgical technique with low complication rates; however, complications have been reported. Farinetti et al[84] reported a minor complication rate of 14.9% and major complication rate of 5%. The most common complication (7.2%) was related to infectious processes including meningitis, acute otitis media, mastoiditis, skin infections, and labyrinthitis. Local skin complications were observed in 2.5% of recipients and included ulceration, infection, or wound dehiscence. Vestibular insult (3.7%), tinnitus (1.7%), and dysgeusia (1.2%) were also reported. Other low-incidence (< 1%) complications include cerebrospinal fluid (CSF) gusher (common in cochlear malformations), transient facial nerve palsy, and device failure. As previously discussed, while loss of residual hearing used to occur essentially 100% of the time, hearing preservation rates are much higher with contemporary electrode arrays and residual cochlear function can often be completely preserved.

12.7 Future Directions

12.7.1 Expansion of Candidacy

The current FDA labeling for standard cochlear implant electrode arrays requires speech recognition ability be defined using sentence materials. As previously described, over time it has become apparent that the initially utilized HINT sentence materials were too simplistic and did not reflect individuals' real-world performance.[16] As a result, the 2011 MSTB evolved to recommend AZ Bio Sentence materials as the sentence material of choice.

More recently, consideration is being given to whether contextual sentence materials are appropriate or whether monosyllabic words would be more appropriate determinants of candidacy. The use of monosyllables is already in place outside of the United States[85] and the most recently labeled device, the Cochlear Nucleus Hybrid electrode array was labeled using CNC words as the candidacy metric for speech recognition. As early as 2010, Gifford et al[85] reported that patient performance should be assessed with respect to individual ear performance and that the current candidacy criteria are set too low and may be excluding appropriate candidates. Specifically, they reported that patients with preimplant CNC scores ranging from 30 to 68% in the best-aided condition—scores that are much higher than scores for the conventional cochlear implant recipient—significantly benefit from a cochlear implant. As cochlear implant technology evolves, measures for assessment of candidacy and longitudinal performance will need to follow suit.

12.7.2 Optimizing Programming

Current programming techniques rely heavily on default parameters and often fail to take into account likely individual differences, such as electrode array insertion depth, presence of cochlear dead regions and neural degradation, variability in cochlear duct length, tonotopic arrangement of the cochlea, and spectral overlap. Researchers have begun to investigate how to optimize programming both within an individual ear and when trying to balance the sound perception between two ears. The application of cochlear implantation in patients with UHL has introduced new opportunities for pitch ranking that were never possible in the past since these recipients have the unique ability to directly compare a normal-hearing ear to one hearing through a cochlear implant. Computed tomography (CT)-guided cochlear implant programming,[37] estimation of cochlear duct length prior to surgery,[86] and personalizing frequency allocation tables[71] are all under investigation as possible methods to optimize cochlear implant outcomes.

12.7.3 Optimizing Acoustic Contributions

The advantages of residual hearing are well documented, but understanding how to optimize the contribution of acoustic hearing is still not completely understood. Recent developments have included Advanced Bionics' launch of the Naida Link hearing aid, the first hearing aid to have binaural streaming capabilities and a proprietary bimodal fitting algorithm that aligns the frequency response, loudness growth, and dynamic compression between the two devices.

Advancements in recommendations for programming an integrated acoustic component, such as determining appropriate electric-acoustic frequency boundaries, are rapidly developing. In the near future, better understanding of how to optimize acoustic hearing in both implanted and contralateral ears as well as the continuing expansion of criteria to include individuals with greater degrees of low-frequency hearing and shorter durations of hearing loss will result in continued improvement in challenging listening conditions such as background noise and music.

12.8 Conclusions

Cochlear implantation has come a long way from its original inception. Implanted devices have evolved from single-channel devices offering little more than sound awareness to multichannel implants using advanced signal processing strategies.[87] From early beginnings as a last resort for patients with bilateral profound SNHL to the current application in patients with significant residual hearing, the benefits offered by cochlear implants continue to improve and the candidacy pool continues to expand. Looking to the future, possible utility in patients with unilateral hearing loss, intractable tinnitus, and significant hearing loss based on word scores instead of sentences offer exciting possibilities. Limitations persist, however, and there is still much to learn regarding optimization of outcomes, perceived sound quality, and candidate identification. Cochlear implantation remains an imperfect, but constantly evolving, combination of art and science that offers the amazing capacity to restore function to a diminished sensory system.

References

[1] Eisen MD. The history of cochlear implants. In: Niparko JK, ed. Cochlear Implants: Principles and Practices. 2nd ed. Philadelphia, PA: Lippincott Williams & Wilkins; 2000:89–93

[2] Sanna M, Free RH, Merkus P, et al, eds. Surgery for Cochlear and Other Auditory Implants. Kindle ed. Stuttgart: Thieme; 2015e

[3] Bilger RC. Evaluation of subjects presently fitted with implanted auditory prostheses. Ann Otol Rhinol Laryngol. 1977; 86(suppl 38):1–176

[4] Hinojosa R, Marion M. Histopathology of profound sensorineural deafness. Ann N Y Acad Sci. 1983; 405:459–484

[5] Lazard DS, Giraud A-L, Gnansia D, Meyer B, Sterkers O. Understanding the deafened brain: implications for cochlear implant rehabilitation. Eur Ann Otorhinolaryngol Head Neck Dis. 2012; 129(2):98–103

[6] Havenith S, Lammers MJ, Tange RA, et al. Hearing preservation surgery: cochleostomy or round window approach? A systematic review. Otol Neurotol. 2013; 34(4):667–674

[7] Wilson BS, Dorman MF. The design of cochlear implants. In: Niparko JK, ed. Cochlear Implants: Principles and Practices. 2nd ed. Philadelphia, PA: Lippincott Williams & Wilkins; 2000:95–135

[8] Wolfe J, Schafer EC, Neumann S. Basic components and operation of a cochlear implant. In: Wolfe J, Schafer EC, eds. Programming Cochlear Implants. 2nd ed. San Diego, CA: Plural; 2015

[9] Carlson ML, Driscoll CLW, Gifford RH, McMenomey SO. Cochlear implantation: current and future device options. Otolaryngol Clin North Am. 2012; 45(1):221–248

[10] Lin FR, Niparko JK, Ferrucci L. Hearing loss prevalence in the United States. Arch Intern Med. 2011; 171(20):1851–1852

[11] Incidence of severe and profound hearing loss in the United States and United Kingdom. American Academy of Audiology Web site. http://www.audiology.org/news/incidence-severe-and-profound-hearing-loss-united-states-and-united-kingdom. Published May 10, 2013. Accessed October 22, 2016

[12] Gifford RH, Driscoll CLW, Davis TJ, Fiebig P, Micco A, Dorman MF. A within-subject comparison of bimodal hearing, bilateral cochlear implantation, and bilateral cochlear implantation with bilateral hearing preservation: high-performing patients. Otol Neurotol. 2015; 36(8):1331–1337

[13] Auditory Potential. Minimum speed test battery (MSTB) for adult cochlear implant users. User manual version 1.0.2011. Available at: Accessed March 29, 2018

[14] Peterson GE, Lehiste I. Revised CNC lists for auditory tests. J Speech Hear Disord. 1962; 27:62–70

[15] Nilsson M, Soli SD, Sullivan JA. Speech recognition materials and ceiling effects: considerations for cochlear implant programs. Audiol Neurootol 2008; 13(3):193–205

[16] Gifford RH, Shallop JK, Peterson AM. Speech recognition materials and ceiling effects: considerations for cochlear implant programs. Audiol Neurootol. 2008; 13(3):193–205

[17] Spahr AJ, Dorman MF, Litvak LM, et al. Development and validation of the AzBio sentence lists. Ear Hear. 2012; 33(1):112–117

[18] Killion M, Niquette P, Revit L, Skinner M. Quick SIN and BKB-SIN, two new speech-in-noise tests permitting SNR-50 estimates in 1 to 2 min (A). J Acoust Soc Am. 2001; 109(5):2502–2512

[19] Firszt JB, Holden LK, Skinner MW, et al. Recognition of speech presented at soft to loud levels by adult co-chlear implant recipients of three cochlear implant systems. Ear Hear. 2004; 25(4):375–387

[20] Roeser R, Clark J. Live voice speech recognition audiometry: stop the madness! Audiol Today. 2008; 20:32–33

[21] Krabbe PF, Hinderink JB, van den Broek P. The effect of cochlear implant use in postlingually deaf adults. Int J Technol Assess Health Care. 2000; 16(3):864–873

[22] Coelho DH, Yeh J, Kim JT, Lalwani AK. Cochlear implantation is associated with minimal anesthetic risk in the elderly. Laryngoscope. 2009; 119(2):355–358

[23] Buchman CA, Joy J, Hodges A, Telischi FF, Balkany TJ. Vestibular effects of cochlear implantation. Laryngoscope. 2004; 114(10 pt 2, suppl 103):1–22

[24] Nordfalk KF, Rasmussen K, Hopp E, Bunne M, Silvola JT, Jablonski GE. Insertion depth in cochlear implantation and outcome in residual hearing and vestibular function. Ear Hear. 2016; 37(2):e129–e137

[25] Santa Maria PL, Gluth MB, Yuan Y, Atlas MD, Blevins NH. Hearing preservation surgery for cochlear implantation: a meta-analysis. Otol Neurotol. 2014; 35(10):e256–e269

[26] Skarzynski H, Lorens A, Matusiak M, Porowski M, Skarzynski PH, James CJ. Cochlear implantation with the nucleus slim straight electrode in subjects with residual low-frequency hearing. Ear Hear. 2014; 35(2):e33–e43

[27] Gifford RH, Dorman MF. The psychophysics of low-frequency acoustic hearing in electric and acoustic stimulation (EAS) and bimodal patients. J Hear Sci. 2012; 2(2):33–44

[28] Nguyen S, Cloutier F, Philippon D, Côté M, Bussières R, Backous DD. Outcomes review of modern hearing preservation technique in cochlear implant. Auris Nasus Larynx. 2016; 43(5):485–488

[29] Hamzavi J, Baumgartner WD, Pok SM, Franz P, Gstoettner W. Variables affecting speech perception in postlingually deaf adults following cochlear implantation. Acta Otolaryngol. 2003; 123(4):493–498

[30] Oh SH, Kim CS, Kang EJ, et al. Speech perception after cochlear implantation over a 4-year time period. Acta Otolaryngol. 2003; 123(2):148–153

[31] Saliba I, Nader ME, El Fata F, Leroux T. Bone anchored hearing aid in single sided deafness: outcome in right-handed patients. Auris Nasus Larynx. 2011; 38(5):570–576

[32] Basura GJ, Eapen R, Buchman CA. Bilateral cochlear implantation: current concepts, indications, and results. Laryngoscope. 2009; 119(12):2395–2401

[33] Choi JE, Moon IJ, Kim EY, et al. Sound localization and speech perception in noise of pediatric cochlear implant recipients: bimodal fitting versus bilateral cochlear implants. Ear Hear. 2017; 38(4):426–440

[34] Galvin KL, Mok M. Everyday listening performance of children before and after receiving a second cochlear implant: results using the parent version of the speech, spatial, and qualities hearing scale. Ear Hear. 2016; 37(1):93–102

[35] Lammers MJW, van der Heijden GJMG, Pourier VEC, Grolman W. Bilateral cochlear implantation in children: a systematic review and best-evidence synthesis. Laryngoscope. 2014; 124(7):1694–1699

[36] Dorman M, Spahr A, Gifford RH, et al. Bilateral and bimodal benefits as a function of age for adults fitted with a cochlear implant. J Hear Sci. 2012; 2(4):EA37–EA39

[37] Labadie RF, Noble JH, Hedley-Williams AJ, Sunderhaus LW, Dawant BM, Gifford RH. Results of postoperative, CT-based, electrode deactivation on hearing in prelingually deafened adult cochlear implant recipients. Otol Neurotol. 2016; 37(2):137–145

[38] Schafer EC, Amlani AM, Seibold A, Shattuck PL. A meta-analytic comparison of binaural benefits between bilateral cochlear implants and bimodal stimulation. J Am Acad Audiol. 2007; 18(9):760–776

[39] Morera C, Cavalle L, Manrique M, et al. Contralateral hearing aid use in cochlear implanted patients: multicenter study of bimodal benefit. Acta Otolaryngol. 2012; 132(10):1084–1094

[40] Morera C, Manrique M, Ramos A, et al. Advantages of binaural hearing provided through bimodal stimulation via a cochlear implant and a conventional hearing aid: a 6-month comparative study. Acta Otolaryngol. 2005; 125(6):596–606

[41] Luntz M, Egra-Dagan D, Attias J, Yehudai N, Most T, Shpak T. From hearing with a cochlear implant and a contralateral hearing aid (CI/HA) to hearing with two cochlear implants (CI/CI): a within-subject design comparison. Otol Neurotol. 2014; 35(10):1682–1690

[42] Brown CA, Bacon SP. Low-frequency speech cues and simulated electric-acoustic hearing. J Acoust Soc Am. 2009; 125(3):1658–1665

[43] Zhang T, Dorman MF, Spahr AJ. Information from the voice fundamental frequency (F0) region accounts for the majority of the benefit when acoustic stimulation is added to electric stimulation. Ear Hear. 2010; 31(1):63–69

[44] Loiselle LH, Dorman MF, Yost WA, Gifford RH. Sound source localization by hearing preservation patients with and without symmetrical low-frequency acoustic hearing. Audiol Neurootol. 2015; 20(3):166–171

[45] Snapp H, Angeli S, Telischi FF, Fabry D. Postoperative validation of bone-anchored implants in the single-sided deafness population. Otol Neurotol. 2012; 33(3):291–296

[46] Newman CW, Jacobson GP, Hug GA, Sandridge SA. Perceived hearing handicap of patients with unilateral or mild hearing loss. Ann Otol Rhinol Laryngol. 1997; 106(3):210–214

[47] Wie OB, Pripp AH, Tvete O. Unilateral deafness in adults: effects on communication and social interaction. Ann Otol Rhinol Laryngol. 2010; 119(11):772–781

[48] Douglas SA, Yeung P, Daudia A, Gatehouse S, O'Donoghue GM. Spatial hearing disability after acoustic neuroma removal. Laryngoscope. 2007; 117(9):1648–1651

[49] Grossmann W, Brill S, Moeltner A, Mlynski R, Hagen R, Radeloff A. Cochlear implantation improves spatial release from masking and restores localization abilities in single-sided deaf patients. Otol Neurotol. 2016; 37(6):658–664

[50] Mertens G, Kleine Punte A, De Bodt M, Van de Heyning P. Binaural auditory outcomes in patients

with postlingual profound unilateral hearing loss: 3 years after cochlear implantation. Audiol Neurootol. 2015; 20(suppl 1):67–72

[51] Zeitler DM, Dorman MF, Natale SJ, Loiselle L, Yost WA, Gifford RH. Sound source localization and speech understanding in complex listening environments by single-sided deaf listeners after cochlear implantation. Otol Neurotol. 2015; 36(9):1467–1471

[52] Kitterick PT, Lucas L, Smith SN. Improving health-related quality of life in single-sided deafness: a systematic review and meta-analysis. Audiol Neurootol. 2015; 20(suppl 1):79–86

[53] Cabral Junior F, Pinna MH, Alves RD, Malerbi AFS, Bento RF. Cochlear implantation and single-sided deafness: a systematic review of the literature. Int Arch Otorhinolaryngol. 2016; 20(1):69–75

[54] Quaranta N, Fernandez-Vega S, D'elia C, Filipo R, Quaranta A. The effect of unilateral multichannel cochlear implant on bilaterally perceived tinnitus. Acta Otolaryngol. 2008; 128(2):159–163

[55] Arts RAGJ, Netz T, Janssen AM, George ELJ, Stokroos RJ. The occurrence of tinnitus after CI surgery in patients with severe hearing loss: a retrospective study. Int J Audiol. 2015; 54(12):910–917

[56] Van de Heyning P, Vermeire K, Diebl M, Nopp P, Anderson I, De Ridder D. Incapacitating unilateral tinnitus in single-sided deafness treated by cochlear implantation. Ann Otol Rhinol Laryngol. 2008; 117(9):645–652

[57] Mertens G, De Bodt M, Van de Heyning P. Cochlear implantation as a long-term treatment for ipsilateral incapacitating tinnitus in subjects with unilateral hearing loss up to 10 years. Hear Res. 2016; 331:1–6

[58] Arts RAGJ, George ELJ, Stokroos RJ, Vermeire K. Review: cochlear implants as a treatment of tinnitus in single-sided deafness. Curr Opin Otolaryngol Head Neck Surg. 2012; 20(5):398–403

[59] Arts RAGJ, George ELJ, Janssen M, Griessner A, Zierhofer C, Stokroos RJ. Tinnitus suppression by intracochlear electrical stimulation in single sided deafness—a prospective clinical trial: follow-up. PLoS One. 2016; 11(4):e0153131

[60] Boisvert I, McMahon CM, Dowell RC, Lyxell B. Long-term asymmetric hearing affects cochlear implantation outcomes differently in adults with pre- and postlingual hearing loss. PLoS One. 2015; 10(6):e0129167

[61] Ryugo D. Auditory neuroplasticity, hearing loss and cochlear implants. Cell Tissue Res. 2015; 361(1):251–269

[62] Connell SS, Balkany TJ. Cochlear implants. Clin Geriatr Med. 2006; 22(3):677–686

[63] Carlson ML, Breen JT, Gifford RH, et al. Cochlear implantation in the octogenarian and nonagenarian. Otol Neurotol. 2010; 31(8):1343–1349

[64] Holden LK, Finley CC, Firszt JB, et al. Factors affecting open-set word recognition in adults with cochlear implants. Ear Hear. 2013; 34(3):342–360

[65] Budenz CL, Cosetti MK, Coelho DH, et al. The effects of cochlear implantation on speech perception in older adults. J Am Geriatr Soc. 2011; 59(3):446–453

[66] Hiel AL, Gerard JM, Decat M, Deggouj N. Is age a limiting factor for adaptation to cochlear implant? Eur Arch Otorhinolaryngol. 2016; 273(9):2495–2502

[67] Finley CC, Holden TA, Holden LK, et al. Role of electrode placement as a contributor to variability in cochlear implant outcomes. Otol Neurotol. 2008; 29(7):920–928

[68] O'Connell BP, Cakir A, Hunter JB, et al. Electrode location and angular insertion depth are predictors of audiologic outcomes in cochlear implantation. Otol Neurotol. 2016; 37(8):1016–1023

[69] Fu Q-J, Shannon RV. Effects of electrode location and spacing on phoneme recognition with the Nucleus-22 cochlear implant. Ear Hear. 1999; 20(4):321–331

[70] Svirsky MA, Silveira A, Neuburger H, Teoh SW, Suárez H. Long-term auditory adaptation to a modified peripheral frequency map. Acta Otolaryngol. 2004; 124(4):381–386

[71] Landsberger DM, Svrakic M, Roland JT, Jr, Svirsky M. The relationship between insertion angles, default frequency allocations, and spiral ganglion place pitch in cochlear implants. Ear Hear. 2015; 36(5):e207–e213

[72] Fu Q-J, Shannon RV. Recognition of spectrally degraded and frequency-shifted vowels in acoustic and electric hearing. J Acoust Soc Am. 1999; 105(3):1889–1900

[73] Fu Q-J, Galvin J, Wang X, Nogaki G. Effects of auditory training on adult cochlear implant patients: a preliminary report. Cochlear Implants Int. 2004; 5(suppl 1):84–90

[74] Barlow N, Purdy SC, Sharma M, Giles E, Narne V. The effect of short-term auditory training on speech in noise perception and cortical auditory evoked potentials in adults with cochlear implants. Semin Hear. 2016; 37(1):84–98

[75] Fu Q-J, Galvin JJ, III. Maximizing cochlear implant patients' performance with advanced speech training procedures. Hear Res. 2008; 242(1–2):198–208

[76] Schumann A, Serman M, Gefeller O, Hoppe U. Computer-based auditory phoneme discrimination training improves speech recognition in noise in experienced adult cochlear implant listeners. Int J Audiol. 2015; 54(3):190–198

[77] Schumann A, Hast A, Hoppe U. Speech performance and training effects in the cochlear implant elderly. Audiol Neurootol. 2014; 19(suppl 1):45–48

[78] Gfeller K, Guthe E, Driscoll V, Brown CJ. A preliminary report of music-based training for adult cochlear implant users: rationales and development. Cochlear Implants Int. 2015; 16(3, suppl 3):S22–S31

[79] Limb CJ, Roy AT. Technological, biological, and acoustical constraints to music perception in cochlear implant users. Hear Res. 2014; 308:13–26

[80] Bruns L, Mürbe D, Hahne A. Understanding music with cochlear implants. Sci Rep. 2016; 6:32026

[81] Hughes ML, Vander Werff KR, Brown CJ, et al. A longitudinal study of electrode impedance, the electrically evoked compound action potential, and behavioral measures in nucleus 24 cochlear implant users. Ear Hear. 2001; 22(6):471–486

[82] Brown KD, Connell SS, Balkany TJ, Eshraghi AE, Telischi FF, Angeli SA. Incidence and indications for revision cochlear implant surgery in adults and children. Laryngoscope. 2009; 119(1):152–157

[83] Battmer RD, Backous DD, Balkany TJ, et al; International Consensus Group for Cochlear Implant Reliability Reporting. International classification of reliability for implanted cochlear implant receiver stimulators. Otol Neurotol. 2010; 31(8):1190–1193

[84] Farinetti A, Ben Gharbia D, Mancini J, Roman S, Nicollas R, Triglia JM. Cochlear implant complications in 403 patients: comparative study of adults and children and review of the literature. Eur Ann Otorhinolaryngol Head Neck Dis 2009; 119(1):152–157

[85] Gifford RH, Dorman MF, Shallop JK, Sydlowski SA. Evidence for the expansion of adult cochlear implant candidacy. Ear Hear. 2010; 31(2):186–194

[86] Mistrík P, Jolly C. Optimal electrode length to match patient specific cochlear anatomy. Eur Ann Otorhinolaryngol Head Neck Dis. 2016; 133(suppl 1):S68–S71

[87] Waltzman SB, Shapiro WH. Cochlear implants in adults. In: Valente M, Hosford-Dunn H, Roeser RJ, eds. Audiology Treatment. New York, NY: Thieme; 2000:537–546

13 Cochlear Implants in Children

Sarah A. Sydlowski

13.1 Introduction

Cochlear implantation in children has rapidly evolved over the past two decades. The introduction of the ability to restore the sense of hearing to children born with profound deafness has had far-reaching impact and has not occurred without fierce debate regarding the ethics of making such a permanent intervention. Proponents of Deaf culture worry that cochlear implants will (or perhaps already have) alter the landscape of their community forever. Families of children born deaf now face options regarding communication mode, educational setting, and access to the auditory world. However, children are not just small adults. Pediatric cochlear implant candidates present a spectrum of challenges that clinicians must navigate in order to facilitate maximum benefit and outcomes. These include how to effectively assess candidacy and outcomes, how to manage decision regarding simultaneous or sequential bilateral, or bimodal, implantation, the probability of future revision surgery during a child's lifetime, deciding on communication mode and educational setting, and managing children with multiple disabilities, among others. The major issues relevant to managing pediatric cochlear implant candidates and recipients is summarized in Chapter 12.

13.2 History of Cochlear Implants in Children

As outlined in Chapter 12, cochlear implants became commercially available in the early 1980s. Although some children experimentally received cochlear implants in the late 1970s and early 1980s, it wasn't until 1990 that the Food and Drug Administration (FDA) approved cochlear implants for use in children. Early investigations focused on providing cochlear implants primarily to prelingually deafened children, many of whom were older and communicated using sign language. As a result, reports of open-set speech understanding were limited and benefits were modest, but measurable. The results were encouraging enough to lead to the pediatric clinical trials that ultimately earned cochlear implants' FDA approval for use in children. In 1990, Cochlear's Nucleus N22 device was approved for use in children ages 2 years and older. Advanced Bionics and MED-EL achieved similar labeling in 1997 and 2001, respectively. Eventually, candidacy was expanded to children as young as 12 months of age. Simultaneous bilateral cochlear implantation has become standard of care for children born with profound deafness and in many centers, implant teams aim to have a child prepared for surgery well before his or her first birthday. Looking to the future, children with greater degrees of residual hearing are receiving cochlear implants, although candidacy criteria continue to be more restrictive than for adults. However, consideration of younger ages and greater residual hearing with expectations for better and better outcomes are certainly on the horizon.

Since the introduction of this technology to the public and despite the tremendous advances, debates have raged about the ethical and moral dilemma of offering children's access to an entirely different auditory experience, many times before they would be old enough to express an opinion relative to the decision. In the earliest days of cochlear implantation, and to some extent even in the modern day, cochlear implantation meant guaranteed intracochlear trauma and loss of any residual hearing. Some individuals opposed cochlear implantation because it prevented the child from potentially benefitting from future technologies. Even today, the question of whether they should "save" one or both ears for advancements is a common question for new parents considering cochlear implantation. As will be discussed later in this chapter, the significant advantages of early, bilateral implantation are now well known and outweigh the potential future benefit of a yet to be developed technology.

13.3 Cultural Issues of Cochlear Implantation

Although cochlear implantation for deaf children is routinely accepted as standard of care in the modern day, in the early days of cochlear implantation in children, debate raged. Perhaps no opponents were more vocal than the Deaf community, who viewed cochlear implantation as an invasive affront to their way of life that prevented children from appreciating and connecting with their Deaf culture. Opponents of cochlear implantation argued that deafness is not an impairment, or a deficiency that needs to be fixed. They also pointed out that individuals with cochlear implants are still, in fact, deaf. On the other side of the debate, proponents argued that because approximately 90% of parents who have deaf child are themselves hearing,[1] cochlear implants were a necessary intervention that was unlikely to specifically impact the Deaf community because these children were born into hearing families and would be unlikely to easily experience Deaf culture.

Although the debate has calmed over the years, the question of viewing deafness as a culture as opposed to a disability remains. Cochlear implants have slowly become more accepted by the Deaf community as a whole, particularly when considered as an option on a spectrum of interventions including use of American Sign Language (ASL).[1] The current National Association of the Deaf (NAD) position statement "recognizes the rights of parents to make informed choices for their deaf and hard of hearing children, respects their choice to use cochlear implants and all other assistive devices, and strongly supports the development of the whole child and of language and literacy."[2] This statement is in stark contrast to the 1991 position statement which stated "(The NAD) deplores the decision of the Food and Drug Administration (to approve implantation in children aged 2 to 17) which was unsound scientifically, procedurally, and ethically.[3]" Continued improvements in patient outcomes have also contributed to changes in perception. Whereas there was concern in the early days of cochlear implantation that children would be trapped in a "no man's land"—unable to communicate with either the deaf or the hearing—modern day outcomes with appropriate intervention and auditory training routinely see children integrated in mainstream classrooms with access to all of the educational and vocational choices of a typically hearing child.

13.4 Candidacy Considerations

As discussed in Chapter 12, cochlear implant candidacy criteria have evolved over time. This evolution was particularly meaningful for children with hearing, for whom cochlear implants weren't an option prior to 1990. When cochlear implants were initially developed, their use was restricted to adult candidates. However, by the mid-1980s, the safety and efficacy of cochlear implants were well established and access to the exciting new technology was extended first to older children then by 2000 to children aged 12 months and younger. Audiological criteria for implantation are based on performance with traditional forms of amplification, such as hearing aids. Children generally must have had access to an adequate trial (at least 3–6 months) with these conventional forms of amplification, as well as adequate training with the aids, before an implant can be considered.

Children being considered for implantation must be using amplification on a daily basis and be enrolled in programs that value audition. Criteria are still disparate for older and younger children, with children younger than 2 years required to have bilateral profound hearing loss before being approved, while children ages 2 to 17 years may demonstrate severe-to-profound audiometric thresholds (▶ Fig. 13.1). As with adult candidacy criteria, there are two primary aspects to approved labeling: audiometric thresholds and auditory skills/speech recognition performance in the best aided condition. Because of the young ages and various development stages of candidates, parental questionnaires are often completed when assessing candidacy and will be discussed in detail shortly. The indications for each manufacturer's devices are summarized in ▶ Table 13.1. It should be noted that while contraindications for cochlear implant are equivalent for pediatric and adult candidates (Chapter 12), candidacy criteria for children is much stricter than for adults. Notably, children must miss 70 to 88% of incoming speech signals before meeting current FDA labeling for cochlear implantation although adults are only required to miss approximately half of the signal. This slower evolution is likely reflective of the medical community's dedication to "do no harm." In very young children, who are still developing speech and language and behavioral responses, an abundance of caution is taken to avoid making incorrect permanent and consequential decisions. However, in recent years, concern that children are being prevented from achieving maximum benefit as a result of this carefulness has occasioned a shifting perspective. Expansion of cochlear implant criteria for children will be discussed later in this chapter.

Perhaps even more important than when considering the candidacy of adult patients is the interdisciplinary composition of pediatric cochlear implant teams. Audiological assessment and intervention

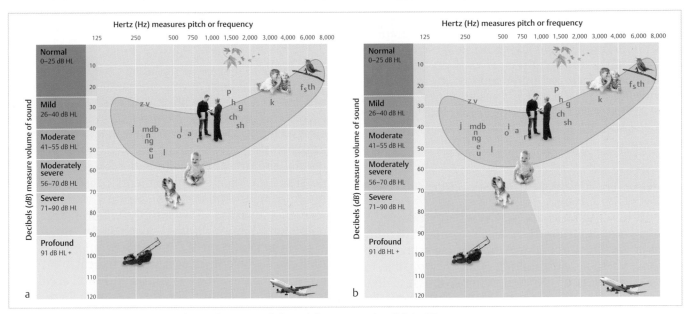

Fig. 13.1 Audiometric criteria for pediatric candidacy. **(a)** <24 months. **(b)** 2–17 yrs.

Table 13.1 Pediatric cochlear implant candidacy criteria

	Unaided audiometric thresholds	Auditory skills and speech recognition (younger children)	Auditory skills and speech recognition (older children)	Amplification requirements
Advanced Bionics HiRes90K HiRes90K Ultra	Severe-to-profound bilateral SNHL (> 70 dB HL)	< 4 y: failure to reach developmentally appropriate auditory milestones per IT-MAIS or MAIS, or < 20% on open-set word recognition test (MLNT) using MLV (70 dB SPL)	> 4 y: < 12% on difficult open-set word recognition (PBK) or < 30% on open-set sentences (HINT-C) using recorded speech (70 dB SPL)	Use of appropriate hearing aids for at least 6 mo (ages 2–17) or at least 3 mo (ages 12–23 mo). Minimum HA use waived in cases of ossification.
Cochlear Americas CI24RE CI512 CI522 CI532	12–23 months: bilateral profound SNHL 24 mo–18 y: bilateral severe-to-profound SNHL	Lack of progress in development of simple auditory skills as quantified on measure like MAIS or ESP	Less than or equal to 30% correct on MLNT or LNT, depending on child's cognitive and linguistic skills	Use of appropriate amplification and participation in an intensive aural habilitation program over 3–6 mo
MED-EL PulsarCI[100] Sonata[100] TI Concert Synchrony	Profound bilateral SNHL with thresholds ≥90 dB HL at 1,000 Hz	Lack of progress in the development of simple auditory skills in conjunction with appropriate amplification	< 20% correct or MLNT or LNT, depending on cognitive ability and linguistic skills	Use of appropriate amplification and participation in intensive aural habilitation over 3–6 months. Radiological evidence of cochlear ossification may justify shorter trial period with amplification

Abbreviations: ESP, Early Speech Perception; HA, hearing aid; HINT-C, Hearing in Noise Test for Children; IT-MAIS, the Infant-Toddler: Meaningful Auditory Integration Scale; MAIS, Meaningful Auditory Integration Scale; MLNT, Multisyllabic Lexical Neighborhood Test; MLV, monitored live voice; PBK, Phonetically Balanced Kindergarten; SNHL, sensorineural hearing loss; SPL, sound pressure level.
Source: Adapted with permission from Cochlear Implant Patient Assessment: Evaluation of Candidacy, Performance, and Outcomes by René H. Gifford. © 2013 Plural Publishing, Inc. All rights reserved.

are key, but the input of parents, teachers, speech language pathologists, auditory verbal therapists, social workers, psychologists, and developmental pediatricians, among others, is critical. Determination of candidacy is rarely centered on a moment in time, but is rather a process that may begin as early of diagnosis of the hearing loss and continues over months or years of consistent evaluation and assessment.

13.4.1 Multidisciplinary Nature of Team

A multidisciplinary approach when considering cochlear implantation is essential to understanding the whole child and making appropriate recommendations. Various team members are responsible for different aspects of the comprehensive assessment. An audiologist will determine the child's hearing levels, confirm the appropriate fitting of amplification, and assess the effect of that amplification on the child's auditory behaviors. The surgeon will review computed tomography (CT) or magnetic resonance imaging (MRI) images to evaluate whether there is an anatomical reason for the hearing loss or a contraindication to surgery. Additionally, the surgeon will review the medical history, family history, and discuss any other disabilities or comorbidities that may be present. A speech language pathologist will assess the child's speech and language development, determine if any deficiencies are related to the hearing loss, and establish a baseline for speech and language skills. Other members of the team may include a psychologist, a social worker, or an educational specialist who will work with the parents to identify any barriers to successful implantation and follow-up, to reinforce the importance of auditory habilitation and training after surgery, and to navigate some of the logistical challenges that they may face when managing the needs of a child with hearing loss. The ability of the team to communicate effectively with one another to cover all of these areas is crucial to the success of a pediatric cochlear implant candidate.

> **Pearl** ✔
>
> The ability of the multidisciplinary team to effectively communicate with one another and thoroughly assess the needs of the child and establish the expectations of the family are key to success.

As will be discussed shortly, time is of the essence when considering cochlear implantation, particularly for a congenitally deaf child, so the ability to orchestrate these evaluations in a timely manner is also an important hallmark of a successful implant team.

13.4.2 Audiological Assessment of Young Children

The ability to assess the auditory capabilities of children is critical both during the candidacy evaluation process and after cochlear implantation. However, there are a number of factors that must be considered including the materials utilized and the manner in which they are presented as well as the developmental abilities of the child being tested. While it is possible to evaluate adult patients consistently over multiple visits, children are generally more difficult to test for a variety of reasons. Attention span, developmental abilities, limited vocabularies, interest in a task (or lack thereof), behavioral differences, and multiple involvement of several medical conditions all influence the ability to consistently and accurately assess their auditory abilities. Despite these challenges, it is critical that every effort be made to capture the auditory progress that is achieved with any hearing device in order to make appropriate clinical recommendations during a critical period of development. Multimodal assessment is necessary and includes evaluation of audibility, speech perception and recognition, and speech and language production. Multiple visits may be necessary as children will frequently fatigue before a comprehensive assessment is complete.

Audibility

The goal of cochlear implant candidacy evaluations and postoperative assessments is to ensure that all critical sounds of speech are both audible and comprehensible. Audibility is related to the ability of the children to detect the presence of sound at soft levels. This audibility is particularly important to children with pre- or perilingual hearing loss as access to these soft sounds of speech is necessary for speech and language development. Audibility can be evaluated by measuring sound-field thresholds in the sound booth. It is recommended to use frequency-modulated (FM) or warbled tones as opposed to narrowband noise both to avoid the impact of standing waves and to elicit threshold estimates that are as frequency-specific as possible.[4] Soft speech is approximately 50 to 56 dBA on average,[5,6] and individual phonemes may be as soft as 15 dB. Thus, clinicians should strive to ensure that any hearing device results in average thresholds of not more than 20 to 25 dB HL.

Speech Perception and Recognition

Audibility alone is not an adequate means of assessment to understand a child's hearing capability. It is necessary to evaluate speech recognition ability as well, once the child is developmentally able to do so. There are several important factors to consider when evaluating speech recognition ability. These include presentation level, speech materials (e.g., recorded or monitored live voice [MLV], ability to assess performance longitudinally), and test condition. Until recently, while a number of linguistically appropriate test measures were available, there were no specific guidelines for assessment and no protocols that easily allowed for comparisons within the same child, across different children, and across different facilities. Recognizing a need to be able to set guidelines and compare performance levels across sites, to encourage realistic expectations for families, and to guide clinical decision making for clinicians,[7] a working group was convened and charged with providing evidence-based recommendations for the development of a standardized test protocol. The result was the Pediatric Minimum Speech Test Battery (P-MSTB).[7] The P-MSTB recommends the following standard guidelines for the assessment of children with hearing loss:

1. Use of recorded materials, if at all possible.
2. Presentation of speech materials at multiple intensities (i.e., conversational speech level, 60–65 dBA; soft speech level, 50 dBA).
3. Presentation of speech materials in multiple listening environments (i.e., quiet; noise, +5 dB signal-to-noise ratio).
4. Use of a ranked array of speech stimuli (i.e., phonemes, words, and sentences).
5. Evaluation of both ears (individually and in tandem) regardless of implantation status.

These guidelines should be incorporated for both determination of candidacy and longitudinal assessment of auditory development post-cochlear implantation.

Pitfall ✕

The use of monitored live voice for presentation of speech materials has the potential to inflate scores and exaggerate the child's ability to hear and communicate, potentially barring them from cochlear implantation when they are good candidates for the procedure. Recorded materials should be used whenever possible.

While the P-MSTB recommends a ranked array of speech stimuli, currently FDA labeling for cochlear implant candidacy incorporates only a single-open set speech recognition test (depending on child's age, this may be the Phonetically Balanced Kindergarten Test [PBK], Hearing in Noise Test [HINT] administered in quiet, the Multisyllabic Lexical Neighborhood Test [MLNT], or Lexical Neighborhood Test [LNT]). Most labeling specifies testing should be conducted MLV at a presentation level of 70 dB SPL. Unfortunately, these arguably outdated labels would likely prevent children who could benefit from cochlear implantation from having access to the technology. In those cases, clinicians may recommend a cochlear implant off-label, or outside of its currently labeled indications.

The dilemma for implant teams remains how to best assess children who are younger than 2 years. In these cases, emphasis is placed on functional gain afforded by hearing aids (audibility) and parental questionnaires that assess observed auditory behaviors. If month-over-month progress with hearing aids is not observed, cochlear implantation may be recommended. The combination of behavioral testing and questionnaires is key, particularly when the child is too young to provide more than threshold information. It is essential to understand what the child is able to do with the speech information he detects in the environment, thus observed responses to auditory stimuli in their own daily environment is of equal relevance and importance.

Parental Questionnaires

For all children, but particularly for children up to 2 years of age who may not be able to offer meaningful responses in the sound booth, parental questionnaires are valuable tools to assist the clinician in understanding the progress that the child is making. There are a number of available questionnaires that provide insight into a variety of aspects of the child's auditory experience.

The Infant-Toddler Meaningful Auditory Integration Scale (IT-MAIS)[8] and the Meaningful Auditory Integration Scale (MAIS)[9] are two of the most commonly administered parental questionnaires and are specifically mentioned in labeling for two of the three U.S. cochlear implant manufacturers. The P-MSTB recommends all families complete a minimum battery of questionnaires (▶Table 13.2); but other questionnaires such as the Early Language Milestones (ELM),[10] Functioning after Pediatric Cochlear Implantation (FAPCI),[11] and Parents' Evaluation of Aural/Oral Performance of Children (PEACH),[12] among others, are also available.

In addition to parental questionnaires, speech/language assessment is very useful for evaluating auditory skills development because it represents the functional outcome of auditory skills development.

Speech and Language Production

Even speech recognition assessment using recorded stimuli in a calibrated environment is not enough to

Table 13.2 Questionnaires recommended in Pediatric Minimum Speech Test Battery

Questionnaire	Ages	Aim	Data source	Length
Auditory Skills Checklist[13]	0–36 mo	Progress through auditory hierarchy	Combination of the family's observations of their child's auditory and language skills and observations of the managing clinician during sessions.	35 items, completed at baseline and every 3 mo
LittlEars (MED-EL)[14,15]	0–24 mo	Assesses auditory development and early speech production development; normative data available	Parental report	35 yes/no items

fully understand the communication capabilities of a patient. Speech recognition testing stops short of the highest level of the auditory hierarchy, comprehension. Although audiological evaluation can quantify the sounds, a child can detect and their ability to identify and discriminate various speech sounds, an evaluation by a speech language pathologist is necessary in order to determine the child's developmental progress and current level of functioning.

Combining the results of the audiological and speech language evaluations may provide the team with the ability to consider the child's current status and to what degree the hearing loss and existing interventions are influencing the child's proficiency. If the child is old enough to participate, the speech language pathologist will conduct assessments of speech production and language development to help inform the team's recommendations regarding implantation. For younger children, the clinician will rely on observation and parental report. The primary aim of the speech language pathologist on the cochlear implant team should be to evaluate how introducing a cochlear implant might change a child's communication development and a secondary aim is to establish a baseline for current speech and language skills.[16] These are both essential components of the candidacy process.

13.4.3 Expanding Criteria for Children

As previously mentioned, children are expected to miss 70 to 88% of incoming speech signals before meeting current FDA labeling for cochlear implantation. This is in disproportionate contrast to adults who are only required to miss approximately half of the signal before their candidacy is confirmed. There is a preponderance of evidence in the adult literature supporting not only the existing adult criteria, but there is also a growing body of evidence to support

expanding the criteria further to utilize word recognition instead of sentence recognition as well as considering ear-specific rather than bilaterally aided results. (see discussion in Chapter 12.) Thus, children, who are in what are arguably some of the most challenging listening environments in the most auditory critical years may be overlooked until well past when they became good candidates for cochlear implantation.

Pitfall

Children, who are in what are arguably some of the most challenging listening environments in the most auditory critical years, may be overlooked until well past when they became good candidates for cochlear implantation. Ironically, the children who are most overlooked tend to be those with more recent progression of hearing loss and more residual hearing; in other words, those children who would do best with cochlear implants.

However, there has recently been the introduction of evidence into the literature on three areas of possible expansion for pediatric candidates: more residual hearing and hearing preservation; asymmetric hearing loss where only one ear meets cochlear implant candidacy; and more specifically, single-sided deafness, where one ear has normal hearing while the other is unaidable.

Residual Hearing and Asymmetric Hearing Loss

Currently, adult candidacy criteria are inclusive of audiometric thresholds as good as moderate to profound (standard cochlear implant) or even normal sloping to profound (hybrid/EAS). However, for children requirements are overly restrictive as thresholds must be severe (ages 2–17 years) or profound

(< 2 years) to meet FDA labeling requirements. Again, the abundance of caution applied to children may initially have been proposed to minimize risk to residual hearing during a time when hearing preservation after cochlear implantation was not expected. In recent years, however, hearing preservation for adult candidates is not only possible, it is more routinely anticipated (see Chapter 12). It is widely accepted that receiving a cochlear implant with more residual hearing may actually be beneficial[17,18] and retaining that residual hearing, particularly in the low frequencies, is beneficial for music appreciation, speech recognition in noise, localization, and overall sound quality.[19,20,21] For the most part, these advantages have been reserved for adults. More recently, however, Bruce et al[22] demonstrated that residual hearing can be consistently preserved and maintained in adolescent recipients. In fact, young age may be a positive prognostic factor for successful hearing preservation.[23] Cadieux et al[24] specifically evaluated the abilities of children with one ear outside of traditional criteria and found that the children who had some residual hearing and auditory experience in the implanted ear prior to implantation all demonstrated measurable benefit. However, those children who had congenital severe-to-profound hearing loss and no hearing aid use still reported subjective improvement over their unilateral hearing aid experience. Similarly, Carlson et al[25] reported that children falling outside of the traditional FDA labeling derive a significant benefit from cochlear implantation. Thus, ironically, the children who are underperforming with hearing aids but exceeding the overly restrictive FDA labeling are likely the candidates who would therefore perform best with a cochlear implant, but may not have access to one.[25]

Single-Sided Deafness

As discussed in Chapter 12, there are myriad negative consequences of unilateral hearing loss. Although a child may have a normal-hearing ear, the negative consequences for academic achievement, localization, speech and language development, and speech recognition in noise are well documented.[26] In recent years, a number of reports have summarized the benefit of cochlear implantation in single-sided deafness (SSD) for adults.[27,28,29] Initially implemented to minimize tinnitus, results have suggested that improvements in speech recognition can also be expected, particularly for shorter-duration hearing losses. There have been reports of objective findings outlining the cortical reorganization that occurs in the presence of a unilateral hearing loss—and more recently, the elimination of this pathological reorganization post-cochlear

implant.[30] While results are still preliminary, it appears that cochlear implantation may be an effective treatment for improving speech recognition and localization ability in children with SSD,[26,31,32] and future investigation is highly anticipated.

13.5 Medical and Surgical Considerations

There are a number of surgical considerations that are unique to the youngest recipients. Although the structures of the inner ear are fully formed at birth, other relevant issues related to cochlear implantation in pediatric patients must be considered. These include surgical time and the safe administration of anesthesia in young children, determination of candidacy for and timing of bilateral cochlear implantation, vestibular impact, and long-term impact of cochlear implantation, including possible revision and hearing preservation.

13.5.1 Critical Window

As with adult cochlear implant recipients, short duration of hearing loss is critical to achieving the best outcomes. Shorter duration of hearing loss and earlier implantation minimizes delayed speech and language development relative to normally hearing peers and yields better outcomes for pediatric cochlear implant recipients. However, unlike for adult cochlear implant candidates, behavioral data necessary for determining candidacy can be difficult to obtain in pediatric patients. Fortunately, thanks to the ubiquity of Universal Newborn Hearing Screening (UNHS) and the ability to identify children with hearing loss as early as the first days and weeks after birth, hearing loss is often known to clinicians very early on. However, evaluation of hearing aid benefit and attainment of typical auditory milestones can be time consuming to assess.

Currently the FDA has approved cochlear implantation in children as young as 12 months of age. A frequent exception to this age limit is in cases of progressive ossification of the cochlea which can occur as the end result of an inflammatory process (e.g., bacterial meningitis). In these cases, cochlear implantation is commonly hurried to ensure an electrode array can be placed before the cochlear scalae are filled with bone and insertion becomes an impossibility. However, for the typical cochlear implant candidate, 12 months remains the labeled indication.

It is well documented that children with hearing loss of a moderate degree or greater are at high risk of negative impact on speech and language development without appropriate intervention.[33] In the same vein, children with a significant degree of hearing loss requiring cochlear implantation benefit from earlier implantation because the period of auditory deprivation is shorter. As discussed in Chapter 12, without appropriate auditory stimulation, structural changes to the auditory nerve, brainstem, and cortex begin[34,35] (▶ Fig. 13.2). The effect of auditory deprivation is even more pronounced in children, who have immature auditory systems. Stimulation of higher-order auditory structures is necessary to simulate maturation of the system. In the absence of appropriate input, structures that were intended to receive and process auditory inputs reorganize. In fact, other sensory inputs (e.g., vision) begin to compete for neural resources and cross-modal organization can occur. In other words, if not being utilized for auditory purposes, neural structures begin to devote their function to other necessary tasks. As a result, the human auditory system can be irrevocably altered by lack of necessary auditory inputs.[33]

Knowing that stimulation is necessary for thorough development of the auditory system, the natural question should be how long the window to restore adequate stimulation may be. The generally accepted guideline has been that the critical window for providing access to sound and speech inputs is greatest in the first 3.5 years of life, decreases significantly by 7 years of age, and may be completely closed by 12 years of age.[33,36] However, the interpretation of the critical window that encouraged use of these guidelines was based primarily on data derived from evoked potentials. When speech and language outcomes are considered, it appears the critical window may be much narrower.

It is important to recognize that by 12 months of age, a deaf baby is already closer to 16 or 17 months behind his or her normally hearing peers. How is this possible? Because embryotic development of the inner ear and rudimentary higher-level auditory system is complete by approximately 25 weeks' gestation, the earliest aspects of speech and language development actually begin in utero.[37] By the time an infant is born, he or she is on the fast track to speech and language development. The first year of life is full of rapid growth including the ability to differentiate familiar speech content in their native language from other speech streams, speech and nonlinguistic segmentation, and identification of multimodal and syntactic patterns.[38] By 12 months of age, infants have already made significant progress in their speech and language development and are beginning to produce first words that are the result of many months of continuous learning.

> **Pitfall** ✕
>
> By the time a deaf child is 12 months old, he or she is already approximately 3,650 hours behind their typically developing peer in terms of auditory experience.

The auditory brain is most plastic at birth and that plasticity declines over time. More current research suggests that the critical window for greatest success with cochlear implantation is probably closer to 12 months,[39,40] not 12 years as was once thought. Specifically, although children implanted before 13 months and children implanted after 13 months may have similar speech perception abilities,[33,41] other language skills such as vocabulary[42] and grammar[43] may be significantly poorer for the later implanted group. In fact,

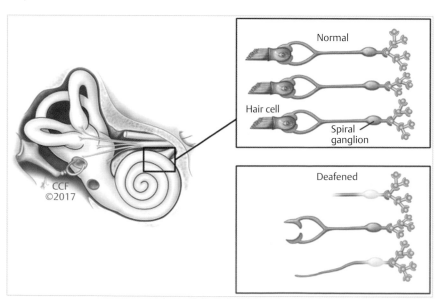

Fig. 13.2 Illustrations of changes to auditory neurons that can occur in the absence of auditory stimulation. Reprinted with permission, Cleveland Clinic Center for Medical Art & Photography © 2017. All Rights Reserved.

Holman et al[44] reported that patients implanted at age 12 months or younger reached age-appropriate speech and language skills by 24 months of age compared with 40 months for children implanted between 13 and 24 months of age. Thus, the earlier a hearing loss that could benefit from cochlear implantation is identified and a cochlear implant is placed, the better the long-term outcomes for the recipient.

13.5.2 How Young Is Too Young?

Given that best outcomes are obtained in very young children, the safety of subjecting children under 12 months of age to surgery and anesthesia has been closely studied recently. While cochlear implantation has been reported in children as young as 2 months of age,[45] most surgeons are hesitant to consider cochlear implantation before a child is old enough to complete a behavioral audiogram (typically 7–10 months). Possible surgical complications in young children include complications with wound healing and device exposure, bradycardia and hypoxia, and facial nerve damage due to the more lateral position of the stylomastoid foramen.[46] Recent reports, however, have suggested that complications in children younger than 12 months of age do not significantly differ from older children,[46,47] although readmission and operative time may be increased.[47]

13.5.3 Vaccination

Another safety consideration is the prevention of pneumococcal meningitis post-cochlear implantation. The incidence of pneumococcal meningitis is greater than 30 times higher for children with cochlear implants than the general U.S. population, although that incidence decreased somewhat after positioners, small silastic wedges that helped position the electrode array more closely to the modiolus, were removed from the market in the early 2000s. As a result of the increased risk of contracting meningitis, the Centers for Disease Control and Prevention (CDC) recommend that all pediatric cochlear implant candidates are up to date on pneumococcal (PCV7 and PPV23) and Haemophilus influenzae type b vaccinations at least 2 weeks before surgery.[48,49]

Pitfall ✕

Cochlear implant recipients are at risk for contracting meningitis because the cochleostomy or opening of the round window creates a possible route for bacteria to travel from the middle ear space to the cerebrospinal fluid (CSF)-filled subarachnoid space via the cochlear aqueduct.

13.5.4 Radiological Assessment

When determining candidacy for cochlear implantation in children, radiological assessment is of utmost importance for identifying cochlear malformations, confirming presence of the cochlear nerve, and confirming that location of the facial nerve allows for drilling of a cochleostomy and uncomplicated placement of the electrode array into the cochlea. However, which imaging modality is preferred has been a topic of debate. High-resolution computerized tomography (HRCT) of the temporal bone and MRI are both valuable, but have different contributions. HRCT and MRI both allow for detection of inner ear malformations, but HRCT is better able to capture bony structures, while MRI is the gold standard for evaluating soft tissue and membranous structures, including cranial nerves. MRI is also valuable for identifying fibrosis, or loss of fluid signal within the cochlea, which can suggest early ossification. Thus, when evaluating pediatric candidates for cochlear implantation, the use of both HRCT and MRI are typically recommended[50] (▶ Fig. 13.3 and ▶ Fig. 13.4).

13.5.5 Cochlear Implant Configuration

In addition to determining whether a child is a candidate for a cochlear implant, it is necessary to determine the configuration that will be recommended to optimize binaural hearing. This recommendation may include bilateral cochlear implantation, bimodal hearing (cochlear implant in the poorer hearing ear and hearing aid in the contralateral ear), and discussion may even need to involve the potential preservation of residual hearing.

Bilateral Cochlear Implantation

Bilateral stimulation of the auditory system is essential and offers a number of binaural benefits which include spatial hearing, head shadow effect, binaural squelch, and binaural summation.[51] The ability of the auditory system to glean binaural benefit requires that auditory inputs are able to be delivered bilaterally, that is, to both ears. It is important to note, however, that the use of the term "binaural" implies a coordination that occurs in the central auditory system. Cochlear implants are somewhat limited in the sense that even when a recipient has two cochlear implants, they are functioning largely independently of one another. Despite this limitation, over time, the practice of providing a cochlear implant for each ear that is a candidate has become more commonplace, especially for children. Bilateral cochlear implants are introduced either simultaneously (in the same

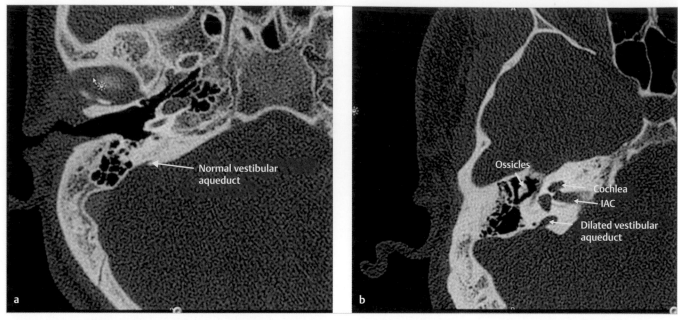

Fig. 13.3   (a, b) Pre-cochlear implant CT scan.

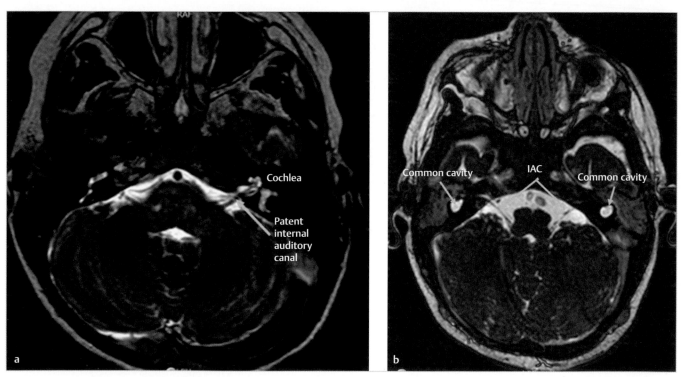

Fig. 13.4   (a, b) Pre-cochlear implant MRI.

surgery) or sequentially (in separate surgeries). Sequential implantations may include short (weeks or months) duration or long (many months or years) duration between surgeries. The practice of introducing bilateral cochlear implants for children varies among clinics; generally, however, simultaneous cochlear implantation is generally offered when the child has no useable residual hearing in either ear, is showing no appreciable benefit from hearing aids,

and does not have a medical or financial contraindication. The duration between sequential cochlear implantations becomes important when considering whether the unimplanted ear is able to be adequately stimulated. The critical window that has previously been described applies to each ear—thus, receiving a single cochlear implant does not eliminate the possibility of auditory deprivation and cross-modal reorganization if the unimplanted ear cannot be adequately stimulated. In these cases, simultaneous or very short-duration bilateral implantation is generally recommended.

Bilateral cochlear implantation has been shown to offer recipients a number of benefits including improved speech recognition and localization ability,[52] enhanced bilateral summation or redundancy,[53,54] and increased speech understanding in noise.[55] Other advantages that are particularly salient for pediatric recipients are the assurance that the "best" candidate ear is always being implanted and the recipient won't be without sound, even if one processor temporarily malfunctioned.[53] Bilateral implantation at a young age in the presence of severe-to-profound hearing loss yields language acquisition with a trajectory for recipients to be on par with their normally hearing peers very quickly.[56] However, for children with some residual hearing, optimal timing of the second cochlear implant must be considered. Choi et al[55] suggest that bilateral cochlear implantation should be considered to enhance overall speech perception ability if speech understanding in noise is worse than the mean bilateral cochlear implant recipient performance on speech perception in multitalker babble. Studies emphasize that improvements are greatest and mismatches are minimized when time between sequential implantations for children with severe-to-profound hearing loss is limited.[57,58] However, for children with low-frequency thresholds better than approximately 90 dB HL,[59] bimodal stimulation may result in better outcomes both before and after sequential implantation.

Bimodal Stimulation

In the early days of cochlear implantation, once a single cochlear implant was placed, it was standard practice to advise discontinuation of a hearing aid on the contralateral ear and the second, unimplanted, ear was left unstimulated. Further, because early cochlear implants were reserved for candidates with bilateral profound hearing loss, having residual hearing was a rare occurrence. As cochlear implant candidacy has continued, and will continue, to expand, more pediatric candidates for cochlear implantation have useable residual hearing in at least one ear. Thus, evidence-based recommendations for the management of the unimplanted ear is of critical importance. As previously discussed, the benefits of binaural hearing are well documented, thus the goal of any clinician is to optimize a child's access to binaural stimulation. It is important to recognize that cochlear implants are most capable of delivering temporal, envelope-based information of speech, but are limited in their ability to process the fine structure information that is necessary for successful

speech comprehension in more challenging listening environments like background noise. Thus, children who use bilateral cochlear implants are relying on a bilaterally degraded signal.[60] While they can be enormously successful, there may be some advantages of incorporating more natural acoustic hearing from at least one side, when possible. Use of a contralateral hearing aid has been shown to improve speech understanding in noise, enhance localization ability, increase music appreciation, and decrease likelihood of cross-modal reorganization or auditory deprivation.[55,61,62] Although much of the literature on bimodal benefits focuses on adult cochlear implant recipients, numerous studies have investigated the benefits for children as well and offer consistent support for the approach.[59,60,63] Beyond simply improving sound quality, bimodal stimulation has been shown offer benefits related to phonemic awareness, working memory, expressive vocabulary, and reading ability.[60]

Hearing Preservation and Electroacoustic Stimulation

As previously discussed, cochlear implantation is now being considered by some clinics for children with residual hearing in the implanted ear. As discussed in Chapter 12, shorter electrode arrays, soft surgical techniques, and electroacoustic stimulation are becoming standard of care for adults with significant residual hearing. Gifford et al[64] reported that bilateral adult cochlear implant recipients with bilateral acoustic hearing preservation achieve the highest levels of performance in challenging noisy environments. Observing such encouraging results in adults with residual hearing begs the question of whether limiting cochlear implantation in children to more significant degrees of hearing loss is unnecessarily strict. However, at the time of this writing, electroacoustic stimulation is not FDA approved for pediatric candidates, although some clinics have begun investigating the benefit for this population. Hearing preservation is possible in children[65,66] and adolescents[22] have demonstrated benefit with shorter-length electrode arrays.[20] Looking forward, it is easy to anticipate that hearing preservation and electroacoustic stimulation in the pediatric population will be of great interest to researchers seeking ways to optimize pediatric outcome data.

13.5.6 Vestibular

Because of the close anatomical relationship between the peripheral auditory and vestibular end organs, children who exhibit significant hearing loss may also exhibit vestibular dysfunction even before cochlear implantation. Etiology is strongly correlated to the presence of vestibular dysfunction, with children with meningitis and cochleovestibular abnormalities most commonly demonstrating the most severe vestibular involvement.[67] As discussed in Chapter 12, there is a strong possibility of transient postoperative vestibular weakness (38% overall and 10% of severe or profound vestibular loss as measured by caloric tests)[68] in adults following cochlear implantation. Thus, the vestibular status of a cochlear implant candidate may be important for selecting an ear to implant. In children, however, it can be cumbersome or even impossible to complete vestibular test batteries. Some have advocated for the use of balance function screening to identify children with vestibular loss.[69] Particularly because many children now receive bilateral cochlear implants, often simultaneously, the potential impact on the vestibular system is highly relevant and must be considered for pediatric cochlear implant candidates. Reassuringly, some research has suggested that cochlear implantation does not seem to pose a substantial risk to pediatric cochlear implant recipients.[68] This may be due in part to the fact that among children with bilateral profound hearing loss (the group that would most commonly receive simultaneous bilateral cochlear implants), approximately half exhibit vestibular end-organ dysfunction before cochlear implantation.[67] In contrast, other studies have suggested that many children have sufficient vestibular function to be at risk for postoperative vestibular weakness or loss, either from involvement of the semicircular canals or otolithic organs, particularly the saccule.[70] In either case, children also seem to be uniquely capable of compensating and participating in many activities that challenge balance, although they may lag behind their normally hearing and balancing peers.[69] Regardless, understanding the vestibular status of a cochlear implant candidate or recipient can be important when considering ear selection and the necessity of early interventional therapy. Furthermore, children with total vestibular loss, either secondary to or unrelated to cochlear implantation, have an increased risk for cochlear implant failure due to propensity for head trauma related to repeated falls.[71]

13.6 Complications and Failures

Cochlear implants are designed to last a lifetime. However, to date, the earliest recipients have had cochlear implants for less than 50 years. As children are implanted at younger ages and life expectancy continues to increase, cochlear implants are being asked to last longer and do more. Realistically, most children implanted today can probably expect to have one or more revision surgeries in their lifetime. Thus, understanding the risks and benefits of revision cochlear implantation is critically important.

One of the primary challenges associated with revision of a cochlear implant is the removal of the existing device and subsequent reinsertion of a new electrode array. After an electrode array is placed, an inflammatory response begins in response to the presence of a foreign body within the cochlea. This response often results in the formation of a fibrous sheath around the electrode array. The development of this sheath can introduce two complications to any revision surgery: difficulty with removal, and possible inability to achieve equivalent depth of insertion, particularly if the newer implant has a different length and diameter.

Cochlear implant revision surgery is most often due to device failure. Implant failure is often classified as hard failure (device related) or soft failure (normal device analysis with decreased performance). Soft failures can be related to subclinical device factors or physiological/medical changes for the patient.[72] Confirmation of soft failure occurs when performance significantly improves after reimplantation. Generally speaking, the incidence of revision cochlear implantation is higher in children than in adults,[73] possibly due to a higher incidence of head trauma, although there is variable support for this theory. Blanchard et al[73] reported that the primary reason for hard failure of a device is typically loss of hermeticity and cracked casing following head trauma. Despite the higher incidence of revision relative to adults, the overall incidence of device failure is relatively low (< 10%).[73,74] Barring difficulty removing the device or achieving a complete reinsertion, postimplantation audiological results are often the same or better postrevision.[73,74]

There are a number of complications that may occur during both primary and revision cochlear implant surgery. These include tinnitus, vestibular insult, loss of residual hearing, infection (skin infection, meningitis, labyrinthitis, acute otitis media, or mastoiditis), CSF leak/gusher, local skin complications (ulcer, infection, wound dehiscence), and transient facial nerve palsy and taste disturbance. Children are more likely to develop infectious complications (most commonly acute otitis media), while adults tend to experience more cochleovestibular complications such as tinnitus and vertigo.[75] However, the overall risk of complications in cochlear implantation is relatively low (approximately 15% minor complications and approximately 5% major complications).[75,76]

13.7 Cochlear Implant Design

The basics of cochlear implant design and function were discussed in Chapter 12. However, when considering structure and function of cochlear implants for use in pediatric recipients, a few key features must be specifically considered. These include reliability and durability, water resistance, and connectivity and compatibility with FM systems and other assistive listening devices.

13.7.1 Durability and Reliability

For pediatric patients, it is essential that available devices be able to stand up to the rough handling to which pediatric recipients subject them. It is to be expected that children who are still just learning to walk will take a tumble from time to time, active children may be involved in sports and outdoor activities, and the foresight to avoid splashes and rainfall won't be consistent. Further, there are many situations in which older devices would have needed to be removed, but where parents cringed to know their child couldn't hear (e.g., swimming, bath time, playing on the beach). Modern day cochlear implant processors are designed to stand up to the rough care they often receive. All vendors now have optional accessories that make their devices completely waterproof, and most are highly water-resistant right out of the box. Cochlear implant reliability has improved over time as well. With the exception of a few specific major recalls, the cumulative survival rate (how many implants remain implanted and functioning) for most implants exceeds 97% or more many years after implantation.

> **Pearl** ✔
>
> Waterproof cochlear implant processors allow parents and caregivers the opportunity to communicate with children during bath time and pool time without worrying.

13.7.2 Connectivity and Compatibility with FM and Other Assistive Listening Devices

Finally, although children with cochlear implants often achieve excellent speech recognition, it is often necessary to supplement their hearing with access to assistive listening devices. These devices have several functions, including the ability to stream audio signals from electronic devices and to improve hearing in situations where background noise, distance, or reverberation threaten to diminish speech understanding. This access is particularly important for children, who are commonly in very challenging environments like classrooms, sporting arenas, and playing fields. The world is increasingly reliant on electronic devices, so ensuring pediatric cochlear implant recipients can effectively stream music, video, and phone calls is equally important. While a thorough discussion of the various configurations and devices that are available for cochlear implant recipients is beyond the scope of this chapter, suffice it to say that modern day cochlear implant systems are well equipped to allow children access to optimal listening conditions using these additional accessories, in many cases automatically and wirelessly. This capability has greatly improved the overall hearing experience for families and, when applied appropriately, significantly increases speech understanding for children in a variety of challenging listening conditions.

13.8 Programming Pediatric Cochlear Implants

Programming the cochlear implant processor of a pediatric recipient is a delicate balance of art and science. For older children, programming may begin to closely follow a similar model as adult programming. However, because many children are not old enough to provide reliable behavioral responses, the ability to balance behavioral observations, history and expectations, and objective measurements becomes essential.

13.8.1 Objective Programming

Following surgical placement of the cochlear implant electrode array, confirmation of appropriate placement and device function is advisable. This confirmation is achievable using the measurement of evoked compound action potentials (ECAP). Each manufacturer has a proprietary version of this measurement (Neural Response Telemetry [NRT] for Cochlear, Neural Response Imaging [NRI] for Advanced Bionics, and Auditory Response Telemetry [ART] for MED-EL). Regardless of the system, an ECAP measurement is a recording of the neural response generated by electrical stimulation of the auditory nerve by the cochlear implant. It is essentially analogous to Wave I of the auditory brainstem response (ABR). These measurements can provide several key pieces of information, including responsiveness of the nerve to electrical stimulation, confirmation of placement of the electrode array within the cochlea, functionality of the implant, and approximation of current levels needed to elicit a response. These measurements are often conducted before the patient leaves the operating room, although they can be obtained postoperatively as well. Other objective measurements that may be obtained, although less commonly, are electrically evoked stapedial reflex tests (eSRT) and electrically evoked auditory brainstem response (eABR). Each is similar to its acoustic counterpart in terms of the recording mechanisms, but the stimulus is electric rather than acoustic.

These objective measurements are particularly useful for pediatric patients because there is a loose correlation between the threshold measurements obtained and the predicted MAP, or current settings, for the cochlear implant programming. Specifically, ECAP suggests current levels that will be audible to the recipient and also suggests minimum levels for the softer end of the MAP (i.e., the threshold levels),[77] while eSRTs tend to suggest approximate upper stimulation levels. These suggested MAP parameters can be invaluable when combined with behavioral observations.

Recently, Noble et al[78] have suggested the possibility of introducing image-guided cochlear implant programming (IGCIP) for pediatric recipients by estimating the position of implanted electrodes relative to the nerve they are stimulating using CT scans. Although preliminary, results suggest that using this advanced technology may allow clinicians of the future to further optimize children's MAPs by deactivating electrodes that introduce high levels of stimulation overlap thereby improving speech recognition and self-reported quality of life.

Datalogging is another objective measure that has improved the ability of a pediatric clinician to optimize care for patients. Several contemporary cochlear implant processors record information about the environments in which the child spends time, how often the processor is on and how often the coil or headpiece is off the head. This information can provide valuable insight and assist a clinician develop appropriate counseling and recommendations for families.

13.8.2 Behavioral Programming

In addition to using objective measurements to program pediatric cochlear implants, behavioral measures can be incorporated, even in children who are too young to specifically guide setting stimulation levels. As previously discussed, speech recognition

measures and detection of FM tones in the sound booth can help guide clinical decision making related to programming.

Feedback from auditory verbal therapists, speech language pathologists, educators, and parents can also be helpful and the continued use of subjective questionnaires should not be underrated. Specifics of the specialized programming techniques necessary for achieving successful outcomes for pediatric recipients are beyond the scope of this chapter, but it is important to recognize the value of specialized pediatric training prior to working with youngest cochlear implant recipients.

13.9 Performance/Expected Outcomes

The most common goal of cochlear implantation in the pediatric population is the development of speech, language, and auditory behaviors on par with normal-hearing peers. The highest performing pediatric cochlear implant recipients are typically children who were implanted at a young age, who have motivated families, and were immersed in auditory-rich environments from early on.[79] This section will discuss factors that can influence expected outcomes and inform parental expectations.

13.9.1 Typical Expected Outcomes

The highest performing children routinely achieve open-set speech recognition comparable to post-lingually deafened adult cochlear implant recipients,[80] on the order of approximately 80% or higher sentence recognition.[81] In addition to the ability to recognize speech, other more complex benefits to cochlear implantation include speech production and language development, reading, and executive functioning.[82] The highest performers are able to catch up to their normally hearing peers in all of these areas; however, variability exists that can be accounted for by a number of factors.

It is important to recognize that children who are now in high school were implanted with different guidelines than children implanted today. Today's adolescents usually received a unilateral cochlear implant, possibly with a long-duration sequential cochlear implant, and were often implanted at older ages. It won't be for another decade or two that we are truly able to assess the outcomes that result from today's recommendations of earlier implantation and the maximization of bilateral inputs.

13.9.2 Factors Affecting Performance

The most common factors affecting cochlear implant outcomes in the pediatric population are summarized in ▶Table 13.3.

Age at Implantation

Children who are identified with severe-to-profound hearing loss early in life and have immediate and appropriate intervention grow up to be highly successful cochlear implant recipients. Arguably, age at implantation, and the related metric of duration of implantation, set the course for the best outcomes. The advantages of implantation before the age of 2, and possibly even before 12 months, have already been discussed. In addition to improved speech recognition ability, early implantation has also been identified as a critical factor in the development of expressive vocabulary, speech production and intelligibility, language development, and academic achievement including reading level.[81] In contrast, long duration severe-to-profound hearing loss with inadequate intervention in the form of appropriate amplification or cochlear implantation has an adverse impact on long-term outcomes.[83] However, the long-term influence age at implantation is not completely understood and it is possible that the influence may not be as pronounced once years of experience with the cochlear implant is more comparable.[84]

Etiology

Cochlear implants are designed as an intervention for cochlear hearing loss. Thus, those etiologies such as Connexin 26 mutations where the impact is isolated to the cochlea itself are likely to have the best outcomes following cochlear implantation, assuming other variables such as early identification and implantation remain constant.[87] Etiologies that threaten the auditory nerve, brainstem, or auditory cortex, or present with other neurologic involvement (e.g., cytomegalovirus [CMV], cerebral palsy) have more guarded expectations. One unique

Table 13.3   Factors influencing pediatric cochlear implant outcomes

Medical/surgical factors	Speech/language factors	Other factors
Age at implantation/auditory deprivation[85,86]	Auditory training[86] and communication mode[85,86]	Education and post-CI rehab and programming services[86] CI Technology[86]
Early implantation results in better speech and language outcomes	*Children who use oral communication have better outcomes than children who use total communication*	*Advancements in processing fine structure and development of noise reduction strategies*
GJB2-related deafness[85]	Cognitive delay[85]	Social factors including socioeconomic status, parent/family expectations, motivation[86]
Positive impact on reading and cognitive outcomes, better speech intelligibility	*May impact degree of benefit, although benefit is observed*	
Inner ear malformations[85,86]	Etiologic factors, delayed milestones[85]	
Less severe malformations have better outcomes; children with severe malformations benefit from cochlear implantation but have poorer outcomes	*No etiologic impact, but children with delayed milestones make slower progress with CI*	*Higher levels of social factors result in better outcomes*
Meningitis[85,86] or other causes of cochlear ossification	Pre-CI speech recognition and discrimination[85,86]	
Significant benefit when implanted early; poorer performance with greater degrees of ossification[b]	*Higher pre-CI performance may result in better outcomes post-CI for postlingually deafened*	
Cytomegalovirus (CMV)	Residual hearing[85,86]	
While not a contraindication, there are usually concomitant neural problems, thus outcomes are poorer	*May result in improved outcomes (more data needed)*	
Multiple disabilities[86]	Binaural hearing[86]	
Potential to impact outcomes with CI; very variable	*Improvements in localization, spatial acuity, speech, understanding over unilateral CI*	

Abbreviation: CI, cochlear implants.

etiology is auditory neuropathy spectrum disorder (ANSD). Children with ANSD demonstrate variable outcomes with cochlear implants. Although ANSD is believed to impact either the junction between the inner hair cell and the auditory nerve, or the auditory nerve itself, reports have suggested that children with isolated ANSD (no other cognitive or developmental disorders) have postoperative outcomes similar to their profound cochlear hearing loss counterparts[88,89] and ANSD is therefore not a contraindication to cochlear implantation. Children with ANSD must be very carefully evaluated, however, to confirm that they present with isolated ANSD with genetic mutations that target a presynaptic site of lesion (OTOF) or postsynaptic site of lesion in the distal auditory nerve (DIAPH3). Other genetic mutations that cause ANSD by specifically targeting the more proximal auditory nerve will likely result in poorer outcomes.[90]

Interestingly, children with cochlear nerve deficiency (cochlear nerve diameter < facial nerve diameter)[91] may be clinically indistinguishable from children with ANSD until MRI scans are reviewed. Walton et al[92] reported that 15 (28%) of their series of 54 children with ANSD actually had cochlear nerve deficiency; further, those children with ANSD and normally developed cochlear nerves demonstrated better outcomes than those children with ANSD and cochlear nerve deficiency. Although a diagnosis of cochlear nerve deficiency increases the probability of less than optimal outcomes, limited success with cochlear implantation has been reported in children who have hypoplastic cochlear nerve(s) and the generally supported recommendation is to consider cochlear implantation before moving to auditory brainstem implant for these children.[91]

Multiple Involvement and Associated Syndromes

Up to 30% of prelingual deafness is due to genetic causes.[93,94] Of the hundreds of genetic syndromes that cause hearing loss, many of the most common syndromes that cause congenital severe-to-profound hearing loss have variable but potentially positive outcomes following cochlear implantation, including Usher's syndrome, Waardenburg's syndrome, Jervell and Lange-Nielson syndrome, and CHARGE syndrome.[94]

Children with medical complexities are increasingly being referred for cochlear complication. For example, children with CMV, cerebral palsy, autism, and global developmental delay may present as candidates for cochlear implantation. Children with multiple developmental and medical conditions present challenges for clinicians as they may be unable to complete behavioral testing and may have neurologic involvement that can limit benefit from cochlear implantation. Furthermore, these children are often late identified with significant hearing loss, or may have serious medical complications that derail the ideal habilitation course. Often, these children do not develop open-set speech recognition abilities; however, families may report significant benefit from sound awareness. These comorbid conditions are not necessarily a contraindication to cochlear implantation; however, clinicians may need to encourage realistic expectations with family members and other caregivers. Because of the variable impact of each of these disorders on outcomes, the input of the multidisciplinary team becomes even more critical during the evaluation, development of clinical expectations, and postoperative follow-ups. A detailed discussion of each of the various associated medical problems that may be encountered in children with cochlear implants is beyond the scope of this chapter, but any pediatric clinician should be sure to consider cochlear implant candidacy and expected outcomes in the context of the child's global medical situation. It is not uncommon the need to redefine expectations based on the child's individual circumstances.[95]

It can be challenging at times to isolate the contribution of hearing loss in a medically complex child, but with a diverse team and effective communication, appropriate recommendations can be made on a case-by-case basis.

Cochleovestibular Anomalies

Approximately 20% of congenital sensorineural hearing loss is related to inner ear malformations.[96] Although these anomalies were initially viewed as a contraindication to cochlear implantation, modern day recommendations have evolved significantly. ▶Table 13.4 summarizes the seven categories of cochleovestibular anomalies in order of severity. Cochlear implantation is only contraindicated in cases of the most severe, Michel malformation and cochlear aplasia, and has been successfully achieved in all other degrees of cochlear malformation, with variable outcomes.[94]

Pearl
Children with cochlear malformations may benefit from the use of straight, fully banded electrode arrays as opposed to a half-banded perimodiolar (precurved) electrode array because of the anomalous configuration and location of the modiolus.

Table 13.4 Classification of cochleovestibular anomalies by severity[95]

Most severe	Complete cochlear and labyrinthine aplasia (Michel's malformation)
	Cochlear aplasia
	Common cavity of the cochlea and vestibule
	Hypoplastic cochlea
	Incomplete partition Type I (< 1.5 turns)
	Incomplete partition Type II (1.5–2.75 turns, Mondini's malformation)
Least severe	Enlarged vestibular aqueduct (EVA)

Cochlear implantation in cases of cochlear malformation offers unique challenges including the ability to achieve a full insertion of the electrode array, maintaining appropriate orientation of the electrode contacts toward the modiolus, aberrant facial nerve course and associated increased risk of facial nerve stimulation, and increased risk of surgical complication including CSF gusher and postoperative infection (meningitis). Despite these challenges, pediatric cochlear implant candidates with mild-to-moderate cochlear malformations can achieve open-set speech recognition.[97,98]

Commitment and Motivation

Those children who rely on their cochlear implant and consistently utilize their device are also the children who typically have better outcomes. With many pediatric cochlear implant recipients being much too young to demonstrate commitment to their device and auditory experience, it often falls to parents, educators, and other caregivers to supply the necessary motivation. Easwar and colleagues[99] reported that children who are in a sound-enriched environment, who had preimplant acoustic hearing, and who have used their cochlear implant longer with fewer episodes of the coil being off their head all contribute to more device use and therefore, improved outcomes. Similarly, Choo and Dettman[100] reported that pediatric patients who attend follow-up appointments 5 years or more after initial activation tend to be more consistent users of their device, while those who stopped attending may be receiving less overall benefit or may be part-time- or nonusers. These results are not surprising and essentially confirm the importance of a demonstrated commitment to device use and an auditory-based environment. As will be discussed shortly, the best speech and language outcomes are enjoyed by those recipients who emphasize the relevance of auditory inputs to the communication needs.

13.10 Habilitation

The primary goals of cochlear implantation are to improve the ability to detect sounds in the environment and subsequently to recognize, discriminate, and understand speech. The development of spoken language skills is also expected. However, the placement of a cochlear implant alone is not sufficient to achieve anticipated speech and language milestones. Rather, the placement and activation of a cochlear implant is merely the first stop in a lengthy process, the end point of which is very much dependent on choices made by parents and caregivers related to communication mode, therapeutic intervention, and educational placements. A spectrum of possibilities exists, from entirely manual communication (e.g., American Sign Language [ASL]) to entirely auditory verbal (e.g., Listening and Spoken Language [LSL]). ▶Table 13.5 summarizes the communication modes available.

It is generally accepted that a family-centered approach is key when determining the best communication options for a child with hearing loss. Chief in consideration should be the environment in which the child will be immersed. All families should receive thorough and unbiased information about all communication options, support, and appropriate resources.[101] Because the vast majority of deaf children are born to hearing parents,[102] considering their ability to support the selected communication strategy is of vital importance. Most parents choose a cochlear implant as an intervention for their child because they desire them to be able to hear and to speak. Research has shown that children who are diagnosed with hearing loss at an early age have early intervention and a high level of family involvement, have better post-cochlear implant language scores than their peers who are diagnosed later or have more limited family involvement, regardless of communication mode.[103] However, best outcomes for speech perception are observed for children using oral modes of communication as compared to children using total communication,[104] or manual communication because they are immersed in an auditory world with constant exposure to auditory stimuli. Further, focused auditory training or auditory-verbal training result in the strongest speech and language outcomes[105,106] because they emphasize hearing as the primary sensory modality when acquiring speech and language. Similarly, mainstream class placement also results in the strongest speech and language outcomes[105] and is most commonly achieved in children implanted at younger than 18 months.[107]

Table 13.5 Available communication modes

Manual communication	Bilingual–bicultural	Manual communication, English-based	Cued speech	Total communication	Auditory–oral	Auditory–verbal
Examples = ASL Has its own grammatical and syntactic structure. Discourages use of hearing devices	Establishment of ASL as first language with secondary introduction of spoken English primarily for use in reading and writing	Examples = Signed Exact English, Seeing English Essentials, Signed English. The simultaneous combination of signed and voiced English	Facilitates lipreading by using simple hand signs near the face to clarify pronunciation of spoken words	Use of all communication modes (manual and auditory) to facilitate interactions	Emphasizes the use of amplified residual hearing, speech and oral language development and encourages speech reading and using visual information	Concentrates on the development of listening and speaking skills using residual hearing or input from hearing devices to the fullest extent possible

Abbreviation: ASL, American Sign Language.

> **Pearl** ✔
>
> Intensive auditory intervention programs are essential for developing open-set speech recognition, expressive and receptive language, vocabulary and reading skills.

13.11 Quality of Life and Cost-Effectiveness

Cochlear implantation has resulted in better outcomes for deaf children in a variety of areas, including academic achievement, quality of life, and employment than for their nonimplanted deaf peers, and in some cases, on par with their normally hearing peers.[80] Kumar et al[108] reported that parents report the cochlear implant–specific health-related quality of life (HRQoL) of their implanted children to be overall very positive, although the possible impact of making such a major choice for their child that could have future psychosocial impact weighed heavily on parents. Parents also assigned lower ratings to the HRQoL in the education domain significantly lower than other domains, suggesting parents perceive academic challenges relative to their expectations. Notably, parents who rated communication abilities higher for their implanted child also rated other domains higher, suggesting that children with better speech and language outcomes may have more perceived benefit in other areas as well.

In terms of cost-effectiveness of pediatric cochlear implantation, Semenov et al[107] reported that even without considering improvements in lifetime earnings, overall cost utility is highly favorable. Younger implantation (< 18 months) results in the greatest increase in quality-adjusted life years (QALYs) with a cost of less than $20,000 per QALY.

13.12 Conclusions and Future Directions

Cochlear implantation in children has changed the future for those with congenital deafness or progressive hearing loss in childhood. Counseling of parents of children with newly diagnosed severe-to-profound hearing loss routinely involves expectations of mainstream classrooms, ability to talk on the telephone, and vocational opportunities unimpeded by hearing loss. The development and implementation of cochlear implantation has rapidly evolved to include considerations for even the youngest recipients. Over less than three decades, candidacy criteria have evolved from "adults only" to children as young as 12 months of age, and research seems to pushing the acceptable age ever lower. Despite the astounding advancements for deaf and hard-of-hearing children, clinical practice for children still lags behind the advancements offered to adults. Children must still wait for greater degree and impact of hearing loss before benefitting from a cochlear implant. Looking to the future, possible consideration of cochlear implantation in younger children and children with more residual hearing offers exciting possibilities.

Continued expansion of pediatric cochlear implantation also presents new challenges in terms of providing pediatric-friendly device options, developing optimization abilities for programming, implementing age-appropriate speech and language assessments, and ensuring that multidisciplinary involvement remains a central focus.

References

[1] Christiansen JB, Leigh IW. Children with cochlear implants: changing parent and deaf community perspectives. Arch Otolaryngol Head Neck Surg. 2004; 130(5):673–677

[2] National Association of the Deaf (NAD). NAD position statement on cochlear implants (2000). http://www.nad.org/about-us/position-statements/position-statement-on-cochlear-implants/. Accessed January 14, 2017

[3] National Association of the Deaf (NAD). Report of the task force on childhood cochlear implants. NAD Broadcaster. 1991; 13:1–2

[4] Gifford RH. Elements of post-operative assessment: pediatric implant recipients. In: René H. Gifford, ed. Cochlear Implant Patient Assessment: Evaluation of Candidacy, Performance, and Outcomes. San Diego, CA: Plural Publishing; 2013:87

[5] Pearson KS, Bennett RL, Fidell S. Speech Levels in Various Noise Environments. (Report No. EPA-600/1–77–025). Washington, DC: US Environmental Protection Agency; 1977

[6] Olsen WO. Average speech levels and spectra in various speaking/listening conditions: a summary of the Pearson, Bennett & Fidel Report. Am J Audiol. 1998; 7(2):21–25

[7] Uhler K, Warner-Czyz A, Gifford R, Working Group P; PMSTB Working Group. Pediatric Minimum Speech Test Battery. J Am Acad Audiol. 2017; 28(3):232–247

[8] Zimmerman Phillips S, Robbins AM, Osberger MJ. Assessing cochlear implant benefit in very young children. Ann Otol Rhinol Laryngol Suppl. 2000; 185:42–43

[9] Robbins AM, Renshaw JJ, Berry SW. Evaluating meaningful auditory integration in profoundly hearing-impaired children. Am J Otol. 1991; 12(Suppl):144–150

[10] Coplan J, Elm Scale: The early language milestone scale. Austin TX: Pro-Ed. 1987

[11] Lin FR, Ceh K, Bervinchak D, Riley A, Mieoh R, Niparko JK. Development of a communicative performance scale for pediatric cochlear implantation. Ear Hear. 2007; 28(5):203-12

[12] Ching TY, Hill M. The parents evaluation of aural/oral performance of children (PEACH) Scale: normative data. J AM Acad Audiol. 2007; 18(3): 220-35

[13] Meinzen-Derr J, Wiley S, Creighton J, Choo D. Auditory Skills Checklist: clinical tool for monitoring functional auditory skill development in young children with cochlear implants. Ann Otol Rhinol Laryngol 2007;116(11):812–818

[14] Weichbold V, Tsiakpini L, Coninx F, D'Haese P. Development of a parent questionnaire for assessment of auditory behavior of infants up to two years of age. Laryngorhinotology 2005;84(5):328–334

[15] Coninx F, Weichbold V, Tsiakpini L, et al. Validation of the LittlEars auditory questionnaire in children with normal hearing. Int J Ped Otorhinolaryngol 2009;73(12):1761–1768

[16] Hammes Ganguly D, Ambrose SE, Cronin Carotta C. The assessment role of the speech-language specialist on the clinical cochlear implant team. In: Eisenberg LS, ed. Clinical Management of Children with Cochlear Implants. 2nd ed. San Diego, CA: Plural Publishing; 2017:276

[17] Rubinstein JT, Parkinson WS, Tyler RS, Gantz BJ. Residual speech recognition and cochlear implant performance: effects of implantation criteria. Am J Otol. 1999; 20(4):445–452

[18] Sadadcharam M, Warner L, Henderson L, Brown N, Bruce IA. Unilateral cochlear implantation in children with a potentially useable contralateral ear. Cochlear Implants Int. 2016; 17(s)(uppl 1):55–58

[19] Driscoll VD, Welhaven AE, Gfeller K, Oleson J, Olszewski CP. Music perception of adolescents using electroacoustic hearing. Otol Neurotol. 2016; 37(2):e141–e147

[20] Gantz BJ, Dunn C, Walker E, Van Voorst T, Gogel S, Hansen M. Outcomes of adolescents with a short electrode cochlear implant with preserved residual hearing. Otol Neurotol. 2016; 37(2):e118–e125

[21] Gifford RH, Dorman MF, Skarzynski H, et al. Cochlear implantation with hearing preservation yields significant benefit for speech recognition in complex listening environments. Ear Hear. 2013; 34(4):413–425

[22] Bruce IA, Felton M, Lockley M, et al. Hearing preservation cochlear implantation in adolescents. Otol Neurotol. 2014; 35(9):1552–1559

[23] Anagiotos A, Hamdan N, Lang-Roth R, et al. Young age is a positive prognostic factor for residual hearing preservation in conventional cochlear implantation. Otol Neurotol. 2015; 36(1):28–33

[24] Cadieux JH, Firszt JB, Reeder RM. Cochlear implantation in nontraditional candidates: preliminary results in adolescents with asymmetric hearing loss. Otol Neurotol. 2013; 34(3):408–415

[25] Carlson ML, Sladen DP, Haynes DS, et al. Evidence for the expansion of pediatric cochlear implant candidacy. Otol Neurotol. 2015; 36(1):43–50

[26] Dornhoffer JR, Dornhoffer JL. Pediatric unilateral sensorineural hearing loss: implications and management. Curr Opin Otolaryngol Head Neck Surg. 2016; 24(6):522–528

[27] Grossmann W, Brill S, Moeltner A, Mlynski R, Hagen R, Radeloff A. Cochlear implantation improves spatial release from masking and restores localization abilities in single-sided deaf patients. Otol Neurotol. 2016; 37(6):658–664

[28] Hoth S, Rösli-Khabas M, Herisanu I, Plinkert PK, Praetorius M. Cochlear implantation in recipients with single-sided deafness: audiological performance. Cochlear Implants Int. 2016; 17(4):190–199

[29] Sladen DP, Frisch CD, Carlson ML, Driscoll CL, Torres JH, Zeitler DM. Cochlear implantation for single-sided deafness: a multicenter study. Laryngoscope. 2017; 127(1):223–228

[30] Sharma A, Glick H, Campbell J, Torres J, Dorman M, Zeitler DM. Cortical plasticity and reorganization

in pediatric single-sided deafness pre- and post-cochlear implantation: a case study. Otol Neurotol. 2016; 37(2):e26–e34

[31] Peters JPM, Ramakers GGJ, Smit AL, Grolman W. Cochlear implantation in children with unilateral hearing loss: a systematic review. Laryngoscope. 2016; 126(3):713–721

[32] Ramos Macías Á, Borkoski-Barreiro SA, Falcón González JC, Ramos de Miguel Á. AHL, SSD and bimodal CI results in children. Eur Ann Otorhinolaryngol Head Neck Dis. 2016; 133(s)(uppl 1):S15–S20

[33] Leigh J, Dettman S, Dowell R, Briggs R. Communication development in children who receive a cochlear implant by 12 months of age. Otol Neurotol. 2013; 34(3):443–450

[34] Gordon KA, Wong DDE, Valero J, Jewell SF, Yoo P, Papsin BC. Use it or lose it? Lessons learned from the developing brains of children who are deaf and use cochlear implants to hear. Brain Topogr. 2011; 24(3–4):204–219

[35] Sharma A, Campbell J, Cardon G. Developmental and cross-modal plasticity in deafness: evidence from the P1 and N1 event related potentials in cochlear implanted children. Int J Psychophysiol. 2015; 95(2):135–144

[36] Sharma A, Dorman MF, Spahr AJ. Rapid development of cortical auditory evoked potentials after early cochlear implantation. Neuroreport. 2002; 13(10):1365–1368

[37] Graven S, Browne J. Auditory development in the fetus and infant. Newborn Infant Nurs Rev. 2008; 8:187–193

[38] Levine D, Strother-Garcia K, Golinkoff RM, Hirsh-Pasek K. Language development in the first year of life: what deaf children might be missing before cochlear implantation. Otol Neurotol. 2016; 37(2):e56–e62

[39] Bruijnzeel H, Ziylan F, Stegeman I, Topsakal V, Grolman W. A systematic review to define the speech and language benefit of early (<12 months) pediatric cochlear implantation. Audiol Neurootol. 2016; 21(2):113–126

[40] May-Mederake B. Early intervention and assessment of speech and language development in young children with cochlear implants. Int J Pediatr Otorhinolaryngol. 2012; 76(7):939–946

[41] Dettman SJ, Dowell RC, Choo D, et al. Long-term communication outcomes for children receiving cochlear implants younger than 12 months: a multicenter study. Otol Neurotol. 2016; 37(2):e82–e95

[42] Houston DM, Miyamoto RT. Effects of early auditory experience on word learning and speech perception in deaf children with cochlear implants: implications for sensitive periods of language development. Otol Neurotol. 2010; 31(8):1248–1253

[43] Caselli MC, Rinaldi P, Varuzza C, Giuliani A, Burdo S. Cochlear implant in the second year of life: lexical and grammatical outcomes. J Speech Lang Hear Res. 2012; 55(2):382–394

[44] Holman MA, Carlson ML, Driscoll CLW, et al. Cochlear implantation in children 12 months of age and younger. Otol Neurotol. 2013; 34(2):251–258

[45] Colletti L, Mandalà M, Colletti V. Cochlear implants in children younger than 6 months. Otolaryngol Head Neck Surg. 2012; 147(1):139–146

[46] O'Connell BP, Holcomb MA, Morrison D, Meyer TA, White DR. Safety of cochlear implantation before 12 months of age: Medical University of South Carolina and Pediatric American College of Surgeons—National Surgical Quality improvement program outcomes. Laryngoscope. 2016; 126(3):707–712

[47] Kalejaiye A, Ansari G, Ortega G, Davidson M, Kim HJ. Low surgical complication rates in cochlear implantation for young children less than 1 year of age. Laryngoscope. 2017; 127(3):720–724

[48] Biernath KR, Reefhuis J, Whitney CG, et al. Bacterial meningitis among children with cochlear implants beyond 24 months after implantation. Pediatrics. 2006; 117(2):284–289

[49] Centers for Disease Control and Prevention (CDC). Advisory Committee on Immunization Practices. Pneumococcal vaccination for cochlear implant candidates and recipients: updated recommendations of the Advisory Committee on Immunization Practices. MMWR Morb Mortal Wkly Rep. 2003; 52(31):739–740

[50] Digge P, Solanki RN, Shah DC, Vishwakarma R, Kumar S. Imaging modality of choice for pre-operative cochlear imaging: HRCT vs MRI temporal bone. J Clin Diagn Res. 2016; 10(10):TC01–TC04

[51] Bronkhorst AW, Plomp R. Binaural speech intelligibility in noise for hearing-impaired listeners. J Acoust Soc Am. 1989; 86(4):1374–1383

[52] Lammers MJW, van der Heijden GJ, Pourier VE, Grolman W. Bilateral cochlear implantation in children: a systematic review and best-evidence synthesis. Laryngoscope. 2014; 124(7):1694–1699

[53] Basura GJ, Eapen R, Buchman CA. Bilateral cochlear implantation: current concepts, indications, and results. Laryngoscope. 2009; 119(12):2395–2401

[54] Galvin KL, Mok M. Everyday listening performance of children before and after receiving a second cochlear implant: results using the parent version of the speech, spatial, and qualities hearing scale. Ear Hear. 2016; 37(1):93–102

[55] Choi JE, Moon IJ, Kim EY, et al. Sound localization and speech perception in noise of pediatric cochlear implant recipients: bimodal fitting versus bilateral cochlear implants. Ear Hear. 2017; 38(4):426–440

[56] Wie OB. Language development in children after receiving bilateral cochlear implants between 5 and 18 months. Int J Pediatr Otorhinolaryngol. 2010; 74(11):1258–1266

[57] Gordon KA, Jiwani S, Papsin BC. What is the optimal timing for bilateral cochlear implantation in children? Cochlear Implants Int. 2011; 12(s)(uppl 2):S8–S14

[58] Reeder RM, Firszt JB, Cadieux JH, Strube MJ. A longitudinal study in children with sequential bilateral cochlear implants: time course for the second implanted ear and bilateral performance. J Speech Lang Hear Res. 2017; 60(1):276–287

[59] Jeong SW, Kang MY, Kim LS. Criteria for selecting an optimal device for the contralateral ear of children

with a unilateral cochlear implant. Audiol Neurootol. 2015; 20(5):314–321

[60] Moberly AC, Lowenstein JH, Nittrouer S. Early bimodal stimulation benefits language acquisition for children with cochlear implants. Otol Neurotol. 2016; 37(1):24–30

[61] Sanhueza I, Manrique R, Huarte A, de Erenchun IR, Manrique M. Bimodal stimulation with cochlear implant and hearing aid in cases of highly asymmetric hearing loss. J Int Adv Otol. 2016; 12(1):16–22

[62] Shiell MM, Champoux F, Zatorre RJ. Reorganization of auditory cortex in early-deaf people: functional connectivity and relationship to hearing aid use. J Cogn Neurosci. 2015; 27(1):150–163

[63] Marsella P, Giannantonio S, Scorpecci A, Pianesi F, Micardi M, Resca A. Role of bimodal stimulation for auditory-perceptual skills development in children with a unilateral cochlear implant. Acta Otorhinolaryngol Ital. 2015; 35(6):442–448

[64] Gifford RH, Driscoll CLW, Davis TJ, Fiebig P, Micco A, Dorman MF. A within-subjects comparison of bimodal hearing, bilateral cochlear implantation, and bilateral cochlear implantation with bilateral hearing preservation: high-performing patients. Otol Neurotol. 2015; 36(8):1331–1337

[65] Brown RF, Hullar TE, Cadieux JH, Chole RA. Residual hearing preservation after pediatric cochlear implantation. Otol Neurotol. 2010; 31(8):1221–1226

[66] Skarzynski H, Matusiak M, Lorens A, Furmanek M, Pilka A, Skarzynski PH. Preservation of cochlear structures and hearing when using the Nucleus Slim Straight (CI422) electrode in children. J Laryngol Otol. 2016; 130(4):332–339

[67] Cushing SL, Gordon KA, Rutka JA, James AL, Papsin BC. Vestibular end-organ dysfunction in children with sensorineural hearing loss and cochlear implants: an expanded cohort and etiologic assessment. Otol Neurotol. 2013; 34(3):422–428

[68] Buchman CA, Jpy J, Hodges A, Telischi FF, Balkany TJ. Vestibular effects of cochlear implantation. Laryngoscope. 2004; 114(10, Pt 2, Suppl103): 1–22

[69] Oyewumi M, Wolter NE, Heon E, Gordon KA, Papsin BC, Cushing SL. Using balance function to screen for vestibular impairment in children with sensorineural hearing loss and cochlear implants. Otol Neurotol. 2016; 37(7):926–932

[70] Cushing SL, Papsin BC. Vestibular assessment. In: Eisenberg LS, ed. Clinical Management of Children with Cochlear Implants. 2nd ed. San Diego, CA: Plural Publishing; 2017:473–510

[71] Wolter NE, Gordon KA, Papsin BC, Cushing SL. Vestibular and balance impairment contributes to cochlear implant failure in children. Otol Neurotol. 2015; 36(6):1029–1034

[72] Battmer RD, Backous DD, Balkany TJ, et al; International Consensus Group for Cochlear Implant Reliability Reporting. International classification of reliability for implanted cochlear implant receiver stimulators. Otol Neurotol. 2010; 31(8):1190–1193

[73] Blanchard M, Thierry B, Glynn F, De Lamaze A, Garabédian EN, Loundon N. Cochlear implant failure

and revision surgery in pediatric population. Ann Otol Rhinol Laryngol. 2015; 124(3):227–231

[74] Sterkers F, Merklen F, Piron JP, et al. Outcomes after cochlear reimplantation in children. Int J Pediatr Otorhinolaryngol. 2015; 79(6):840–843

[75] Farinetti A, Ben Gharbia D, Mancini J, Roman S, Nicollas R, Triglia J-M. Cochlear implant complications in 403 patients: comparative study of adults and children and review of the literature. Eur Ann Otorhinolaryngol Head Neck Dis. 2014; 131(3):177–182

[76] Googe BJ, Carron JD. Analyzing complications of minimally invasive pediatric cochlear implantation: a review of 248 implantations. Am J Otolaryngol. 2016; 37(1):44–50

[77] Wolfe J, Schafer EC. Programming cochlear implants in children. In: Eisenberg LS, ed. Clinical Management of Children with Cochlear Implants. 2nd ed. San Diego, CA: Plural Publishing; 2017:105-151

[78] Noble JH, Hedley-Williams AJ, Sunderhaus L, et al. Initial results with image-guided cochlear implant programming in children. Otol Neurotol. 2016; 37(2):e63–e69

[79] Yoon PJ. Pediatric cochlear implantation. Curr Opin Pediatr. 2011; 23(3):346–350

[80] Russell JL, Pine HS, Young DL. Pediatric cochlear implantation: expanding applications and outcomes. Pediatr Clin North Am. 2013; 60(4):841–863

[81] Davidson LS, Geers AE, Blamey PJ, Tobey EA, Brenner CA. Factors contributing to speech perception scores in long-term pediatric cochlear implant users. Ear Hear. 2011; 32(s)(uppl)(1):19–26

[82] van Wieringen A, Wouters J. What can we expect of normally-developing children implanted at a young age with respect to their auditory, linguistic and cognitive skills? Hear Res. 2015; 322:171–179

[83] Kang DH, Lee MJ, Lee KY, Lee SH, Jang JH. Prediction of cochlear implant outcomes in patients with prelingual deafness. Clin Exp Otorhinolaryngol. 2016; 9(3):220–225

[84] Dunn CC, Walker EA, Oleson J, et al. Longitudinal speech perception and language performance in pediatric cochlear implant users: the effect of age at implantation. Ear Hear. 2014; 35(2):148–160

[85] Black J, Hickson L, Black B, Perry C. Prognostic indicators in paediatric cochlear implant surgery: a systematic literature review. Cochlear Implants Int 2011;12(2):67–93

[86] Cosetti MK, Waltzman SB. Outcomes in cochlear implantation: variables affecting performance in adults and children. Otolaryngol Clin N Am 2012;45:155–171

[87] Varga L, Kabátová Z, Mašindová I, et al. Is deafness etiology important for prediction of functional outcomes in pediatric cochlear implantation? Acta Otolaryngol. 2014; 134(6):571–578

[88] Budenz CL, Starr K, Arnedt C, et al. Speech and language outcomes of cochlear implantation in children with isolated auditory neuropathy versus cochlear hearing loss. Otol Neurotol. 2013; 34(9):1615–1621

[89] De Carvalho GM, Ramos P, Arthur C, Guimaraes A, Sartorato E. Performance of cochlear implants in

pediatric patients with auditory spectrum disorder. J Int Adv Otol. 2016;12(1): 8-15

[90] Santarelli R. Information from cochlear potentials and genetic mutations helps localize the lesion site in auditory neuropathy. Genome Med. 2010; 2(12):91

[91] Young NM, Kim FM, Ryan ME, Tournis E, Yaras S. Pediatric cochlear implantation of children with eighth nerve deficiency. Int J Pediatr Otorhinolaryngol. 2012; 76(10):1442-1448

[92] Walton J, Gibson WPR, Sanli H, Prelog K. Predicting cochlear implant outcomes in children with auditory neuropathy. Otol Neurotol. 2008; 29(3):302-309

[93] Cohen M, Phillips JA, III. Genetic approach to evaluation of hearing loss. Otolaryngol Clin North Am. 2012; 45(1):25-39

[94] Hang AX, Kim GG, Zdanski CJ. Cochlear implantation in unique pediatric populations. Curr Opin Otolaryngol Head Neck Surg. 2012; 20(6):507-517

[95] Wakil N, Fitzpatrick EM, Olds J, Schramm D, Whittingham J. Long-term outcome after cochlear implantation in children with additional developmental disabilities. Int J Audiol. 2014; 53(9):587-594

[96] Jackler RK, Luxford WM, House WF. Congenital malformations of the inner ear: a classification based on embryogenesis. Laryngoscope. 1987; 97(3, Pt 2, Suppl 40):2-14

[97] Adunka OF, Teagle HFB, Zdanski CJ, Buchman CA. Influence of an intraoperative perilymph gusher on cochlear implant performance in children with labyrinthine malformations. Otol Neurotol. 2012; 33(9):1489-1496

[98] Pakdaman MN, Herrmann BS, Curtin HD, Van Beek-King J, Lee DJ. Cochlear implantation in children with anomalous cochleovestibular anatomy: a systematic review. Otolaryngol Head Neck Surg. 2012; 146(2):180-190

[99] Easwar V, Sanfilippo J, Papsin B, Gordon K. Factors affecting daily cochlear implant use in children:

datalogging evidence. J Am Acad Audiol. 2016; 27(10):824-838

[100] Choo D, Dettman SJ. What can long-term attendance at programming appointments tell us about pediatric cochlear implant recipients? Otol Neurotol. 2017; 38(3):325-333

[101] Bobsin LL, Houston KT. Communication assessment and intervention: implications for pediatric hearing loss. Otolaryngol Clin North Am. 2015; 48(6):1081-1095

[102] Mitchell RE, Karchmer MA. Chasing the mythical ten percent: parental hearing status of deaf and hard of hearing students in the United States. Sign Lang Stud. 2004; 4:138-163

[103] Yanbay E, Hickson L, Scarinci N, Constantinescu G, Dettman SJ. Language outcomes for children with cochlear implants enrolled in different communication programs. Cochlear Implants Int. 2014; 15(3):121-135

[104] Dunn CC, Walker EA, Oleson J, et al. Longitudinal speech perception and language performance in pediatric cochlear implant users: the effect of age at implantation. EarHear, 2014;35(2): 148-160

[105] Geers AE, Nicholas JG, Sedey AL. Language skills of children with early cochlear implantation. Ear Hear. 2003; 24(suppl 1): S46-S58

[106] Roman S, Rochette F, Triglia JM, Schön D, Bigand E. Auditory training improves auditory performance in cochlear implanted children. Hear Res. 2016; 337:89-95

[107] Semenov YR, Yeh ST, Seshamani M, et al; CDaCI Investigative Team. Age-dependent cost-utility of pediatric cochlear implantation. Ear Hear. 2013; 34(4):402-412

[108] Kumar R, Warner-Czyz A, Silver CH, Loy B, Tobey E. American parent perspectives on quality of life in pediatric cochlear implant recipients. Ear Hear. 2015; 36(2):269-278

14 Bone Conduction Hearing Solutions

William Hodgetts

14.1 Introduction

The pathway to hearing help for an adult with less than severe inner ear hearing loss typically requires very little medical involvement. A person may decide to seek help, contact the first private clinic he/she finds on the Internet, get an appointment, decide whether he/she likes the audiologist, and start a journey toward better hearing. There are, of course, many challenges about the individual and his/her expectations of hearing help. There can also be confusion and concerns about costs associated with interventions and what the individual is actually paying for (bundled services). However, when family or other significant communication partners are included in the treatment pathway and there is a genuine, knowledgeable, and trusting relationship with an audiologist, the pathway is not terribly complex, nor it is difficult to access. Typically, it will involve counseling, assessment, technology provision, outcome measurement, and follow-up. In contrast, the pathway for a patient with conductive, mixed, or single-sided hearing loss can be much more complex.

14.2 Case Vignette

Consider a 35-year-old woman with a lifetime of bilateral, chronic draining ears and hearing loss as a result of poor eustachian tube function. For the first many years of her life, the family physician did his best to manage the infections. Eventually, she was sent to an otolaryngologist for tubes. The tubes did help, for as long as they would stay in. When they fell out, the tympanic membrane would temporarily heal and then the middle ear would again cause problems. A cycle of repeated ear infections and fluctuating hearing loss led to struggles throughout school and into adulthood. Eventually she decided

to just "live with it." After years of persistent nudging, the people in her life convinced her that it might be helpful for her to try hearing aids. She went back to an otolaryngologist who placed pressure equalization tubes that were designed to stay in for a long time. He also recommended that she see an audiologist about getting hearing aids. Unfortunately, neither the otolaryngologist nor the audiologist was up to date on bone-conduction intervention and both were likely just hoping that the person's history of chronic draining ears would not be an issue. After the patient's initial fitting, the chronic draining ears were the last things on her mind. She had no idea that it was possible to hear as well as she was hearing. She was thrilled. However, it took only a matter of days for her ears to begin a new cycle of infections, and soon enough, the hearing aids were mostly ineffective, and now were exacerbating infections and medical risk. The hearing aids ended up in a drawer and the woman went back to struggling with hearing loss. The above story is true, but incomplete. We will return to it later.

Unfortunately, for many people working in the field of bone-conduction amplification, this story is far too common. The pathway for a person to get to our institute, and many centers like ours, is complicated. It usually involves more professionals, more resources, more choices, and more time. There are many more points along the journey where the patient may be told (or come to the conclusion) that she is going to have to "live with it." There are many chances for the patient to be given a less than ideal solution. Even if this patient gets to a center that offers bone-conduction treatment, the explosion of options in recent years makes deciding which one to choose extremely challenging. Not all options cost the same and often we do not know enough about new technologies to justify their use. There are necessary and important surgical and audiological alliances around the patient that can help to guide

under the age of 5 (in the United States, the Food and Drug Administration [FDA] requires the child to be 5 years before surgery for bone-conduction devices). ►Fig. 14.2 shows a young child wearing a soft band and a Ponto device from Oticon Medical. Many children lack good-quality bone and sufficient thickness until they are around 5 years of age.[14,16]

The other skin drive solutions are the Baha Attract from Cochlear[17,18] and the Alpha 2 from Sophono.[19] For these devices, the surgeon implants a magnet under the skin. These transcutaneous devices are considered "passive" because the magnet under the skin doesn't actively vibrate. Instead the vibrations from the processors are sent across the skin. There is a loss of energy to skin with both of these systems. This has been studied extensively.[20,21,22] Unfortunately, the amount of energy lost on average is greatest in the high frequencies and the amount lost is highly individual.

14.6.2 Direct Drive

There are two types of direct drive bone-conduction solutions: percutaneous and active transcutaneous solutions. The percutaneous solutions are the most common in the field with estimates of over 100,000 devices on the market. A percutaneous solution involves implanting a titanium screw (usually 4 mm in length) into the parietal mastoid region of the skull behind the ear. The implant has an attachment referred to as an "abutment" that goes through the skin and provides an anchor for the processor (either the Ponto or the Baha). Because the implant, abutment and processor are all rigidly connected, and the skin is no longer a part of the vibration pathway, these devices directly vibrate the skull. In contrast to the skin drive solutions, there is an advantage to stimulating the skull directly and this advantage is most prominent in the high frequencies. Again, the size of the advantage varies considerably for each individual and is not predictable. ►Fig. 14.3 shows the difference between transcutaneous passive (Attract) and percutaneous Baha (Connect) both from Cochlear. The Attract (►Fig. 14.3a) shows the intact skin and the passive magnet, while the Connect is a rigid skin bypass system.

The most recent bone-conduction hearing solutions are called active transcutaneous solutions. The principle behind these devices is that the vibrator is implanted under the skin in direct contact to the bone. The processor is magnetically connected to

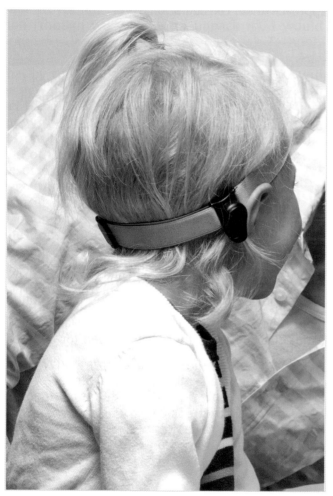

Fig. 14.2   Image of a young child wearing a soft band and a Ponto device.

> **Pitfall**
>
> We often need to make candidacy decisions from transcutaneous thresholds and we cannot predict on a case-by-case basis how much better someone will hear by direct bone conduction.

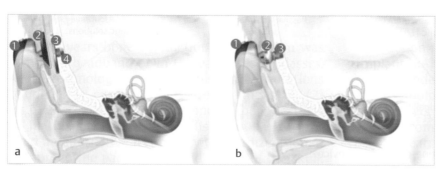

a   b

Fig. 14.3   (a, b) Image depicting the difference between (a) a transcutaneous passive and a (b) percutaneous bone-conduction solution. For the transcutaneous solution 1 = processor, 2 = external magnet, 3 = internal magnet, 4 = implant. For the percutaneous solution 1 = processor, 2 = abutment, 3 = implant. Image courtesy of Cochlear Bone Anchored Solutions.

the patient. However, the information from the processor is passed inductively to a coil that converts the signal into direct drive vibration. In other words, while the skin is still intact, there is almost no loss of energy across the skin. There are currently two such devices on the market, the BONEBRIDGE from MED-EL and the BCI, which have been extensively presented in the literature and are undergoing clinical trials.[1,13,23,24,25,26,27,28,29,30] For the BONEBRIDGE, the candidacy and availability for this device ranges from country to country. At the time of writing, the device is not yet approved for sale in the United States. However, Canada and many European countries have been using the device for several years. In Canada, the device is approved from 5 years of age; however, the current transducer is quite large and requires very careful planning with respect to candidacy and surgery.[25]

14.7 Output Considerations

As indicated above, there are significant differences between skin drive and direct drive technologies. However, there are methods that can be used to compare the output capabilities of these devices for both the maximum pure tone average thresholds suitable for the device in question and the maximum dynamic range available with each device. Zwartenkot[31] and Reinfeldt[13] used the results of published studies to define the maximum dynamic range of output across a number of bone-conduction devices. They also proposed aided pure tone average thresholds of 35 dB HL (500, 1,000, 2,000, and 4,000 Hz) to be a reasonable target since word recognition scores of approximately 75% could be predicted from the articulation index.[32] These values together can be used to derive maximum inclusion criteria by device. While there may be challenges with these assumptions, they at least provide a metric against which some compari-

sons can be made (see Zwartenkot[31] and Rienfeldt[13] for a detailed explanation).

▶Fig. 14.4 shows the maximum dynamic range of hearing (in dB HL) and the maximum recommended pure tone average unaided bone conduction thresholds for a number of bone-conduction devices. Notably the Baha Attract is likely to have similar values as the Sophono. Also, the maximum power output (MPO) of the Divino is similar to the MPO of recent devices (the Ponto Plus from Oticon Medical and the Baha 5 from Cochlear Corporation). More powerful devices from both companies (Ponto 3 SuperPower from Oticon Medical and Baha Superpower from Cochlear) have been released and have MPOs similar to the Cordelle. Those familiar with this field may notice that the maximum unaided thresholds in ▶Fig. 14.4 differ slightly from many of the manufacturers' recommendations. These lower values are a conservative guide to ensure that sufficient output is available for a given user with a given bone-conduction device.

14.8 Other Considerations

▶Fig. 14.4 shows that the skin drive solution (Sophono in this case) loses some energy to the skin. From an audiological perspective, this does not seem like an ideal solution. Why would we limit our available maximum thresholds and maximum dynamic range? As I indicated at the beginning of this chapter, the pathway to bone conduction hearing is a much more complicated pathway (involving many more people and many more decisions and often a great deal more distance) than a typical air-conduction pathway. Perhaps the individual has perfectly normal bone-conduction thresholds and lives a plane ride away from the center where the surgery and after care of the tissue are performed. Perhaps the risk of having an abutment through the skin is more complicated for the person's life.

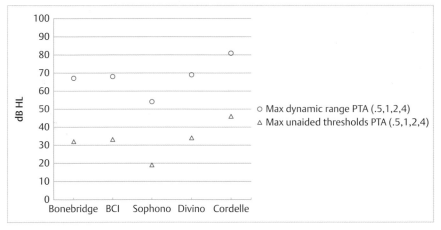

Fig. 14.4 Maximum dynamic range of hearing and maximum recommended bone-conduction thresholds for a variety of bone-conduction devices.

However, then what happens if a decision is made in favor of tissue preservation only to find that the device is not powerful enough? Would another surgery be necessary? Who is paying for these devices and the operating room time? Can we honestly say that one device is just as good as another if, while giving roughly equivalent "audiological results" but cost more in terms of device, components, and operating room time? How do we navigate the complex space where multiple team members may have competing interests for the same case? It is entirely conceivable that the patient might want one type of solution for aesthetic reasons, the surgeon might want a different solution for surgical interests, the audiologist might want a different solution for audibility considerations and the administrator or third-party payer might want a different solution for cost reasons. How are we able to make these decisions?

> **Controversial Point**
>
> Often the bone-conduction solutions available in a certain clinical environment/setting are influenced by factors beyond the technology and the output capabilities of given devices.

14.9 Understanding your Own Environment

These hypothetical questions underscore a very important point. Wherever and with whomever we are working, there is likely to be a unique environment that has local, state, province, and federal considerations to be navigated. No chapter that summarizes the literature showing a certain amount of decibels' advantage for one device over another is necessarily going to help the reader easily navigate their unique environment. Rather, it is important to form strong and collaborative partnerships with the surgeons that are interested in the bone-conduction options and the health care/hospital/insurance administrators supporting the provision of bone-conduction solutions. You will need to be prepared to lobby for or defend against certain solutions for certain individuals.

14.10 Outcome Measures in Bone Conduction

One of the significant challenges in summarizing the literature in the field of bone conduction has to do with how we measure outcomes. For example,

because there are many challenges with performing "real-ear" verification, many studies still report aided sound field thresholds when comparing aided to unaided performance or when comparing one device to another. However, it has been well documented that aided sound field thresholds have significant limitations that render them insensitive to some of the differences we might be trying to identify.[33,34,35,36] Another frequently reported, though not particularly audiological, outcome measure is the Holger's Index for skin response.[37,38] This measure is used to compare the skin reactions and outcomes of various surgical approaches and incision techniques when considering the follow-up care of percutaneous abutments. Unfortunately, the scale is quite subjective and, depending on who is rating the score (e.g., a resident grading a senior surgeon's technique or surgeon grading their own technique), there may be considerable bias in the literature with respect to this outcome measure. Both of these outcome measures are illustrative of an even more important issue with our field in general: neither one is directly relevant to the patient. Has anyone ever met a patient who comes to clinic and says, "I'd really like to hear soft warble tones better in a quiet room" or "I'm really hoping for a Holger's skin response that is a 2 or less following surgery"? I am not arguing that clinician-derived outcome measures are unimportant. However, if we are going to use them, they should at least provide greater sensitivity and less bias. Hodgetts[39] and Hodgetts and Scollie[40] describe an approach to verifying output for percutaneous bone-conduction devices using a skull simulator in combination with a Desired Sensation Level (DSL) m[i/o] prescriptive algorithm for bone. This approach is a logical parallel to real-ear verification with air-conduction hearing aids and is much more sensitive to small changes in device output. Recently, Oticon medical has included this DSL-BC prescription in their Genie medical software. Clinicians fitting Ponto devices can now choose to view the fitting in a format that is very familiar. Instead of viewing the fitting as an SPL-o-gram, clinicians can view the fitting as a force-level FL-o-gram. That is, the patient's thresholds (measured directly through the device) are plotted as force-level thresholds. The targets for DSL are plotted above the thresholds and represent a starting point for the fitting consideration.

There is also a module within the Genie Medical software that allows for communication with an interacoustics affinity test box. Clinicians who have a skull simulator can then directly measure the output of the device on the skull simulator to see how the output compares to the individual's thresholds and the targets all in force-level decibel. More details about the prescriptive approach can be found in

Hodgetts and Scollie.[40] We are currently working to get DSL prescription into other manufacturers' software as well.

In recent years, a group of clinicians and researchers formed the Auditory Rehabilitation Network (AURONET) to try to address some of the challenges with outcome measures in the field of bone conduction.[41] The goal for AURONET is to review all outcome measures (surgical, audiological, financial, etc.), and subject them to a filtering process adopted from the Outcome Measures in Rheumatology (OMERACT) group. In order to be considered a relevant (not necessary recommended) outcome measure, it should meet the following three criteria:

1. Truth: Does the outcome measure what it intends to? Are the results unbiased?
2. Discrimination: Does the outcome measure distinguish change between groups? Is it stable with test–retest reliability?
3. Feasibility: Can the outcome measure be easily used in different health care settings without great expense in terms of time and money?

Those outcome measures that remain after this filtering process will be further subjected to filtering and consensus voting by the AURONET members for inclusion into a "Core Set" of outcome measures. Where no outcome measure exists for a particular domain, recommendations will be made for the development of a new outcome measure to address the gap. A core set of measures that we all take in our clinics and in our studies will greatly facilitate our ability to compare devices across different health care contexts, centers, and countries.

14.11 Case Vignette

I promised to return to the case vignette. Finally, after nearly 33 years of struggling with her ears, the individual met the right audiologist who referred her to our institute. Our team (audiologist and surgeon) jointly decided with the patient that we would treat her left side first with a percutaneous Ponto device. This ear had a slightly larger conductive hearing loss. She was fitted with that device in 2014 and has been extremely satisfied with it ever since. In 2016 we were able to treat her right ear with a BONEBRIDGE. Our expectation in doing this was, first and foremost, an opportunity to give her bilateral hearing. However, the ability within a single subject to compare her experiences using both devices was also of great interest. As expected, surgery for and recovery from the BONEBRIDGE was much more complicated

than the Ponto. The site remains numb and there has been a need to reduce the magnet strength to the point where the device gets knocked off easily. Performance-wise, I think the most fascinating thing she has said is, "when I close my eyes, it isn't obvious which device is better. When I go back and forth, I can't really tell which one I like more. What I can tell, immediately, is that having two devices is a massive improvement over either one and I feel like, with both, I have more resources at my disposal."

14.12 Conclusion

It is easy to get lost in some of the technical detail of device A versus device B and it can be easy to forget the simple things about why someone came to us in the first place. This case illustrates the point I've been making this whole chapter. The question "which device is better" is a complex, difficult to navigate, environment- and relationship-dependent question that requires sensitive core outcome measures that matter to the patient. To be a successful clinician in the field of bone conduction requires you to surround the patient with a team of collaborative decision makers that understand the context in which you are working. There are often significant differences between centers that might make one device easier to prescribe than another. There are different funding situations for different groups. There are many biases for both the clinician and the patient that need to be understood and carefully checked. With this backdrop then, it should be fairly clear to the reader that there is not likely to be a "best" solution for a given person. Instead you should strive for the best decision you can make as a team in the environment in which you practice to give a person the best chance to hear well again.

References

[1] Reinfeldt S, Östli P, Håkansson B, Taghavi H, Eeg-Olofsson M, Stalfors J. Study of the feasible size of a bone conduction implant transducer in the temporal bone. Otol Neurotol. 2015; 36(4):631–637
[2] Håkansson B, Tjellström A. Bone conduction implants for amplification: comparison of results. Ear Nose Throat J. 1998; 77(2):144–145
[3] Tjellström A, Håkansson B. The bone-anchored hearing aid. Design principles, indications, and long-term clinical results. Otolaryngol Clin North Am. 1995; 28(1):53–72
[4] Håkansson B, Lidén G, Tjellström A, et al. Ten years of experience with the Swedish bone-anchored hearing system. Ann Otol Rhinol Laryngol Suppl. 1990; 151:1–16

[5]   Håkansson B, Tjellström A, Rosenhall U, Carlsson P. The bone-anchored hearing aid. Principal design and a psychoacoustical evaluation. Acta Otolaryngol. 1985; 100(3–4):229–239

[6]   Dumper J, Hodgetts B, Liu R, Brandner N. Indications for bone-anchored hearing AIDS: a functional outcomes study. J Otolaryngol Head Neck Surg. 2009; 38(1):96–105

[7]   Snik AF, Mylanus EA, Proops DW, et al. Consensus statements on the BAHA system: where do we stand at present? Ann Otol Rhinol Laryngol Suppl. 2005; 195:2–12

[8]   Nelissen RC, Mylanus EA, Cremers CW, Hol MK, Snik AF. Long-term compliance and satisfaction with percutaneous bone conduction devices in patients with congenital unilateral conductive hearing loss. Otol Neurotol. 2015; 36(5):826–833

[9]   Mertens G, Desmet J, Snik AF, Van de Heyning P. An experimental objective method to determine maximum output and dynamic range of an active bone conduction implant: the Bonebridge. Otol Neurotol. 2014; 35(7):1126–1130

[10] Hol MK, Bosman AJ, Snik AF, Mylanus EA, Cremers CW. Bone-anchored hearing aids in unilateral inner ear deafness: an evaluation of audiometric and patient outcome measurements. Otol Neurotol. 2005; 26(5):999–1006

[11] Hol MK, Bosman AJ, Snik AF, Mylanus EA, Cremers CW. Bone-anchored hearing aid in unilateral inner ear deafness: a study of 20 patients. Audiol Neurootol. 2004; 9(5):274–281

[12] Bosman AJ, Hol MK, Snik AF, Mylanus EA, Cremers CW. Bone-anchored hearing aids in unilateral inner ear deafness. Acta Otolaryngol. 2003; 123(2):258–260

[13] Reinfeldt S, Håkansson B, Taghavi H, Eeg-Olofsson M. New developments in bone-conduction hearing implants: a review. Med Devices (Auckl). 2015; 8:79–93

[14] Priwin C, Granström G. A long-term evaluation of bone-anchored hearing aid (BAHA) in children. Cochlear Implants Int. 2005; 6(suppl 1):81–83

[15] Hol MK, Cremers CW, Coppens-Schellekens W, Snik AF. The BAHA Softband. A new treatment for young children with bilateral congenital aural atresia. Int J Pediatr Otorhinolaryngol. 2005; 69(7):973–980

[16] Priwin C, Granström G. The bone-anchored hearing aid in children: a surgical and questionnaire follow-up study. Otolaryngol Head Neck Surg. 2005; 132(4):559–565

[17] Briggs R, Van Hasselt A, Luntz M, et al. Clinical performance of a new magnetic bone conduction hearing implant system: results from a prospective, multicenter, clinical investigation. Otol Neurotol. 2015; 36(5):834–841

[18] Kurz A, Flynn M, Caversaccio M, Kompis M. Speech understanding with a new implant technology: a comparative study with a new nonskin penetrating Baha system. BioMed Res Int. 2014; 2014:416205

[19] Nelissen RC, Agterberg MJ, Hol MK, Snik AF. Three-year experience with the Sophono in children with congenital conductive unilateral hearing loss:

tolerability, audiometry, and sound localization compared to a bone-anchored hearing aid. Eur Arch Otorhinolaryngol. 2016; 273(10):3149–3156

[20] Carlsson P, Håkansson B, Ringdahl A. Force threshold for hearing by direct bone conduction. J Acoust Soc Am. 1995; 97(2):1124–1129

[21] Håkansson B, Tjellström A, Rosenhall U. Acceleration levels at hearing threshold with direct bone conduction versus conventional bone conduction. Acta Otolaryngol. 1985; 100(3–4):240–252

[22] Håkansson B, Tjellström A, Rosenhall U. Hearing thresholds with direct bone conduction versus conventional bone conduction. Scand Audiol. 1984; 13(1):3–13

[23] Zernotti ME, Sarasty AB. Active bone conduction prosthesis: Bonebridge(TM). Int Arch Otorhinolaryngol. 2015; 19(4):343–348

[24] Bento RF, Lopes PT, Cabral Junior FdaC. Bonebridge Bone Conduction Implant. Int Arch Otorhinolaryngol. 2015; 19(4):277–278

[25] Sprinzl GM, Wolf-Magele A. The Bonebridge Bone Conduction Hearing Implant: indication criteria, surgery and a systematic review of the literature. Clin Otolaryngol. 2016; 41(2):131–143

[26] Rahne T, Seiwerth I, Götze G, et al. Functional results after Bonebridge implantation in adults and children with conductive and mixed hearing loss. Eur Arch Otorhinolaryngol. 2015; 272(11):3263–3269

[27] Taghavi H, Håkansson B, Reinfeldt S, et al. Technical design of a new bone conduction implant (BCI) system. Int J Audiol. 2015; 54(10):736–744

[28] Reinfeldt S, Håkansson B, Taghavi H, Fredén Jansson KJ, Eeg-Olofsson M. The bone conduction implant: clinical results of the first six patients. Int J Audiol. 2015; 54(6):408–416

[29] Reinfeldt S, Håkansson B, Taghavi H, Eeg-Olofsson M. Bone conduction hearing sensitivity in normal-hearing subjects: transcutaneous stimulation at BAHA vs BCI position. Int J Audiol. 2014; 53(6):360–369

[30] Eeg-Olofsson M, Håkansson B, Reinfeldt S, et al. The bone conduction implant—first implantation, surgical and audiologic aspects. Otol Neurotol. 2014; 35(4):679–685

[31] Zwartenkot JW, Snik AF, Mylanus EA, Mulder JJ. Amplification options for patients with mixed hearing loss. Otol Neurotol. 2014; 35(2):221–226

[32] Mueller HGK, Killion MC. An easy method for calculating the articulation index. Hear J. 1990; 43(9):14

[33] Hodgetts WE, Håkansson BE, Hagler P, Soli S. A comparison of three approaches to verifying aided Baha output. Int J Audiol. 2010; 49(4):286–295

[34] Hawkins DB. Limitations and uses of the aided audiogram. Semin Hear. 2004; 25:51–62

[35] Zelisko DL, Seewald RC, Gagné JP. Signal delivery/real ear measurement system for hearing aid selection and fitting. Ear Hear. 1992; 13(6):460–463

[36] Seewald RC, Hudson SP, Gagné JP, Zelisko DL. Comparison of two methods for estimating the sensation level of amplified speech. Ear Hear. 1992; 13(3):142–149

[37] Holgers KM. Characteristics of the inflammatory process around skin-penetrating titanium implants for aural rehabilitation. Audiology. 2000; 39(5):253–259

[38] Holgers KM, Tjellström A, Bjursten LM, Erlandsson BE. Soft tissue reactions around percutaneous implants: a clinical study of soft tissue conditions around skin-penetrating titanium implants for bone-anchored hearing aids. Am J Otol. 1988; 9(1):56–59

[39] Hodgetts WE. Other hearing devices: bone conduction. In: Tharpe AMS, ed. Handbook of Pediatric Audiology. 2nd ed. Abingdon: Plural Publishing; 2015

[40] Hodgetts WE, Scollie SD. DSL prescriptive targets for bone conduction devices: adaptation and comparison to clinical fittings. Int J Audiol. 2017; 56(7):521–530

[41] Tysome JR, Hill-Feltham P, Hodgetts WE, et al. The Auditory Rehabilitation Outcomes Network: an international initiative to develop core sets of patient-centred outcome measures to assess interventions for hearing loss. Clin Otolaryngol. 2015; 40(6):512–515

15 Hearing Assistive and Related Technology

Samuel R. Atcherson

15.1 Introduction

Assistive technology, in a broad sense, is "any item, piece of equipment, software program, or product system that is used to increase, maintain, or improve the functional capabilities of persons with disabilities."[1] This description in mind, it is generally not difficult to come up with a list of technologies (or devices) that help individuals with various sensory or physical challenges. For those with visual impairments we tend to think of braille and walking canes. For those with mobility impairments, we tend to think of motorized wheelchairs. For those with severe speech impairments, we tend to think of speech-generating communication boards. And for those with hearing loss, we tend to think of hearing aids, and possibly implantable devices such as a cochlear implant. Each of these examples is a technology that individuals with disabilities may use for daily living, education, employment, and recreation in order to function as independently as possible while enjoying a reasonably good quality of life.

One of the biggest challenges for consumers and professionals alike is an understanding of the purpose and types of a broad range assistive technology for individuals with hearing loss. That is, there is a technology for almost every conceivable life situation, yet each has both advantages and disadvantages. Moreover, technological advances have often combined two or more technologies, and there may be compatibility for some systems while others have become proprietary with limited compatibility. Some technologies are specific to hearing augmentation, some provide access *via* alternative modalities (e.g., visual or tactile), and some provide access through more than one modality (e.g., auditory, visual, and tactile). Thus, the purpose of this chapter is to provide a broad overview of existing hearing assistive and related technologies. The chapter is organized in a way that, hopefully, helps the reader appreciate the various types of technology and their benefits. It should be noted that there are quite a few manufacturers of hearing assistance (or assistive) technologies (HATs), and examples provided in this chapter do not constitute direct endorsement by the author.

15.2 Establishing the Need for Hearing Assistive and Related Technology

Audiologists must understand at the outset that while hearing aids and implantable devices are wonderful technologies: (1) their maximum effectiveness remain at the mercy of the physical and physiological conditions of the patient's ears and/or brain, (2) they oftentimes cannot meet the demands of every possible listening need, (3) some needs do not require augmentation for hearing, and (4) available technologies are not always adopted by patients.

Although hearing aids and implantable devices have unique features to help patients in complex listening situations, they cannot help with all listening situations. Physical proximity to the sound of interest is one important consideration. When sounds are close, they are audible and there is greater likelihood that it will be heard over other competing sounds, such as noise and reverberation. When sound travels, its power is spread over an ever-increasing area, which causes it to become softer and weaker with distance. The further away the sound of interest, the more likely it will become drowned out by noise and reverberation. This leads to a second important consideration: **signal-to-noise ratio (SNR)**. When the sound of interest (signal) is louder than other sounds (noise), the SNR will have a positive value (e.g., + 6 dB). Conversely, when the noise is louder than the signal, the SNR will have a negative value (e.g., − 6 dB). To maintain a positive SNR, patients will need to make sure they are of reasonably close proximity to what they want to hear. That is, with hearing aids and implantable devices, they must be within some **critical distance** within which the SNR is never 0 dB or negative. It is much easier to control one's listening environment at home, but oftentimes it is far more difficult to control at school, work, and out in public.

Second, sound processed by the hearing aid can be distorted in some way by the ear pathology on its way to the brain. As another example, cochlear implants rely on the integrity and relationship between stimulation electrodes and the auditory nerve. While the programming of hearing aids implantable devices can be customized for highest possible outcome, their maximum effectiveness will ultimately depend on the individual capacities related to the auditory brain, higher-order cognitive resources, training/intervention, as well as self-motivation and support.

Third, there are some individual or daily-life circumstances that do not require increased access to sound. Instead, assistive technology may be desired that takes the place of acoustic technology, or uses acoustic technology to convert environmental sounds into a different sensory form or modality (e.g., flashing light or vibration). Furthermore, there are assistive technologies (and associated services) available that convert spoken language into readable text.

Finally, it is inevitable that some patients may not adopt hearing aids or implantable devices for a variety of reasons, yet they still desire to have some level of independence by relying on other beneficial technologies or strategies. For example, individuals with mild hearing loss (or even normal hearing) may not want to wear hearing aids, but they would appreciate something to hear better in noisier environments. Other individuals with severe hearing loss may use sign language as his or her communication and have little to no desire to wear hearing aids or implantable device, yet still want to be able to wake up in the morning and to be able to make a phone call.

In summary, the sooner we accept that hearing aids and implantable devices are unable to help in every listening or daily-life situation, it becomes much easier to learn about, explore, and recommend assistive technology to others. While **assistive listening devices (ALD)** have been around for over 40 years, Thibodeau[2] argues that the term ALD is not inclusive of many other assistive technologies that can also provide access to communication. She advocated for the use of the term **hearing assistance (or assistive) technology (HAT)**, which is increasingly being adopted by others. Thus, HAT may be better described as "any

device that helps to overcome hearing loss whether it is to provide or enhance sound, or to provide sound-based information in an alternate modality such as a visual or tactile cue."[3] Regardless of the terminology used, the goal of assistive technology for individuals with hearing loss is to provide *assistance* and *access* in an otherwise auditory world. It should be remembered that equal access and equal opportunities may be provided, but equal outcome is never guaranteed.

Pearl

In several instances, technologies developed for the general population have been readily adopted by individuals with hearing loss, which this author likes to refer as "great equalizers." Examples of great equalizers include cellular short message service (SMS, or text message), instant messaging (e.g., internet chat), and electronic mail (e-mail). Conversely, scores of normal-hearing listeners have benefitted from the use of closed captioning and subtitles in noisy public places.

As suggested by Bankaitis,[4] there is an inherent absence of standardized categories for HATs. They could be categorized: (1) by modality, such as auditory, visual, and tactile; (2) by functional purpose, such as ALD, telecommunication, and environmental sound awareness; (3) by location, such as education, employment, or entertainment and recreation; (4) by hardwired or wireless transmission, (5) by whether they are personal or public, (6) by severity of hearing loss, or (7) by language-communication modality. The problem with any of these specific categories is that they are highly restrictive and they ignore the versatility and overlapping features in many of today's modern day devices. In this chapter, the following *loose* categories will be used: assistive listening device, telecommunication technology, speech-to-text technology, and alerting technology. In addition, brief discussion is also provided on assistive technologies available for health professionals with hearing loss and mobile device applications potentially useful for individuals with hearing loss. ▶**Table 15.1** provides a list of common hearing assistive and related technologies.

15.3 Target Populations and Groups Who May Benefit from Hearing Assistive and Related Technology

The World Health Organization[5] reviewed several population-based studies and estimated that

Table 15.1   List of common hearing assistive and related technologies

Technology	Description	Hearing, related, or both
Frequency-/digital-modulation (FM/DM) system	Assistive listening device; usually describes a wireless transmitter microphone and receiver system that uses radio broadcast transmission via analog or digital means	Hearing
Electromagnetic induction system	Assistive listening device; usually describes wireless transmitter microphone and receiver system that uses electromagnetic induction and a telecoil	Hearing
Infrared (IR) system	Assistive listening device; usually describes a wireless transmitter microphone and receiver system that uses a restricted, invisible portion of the light spectrum.	Hearing
Amplified stethoscope	Assistive listening device; a stethoscope with built-in amplifier to overcome noise and augment auscultation-related sounds	Hearing
Amplified phone	Telecommunication device; a corded or coreless telephone with built-in volume and tone controls, and may have larger displays and buttons for those with visual dexterity issues	Hearing
Captioned phone	Telecommunication device; a telephone that allows a user to simultaneously hear and read what is said by the other caller, while allowing the user to use his or her own voice to respond back	Both
Voice carry over (VCO)	Telecommunication device; a telephone (or accessory) that allows a user to read what is said by the other caller and use his or her own voice to respond back	Both
Teletypewriter (TTY)	Telecommunication device; a telephone-type device with keyboard that uses a phone line or Internet protocol (IP) network to allow two TTYs to share typed text, or to use a TTY and relay service to call a non-TTY user	Related
Videophone (VP)	Telecommunication device; a telephone with video display that uses typically uses an Internet protocol (IP) network to allow two TTYs to share typed text, or to use a TTY and relay service to call a non-TTY user	Both
Captioning (various)	Telecommunication and speech-to-text device; a device that produces live or prerecorded text on a television, monitor, or mobile device, or is embedded in an open or closed format within digital media	Related
Automatic speech recognition (ASR)	Speech-to-text device; an independent, computer-driven transcription of speech into readable text	Related
Phone signaler	Alerting device; a monitoring device that provides visual and/or vibrotactile awareness of a landline telephone ringing	Related
Sound signaler	Alerting device; a monitoring device that provides visual and/or vibrotactile awareness of sounds (e.g., baby cry)	Related
Fire, smoke, and carbon monoxide alarms	Alerting device; a device that provides visual, vibrotactile, and/or auditory alarm for environmental hazards in the home and public areas	Both

Table 15.1 *(Continued)* List of common hearing assistive and related technologies

Technology	Description	Hearing, related, or both
Door and window signaler	Alerting device; a device that provides visual and/or vibrotactile awareness of an opening of a door or window, or a knock at the door	Related
Motion signaler	Alerting device; a device that provides a visual and/or vibrotactile awareness of a person entering a space	Related
Weather alert	Alerting device; a severe weather alert system with a radio receiver that provides audible warnings and, with optional accessories, visual and vibrotactile awareness	Both
Clocks and watches	Alerting device; desktop, portable, and wearable timekeeping devices with audible, visual, and/or vibrotactile alarms	Both

there were approximately 360 million individuals worldwide (about 5.3%) with average hearing loss (0.5, 1, 2, and 4 kHz) in both ears. Of the 360 million, about 32 million (9%) are children. In the United States, it is estimated that as many as 30 million (12.7%) of Americans aged 12 years or younger have bilateral hearing loss, and that number is estimated to increase to about 48.1 million (20.3%) if there is hearing loss in at least one ear[6] which translates to about 1 in 5 Americans. Also, in the United States, it is estimated that 1 to 6 in 1,000 children will be diagnosed with hearing loss,[7] and neonatal hearing loss is about 1.1 in 1,000 infants.[8]

Based on these various estimates, the patients encountered will not only be quite diverse in terms of the type, degree, and configuration of hearing loss, but they will also be quite diverse in terms of their demographics, background, available resources, and, ultimately, which technologies are recommended or adopted. While assistive technologies are essentially the same for both children and adults, it is helpful to consider the actual purpose and needs. Below are but a few examples of target demographics:

- **Young Children:** Young children with hearing loss may need communication access to promote language development. As such, hearing aids and/or implantable device will often be the first step for audibility, but an ALD may be helpful in a variety of listening conditions in which the SNR is less than ideal (e.g., day care, in the car seat, etc.).
- **School-aged Children and Adult Learners:** School-aged children with hearing loss may need improved access to their teachers and classmates, particularly to minimize fatigue and to overcome less than ideal SNR. From vocation schools to professional development opportunities, adults with hearing loss, as

with school-aged children, often benefit from improved access to instructors and other learners to maximize learning.

- **Home and Social Network:** To increase independence and self-reliance for face-to-face and other communication needs.
- **Employees and Other Workers:** To increase independence and self-reliance to meet workplace demands.
- **Consumers and Travelers:** To promote public access to consumers of recreation and entertainment media, as well as places of worship, there are both ALD and caption options. Similarly, travel solutions are available for individuals with hearing loss if they are away from their usual comforts and technologies.
- **Other Individuals with Auditory and/or Language Compromise:** Individuals such as those with hidden hearing loss, (central) auditory processing disorders, learning and language impairments, and brain injuries may benefit from ALDs and caption options as well.

15.4 Assistive Listening Devices

In this section, an overview is provided primarily on wireless ALDs (i.e., remote microphone systems) to overcome the deleterious effects of soft/inaudible sounds, background noise, and/or distance. An oft-cited analogy for ALDs is that they act like a magnifying lens system (e.g., binoculars). For example, when an object of interest is too far or too small to be seen with the naked eye, binoculars can provide a sense of nearness because of the magnification produced by the lenses. Similarly, an ALD will provide a sense of nearness by making the sound of interest appear much louder or closer than it would otherwise be. Many have experienced the benefits of a well-designed public address (PA) system, which allows sound to be projected from loudspeakers connected to an amplifier and microphone, or some other audio device. There are also systems that allow wireless transmission of auditory information to personal receivers from a microphone or audio device. The former is a type of sound field system where sound is projected through the air and virtually all individuals within a given space will hear the sound. The latter is fundamentally more in line with a personal ALD that oftentimes provides clearer (more direct) access to sound. Three broad categories of ALDs will be described here: **frequency-modulation (FM) and digital-modulation (DM) systems**, **induction systems**, and **infrared systems**. ▶ Table 15.2 briefly summarizes the key components and transmission technology for the three categories of ALDs.

Pearl ✔

Assistive listening devices that are truly "wireless" are also commonly known as **remote microphone systems**.

15.4.1 Frequency-Modulation and Digital-Modulation Systems

In this category are ALDs that rely on one-way radio wave transmission from a microphone transmitter to a receiver. For example, acoustic information that is picked up by the microphone transmitter (e.g., worn by a teacher) is wirelessly sent to a receiver (e.g., worn by a student). There are two different types of transmission available commercially: FM and DM.

Table 15.2 Remote microphone systems (wireless assistive listening devices)

Remote microphone system	Key components	Transmission technology
Frequency-/digital-modulation system	Microphone/audio source, transmitter, receiver	72–76 MHz (analog) 216–217 MHz (analog) 900 MHz (digital) 2.45 GHz (digital)
Induction system	Microphone/audio source, amplifier, wire loop, telecoil	Magnetic field (audio frequencies 0.1–5 kHz ±3 dB re: 1 kHz)
Infrared system	Microphone/audio source, transmitter, emitter, receiver	95 kHz 250 kHz 2.3 MHz 2.8 MHz

The former is analog and the latter is digital. With FM, the sound that is picked up by the microphone is converted into a "frequency-modulated" radio signal. When the FM radio signal is "received" by the receiver, the FM signal is demodulated and converted back into an acoustic signal. With DM, the sound that is picked up by the microphone undergoes analog-to-digital (A/D) conversion (binary code of 0s and 1s) and is converted into a "digitally modulated" ultra-high-frequency radio signal. When the DM radio signal is "received" by the receiver, it undergoes digital-to-analog (D/A) conversion to reproduce the original acoustic signal. ▶ **Fig. 15.1** shows a schematic of the differences between FM and DM, and ▶ **Fig. 15.2** shows a commercial example of a 72-MHz FM microphone transmitter and receiver.

Pearl ✔

Both FM and DM bands can be divided into wide- and narrow-bands, usually 10 and 40 bands, respectively. The actual bandwidth does not determine sound quality. Rather, narrow-bands can yield greater channel separation to avoid interference by other bands. In contrast to the 72 to 76 and 216- to 217-MHz FM bands, DM bands plus channel-hopping (key shifting) reduces the chance for interference further. The 2.45-GHz DM band has broad utility for industry, science, and medical (ISM) applications.

In the United States, for example, the Federal Communications Commission (FCC) has set aside two FM bands specifically for hearing instruments: 72 to 76 MHz and 216 to 217 MHz. The DM lives in a band that ranges from 2,400 to 2,483.5 MHz, which gives rise to the 2.4-GHz band (or more precisely, the 2.45-GHz band). Although not as common, some DM devices live on the 900-MHz band. The two DM bands are not exclusive to hearing instruments, however. Just as music radio stations can be found on different channels (subbands), FM/DM systems can also be confined to different channels (wide- or narrow subbands) within their respective frequency bands.

Advantages of FM and DM Technology

The biggest advantage of FM/DM technology is that the radio signal transmission can penetrate walls, the devices can be highly portable, it can be used indoors or outdoors, and it can have transmission ranges varying from 100 (personal systems) to 1,000 ft (commercial systems). As a remote microphone system, the uses for FM/DM are numerous. For example, multiple FM/DM microphone and receiver systems

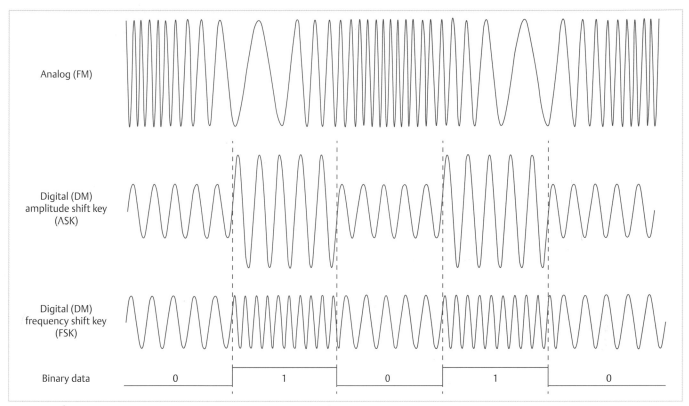

Fig. 15.1 Schematic differences between frequency modulation and digital modulation for transmission of signals from a microphone transmitter to a receiver.

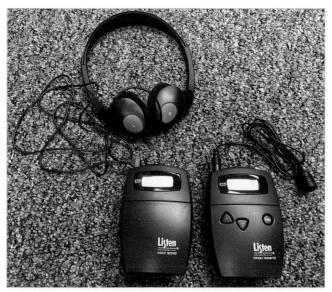

Fig. 15.2 Commercial example of a frequency-modulation microphone transmitter and receiver system. By design, this system has a plug-in, lapel-style microphone transducer and a pair of headphones.

can be used in the same building so long as each system is on its own channel. Conversely, multiple receivers can be used with a single microphone so long as they are all on the same channel. They can be used in a classroom environment, in the car, and out on tours to name a few. DM technology has some additional advantages over FM technology, such as greater digital control for sound precision and manipulation and enhanced connectivity to personal consumer electronics (e.g., mobile phones and tablets).[9]

Disadvantages of FM and DM Technology

Although the advantages far outweigh the disadvantages for FM/DM technology, there are a few disadvantages worth mentioning. The receiver must be appropriately paired with the transmitter, which can result in some compatibility issues. The FM can be susceptible to interference, though rare. Both FM/DM require that the microphone transmitter be strategically placed (e.g., usually within 6 inches of the sound source).

15.4.2 Induction Systems

Induction systems (also known as electromagnetic induction or induction loop system) is a wireless ALD that involves harnessing the magnetic field produced by an alternating current within audio systems. As an alternating current moves throughout a conducting wire, a magnetic energy by-product occurs whereby

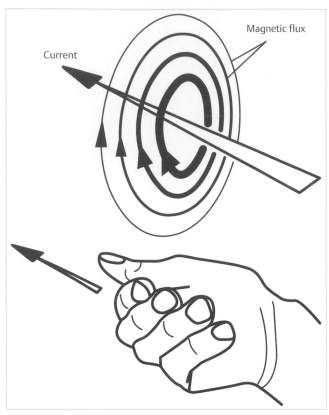

Fig. 15.3   Lines of magnetic flux flowing around a conductor carrying a current and the right hand rule showing how the curled fingers help to visualize the direction of the magnetic field caused by current flowing in the direction in which the thumb points. Image courtesy of Thieme Medical Publishers.

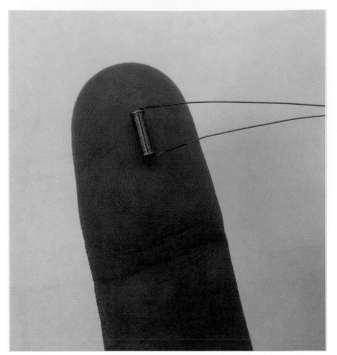

Fig. 15.4   Example of a telecoil, which looks like a miniature spool of copper wire (adult finger for size reference). Image courtesy of Jason A. Galster.

concentric flux lines perpendicular to the conducting wire is produced (▶**Fig. 15.3**). A **telecoil** is made up of a small metal rod encircled many times by a thin copper wire (two examples are shown in ▶**Fig. 15.4**). When a properly oriented telecoil is placed in the magnetic field, it becomes sensitive to the changes in the magnetic field thus reproducing the alternating current in the circuitry of a hearing aid, implantable device, or an external receiver-headphone unit. As alternating current moves through the conducting wire (or loop) it acts as the transmitter, while the telecoil acts as the receiver (▶**Fig. 15.5** for the magnetic loop induction system chain). In contrast to FM/DM and infrared systems, induction is analog and there are no carrier radio signals or light waves involved.

Advantages of Induction Systems

With induction systems, the options are almost limitless in terms of ways to produce and capture magnetic signals: (1) area (e.g., large or small rooms), (2) service desk or station (e.g., countertops, tellers, windows, and elevators), (3) transportation (e.g., personal vehicles and taxis), (4) neckloop connected to an audio device or other ALD, (5) a pair of headphones, and (6) compatible telephones and mobile phones. At its simplest, it could be nothing more than a microphone, amplifier with power supply, and a spool of wire that is easy to install (▶**Fig. 15.6**). For larger rooms or public spaces with complex arrangements, there are multiloop configurations that can help improve the overall

Pearl

Many headphones produce a magnetic field that is easily detected by telecoils. This may be a great option for those who want to wear headphones over their hearing aid or implant device. As an example, pilots who have telecoils in their hearing instruments are able to use aviation headsets.

Special Consideration

Telecoils have wide application for use, not only with assistive listening device systems, but also for telephone use. During use, the telephone may need to be rotated forward or backward slightly around the hearing instrument to find the "sweet spot" at which time the signal intensity and clarity will be maximal.

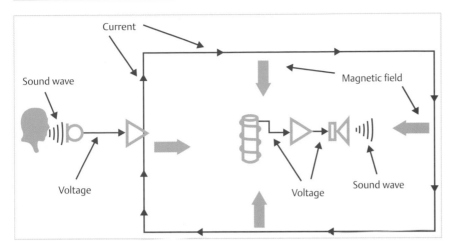

Fig. 15.5 The complete chain, from sound wave in to sound wave out, for a magnetic loop induction system. Image courtesy of Thieme Medical Publishers.

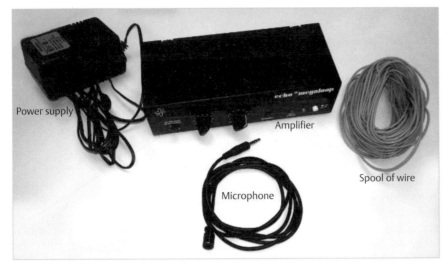

Fig. 15.6 Commercial example of a small, easy-to-install induction loop system.

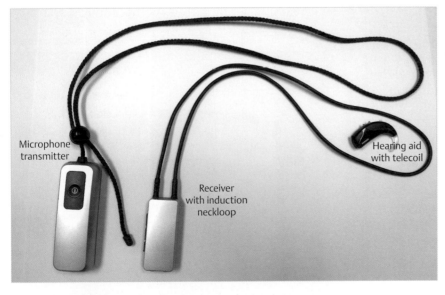

Fig. 15.7 Commercial example of a digital-modulation microphone transmitter and receiver system. By design, this particular DM system also incorporates an induction neckloop that communicates with the built-in telecoil of a hearing aid. Thus, two different wireless technologies are demonstrated.

magnetic signal strength and/or form clear magnetic field boundaries (to avoid magnetic spillover). For very large areas, such as a basketball stadium, professional audio installation is best. (Interested readers are encouraged to consult with the William Sound Design Guide for Induction Loop Systems.) Induction loops could also be in the form of a neckloop to be used with an ALD or coupled with an audio source. For example, ▶**Fig. 15.7** shows a combination system of a DM system with a neckloop receiver. Induction loops can also be highly constrained to a very small area, such as in a chair (using a looped chair pad) and in front of a service counter (using a portable or permanent fixture). An alternative to a neckloop is a silhouette coil that can be worn adjacent to a hearing aid or implant device. Since the telecoil is the receiver, it is a very cost-effective wireless ALD that can be readily designed into many hearing aids and implantable devices, which doubles the functionality of these devices as both hearing instrument and ALD.

Disadvantages of Induction Systems

As would be expected, the magnetic field and/or telecoil can be affected by interference from stray magnetic fields and other digital devices. During interference, the user perceives a constant buzzing sound. For this reason, induction loop systems to be used in the educational or public environments ought to be professional installed and tested for interference. The telecoil generally works well within the parameters of the induction loop. However, there are times when there is a mismatch between the orientation of the telecoil and the direction of the magnetic flux lines. Recall from ▶ Fig. 15.3 shows that the magnetic flux lines form concentric rings that are perpendicular to the wire(s) of the loop. If a loop is installed on the floor around the room, the magnetic flux line will be vertical within and toward the center of the room. In contrast, the magnetic flux lines will be horizontal directly over the wire. The goal is for the telecoil to be placed in parallel (vertical) to the magnetic flux line for maximum signal pickup. Thus, a clear disadvantage of induction loops is either poor installation and/or poor hearing instrument design in the placement of the telecoil. Telecoils have pronounced low-frequency roll-off beginning at 1 kHz. Because of this, sound quality for music may be less than satisfactory because of the attenuation of bass tones.

Pitfall ✕
Telecoils have pronounced low-frequency roll-off beginning at 1 kHz. Because of this, sound quality for music may be less than satisfactory because of the attenuation of bass tones.

15.4.3 Infrared Systems

The use of infrared (IR) is a common occurrence in many households with a remote control (transmitter and light-emitting diode) to operate a televi-

sion, cable box, and DVD/Blue-ray player (houses receiver unit). Similarly, there are ALDs that utilize IR technology. In IR technology, the processing and transmission of information is similar to FM/DM technology. What makes IR different from FM/DM is that IR operates using invisible light that is just below the visible light range. What also makes IR different from FM/DM is that the transmission of IR light cannot penetrate walls, limiting its use to a single room. The functional use of IR should be familiar since television remote controls operate on the same principle.

A typical audio IR system has a transmitter, emitter, and receiver. The transmitter can be connected directly to an audio output jack, or a microphone can be used. The transmitter causes the audio signal to be emitted and carried on the IR wave by a series of pulses. The receiver picks up the IR carrier wave and demodulates the pulses back into an audio signal. Typically, a pair of headphones is coupled to the output of the receiver. ▶ Fig. 15.8 shows an example of a home IR system used often with televisions.

Advantages of Infrared Systems

The primary advantage of an IR system is that its transmission does not pass through walls and can be reflected off of lighter colored, flat surfaces. It can be used in the dark and is not interfered by radio or magnetic fields. In a building with multiple rooms, separate IR systems can be operated simultaneously without interference from another room. If all trans-

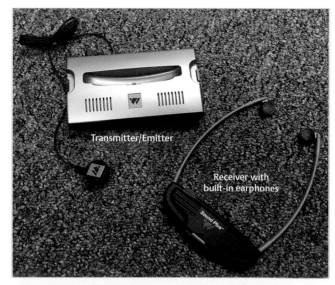

Transmitter/Emitter

Receiver with built-in earphones

Fig. 15.8 Infrared listening system with transmitter/emitter base and receiver with built-in earphones. The transmitter/emitter box can be connected to an audio system output, such as a television, for personal listening.

mitters/emitters and receivers are all the same (or on the same carrier frequency), one can use one receiver in multiple rooms.

Disadvantages of Infrared Systems

The two primary disadvantages of infrared systems are: (1) the requirement of direct line of sight between the emitter and receiver and (2) they are largely restricted to the indoors because of potential interference by visible light.

15.4.4 Other Wireless Assistive Listening Devices

Modern day hearing aids and implantable devices are taking advantage of some additional wireless technologies that do not strictly fall under, but sound similar to, the FM/DM description. For example, there has been a rise in connectivity between hearing aid and implantable devices with a variety of digital media devices and hearables. Examples include near-field magnetic induction (NFMI) and Bluetooth (a 2.4-GHz technology). For these types of connectivity options, interested readers are referred Galster.[10,11]

As mentioned earlier, sound field systems using loudspeakers are also available. In the classroom environment, they are known as *Classroom Audio Distribution Systems (CAD system or CADS)*. The basic components of a CAD system are a wearable or handheld microphone transmitter and one or more loudspeaker receiver room installations. The manner in which the microphone transmitter and loudspeakers communicate varies, but generally fall into the DM or IR categories. As indicated earlier, CADS is useful for amplifying signals for wide distribution throughout the room and virtually all individuals in the room can benefit from amplification.

15.5 Telecommunication Technology

Telecommunication is a universal term used to describe a wide range of information-transmitting technologies. In the case of HATs, there are a number of telecommunication devices and associated services that make it possible for individuals with hearing loss to use the telephone or technology that serves a similar purpose as the telephone.

15.5.1 Amplified Phones

Amplified phones work much like standard landline telephones, except they have one or more additional features that make them useful for many individuals with hearing loss. The most sought-after feature is the amplification (< 50 dB). Many also offer a tone control to shape the frequency response (e.g., adding a high-frequency boost to speech sounds). Other acoustic features that may be found on an amplified phone include a loud ringer (< 95 dB), a flashing light ring signaler, and speakerphone option. Many amplified phones have wide appeal that they are often made to have larger buttons and large visual displays for those with manual dexterity and vision issues as well. In some cases, a vibrating bed shaker unit can be connected to the phone as well. ▶ **Fig. 15.9** shows examples of corded and cordless amplified phones.

Pearl

Using a special adapter (VEC TRX-20 3.5-mm direct connect telephone record device) with a landline telephone and an induction loop amplifier, the telephone audio signal can be transmitted directly to the hearing aid or implant device telecoils in a hands-free manner. Secondly, if there is a telecoil on both ears, telephone use can be binaural!

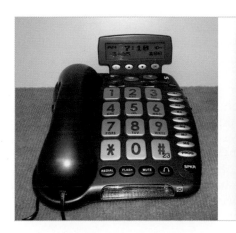
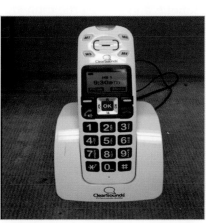

Fig. 15.9 Examples of corded (*left*) and cordless (*right*) amplified telephones.

15.5.2 Captioned Phones

As with amplified phones, captioned phones can offer many of the same features. However, captioned phones utilize a third-party communication service that translates speech into readable text. For example, when an individual with hearing loss places a call, everything that is said by the person being called is made accessible *via* readable text scrolling on a display screen. The individual with hearing loss can continue to listen through the handset, or may be able to add an induction neckloop or hands-free headset with microphone. Captioned phones have three basic requirements to work: (1) telephone service, (2) internet service, and (3) wall AC power jack. In addition, the captioned phone service will need to be registered In the United States, captioned phones are made available to qualifying individuals with hearing loss for a greatly reduced fee or possibly free, depending on the services or government programs available to the individual. Examples of certified captioned phone companies are *CapTel*, *CaptionCall*, and *ClearCaptions*. ▶ **Fig. 15.10** shows one example of a captioned phone.

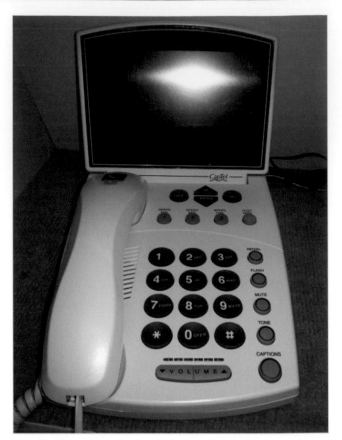

Fig. 15.10 Example of a captioned phone with large visual display for reading captions.

> ### Special Consideration
>
> To avoid misuse and abuse of the captioned telephone services by nonqualifying individuals, United States users are required to register (and activate) their captioned phones with the FCC. Although a pitfall, this offers a level of protection and increases accountability of third-party caption services.

15.5.3 Teletypewriter

The **teletypewriter (TTY)**, also known as a **telecommunication device for the deaf (TDD)**, is been around for a long time. However, except for a very small segment of the population, they are largely in disuse with the advent of another, more efficient telephone and electronic communication options. Nevertheless, the TTY continues to exist for use in some public areas and in service- and emergency-related agencies. A TTY is an electromechanical typewriter, or text telephone with keyboard. It receives and sends electrical signals over a phone line using acoustic coupler technology. The individual with hearing loss using a TTY will type messages using the keyboard and read receiving messages on the display, somewhat similar to an internet chat. The difference, however, is that TTY conversations require a particular etiquette. That is, only one person communicates at a time and must signal to the person on the other line that they are finished. For example, at the end of a message, the TTY user must type "GA" which stands for "Go Ahead." The person on the other line must do the same. As the conversation comes to an end, both users will type "SK" which stands for "Stop Keying." When the call is terminated, one or both parties will type "SKSK." A TTY can call a non-TTY user using the telecommunications relay service (TRS), which is a third-party communication service. The communications assistant will use a TTY and speak the message to the person on the other end of the line. Whatever that person says, the communications assistant will type into the TTY to be read by the individual with hearing loss. At the beginning of a relay call, the communications assistant provides brief instructions to the non-TTY user. The etiquette remains the same, requiring that only one person communicate at a time, and the non-TTY user must say "Go Ahead" to signal the end of their message. TTY conversations can be awkward and time consuming because interruptions are not permitted by either party. A technical variation of the TTY is the use of **voice carry over (VCO)**, which has been beneficial to individuals with hearing loss who have intelligible speech but still have difficulty understanding over the phone. In a VCO call, the individual with hearing loss will speak normally, and anything the person on the other end of the line says will be converted to text using similar TTY technology. An advantage the VCO over the TTY is a slightly more natural flow of conversation. As with TTY, there is decline in the use of VCO in favor of other communication options, particularly captioned phones and videophones (VPs).

Pearl ✔

Telecommunications relay services (TRS) permit persons with a hearing or speech disability to use the telephone system via a text telephone (TTY) or other device to call persons with or without such disabilities. To make using TRS as simple as possible, you can simply dial 711 to be automatically connected to a TRS operator. It is fast, functional, and free. Dialing 711, both voice and TRS users can initiate a call from any telephone, anywhere in the United States, without having to remember and dial a seven or 10-digit access number.

15.5.4 Videophones

VPs, as with the TTY and captioned phones, rely on a third-party communication service (i.e., video relay service [VRS]) when calling a non-videophone user. Or, they can be used to call another videophone user direct (similar to *Apple FaceTime* or *Skype*). As with captioned phones, users need to register. VPs have three basic requirements to work: (1) television set, (2) internet service, and (3) wall AC power jack. The videophone itself has a processing unit with a camera. There may be even options to use VRS technology on a desktop or smartphone device as well. VPs are primarily used by individuals with hearing loss who use sign language. Example VRS companies available include, *Sorenson VRS*, *Purple Communications*, and *ConvoRelay*.

15.5.5 Some Notes on Cellular Phones

Although not classified as an assistive technology *per se*, there are cellular phones on the market that are **hearing aid compatible (HAC)**. This means that these phones should be (1) relatively immune to radiofrequency interference and (2) offer inductive coupling to a telecoil. In the spite of the name, HAC phones should also permit use by those with implantable devices with built-in or add-on telecoils. Generally speaking, manufacturers of HAC phones will provide this information on the packaging, in the instruction manual, or in the specifications sheet. Users should look for HAC phones with a microphone (M) and telephone (T) mode minimum rating of 3 or a

maximum rating of 4 (e.g., M3/T4). In the M mode, the hearing instrument microphone is being used. In the T mode, the hearing instrument telecoil is being used. A good source for browsing and shopping for HAC phones ahead of purchase is www.phonescoop.com. Additionally, cellular customers are encouraged to "try before you buy."

Special Consideration

Cellular service providers may provide a text- and internet-only plan for those who will not be using the acoustic portion of the phone.

15.6 Speech-to-Text Technology

Transcription or translation technologies are ways in which spoken (or even signed) language is provided in the form of text. In today's world, we have become familiar with closed captioning on television and subtitles in digital media. However, there are many more speech-to-text technologies out there of benefit to individuals with hearing loss. Speech-to-text technologies can be broadly grouped into three areas: (1) real-time transcription, (2) off-line transcription, and (3) automatic speech recognition.

15.6.1 Real-Time Transcription

Real-time transcription is often found in court rooms where details of the deliberations are captured in "real time" and in print for documentation. Outside of the court room, real-time transcription is also found during live television programming and in large convention halls. During live television programming, for example, you can notice an occasional error made by the stenographer, which may or may not be corrected. Real-time transcription is made possible by trained stenographers or captioners who use specialized or traditional keyboards to transcribe speech into readable text. The term **captioning** may be more familiar to others than transcription. In the education and convention environment, stenographers/captioners can be found in the room, or be listening in remotely, and what they transcribe will be displayed on a laptop computer or mobile device. Example captioning services include *C-Print*, *Typewell*, and *CART* (Communication Access Real-time Transcription). Whereas CART is transcribed word-for-word (verbatim), C-Print and Typewell are transcribed meaning-for-meaning. There are some pros and cons to each. With CART, a copy of the transcript can be provided which leaves nothing out, and the transcript will be much longer in duration for later review. C-Print and Typewell, on the other hand, will have shorter transcripts, but every effort is made to preserve intent and meaning.

15.6.2 Off-line Transcription

Off-line transcription is similar to real-time transcription except that the transcription is being made after the event has already taken place. This is useful for historic media that predates transcription technology, or it can also be used today to caption digital media such as YouTube videos and instructional or promotional videos. This type of captioning is different from entertainment captioning (e.g., television shows and movies, *Netflix*, and DVD/Blue-ray discs) in which entire scripts are time-locked. With proper software, these scripts can be merged into digital media and turned on and off.

15.6.3 Automatic Speech Recognition

Automatic speech recognition (ASR) is a rapidly developing technology making it possible to convert speech directly to text using sophisticated speech detection and analysis algorithms. Many are familiar with smartphones having built-in ASR, such as "Siri" on Apple iPhone devices. ASR technology is becoming increasingly promising for communication purposes for individuals with hearing loss.

15.7 Alerting Technology

Each and every day, we rely on any number of alerts or signals, many of which are acoustic. For individuals with hearing loss, failure to hear mainstream alerts and signals may be a matter of the overall intensity or frequency, a matter of location and distance, or simply because hearing aids or implant devices are not worn 24-hours a day. For home and office use, there are a variety of small alerting technologies sensitive to sound (e.g., baby cry) and motion and is converted to a vibratory or flashing signal. There are alarm clocks (and watches) as well as home devices (e.g., doorbell, smoke, and carbon monoxide alarms) that when activated can be made louder and with a lower tone frequency, as well as converted into a vibratory or flashing signal. For emergency preparedness related to the weather, a National Weather Radio (NWR) system can be acquired. Using an adapter or accessory package, these systems can be assembled to provide audible, visual, or vibrotactile alerts, and readable display messages for weather-related warnings.

Special Consideration

Consumers looking to purchase emergency products should ensure that meet standards published by the National Fire Protection Association (NFPA). A great resource that the NFPA provides is a list of products that meet the performance and evaluation standards of Underwriters Laboratories standard[12] 1971, and will be appropriately marked on the product.

15.8 Devices for Health Professionals

15.8.1 Amplified and Visual Stethoscopes

A common issue for many health care professionals with hearing loss is auscultation. That is, using a stethoscope to listen to heart, lung, and other organs. Compared to conventional (nonelectronic) stethoscopes, there are commercially available stethoscopes that depend on additional (usually digital) technology to provide further amplification and/or convert auscultation sounds into readable and recordable waveforms. Based on anecdotal reports, there are three amplified stethoscopes in common use and manufacture today. They include (1) *Thinklabs One* (100× amplification), (2) *Cardionics E-Scope II* (two different models; 30× amplification), and (3) *3M Littmann 3100/3200 Electronic Stethoscope* (24× amplification). There are a few caveats when considering amplified stethoscopes:

- Unlike hearing aids, amplified stethoscopes' specifications do not currently have uniform measurement standards (e.g., American National Standards Institute). Thus, when statements are made that a product provides "(number) times amplification" or "(number) dB of amplification," it may not be clear relative to "what." A commonly used reference is the conventional (nonelectric) stethoscope, which may also have differences based on design. As a general point of reference, 24 times amplification is about 27 dB SPL, while 100 times amplification is about 40 dB SPL.

- Many amplified stethoscopes still have conventional ear tips, but that may not be useful for health professionals with severe hearing loss or for those who use hearing aids or other implantable devices. When an amplified stethoscope is coupled in some way to a hearing aid or implant device, the frequency-gain response of the auscultation sound will be further shaped, for better or for worse. For example, hearing aids and implant devices generally have a high-pass filter primarily for speech frequencies, which could diminish overall intensity of very-low-frequency heart and lung sounds. Oftentimes, a customized programs or map for auscultation can be made by the audiologist. One of the least effective coupling methods, however, is electromagnetic induction via telecoil because of the greater low-frequency attenuation by telecoil for sounds below about 1,000 Hz.

To date, there is only one stand-alone visual stethoscope on the market, *ViScope*. Not only does it have a handheld display of auscultation waves, but it also offers about 30× amplification.

> **Pitfall** ✕
>
> Hearing aids and implantable devices are primarily designed with speech frequencies in mind and may have a high-pass filter that can be problematic for low-frequency auscultation. Furthermore, telecoils have a characteristic low-frequency roll-off below 1,000 Hz. For this reason, the use of electromagnetic induction is not recommended for auscultation.

15.8.2 Face Masks

In many areas of health care, face masks are often used as a protective barrier against liquid and airborne particles. The most commonly used face masks are those loose-fitting, disposable devices that cover the nose and mouth, and may also have a shield for the eyes. For individuals with hearing loss who depend on visual speech cues, a low-tech transparent face mask could prove beneficial for communication access.[13,14] Two start-up companies working hard to try to mass produce these products that meet health and safety standards include *FaceView Mask* and *Safe'N'Clear*. Until these face masks become readily available, disposable transparent face shields (e.g., Guardall visors) and face shield systems (e.g., *Stryker T5 Personal Protection System*) are also available, each with both advantages and disadvantages.

15.9 Mobile Applications

The advent of smartphones and tablet devices have opened up some new and innovative assistive technology possibilities for individuals with hearing

loss. These are powerful mobile devices with both cellular and internet capabilities for a variety of applications (or, for short, **apps**). The best up-to-date source on apps for children and adults with hearing loss is a spreadsheet maintained by audiologist, Dr. Tina Childress: http://bit.ly/Apps4FL. Apps do come and go, and a particular app, by name, may not be available on all platforms (e.g., *Apple Store* vs. *Google Play*). If a particular app cannot be located, use keyword search to identify similar apps. Below are but a few examples in keeping with the types of technologies described earlier in this chapter.

15.9.1 Personal Amplifiers

By taking advantage of the built-in microphone and audio output jack, a smartphone and a pair of hard-wired or wireless headphones could be turned into a personal amplifier. More recently, we are beginning to see the emergence of **hearables**, of which smartphone-based amplifying apps are included.[15] A hearable is a hybrid of the terms *wearable* and *headphone* coined by Apple in 2014. While there are many personal amplifier apps available, they are not all created equally, many with poor sound quality and acoustic delays. Three to check out are *EarMachine*, *SoundAMP*, and *Hearing Aid with Replay*. As one audiologist cautions, these apps are not meant to replace professional services, rather may help some listeners as a starter or stopgap amplification.[16]

15.9.2 Telecommunication

One of the most exciting telecommunications innovations is having captioned telephone calls on a smartphone or tablet device. The individual with hearing loss can place a call to virtually anyone using a mobile device and a professional stenographer will transcribe what is said. As with captioned phones, these services require registration with the FCC. *InnoCaptions*, *WebCapTel*, and *ClearCaptions* are a few examples of companies offering this service, which have made it possible for individuals with hearing loss to carry on nearly seamless conversations over a smartphone. *CaptionCall* has an app that can be used with an Apple iPad 2 or higher.

15.9.3 Alerting

A smartphone device can double as a signaler for environmental sounds with an app that takes advantage of the built-in microphone. Depending on the app, it may be able to learn (preprogramed) specific sounds in one's environment through sound recognition (e.g., doorbell, oven timer, smoke alarm, etc.) and provide flash, vibration, and third-party notification (e.g., SMS text). One example of this type of app is *Otosense*. Simpler apps, like *FlashAlert2* and *AppForTheDeaf*, serve to alert the user of any environmental sound using a sensitivity-based toggle and can provide flash and vibration alerts.

Though not an actual app, there is a wonderful service available when 9-1-1 is dialed from a mobile phone in case of emergency. This is a service whereby the caller is registered with www.smart911.com and anytime 9-1-1 is called from that mobile number; the operator will have access to any information provided including communication alternatives (e.g., SMS text messaging).

15.9.4 Song Recognition

Learning new songs can be a challenge for some individuals with hearing loss. Music recognition apps are available that link to lyric libraries for a more sing-a-long experience. Once a song is recognized by the app, the lyrics are displayed on the display and may even be synchronized in time like a karaoke machine. Examples of these apps include *SoundHound*, *Shazam*, and *Musixmatch*.

15.9.5 Television or Movie Captions

Television and movies have scripts that are often publicly available and easy to access online. Several apps have been developed that take advantage of these scripts so that they can be activated while watching a prerecorded television show or movie at home or at the theater. Examples include *Captionfish* and *Subtitle Viewer*. Alternatively, one can subscribe to a streaming service such as *Netflix*, *ABC*, or even *The Disney Channel* and activate the subtitles or closed caption ("CC").

15.9.6 Automatic Speech Recognition

In place of typing or writing, there are apps that utilize automatic speech recognition (ASR) technology. The most popular (and reliable) app on the market appears to be *Dragon Dictation*. This app may be a better alternative to writing notes.

15.10 Incorporating Hearing Assistive and Related Technology into Clinical Practice

There is no one-size-fits-all approach for incorporating hearing assistive and related technology into clinical practice. At the outset, audiologists are in a unique position, not only to treat hearing loss, but they also bear the responsibility of being health care providers who view individuals with hearing loss more broadly and holistically with respect to their overall quality of life. As seen in this chapter, technologies are available for almost every aspect of daily life. The problem, however, is the vastness and variety of technologies, the manner in which they work, and the technical requirements.

A useful clinical tool to help individuals with hearing loss select hearing assistive and related technologies is the TELEGRAM questionnaire developed and proposed by Thibodeau.[2] The acronym stands for (T)elephone, (E)mployment, (L)egislation, (E)ntertainment, (G)roups, (R)ecreation, (A)larms, and (M)embers of the House. Although these categories appear limited, they are tied to specific life scenarios such as cell phone (telephone), job (employment), meetings (groups), and television (entertainment) to name a few. The TELEGRAM is one-page assessment tool that helps the audiologist and individual with hearing loss begin a conversation about the level of perceived difficulty (Likert scale 1–5) with and without hearing aids or implantable devices, and the members of the household with whom they live (e.g., normal hearing adult, teenagers, live alone, etc.). The results are plotted on the grid of the TELEGRAM and from there potential solutions can be made for each scenario in which there is perceived difficulty. It can also be used as a prefit and postfit assessment tool to examine outcomes. The TELEGRAM questionnaire is and rating scale key are shown in ▶ Fig. 15.11 and ▶ Fig. 15.12. A pediatric version of the TELEGRAM is available from Dr. Thibodeau's website: http://www.utdallas.edu/~thib/.

Audiologists should consider methods that increase awareness of hearing assistive and related technologies among their patients. One way to achieve this is to have a small-scale area of a few hearing assistive and related technologies in the office and resource materials for how to locate, acquire, and/or purchase these technologies. The TELEGRAM questionnaire can help with anticipation, but demonstration and experience are activities that can take place within or outside the

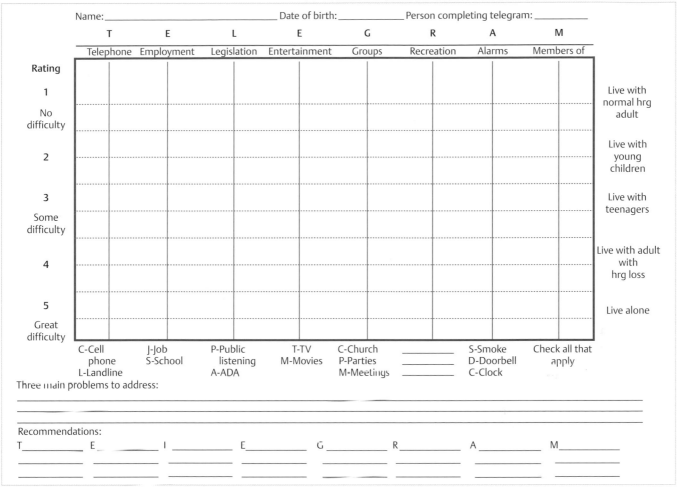

Fig. 15.11   The TELEGRAM questionnaire created by Linda Thibodeau. (Reprinted with permission.) See ▶Fig. 15.12 for key questions.

office before, during, or after hearing instrument fitting. Purchase and install a few technologies for the office (e.g., active induction loop for the clinic lobby and a few alerting devices), communicate with government-sponsored programs or third-party services about available technologies specific to individuals with hearing loss (e.g., amplified and captioned telephones), and ask vendors or manufacturers about demonstration units (e.g., FM/DM systems). Be prepared to demonstrate and have patients experience how these various technologies work. Instead of just asking patients about their needs, find out from experienced users what technologies they have come across and find benefit to them. Over time, the culture of one's practice and patient population may become savvier with respect to assistive technologies beyond hearing aid and implantable devices.

15.11 Summary

The array of hearing assistive and related technology options is both exciting and intimidating. If that is the case for the audiologist, it most surely will be the case for individuals with hearing loss. Audiologists are uniquely positioned (and trained) to help individuals with hearing loss with a variety of communication and daily living needs. In this chapter, we covered three broad categories of assistive listening devices: FM and DM systems, induction systems, and infrared systems, intended to augment hearing. We also covered a wide variety of technologies with respect to telecommunication, speech-to-text technologies, and alerting needs. Special attention was drawn to health professionals with hearing loss who may benefit from amplified or visual stethoscopes, and transparent

	Telegram rating scale key	
Topic	Question	Rating
T	Are you having difficulty with communication over the **telephone**?	Difficulty 1 = None, 2 = Occasional, 3 = Often, 4 = Always, 5 = Can't use the phone *Use "L" to designate landline and "C" to designate cellphone*
E	Are you having any difficulty with communication in your **employment** or **educational** environment?	Difficulty 1 = None, 2 = Occasional, 3 = Often, 4 = Always, 5 = Stopped working
L	Do you know about **legislation** that provides assistance for you to hear in public places or in hotels when you travel?	Knowledge 1 = Vast, 2 = Considerable, 3 = Some, 4 = Limited, 5 = None
E	Are you having difficulty with hearing during **entertainment** activities that you enjoy such as television, movies, or concerts?	Difficulty 1 = None, 2 = Occasional, 3 = Often, 4 = Always, 5 = Stopped going
G	Are you having difficulty with communication in **group** settings?	Difficulty 1 = None, 2 = Occasional, 3 = Often, 4 = Always, 5 = Can't hear at all in groups
R	Are you having difficulty with hearing during **recreational** activities such as sports, hunting, or sailing?	Difficulty 1 = None, 2 = Occasional, 3 = Often, 4 = Always, 5 = Stopped the activity
A	Are you having difficulty hearing **alarms** or **alerting** signals such as the smoke alarm, alarm clock, or the doorbell?	Difficulty 1 = None, 2 = Occasional, 3 = Often, 4 = Always, 5 = Can't hear alarm *Use "S" for smoke alarm, "D" for doorbell, and "A" for alarm clock*
M	Are you communicating with **members** of your family?	1 = Live with normal hrg adult, 2 = Live with young children, 3 = Live with teenagers, 4 = Live with adult with hrg loss, 5 = Live alone *Check all that apply*

Fig. 15.12 Key questions to ask patients when completing the TELEGRAM are listed in the left column. The 1 to 5 rating scale is listed in the right column.

face mask options. Finally, the advent of smartphones and tablets has led to a variety of mobile applications as well. It is hopeful that the information in this chapter helps to break down barriers to knowledge and accessibility with respect to hearing assistive and related technology and to encourage a brighter future with prospects for a high quality of life and independence for individuals with hearing loss.

References

[1] Assistive Technology Industry Association. What is AT? n.d.; Available from: https://www.atia.org/at-resources/what-is-at/#what-is-assistive-technology. Accessed March 21, 2018

[2] Thibodeau LM. Hearing assistance technology (HAT) can optimize communication. Hear J. 2004; 57(11):11

[3] Atcherson SR, Franklin CA, Smith-Olinde L. Hearing Assistive and Access Technology. San Diego, CA: Plural Publishing, Inc; 2015

[4] Bankaitis AU. Hearing assistance technology (HAT). In: Valente M, Hosford-Dunn H, Roeser RJ eds. Audiology: Treatment. 2nd ed. New York, NY: Thieme Medical Publishers; 2007:400–417

[5] World Health Organization. Prevention of blindness and deafness. Estimates. 2012. http://www.who.int/pbd/deafness/estimates/en/. Accessed June 27, 2016

[6] Lin FR, Niparko JK, Ferrucci L. Hearing loss prevalence in the United States. Arch Intern Med. 2011; 171(20):1851–1852

[7] Bachmann KR, Arvedson JC. Early identification and intervention for children who are hearing impaired. Pediatr Rev. 1998; 19(5):155–165

[8] Mehra S, Eavey RD, Keamy DG, Jr. The epidemiology of hearing impairment in the United States: newborns, children, and adolescents. Otolaryngol Head Neck Surg. 2009; 140(4):461–472

[9] Wolfe J, Lewis D, Eiten LR. Remote microphone systems and communication access for children. In Tharpe AM, Seewald R, eds. Comprehensive Handbook of Pediatric Audiology. 2nd ed. San Diego, CA: Plural Publishing, Inc.; 2016:677–711

[10] Galster JA. A new method for wireless connectivity in hearing aids. Hear J. 2010; 63(10):36–39

[11] Galster JA. Awash in a stream of wirelesss solutions. Audiology Practices. 2011; 3(2):26–29

[12] Underwriters Laboratory (UL 1971). Standard for Signaling Devices for the Hearing Impaired. 2013. Available from: https://standardscatalog.ul.com/standards/en/standard_1971_3. Accessed March 21, 2018

[13] Atcherson SR, Mendel LL, Baltimore WJ, et al. The effect of conventional and transparent surgical masks on speech understanding in individuals with and without hearing loss. J Am Acad Audiol. 2017; 28(1):58–67

[14] Mendel LL, Gardino JA, Atcherson SR. Speech understanding using surgical masks: a problem in health care? J Am Acad Audiol. 2008; 19(9):686–695

[15] Taylor B. Hearables: the morphing of hearing aids consumer electronic devices. Audiol Today. 2015; 27(6):22–30

[16] Amlani AM. Apps for the ears. ASHA Leader. 2014; 19:34–35

Suggested Readings

American Academy of Audiology. Clinical Practice Guidelines. Remote Microphone Hearing Assistance Technologies for Children and Youth from Birth to 21 Years. (Includes Supplement A). 2011. https://audiology-web.s3.amazonaws.com/migrated/HAT_Guidelines_Supplement_A.pdf_53996ef7758497.54419000.pdf. Accessed June 21, 2016

American Academy of Audiology. Clinical Practice Guidelines. Remote Microphone Hearing Assistance Technologies for Children and Youth from Birth to 21 Years. Supplement B: Classroom Audio Distribution Systems—Selection and Verification. 2011. https://audiology-web.s3.amazonaws.com/migrated/HAT_Guidelines_Supplement_A.pdf_53996ef7758497.54419000.pdf. Accessed June 21, 2016

American Speech-Language-Hearing Association. Guidelines for Fitting and Monitoring FM Systems [Guidelines]. 2002. https://www.asha.org/policy. Accessed 2nd February, 2018

Atcherson SR, Franklin CA, Smith-Olinde L. Hearing Assistive and Access Technology. San Diego, CA: Plural Publishing, Inc.; 2015

Morris R. On the Job with Hearing Loss: Hidden Challenges. Successful Solutions. Garden City, NY: Morgan James Publishing; 2007

Smaldino J, Flexer C. Handbook of Acoustic Accessibility. New York, NY: Thieme Medical Publishers; 2012

16 Hearing Protection Devices

Brian J. Fligor

16.1 Introduction

Where the physician prescribes medications (chemicals) to treat a disease, the audiologist prescribes sound in a similar fashion. Like the medications that are dosed according to an amount necessary to be therapeutic, but not so high as to cause chemical toxicity, so too can sound be therapeutic at a certain dose, and toxic if overdosed. In an individual requiring amplification to mitigate the negative effects of sensorineural hearing loss, hearing aids must have adequate gain to provide a therapeutic effect, without overamplifying and causing a cochlear toxicity (noise-induced hearing loss [NIHL]). Underdosing with medication is also deleterious, as the disease continues unabated. Hearing aids that underamplify relative to the degree of hearing loss fail to provide adequate benefit, and the deleterious effects of untreated hearing loss continue. The analogy drawn between the use of chemicals to treat disease and the use of sound to treat hearing loss extends to the use of hearing protection devices (HPDs) to mitigate the dose of noise that would cause NIHL. HPDs are a last line of defense to protect an individual's cochleas from an environmental toxin, with the intent to decrease the noise dose to below the toxic threshold.

In the hierarchy of occupational health exposure controls (▶Table 16.1), the most desired approach to controlling hazardous exposures (to chemicals, noise, radiation, etc.) is to eliminate the hazard altogether (as this is the most reliable way to protect the individual). Failing to eliminate the hazard, the next most reliable and desirable control is to substitute a less hazardous source; for instance, a piece of equipment that emits a hazardous level of noise could be replaced with a quieter piece of equipment. If the hazardous source cannot be substituted, perhaps engineering controls (such as a muffler or sound enclosure) can mitigate the level of noise reaching the individual. If engineering controls have been exhausted, administrative controls

can reduce the overall noise dose (i.e., the level integrated over time) by job sharing/rotating workers between noisier and quieter activities. Finally, personal protective equipment (PPE), is the last line of defense against a hazardous exposure; this puts the individual at greatest risk, as the responsibility for correct use of the PPE falls to the individual. In the case of HPDs, the noise-exposed individual must know how to use the devices correctly (to achieve the prescribed amount of noise attenuation) and consistently; even small amounts of time in which an individual chooses to not use HPDs, resulting in exposure at unprotected levels, can negate the protection of the HPD altogether. Additionally, too much attenuation ("overprotection") is potentially dangerous, as the sense of hearing is one of our most important senses for survival. HPDs that provide too much sound attenuation interfere with situational awareness (detection of warning signals, localization of important auditory cues) and speech intelligibility. More attenuation is *not* better. The right HPD is the one that (1) is comfortable enough to wear for the intended duration; and (2) consistently reduces the sound level under the hearing protector to 70 to 75 dBA.

Pearl ✔

The right HPD is the one that is comfortable enough to wear for the intended duration, and consistently reduces the sound level under the hearing protector to 70 to 75 dBA. More is *not* better.

The concept "more attenuation is not always better" may seem antithetical to the concept of safety. However, it is vital for the audiologist to base HPD recommendations on the available noise exposure data, rather than find the hearing protector that provides the most attenuation. Typical sound exposures across all industries are less than 95 dBA for an 8-hour time-weighted average (TWA): that is,

Table 16.1 Hierarchy of occupational health exposure controls

Elimination	Most reliable and desirable
Substitution	
Engineering controls	
Administrative controls	
Personal protective equipment (PPE)	Least reliable and desirable

Table 16.2 Elements of a hearing conservation program

Noise survey
Engineering controls
Audiometric monitoring
Education and motivation
Hearing protection devices (HPDs)

roughly 95% of all workplace noise exposures are less than or equal to 95 dBA (for a daily equivalent continuous level of exposure).[1] Sound levels of 75 dBA (for an 8-hour TWA) are known to not contribute to noise-induced permanent threshold shift, even in highly susceptible individuals.[2] Thus, HPDs that provide 20 dB attenuation are adequate for the vast majority of workplace noise exposures. However, there are some noise exposures that require more attenuation than can be achieved with conventional, passive HPDs; for instance, naval personnel who work on the flight deck of an aircraft carrier are typically exposed to levels of 150 dBA.[3] A combination of active noise cancelation, deeply fitting custom hearing protection, and custom-fitted helmet (to attenuate the level of the noise reaching the cochlea through bone conduction) are necessary to protect the hearing of the flight deck crew. Other extremely noisy jobs reflecting the 5% with exposures greater than 95 dBA, 8-hour TWA include mining, metalworking, and pit crew worker in motorized sports.[4]

There are a variety of occupational noise exposure limits enacted around the world. The majority of industrialized countries (with the notable exception of the United States and China) have adopted an 85 dBA 8-hr TWA as the maximum permissible exposure limit (PEL), with a 3 dB time-intensity trading ratio (85 dBA for 8 hours; 88 dBA for 4 hours; 91 dBA for 2 hours; etc.). According to Prince, et al,[5] 8% of workers exposed to this PEL will sustain a material hearing impairment after a 40-year working lifetime (with 92% protected from this degree of NIHL). The Occupational Safety and Health Administration (OSHA) enforces the regulations promulgated by the Hearing Conservation Act[6] and Hearing Conservation Amendment[7], which indicate a maximum PEL of 90 dBA 8-hr TWA with a 5 dB time-intensity trading ratio (90 dBA for 8 hours; 95 dBA for 4 hours; 100 dBA for 2 hours; etc.). Prince, et al,[5] predicted 25% of workers exposed to this more relaxed 90 dBA 8-hr TWA PEL would sustain a material hearing impairment after a 40-year working lifetime. However, regulations in the United States indicate an "action level" where workers exposed to 85 dBA (i.e., 85–89.9 dBA) must be enrolled in

a hearing conservation program, which includes provision of HPDs.

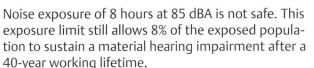

Pearl ✔

Noise exposure of 8 hours at 85 dBA is not safe. This exposure limit still allows 8% of the exposed population to sustain a material hearing impairment after a 40-year working lifetime.

Workers exposed to potentially hazardous levels of noise must be enrolled in a hearing conservation program (▶**Table 16.2**) that is akin to the hierarchy of occupational health exposure controls.[6] The noise survey determines if worker exposure exceeds the Action Level, or PEL. Engineering controls are investigated to determine if the noise can be mitigated at the source. If engineering controls cannot reduce the noise to less than the Action Level (85 dBA 8-hour TWA in the United States), then workers in the Hearing Conservation Program must undergo baseline and annual audiometric testing. Workers must receive workplace safety training that includes education regarding the risks of noise and deleterious effects of noise on hearing and quality of life, and motivation to take personal responsibility to lessen noise exposures (on and off the job). Finally, workers must be provided with a variety of HPDs; that is, employers cannot provide workers with a single type of HPD, since no hearing protector is appropriate for all individuals.

16.2 Types of Hearing Protection Devices, Attenuation Characteristics

HPDs are available in a variety of shapes, sizes, and models with different attenuation characteristics and purposes; the National Institute for Occupational Safety and Health (NIOSH) maintains a compendium of hundreds of commercially available HPDs.[8] There are essentially two major types of HPDs: earplugs and earmuffs. Earplugs are usually one-size-fits-most and can be made of closed-cell foam or premolded silicone or thermoplastic elastomer.

Table 16.3 Noise reduction ratings of four HPDs along with their octave-band attenuations and associated standard deviations

	NRR (dB)	Frequency (Hz)	125	250	500	1,000	2,000	3,150	4,000	6,300	8,000
3M E-A-R Classic Soft earplug	31	Mean attenuation	35.7	41.5	46.2	42.4	37.7	42.5	44.7	47.2	46.4
		SD	7.4	8.5	6.2	5.3	2.4	2.8	3.5	5.4	4.5
Model 3000 earmuff (overhead position)	25	Mean attenuation	16.5	21.8	33.8	40.4	35.1	36.2	38.4	38.3	39.7
		SD	2.5	2.7	3.0	3.9	3.4	3.4	3.2	2.2	2.8
"Combat Arms" earplug (open position)	7	Mean attenuation	4.1	4.5	11.0	18.7	24.9	29.8	25.8	18.7	22.2
		SD	2.7	2.8	3.9	3.2	3.3	2.7	3.3	3.6	4.7
Etymotic Research Musicians Earplug (15 dB filter)	9	Mean attenuation	15.8	14.9	16.7	17.1	16.6	16.9	17.9	19.1	22.8
		SD	3.6	4.4	4.3	2.8	3.5	3.9	4.3	3.8	4.5

Abbreviations: HPD, hearing protection device; NRR, noise reduction rating; SD, standard deviation.
Source: Data courtesy of Lantos Technologies, Inc. (Wakefield, MA).
Note: The E-A-R Classic Soft earplug (3M Corp., St. Paul, Minnesota) is a typical industrial foam earplug HPD. The Model 3000 earmuff (3M Corp., St. Paul, Minnesota) is commonly used in industry. The "Combat Arms" earplug (3M Corp., St. Paul, Minnesota) is a premolded HPD for military use that has an "open" and "closed" position of a rocker switch which provides hearing protection to high-level sound while allowing users to hear many environmental noises. Source: Data courtesy of 3M Corp (St. Paul, MN) http://multimedia.3m.com/mws/media/1087607O/attenuation-data-for-3m-hearing-protection.pdf. Accessed February 15, 2017.).
Etymotic Research Musicians Earplug is a custom-fitted "flat" frequency attenuating earplug with a filter that can be interchangeable between 9-, 15-, and 25 dB.

Closed-cell foam earplugs are intended to be rolled up, inserted into the ear canal and held in place, and allowed to expand once inserted in the user's ear. Depending on how deeply these earplugs are seated in the ear canal, varying degrees of attenuation (and occlusion effect) will be observed. Premolded plugs can be seated deeply or in a more shallow position in the ear canal; this relates more to the size of the ear canal than to insertion depth per se. For these reasons, earplug HPDs tend to have more variability in attenuation than earmuffs. In contrast, earmuff HPDs are circumaural and are connected either to a spring-loaded headband or to a safety helmet. Because insertion depth and individual variability in ear canal size are not factors with earmuffs, the attenuation variability is not as great as that with earplug HPDs (►Table 16.3).

16.3 Attenuation Characteristics

Considerable research has been focused on refining the attenuation properties of HPDs.[9,10,11] The degree to which HPDs attenuate environmental sound energy across frequencies can be affected by many factors. Such factors pertain not only to the thickness and density of the material used in hearing protectors but also to the level of bone-conducted sound transmission.

Typical (passive-attenuating) HPDs reduce high-frequency sounds more effectively than low-frequency sounds. Illustrated in ►Table 16.3 are the frequency-dependent characteristics of a typical industrial foam plug inserted deeply into the ear canal. As frequency increases, attenuation increases and is essentially asymptotic above 2,000 Hz. Without deep insertion, low-frequency attenuation (up to 750 Hz) would be compromised relative to the numbers reported in ►Table 16.3. This is because low-frequency sound energy would more freely enter a slit-leak/gap between the ear canal wall and the earplug. This would be expected to be less of an issue with circumaural earmuff HPDs. ►Fig. 16.1a shows the attenuation that can be achieved by an ideal-fit, widely available foam earplug, shown in ►Fig. 16.1b.

Berger et al,[9] ascertained the upper limits of passive sound isolation that can be provided by HPDs. They noted that the bone-conduction limit for hearing protection was the lowest at 2,000 Hz (40 dB). At this input level, sound is conducted through the temporal bone directly to the cochlea, bypassing the air-conduction route. Shown in ►Fig. 16.2 are the bone-conduction limits across frequency for passive hearing protector attenuation.

The performance of HPDs (i.e., the attenuation expected to be achieved) is typically reported by a

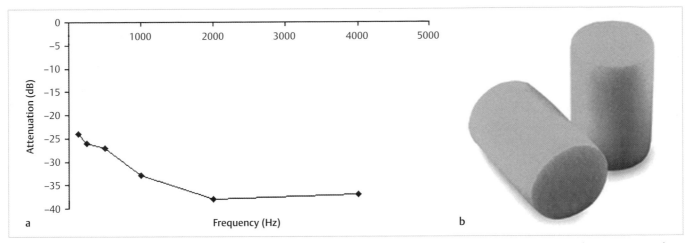

Fig. 16.1 (a) Attenuation of a deeply inserted 3M Classic Soft foam earplug. Note that the attenuation is the greatest in the higher-frequency region. (b) Photograph of 3M Classic Soft foam earplug. Courtesy of Elliott Berger.

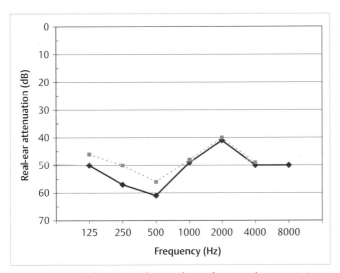

Fig. 16.2 The bone-conduction limits for sound transmission for hearing protection devices indicating that the maximum attenuation is 40 dB at 2,000 Hz. The dotted line represents previous data. Adapted from Berger EH, Kieper RW, Gauger D. Hearing protection: surpassing the limits to attenuation imposed by the bone-conduction pathways. J Acoust Soc Am 2003;114(4 part 1):1955–1967, with permission.

single number rating system. In the United States, all HPDs are required by law to be labeled with a noise reduction rating (NRR), which is a single-number rating (in dB) of the amount of attenuation a trained user can expect while wearing a specific HPD. The NRR was established by the U.S. Environmental Protection Agency (EPA)[12] in 1979 through a rule titled "Noise Labeling Standards for Hearing Protection Devices." (http://www.gpo.gov/fdsys/pkg/FR-2009-08-05/pdf/E9-18003.pdf, accessed 12/24/16), adopting ANSI Standard S3.19.[13] Prior to this regulation, there had been no requirement for standardized testing procedures and labeling approaches for HPDs, and adoption of the rule created a powerful new tool by which users could compare attenuation across different HPDs. However, users commonly misinterpret a larger NRR value as indicating the HPD is "better." Such is not the case, as there are safety risks for too much attenuation that may exceed the benefits of lessening risk for NIHL.

The NRR is a simplified interpretation of the expected attenuation of a given HPD across nine different frequency bands between 125 and 8,000 Hz when the HPD is fitted on a trained subject by an experimenter under laboratory test conditions. The experimental technique used to determine the attenuation as a function of frequency is real-ear attenuation at threshold (REAT). A sound field audiogram is performed with the subject's ears unoccluded, and again with the HPD placed by an expert fitter (the experimenter). The NRR is computed from test data taken across ten test subjects, and then subtracts twice the standard deviation from the mean attenuation at each frequency to account for individual user variability. This subtraction exercise is intended to result in a predicted attenuation that can be achieved by 98% of users of the HPD. Mathematically, the NRR is calculated by:

NRR = N (C-weighted) – N (A-weighted) + attenuation (A-weighted) – 3 dB – 2 SDs
(where N = noise level)

As can be seen in this equation, if the true noise spectrum has no low-frequency energy, then the first two terms are identical (A-weighted and C-weighted noise levels would be the same), and the NRR is the attenuation determined by REAT, subtracting two standard deviations and an additional safety factor of 3 dB. For a musician's ER-15 "flat" (uniform attenuator) earplug, the octave-band attenuation is approximately 15 dB (125–8,000 Hz), with the calculated NRR being only 9 dB (▶**Table 16.3**). Johnson and Nixon[14] noted that the NRR tends to be artificially high if there is minimal low-frequency attenuation and artificially low if there was a flat attenuation characteristic.

Four examples of the attenuation characteristics and consequent NRRs of four different HPDs are shown in ▶Table 16.3.

While the NRR labeling requirement provides some level of guidance for the user, the NRR itself has been heavily criticized. A large body of research on attenuation achieved by actual users in the field, as opposed to trained test subjects in a laboratory setting, is substantially lower than the NRR suggests.[15] The poorer observed performance stems from a variety of causes, most notably poor hearing protector fit among users in field studies. Generally, the discrepancy between NRR and field measurements of attenuation are larger for earplugs than for earmuffs, as earmuffs are generally much easier to fit correctly. The U.S. EPA has acknowledged the limitations with the current approach to measuring and labeling NRRs, and has for some years been considering an update to the NRR regulation. Other standards for providing HPD performance labeling have been proposed,[16] but none have yet replaced the NRR.

While the actual attenuation of a given HPD is known to vary widely across individuals, use of the NRR to estimate the attenuated (i.e., the level underneath the HPD) noise exposure for workers is nevertheless common. The nominal approach for computing attenuated noise exposures for workers, whose A-weighted, 8-hour TWA noise levels is known, is shown in the equation:

Nominal attenuated exposure (dBA) = TWA (dBA) − (NRR − 7)

The subtraction of 7 dB in the equation is a spectral correction factor required to account for differences in the way noise is measured during the NRR test (using C-weighted decibels [dBC]) versus measurements made in the workplace (using dBA). However, the equation above does not take into account variability in achieved attenuation, rather assumes that all users of a hearing protector will achieve the labeled NRR. As described above, this is an unrealistic expectation. There are two approaches for accounting for expected differences between labeled and achieved attenuation. The first is recommended by OSHA, and involves derating the labeled NRR of an HPD by 50%:

OSHA attenuated exposure (dBA) = TWA (dBA) − ([NRR − 7] × 50%)

The second approach is recommended by the NIOSH, given by:

NIOSH attenuated exposure (dBA) = TWA (dBA) − (NRR$_d$ 7)

Where NRR$_d$ is the *derated* NRR for the type of earplug being considered. NIOSH's recommended derating (penalty) of a HPD is to subtract 25% of the NRR for earmuffs, 50% for foam earplugs, and 70% from all other earplugs (such as preformed earplugs). So, as an example, if a worker uses a foam earplug with an NRR of 30 dB, the NIOSH NRR$_d$ would be 30 − (30 × 70%) = 9 dB. It should be noted that OSHA attenuated exposure and NIOSH attenuated exposure equations do not consider the lack of discrepancy between laboratory tested NRR and field-measured attenuation in custom-fit HPDs. If one were to use such derating schemes with custom HPD, users of the custom devices would be inappropriately labeled underprotected, when, in fact, they might be overprotected.[17]

Workers with very high exposures (> 100 or 105-dBA TWA) should be fit with dual protection—that is, a pair of earmuffs over earplugs. The general rule of thumb for estimating attenuation for dual protection is to add 5 dB to the attenuation of the HPD with the higher NRR.[4]

While the NRR is the required standard for testing and labeling HPDs in the United States, there are other standards in use around the world. Common testing and labeling schemes include the single number rating (SNR, used in the European Union [EU]) and the sound level conversion (SLC$_{80}$) used in Australia and New Zealand. There are several differences between the NRR, SNR, and SLC$_{80}$, including the fact that the NRR calculation subtracts 2 SD to account for user variability, whereas the other two schemes subtract only 1 SD, and that the test frequencies are somewhat different. The SNR rates protectors for specific types of noise environments, with different ratings for high-frequency (H), mid-frequency (M), and low-frequency (L) spectra. The SLC$_{80}$ value is used to assign a classification to the tested HPD; for example, "Class 1" is valid for use up to 90 dBA, "Class 2" to 95 dBA, and so on.[18]

16.4 Limitations of Standard HPDs

As previously suggested, the right HPD is the one that the individual will use; that is, an earplug that provides a remarkable amount of attenuation, but is uncomfortable and interferes with ability to hear the backup alarm of a forklift and coworkers' speech is unlikely to be consistently used. When workers opt to remove HPDs in violation of workplace safety rules, the employer is economically liable for the hearing loss sustained on the job. If an OSHA inspector observes noncompliance with mandatory HPD use, the company may be issued a warning, or monetary fine. While the worker's compensation payments and the OSHA fine typically are not burdensome to the employer, such penalties do raise workplace insurance annual premiums, which can become high enough to influence a culture of safety. Thus, it is in everyone's best interest to identify and mitigate the limitations of HPDs.

These limitations include, but are not limited to, comfort (over the duration of the work-shift where HPD is required), interference with situational awareness, occlusion effect, and interference with speech communication. Each of these potential limitations will be taken in turn.

Pearl ✔

Challenges associated with using HPDs include comfort, interference with situational awareness, occlusion effect, and interference with speech communication.

The ear is an exquisitely sensitive area of the body, being innervated by the facial nerve (CNVII) and the vagus nerve (CNX). The outer ear has a generous blood supply, and each external ear is as different as a fingerprint. Additionally, the front wall of the outer one-third of the ear canal is in direct communication with the condyle of the mandible. In roughly 50% of ear canals, the opening of the jaw results in a shape change in the area between the first and second bends of the ear canal (an area understood to be important for achieving adequate acoustic seal for a HPD).[19] This shape change might result in a compression of the canal (in roughly 10% of ears) potentially resulting in the ear feeling a rub or a pinch if a HPD is in place. The shape change is more likely to be an expansion of the ear canal (roughly 45% of ears) potentially resulting in a loss of acoustic seal of a HPD. It would be reasonable to assume that not using a HPD is more comfortable than using *any* HPD. Thus, the question of comfort is "what HPD is the *least uncomfortable*?"

Park and Casali[20] developed, and validated, a standardized survey entitled the Comfort Index (CI), which is a list of 14 questions with respondents answering the question "How does the hearing protector feel now?" on a seven-point Likert scale between two extremes. Davis et al,[21] updated the CI, using the same 14 questions, but reduced the response scale to a five-point Likert scale. Exemplar responses to the question "How does the hearing protector feel now?" are "painful to painless" (with five-point scale between extremes) and "smooth to rough" (with same five-point scale between extremes). The respondent's report for each question is assigned a value (1 = most comfortable; 5 = least comfortable), and a total "CI" score is reported. The smaller the CI, the more comfortable is the feeling. With the Davis et al,[21] five-point Likert scale modification, responses will range from a CI score of 14 (extremely comfortable) to 70 (extremely uncomfortable). The CI was validated across both earplugs and earmuffs, but only for passive devices.

Workers have been killed as a result of not hearing important audible safety alerts, such as the backup alarm of a forklift or other motor vehicle, due to being overprotected by the HPD.[22] Workers will report lack of compliance with using HPD due to fears of losing situational awareness. This is a rampant challenge in the military during active combat, where the soldier's survivability and lethality depend on excellent situational awareness.[23] Unfortunately, the report of a single shot from an assault rifle could result in immediate, permanent sensorineural hearing loss and tinnitus in an unprotected ear. To assist with the challenge associated with overprotection, some earplugs have been manufactured to attenuate high frequencies, but let low frequencies pass through relatively unattenuated. Other earplugs (for instance, the Combat Arms Earplug, ▶ **Table 16.3**) have been acoustically tuned to create a turbulence in the constricted sound channel, such that very high sound pressures will be attenuated, while lower-level sound waves are not restricted. In addition to passive (nonelectronic) devices, many different technologies have been developed and commercialized to mitigate interference with situational awareness (e.g., active/electronic HPDs, active noise reduction [ANR], low sound-level amplification devices, etc.).

One challenge with any device placed in the ear (hearing protection, consumer audio headphone, or hearing aid earmold) is the relative amplification of the fundamental frequency of one's voice when the ear canal is closed on both ends. This is known as the *occlusion effect*. With no device placed in the ear canal, low frequencies emanate from the open aperture of the ear canal. When the ear canal is closed (such as by placing one's fingers in the aperture, or by placing a device in the ear canal), the low-frequency energy is trapped in a confined space, and is therefore amplified. Two approaches to mitigating the occlusion effect are: (1) vent the earpiece so that low-frequency sound can escape, and (2) place the device as deeply in the canal as possible, such that the wall of the ear canal through which sound from the vocal tract is traveling is in contact with a device into the bony region (at or past the second bend). The combination of increased impedance of a device against the full area of the soft tissue portion of the ear canal, and the smaller volume of air trapped between the device and the eardrum, greatly reduces the low-frequency boost that is the characteristic of the occlusion effect.[24] Venting is a reasonable (and often desirable) approach to managing the occlusion effect with hearing aids, but venting would essentially negate the performance of a HPD, except in rare circumstances where the venting is done purposely (such as in a vented-tuned plug for an offending noise that has only very-high-frequency sound energy).

A final limitation of typical HPDs, reviewed in this chapter, is the interference with speech communication caused by a HPD. Often, the reason an individual will remove his or her HPD is to talk with a coworker. There is general agreement that as the noise level is increased (with a subsequent degradation in signal-to-noise ratio [SNR]), speech communication ability decreases. In most cases, it is the SNR that is the primary factor in determining speech intelligibility, although other extrinsic and intrinsic factors, such as reverberation and auditory processing skills, can be equally important. In industry, the SNR is inherently poor, and the presence of reverberation further decreases speech recognition. An early study by Abel et al[25] demonstrated that while speech recognition decreased as the SNR decreased, HPDs had minimal effect on normal-hearing subjects. Casali et al[22] also reported that there was no evidence that for normal-hearing workers in relatively quiet occupational settings HPDs compromise their ability to understand. It should be noted, however, that many workers in occupational settings do have some sensorineural hearing loss, whether from noise exposure, presbycusis, or other causes. In contrast to Abel et al,[25] and Casali et al,[22] Tufts and Franks[26] demonstrated that communication difficulty in noisy environments is further exacerbated when earplugs are worn, as a speaker's voice is typically less intense (perhaps due to the occlusion effect), and has correspondingly less high-frequency speech energy. They concluded that "talkers wearing earplugs (and consequently their listeners) are at a disadvantage when communicating in noise."

As another example of speech communication limitations of HPDs, musical performers on stage will often be seen removing the in-ear monitor in one ear, leaving the monitor in the other ear. The reason for this is the musician needs to continue to hear the content presented in the monitoring ear (for instance, hearing the drums to keep time), but wants to have unfettered interaction with the crowd, or to hear bandmates between songs. Such approaches to improve speech communication by removing the HPD all but eliminates the benefits of HPD use. For example, in a study by Neitzel and Seixas,[27] construction workers used hearing protection less than one-quarter of the time that they were exposed to noise greater than 85 dBA. Despite a high NRR label on the HPD, the limited time of use resulted in the construction workers receiving less than 3 dB of effective protection from their HPDs.

16.5 Custom-Fit HPDs

Custom-fit HPDs are one approach to mitigate the comfort limitations of typical, passive HPD, as well as the variability between laboratory tested and field-measured attenuation in all HPDs (active as well as passive). With essentially no exception, custom-fit HPDs are earplugs, which either fill the entire concha through the cymba concha (helix lock) and some distance into the ear canal, or occupy the lower (cavum) concha and some distance into the ear canal. The amount of attenuation achieved is a function of the snugness of the earplug in the aperture through the first bend, and how deep the device goes into the ear canal.[28] The deeper the device goes into the ear canal, the higher the achieved attenuation (and the lower the occlusion effect). The larger the earplug is, relative to the ear canal, the greater the attenuation. However, there is a trade-off between snugness and depth in the ear canal, and comfort. If the device stretches the ear canal, and/or applies radial pressure deep in the ear canal in the bony region, the custom-fit HPD will have *worse* comfort than noncustom HPD. However, such a device could provide attenuation at the limits of bone conduction.

With custom-fit HPDs, the devices are either inserted correctly, or they are not really inserted at all (and are grossly uncomfortable and hanging out of the ear canal). Neitzel et al,[17] showed that custom-fit HPD had nearly the same attenuation in field measurement as the labeled NRR, while non-custom earplugs had a large deviation in field measurement as the labeled NRR. Basically, the customization of the earplug greatly reduced the variability in earplug attenuation from one fitting to the next. Custom-fit HPDs require an earmold impression (or, more recently, direct ear scan), which is then sent to an earmold laboratory for manufacture of the custom HPD. Most often, the custom-fit HPD is made of a soft material (such as a biocompatible silicone) to accommodate ear canal shape changes due to jaw movement, but can be made of hard material (like acrylic). Cost of passive custom-fit HPDs in 2017 range from $80 per pair to $225 per pair. For a stable workforce (low worker turnover), the cost to the company per employee for custom HPD is less than the cost of disposable HPDs at 20 cents per pair, after 2 to 3 years (depending how many times per day workers throw out their disposable plugs and get a new pair).

16.6 Passive Acoustically Tuned HPDs

An approach to mitigate the limitation of overattenuation is the development of passive, acoustically tuned HPDs. One example of this is the Etymotic Research (Elk Grove Village, Illinois) Musicians Earplug. This earplug is available as a custom-fit device (shown in Fig. 16.3a), and there are off-the-shelf one-size-fits-most versions (e.g., the ER20Xs) that are less expensive, but have less uniform attenuation across the frequency spectrum. The Musicians Earplug is an acoustically tuned product that was first invented by electrical engineer, Elmer Carlson, in the 1970s, and licensed to Etymotic Research by Mr. Carlson's employer, Knowles Electronics (Itasca, Illinois).[29] Shown in ▶ **Fig. 16.3** is an illustration of the two parts of the Musicians Earplug (the hollow "sleeve" and the button filter), with acoustical circuit components analogous to an electrical circuit. The filters are available in 9-, 15-, and 25 dB attenuators, all of which are nominally equal in the amount of attenuation provided across frequencies 125 to 8,000 Hz, so long as the earmold impression or direct ear scan captures ear canal anatomy past the second bend, and the sound bore of the sleeve is of sufficient size to provide an appropriate acoustical mass meeting manufacturer specification. Etymotic Research certifies individual earmold laboratories that wish to manufacture the Musicians Earplug, with all custom sleeves being tested for appropriate acoustic mass using an acoustic mass meter.

The Musicians Earplug was commercialized in 1988 following studies of sound exposures and hearing sensitivity of members of the Chicago Philharmonic Orchestra,[30] which demonstrated the need for a high-fidelity HPD. As with most industrial noise exposures, most musical exposures do not exceed 95 dBA for an 8-hour TWA. Therefore, modest attenuation would be prudent, particularly for individuals for whom the offending sound is not noise, but music. Rather than attempt-

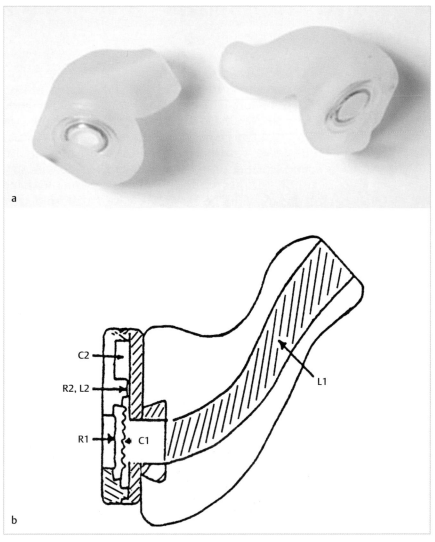

Fig. 16.3 **(a)** Photograph of a pair of custom-fitted silicone Etymotic Research Musicians Earplugs. © Copyright Iantos Technologies, Inc. Used with permission. **(b)** A cross-sectional schematic of the ER-15 earplug with a custom earmold showing capacitances (C), resistances (R), and inductances (L). © Copyright Etymotic Research Inc. Used with permission.

ing to block out as much unwanted signal (noise) as possible, the potentially hazardous signal (music) is the *purpose* of the activity for musicians and music consumers. An acceptable HPD would be one that interferes the least with the musical signal, while still providing a level under the attenuator that is less than 75 dBA 8-hour TWA; the reader is cautioned to note this 75 dBA is integrated over an 8-hour TWA, so should not be misconstrued to think more than 15 dB attenuation is typically needed, if a performance is 2 hours or less. Only under rare circumstances would a musician or music consumer require a 25 dB filter; less sound is often not more protection, if the user is overprotected and chooses to not use the HPD.

Other passive "musicians'" earplugs have been commercialized in recent years, but these devices have not been studied nearly to the level of the Etymotic Research branded product, and less is available on the frequency response expected with the different levels of filter attenuation. If the audiologist chooses to fit a patient with an earplug claiming to be flat, it would be in the audiologist's and patient's best interest to perform verification measures (such as a REAT in the sound field, using 1 dB step sizes) to determine if the HPD is "flat" as it may claim to be.

Other passive, acoustically tuned HPDs include devices such as the Combat Arms earplug (illustrated in ▶Table 16.1). The intent of this HPD is to allow softer-level sounds (such as speech, important environmental acoustic cues) to pass through the HPD relatively unimpeded, while significantly reducing (peak-clipping) the sound level of the report of a firearm. For a noncustom HPD, the effectiveness of such a device depends on how well the HPD is sealed in the ear canal. Other acoustically tuned HPDs include earplugs with filters such as the Hocks filter, which is a hard plastic insert with a very-small-diameter lumen, placed into a drilled-out sound canal in an otherwise occluding earplug. The intent of this very narrow sound channel is to allow very-low-frequency sound (with very long wavelengths) through relatively unattenuated, while attenuating higher-frequency sound as much as a solid, occluding earplug. Examples when this type of filtered earplug are useful are when the offending noise in an environment is limited to high frequency, but speech communication is necessary.

16.7 Active Electronic HPDs

A number of HPDs with embedded electronics have entered the market, benefiting from the miniaturization of electrical components, excellent performance and stability of hearing aid microphones, and good battery life for button-sized (hearing aid) batteries. These "active" electronic HPDs can be custom-fitted,

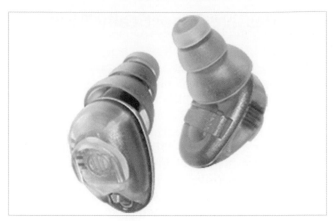

Fig. 16.4 Photograph of Etymotic Research Music-PRO electronic, nonlinear HPD. This earphone has two settings: a "15 dB" mode and a "9 dB" mode. In 15 dB mode, the ambient signal picked up by the microphone is presented into the ear canal at unity gain up to 70 dB SPL, then gradually compresses the output signal when inputs are 70- to 100 dB SPL. For input signals 100 to 120 dB SPL, there is a uniform 15 dB attenuation across frequencies. At inputs of 120 dB SPL and higher, the output is limited at 105 dB SPL. Other PRO series electronic hearing protection devices are the same form factor, but have different input–output characteristics.

or off-the-shelf. Examples include the Westone DefendEar and the Etymotic Research PRO Series (Music-PRO, GunSport-PRO, etc.). An example of an Etymotic Research Music-PRO electronic HPD is shown in ▶Fig. 16.4. This device can be retrofitted with a custom sleeve, which may give more consistent passive sound isolation in the low frequencies (as with any custom vs. noncustom HPD), depending on the shape of the individual's ear canal. Given that soft- and modest-level sound need not be attenuated to protect hearing, and these sounds are often important to hear, active/electronic HPDs allow these nonhazardous sounds through at unity gain (or, depending on the device and setting, may provide a modest gain for soft-input sound). These devices go into compression and/or peak clipping for sound that exceeds a criterion high level determined by the circuit. It is important to note that standard REAT testing to determine the NRR is not possible with these types of active, level-dependent devices, so alternative test methods are used to provide NRR product labeling.

16.8 Active HPD for Communication-Critical Applications

In communication-critical uses, the use of HPD is considered to interfere with productivity and safety. Specific to mitigating the deleterious effects of HPD use on speech communication, here are three technological strategies to improve speech communication (and localization of warning signals) in noise: ANR, use of HPDs with built-in communication systems, and use of HPDs with less high-frequency attenuation (i.e., attenuation properties that are more uniform across the speech spectrum, rather than more attenuation in the high frequencies than in the low frequencies). In general, ANR uses phase cancellation to attenuate ambient sound in the environment. ANR devices have found wide acceptance in a range of nonoccupational listening environments, particularly on airplanes where the ambient noise is fairly high (75–80 dBA[31]) and constant. Because ANR uses phase cancellation (generating a sound that is 180 degrees out of phase so that cancellation occurs), it requires less signal processing resources for low-frequency sounds (i.e., frequencies below 1,000 Hz), although the technology exists to provide wideband ANR. Often, HPDs using ANR will incorporate passive sound isolation to provide attenuation in the high frequencies, which lessens the necessity for ANR to act on the high frequencies. Typical low-frequency attenuation using these devices is 10 to 15 dB. Using such devices would significantly improve the SNR by reducing the low-frequency environmental noise while maintaining the mid- to high-frequency consonant sounds that are so crucial to speech recognition. ANR HPDs have not yet gained widespread acceptance in industry primarily because of cost, yet studies such as Casali et al[22] attest to the potential benefits in terms of improved speech recognition and vehicle backup alarm detection in noise.

> **Pearl** ✔
>
> HPDs using active noise reduction (ANR) uses a combination of phase cancelation to attenuate low-frequency sound, and passive sound isolation to attenuate the high-frequency sounds.

16.9 Hearables: An old, and New, Use for Ears

A new class of wearable technically, for use in the ear, has been termed "hearable." Such devices are considered "convergent" devices, as they may act as a HPD (typically an active, level-dependent device), as a hearing enhancement device (e.g., provide some gain for soft- and modest-level input), entertainment (stream music or other audio content from a wirelessly connected smartphone), and may offer other functionalities, such as heartrate monitoring/fitness tracking using a photoplethysmogram (PPG)

sensor that is in contact with the skin of the ear. The ear happens to be a very good location for measuring biometric data using a PPG sensor, given it the ear is well-vascularized and (relative to the wrist) is better protected from ambient light (which interferes with the light-based signal the PPG receives from the color of the perfused skin). Whether or not these hearables are a new wave in technology to be used in the ear, or are a fad, is yet to be seen. However, if technology analysts are to be believed, the hearables market is expected to grow to $45 billion in 2020.[32]

16.10 Assessment Techniques

There are multiple approaches to verification of HPDs, although three methods are currently the most popular: REAT, microphone in real ear (MIRE), and acoustical test fixtures (ATF). Each method has its strengths and weaknesses, and some methods are more appropriate than others for specific types of HPDs.[33]

16.11 Real-Ear Attenuation at Threshold Method

As noted previously in defining the NRR, the REAT method requires the user's hearing to be tested across a specified range of frequencies without earplugs in place, and again with the plugs in place. This method can be conducted via sound field audiometry or under circumaural earphones (as long as these earphones are large enough that they do not distort the shape of the pinna). Often, 1 dB step sizes are used to narrow the standard deviation in the measure. The REAT method is considered the gold-standard method for verifying HPD, although it has its drawbacks. For one, it requires a behavioral response (and so an introduction of subjectivity in the measure) which is a source of variability in the measure. NRR is measured only in adults, whereas REAT measures with sufficiently small variability using pediatric test techniques (conditioned play audiometry or visual reinforcement audiometry) have not been established. Additionally, it is relatively slow and requires appropriate test equipment and a professional capable of performing audiometry; it requires more time than is typically allotted for fitting a person with earplugs or earmuffs and may not be possible (due to equipment limitations) in the field. Finally, level-dependent (e.g., ANR and passive nonlinear) HPDs that are designed to provide little-to-no attenuation at low-input levels (such as used when measuring

REAT) and so would purposely show a REAT value of 0- (or near zero) dB attenuation.

16.12 Microphone in Real-Ear Method

The MIRE method uses a probe microphone placed near the eardrum and is equivalent to real-ear measures (REM) in measuring hearing aid output with hearing aid verification equipment. The difference is that REM is intended to document increase in sound reaching the eardrum when the device is in place and functioning (to bring sound into the residual auditory area of the person with hearing loss), whereas the MIRE technique is intended to document the insertion loss (i.e., attenuation) between the diffuse field and the eardrum when the device is in place and functioning. Benefits over REAT include (1) this measure is more objective (no subject response required) and it is considerably faster. A principal challenge, however, is placement of the microphone in the ear canal or through the HPD in a way that does not influence the performance of the HPD. A leak between the HPD and wall of the ear canal due to presence of a probe tube introduces a measurement artifact that greatly reduces the amount of low-frequency attenuation. Commercially available MIRE systems have managed this challenge using different techniques, such as inserting microphones through a valve in the HPD.

16.13 Acoustical Test Fixture Method

The ATF method involves the use of a mannequin that acts as a surrogate for the human head and ears. The most readily recognized ATF for audiologists is likely Knowles Electronics Mannequin for Acoustic Research (KEMAR). To be an appropriate surrogate, the ear canals, pinnae, head, etc., should be equivalent to the size of the intended user and have characteristics (such as skin simulation) for testing the HPD of interest. A static model ATF lacks the wide variability in the dimensions of adults, and therefore gives data that have limited inference to the real world. An ATF can be used for applications that are unsuitable for using human subjects, such as measuring nonlinear response of HPD to gunshots and explosions. More sophisticated ATFs can incorporate characteristics of sound transmission through bone conduction to avoid some of the errors with exceeding maximum possible attenuation.

Pearl

There are three different methods to evaluate the sound attenuation provided by HPDs. Each has strengths and weaknesses, but field attenuation evaluation can be done in the field, using commercially available equipment.

16.14 Summary

HPDs are the last resort to protect the hearing of noise-exposed persons, when the other efforts outlined in the hierarchy of exposure control have not succeeded in eliminating the NIHL risk. HPDs are an imperfect solution to noise control, as there are several limitations, including interference with speech communication, poor situation awareness, comfort, and occlusion effect. Perhaps even more concerning, the labeling that indicates the HPD "effectiveness" can be deceiving (as seldom does a user achieve the labeled noise reduction of a noncustom HPD), and misinterpreted (users misunderstanding that more attenuation is not necessarily better). Custom HPD, active/electronic HPD, filter/tuned HPDs, and communication-enabled devices are technological solutions that can help the user overcome the limitations of off-the-shelf, passive HPDs, and it is the role of the audiologist to advocate to the end user how best to address his or her hearing protection needs, as part of an overall hearing conservation program.

References

[1] Cheng W, Roberts B, Mukherjee B, Neitzel RL. Meta-analysis of job-exposure matrix data from multiple sources. J Expo Sci Environ Epidemiol. 2017

[2] American National Standards Institute (ANSI). Determination of Occupational Noise Exposure and Estimation of Noise-Induced Hearing Impairment (ANSI S3.44–1996). New York, NY: Acoustical Society of America; 1996

[3] Yankaskas K. Prelude: noise-induced tinnitus and hearing loss in the military. Hear Res. 2013; 295:3–8

[4] National Institute for Occupational Safety and Health. Criteria for a Recommended Standard: Occupational Noise Exposure, Revised Criteria 1998. DHHS (NIOSH) Publication No. 98–126. Cincinnati, OH: National Institute for Occupational Safety and Health; 1998

[5] Prince MM, Stayner LT, Smith RJ, Gilbert SJ. A reexamination of risk estimates from the NIOSH Occupational Noise and Hearing Survey (ONHS) J Acoust Soc Am. 1997; 101(2):950–963

[6] Occupational Safety and Health Administration. Occupational noise exposure: Hearing Conservation Amendment. Fed Regist. 1981; 46:4078–4179

[7] Occupational Safety and Health Administration. Occupational noise exposure: Hearing Conservation Amendment: final rule. Fed Regist. 1983; 48:9738–9785

[8] National Institute for Occupational Safety and Health. The NIOSH Compendium of Hearing Protection Devices. Updated version. Publication No. 95–105. Cincinnati, OH: US Department of Health and Human Services/Centers for Disease Control, National Institute for Occupational Safety and Health; 2003

[9] Berger EH, Kieper RW, Gauger D. Hearing protection: surpassing the limits to attenuation imposed by the bone-conduction pathways. J Acoust Soc Am. 2003; 114(4 pt 1):1955–1967

[10] Shaw EAG, Theissen GJ. Improved cushion for ear defenders. J Acoust Soc Am. 1958; 30:24–36

[11] Zwislocki J. In search of the bone-conduction threshold in a free sound field. J Acoust Soc Am. 1957; 29:795–804

[12] Environmental Protection Agency (EPA). Noise Labeling Standards for Hearing Protection Devices; 1979. http://www.gpo.gov/fdsys/pkg/FR-2009-08-05/pdf/E9-18003.pdf. Accessed December 24, 2016

[13] American National Standards Institute (ANSI). Method for the Measurement of Real-Ear Protection of Hearing Protectors and Physical Attenuation of Earmuffs. (ANSI S3.19–1974) (ASA STD1–1975). New York, NY: Acoustical Society of America; 1974

[14] Johnson DL, Nixon CW. Simplified methods for estimating hearing protector performance. J Sound Vibrat. 1974; 7:20–27

[15] Berger EH, Franks JR, Lindgren F. International review of field studies of HPD Atten. In: Axlesson A, Borchgrevink H, Hamernik RP, Hellstrom P, Henderson D, Sanvi RJ, eds. Scientific Basis of NIHL. New York, NY: Thieme Medical Publishers. 1996;361–377

[16] American National Standards Institute (ANSI). Method for the Measurement of Real-Ear Attenuation of Hearing Protectors. (ANSI S12.6–1984). New York, NY: Acoustical Society of America; 1984

[17] Neitzel R, Somers S, Seixas N. Variability of real-world hearing protector attenuation measurements. Ann Occup Hyg. 2006; 50(7):679–691

[18] Williams W. A proposal for a more refined single number rating system for hearing protector attenuation specification. Noise Health. 2012; 14(59):210–214

[19] Pirzanski C, Berge B. Ear canal dynamics: facts versus perception. Hear J. 2005; 58(10):50–58

[20] Park MY, Casali JG. An empirical study of comfort afforded by various hearing protection devices: laboratory versus field results. Appl Acoust. 1991; 34(3):151–179

[21] Davis RR, Murphy WJ, Byrne DC, Shaw PB. Acceptance of a semi-custom hearing protector by manufacturing workers. J Occup Environ Hyg. 2011; 8(12):D125–D130

[22] Casali JG, Robinson GS, Dabney EC, Gauger D. Effect of electronic ANR and conventional hearing protectors on vehicle backup alarm detection in noise. Hum Factors. 2004; 46(1):1–10

[23] Casali JG, Ahroon WA, Lancaster JA. A field investigation of hearing protection and hearing enhancement in one device: for soldiers whose ears and lives depend upon it. Noise Health. 2009; 11(42):69–90

[24] Killion MC, Wilber LA, Gudmundsen GI. Zwislocki was right... A potential solution to the "hollow voice" problem. Hear Instr. 1988; 39(1):14–18

[25] Abel SM, Alberti PW, Haythornthwaite C, Riko K. Speech intelligibility in noise: effects of fluency and hearing protector type. J Acoust Soc Am. 1982; 71(3):708–715

[26] Tufts JB, Frank T. Speech production in noise with and without hearing protection. J Acoust Soc Am. 2003; 114(2):1069–1080

[27] Neitzel R, Seixas N. The effectiveness of hearing protection among construction workers. J Occup Environ Hyg. 2005; 2(4):227–238

[28] Tufts JB, Chen S, Marshall L. Attenuation as a function of the canal length of custom-molded earplugs: a pilot study. J Acoust Soc Am. 2013; 133(6):EL446–EL451

[29] Killion MC. Elmer Victor Carlson: a lifetime of achievement. Bulletin Am Auditory Soc. 1992; 17(1):10–13

[30] Royster JD, Royster LH, Killion MC. Sound exposures and hearing thresholds of symphony orchestra musicians. J Acoust Soc Am. 1991; 89(6):2793–2803

[31] Portnuff CDF, Fligor BJ, Arehart KH. Teenage use of portable listening devices: a hazard to hearing? J Am Acad Audiol. 2011; 22(10):663–677

[32] Hunn N. Hearables sales could reach $45 billion in 2020; 2016. https://www.nickhunn.com/hearables-sales-could-reach-45-billion-in-2020/. Accessed February 15, 2016

[33] Berger EH. Preferred methods for measuring hearing protector attenuation, in Proceedings of Inter-Noise 07–10 August. Rio de Janeiro, Brazil; 2005

17 Tinnitus and Sound Sensitivity

Christopher Spankovich

17.1 Introduction

Tinnitus (pronounced tin-it-us or tin-night-us) is the perception of a sound without an external source. Tinnitus, often described as ringing, buzzing, humming, and other sounds is a familiar experience commonly associated with hearing loss and is often reported even in normal-hearing individuals in artificially low-noise environments (e.g., sound-treated room, anechoic chamber). There is not one type, cause, mechanism underlying tinnitus, or effect on the patient's quality of life; rather the phenomenon is heterogeneous. Prevalence estimates are mixed, but larger epidemiological studies in the United States (e.g., National Health and Nutrition Examination Survey [NHANES] and the Epidemiology of Hearing Loss Study) show prevalence between 4 to 25% of the U.S. adult population.[1,2,3,4,5] Similar prevalence estimates have been seen in other sampled populations across the globe.[6,7,8,9,10,11,12,13,14] The variability in reported prevalence is directly related to how tinnitus is defined, such as the inclusion of only "clinically relevant" tinnitus (i.e., bothersome), as well as the sample's demographics. Higher prevalence estimates (> 20%) are commonly reported if tinnitus is defined as the experience of tinnitus "ever" in the past year. Lower prevalence reports (4–12%) are commonly reported when tinnitus is defined by higher occurrence (i.e., daily or weekly) or include report of a bothersome nature.

Contrary to the high prevalence of tinnitus (conservatively 1 in 10 U.S. adults)[1] and relationship to hearing loss, a minority of individuals with tinnitus experience significant impact on their quality of life. It is estimated that approximately 20 to 25% of patients with tinnitus consider the symptom to be a significant problem.[1,15] However, for these patients, tinnitus can be quite debilitating, leading to psychological distress, social isolation, and deleterious impact on daily life activities.[16,17,18,19] A factor that contributes to the negative effect and experience often associated with tinnitus is the unknowns regarding pathophysiology and lack of evidence-based medical and nonmedical interventions. Individual variability and susceptibility to tinnitus and the affiliated negative reaction are not well understood. Nonetheless certain determinants have been identified related to increased report of tinnitus, including being a non-Hispanic white male, increased age, presence of hearing loss, history of noise exposure, history of cardiovascular disease, history of head/neck injury, history of depression, history of anxiety, former or current smoker, history of diabetes, history of arthritis, higher body mass index, and use of nonsteroidal anti-inflammatory drugs.[3,4,5,10,20,21,22,23]

Tinnitus is currently the most prevalent service-connected disability among veterans in the United States (23% of total cases of service-connected disability). The VA 2014 Annual Benefits Report showed 293,876 new service-connected recipients for the year. Of those, 140,288 (48%) received compensation for tinnitus. The total number of veterans receiving compensation benefits was 3,949,066 with 1,276,456 (32%) of total veterans receiving compensation for tinnitus.[24] In 2012, the VA spent $1.2 billion on hearing-tinnitus related compensation to veterans. A recent meta-analysis suggested a prevalence of tinnitus among military personnel deployed to Iraq or Afghanistan at a point estimate of 30.8%, however, restricted samples in personnel with deployment-related blast exposure and traumatic brain injury reported prevalence from 6.1 to 75.7% (Theodoroff et al[25]).

Children and teenagers also report tinnitus. Mahboubi et al[2] analyzed NHANES data and reported that 7.5% of 12 to 19 year olds in the United States reported experiencing tinnitus lasting at least 5 minutes in the preceding 12 months. Chronic tinnitus, defined as bothered by tinnitus for more than 3 months, was found to effect 4.7% of the population. Increased odds or report were associated with being female, low income, exposure to passive smoke, ear infections, history of tympanostomy tubes, and report of noise exposure. Even higher prevalence was reported from the Korean versions of the NHANES at 17.7% in the same age category, however, only 0.3% reported severe discomfort.[26] Other prevalence estimates in children and teenagers have varied from 4.7 to 62.2%, but are highly influenced by study population and how tinnitus was estimated.[27] The general prevalence of persistent tinnitus in children and teenagers is likely consistent with the lower end of these estimates. There is also suggestion that childhood hearing disorders including recurrent ear infections increase the risk for report of tinnitus as an adult.[28]

Limitations to obtaining accurate epidemiological descriptives of tinnitus are related to lack of knowledge of mechanism and inability to measure tinnitus objectively.

Pearl

The term tinnitus is derived from the Latin word tinnire, meaning to ring.

17.2 Types of Tinnitus

Through the years numerous classification systems have been applied to tinnitus.[29,30,31] A simple nomenclature dichotomizes tinnitus as either objective or subjective tinnitus. Alternative terms include somatosound or sensorineural/neurophysiological tinnitus, respectively. Here we will use the terms somotosound and neurophysiological tinnitus.

Somatosound tinnitus refers to a sound that is an identifiable within-body sound generated by a mechanical (somatic) process. For example, the perception of a heartbeat-like sound that is consistent with the individual's pulse is often related to a vascular source and called pulsatile tinnitus. Somatosounds in some cases can be objectively heard, measured, or the source visualized. However, in many cases, these somatosounds are subjective and not able to be detected by an observer.

Neurophysiological tinnitus accounts for the vast majority of tinnitus. Currently, there is no way to objectively measure neurophysiological tinnitus and rarely this type of tinnitus can be observed by an examiner; it is almost always subjective in nature (rare cases of objective neurophysiological tinnitus have been reported associated with spontaneous otoacoustic emission). Though confined to the individual, many patients describe similar auditory percepts including ringing, buzzing, humming, hissing, etc. Neurophysiological tinnitus is commonly associated with hearing loss, noise exposure, and ototoxic drug exposure. The exact mechanisms underlying neurophysiological tinnitus remains elusive, but likely involves multiple peripheral and central auditory and nonauditory components, further complicated by multiple means of pathogenesis. Neurophysiological tinnitus does not represent one entity rather it is a spectrum-based pathology. Many individuals with neurophysiological tinnitus can modulate perception through movement. This phenomenon has been called somatic tinnitus and implies interaction between somatosensory neurons and the auditory system. A study by Simmons et al[32] suggested that 78% of patients with tinnitus could modulate perception of their tinnitus through some type of head, neck, or eye movement. However, this should not be confused with somatosound tinnitus.

Another variation of tinnitus is referred to as idiopathic transient ear noise. Virtually everyone experiences an episode of idiopathic transient ear noise, which is usually described as a high-pitch sound accompanied by a brief fullness sensation. These episodes are usually unilateral, and often accompanied by a feeling of ear blockage (i.e., aural fullness); the sensation usually resolves within seconds to minutes. Differentiation of tinnitus and idiopathic transient ear noise is based on duration, frequency, and known cause. If the sound lasts at least 5 minutes and occurs at least twice a week, it is considered tinnitus.[33] The exact mechanism underlying transient ear noise is not understood.

The experience of tinnitus in normal-hearing individuals without chronic tinnitus perception was first reported by Heller and Bergman[34] and sometimes referred to as subaudible tinnitus. In this classic study, participants with self-reported normal hearing (n = 80) and hearing loss (n = 100) entered a sound-treated room with an ambient noise level between 15 and 18 dB for 5 minutes (accurate measure of level were limited by period technology). The participants were instructed to take note of any sounds they may hear. Approximately 94% of the normal-hearing group reported hearing a sound, most commonly described as a buzz, hum, and ring. Attempts at replicating Heller and Bergman's experiments have been less sensational with only 64 to 68% of participants experiencing tinnitus in a sound-treated room.[35,36] Del Bo et al[37] in the most recent replication study investigated the prevalence of subaudible tinnitus in individuals with audiologically confirmed normal hearing and its relationship to presence of otoacoustic emissions in an anechoic chamber. Up to 92% of the participants reported sound perception, however, there was no association with otoacoustic emissions. These findings suggest that the vast majority of people will experience a sound percept in settings with artificially low-noise floors, such as a sound-treated room or anechoic chamber. Tinnitus perception has also been reported with extended use of hearing protection devices. Eighteen subjects wore an earplug in one ear continuously for 7 days. Fourteen out of the 18 reported tinnitus perception which disappeared once the use of the earplug was discontinued.[38]

Auditory hallucinations also represent an experience of sound without an external source, but the phenomenological boundaries with tinnitus are blurred and in general, auditory hallucinations tend to be more complex in nature. Auditory hallucinations are generally divided into two categories, verbal auditory hallucination and nonverbal auditory hallucinations. Auditory verbal hallucinations may consist of human or nonhuman voice and maybe intelligible or unintelligible. These hallucinations can be benign or malignant in nature, in the sense that they may be pleasant or negative. Nonverbal auditory hallucinations are also known as acoasms, which includes nonhuman sounds and music. Musical hallucinations are characterized by songs, tunes, and melodies that resemble music; the content can be familiar or unfamiliar.[39] These experiences are often related to medications or focal neural injury.

Almost all individuals have experienced tinnitus or idiopathic ear noise in their lifetime. In addition, most people will experience a tinnitus-like percept when in an artificially quiet environment. These elements of tinnitus raise the question if tinnitus is a disruption of regular function (i.e., a disorder) or normal state related to reduced auditory input. Often, providers will tell patients tinnitus is not a disease or a disorder, rather a side effect of some other disruption, such as hearing loss. A logical correlate to the experience of tinnitus is pain. Pain is a normal response to damaging stimuli and serves a role to motivate withdrawal from the causative stimulus; there are numerous categories of pain, complex mechanisms at play, and a wide spectrum of tolerance and effect on the patient. Pain can become a disorder, when it becomes chronic and disables the patient. In the same sense, tinnitus may be viewed as a normal experience, but can become a disorder when it becomes chronic and/ or disables the patient in some way.

17.3 Neuroscience of Tinnitus (Limited to Neurophysiological Tinnitus)

Our understanding of the pathophysiology of tinnitus has grown exponentially over the past 20 years. Although numerous pathophysiological models have been proposed, none are complete. This reflects the heterogeneous nature of tinnitus and supports the probable existence of multiple mechanisms at play that are not always interdependent on each other. The development of animal models of tinnitus and advances in imaging and electrophysiological technologies has helped accelerate the formation of a theoretical framework for tinnitus.

Prior to animal models and advances in imaging, study of tinnitus was limited to psychophysical assessment and attempts to correlate electrophysiological findings to the tinnitus percept. However, in general, psychophysical assessments lack correlation to subjective measures of tinnitus severity and electrophysiological measures (usually showing prolonged latencies and reduced amplitudes) are confounded by peripheral hearing loss and hyperacusis often not replicated or not clinically significant (meaning difference can be statistically significant, but individual findings fall within clinical normative data). The introduction of animal models introduced the ability to perform more invasive experiments to provide evidence to accumulating theoretical models of tinnitus. The first published animal model of tinnitus (rat) was reported in Jastreboff et al.[40] In this case, the rat was trained in a conditioned suppression paradigm, to not lick when a continuous background noise was interrupted with a silent period; this was accomplished by a mild shock when the animal drank during a silent period. Subsequently, a group of the rats were injected with a high dose of salicylate (300 mg/kg). Salicylate, congener of aspirin, almost invariably produces temporary tinnitus in such high doses in humans. The rats that received the salicylate continued licking through the experiment, that is, they behaved as if they did not hear the silent periods, as if tinnitus was filling the silent gap. In contrast, the control animals (no salicylate) stopped licking during silent periods. The effect would distinguish as the animal metabolized the salicylate. Numerous other models also exist including interrogative and reflexive.[41,42,43,44] The generation of animal models of tinnitus has allowed more invasive studies and groundwork for an evidence-based theoretical framework. For example, the first published animal model of tinnitus by Jastreboff et al[40] findings led to the development of the neurophysiological model of tinnitus used in tinnitus retraining therapy.[45]

Advances in neuroimaging have also led to significant advances in understanding neural regions implicated in tinnitus. The application of positron emission testing (PET), functional magnetic resonance imaging (fMRI), diffusion tensor imaging (DTI), and magnetoencephalography (MEG) have been critical in revealing neural networks underlying tinnitus. Imaging studies have generally focused on two broad theses: (1) correlation between auditory and nonauditory brain networks and (2) increased correlation between the limbic system and other brain regions. Much of the early work in imaging of tinnitus was performed with patients that were able to modulate their tinnitus through voluntary movements; this self-modulation allowed patients to serve as their own control. The ability to modulate tinnitus has been referred to as somatic tinnitus, described previously. Lockwood et al[46] using PET imaging performed one of the first imaging studies in tinnitus. Subjects were recruited that could alter their tinnitus by performing oral facial movements. The PET imaging showed increases in activity in the temporal lobe (Brodmann's areas 21 and 41), hippocampus, and medial geniculate body of the thalamus, supporting suggestions of limbic system role in tinnitus. The activity was localized to the hemisphere contralateral to the ear, which the tinnitus was perceived. Many studies have since followed using other forms of somatic modulation (e.g., gaze-evoked tinnitus, cutaneous-evoked tinnitus) and drugs such as lidocaine, which can suppress tinnitus in some individuals. Other approaches have used masking noise to alter tinnitus loudness[47] or using matched controls.

Animal-based models and human neuroimaging studies of tinnitus over the past two decades have demonstrated changes associated with tinnitus at the level of the cochlea, synapse of the auditory nerve, cochlear nucleus, inferior colliculus, medial geniculate body of thalamus, and auditory cortices. In addition, nonauditory structures such as somatosensory pathways, prefrontal cortex, parietal cortex, cingulate cortex, amygdala, hippocampus, nucleus accumbens, insula, cerebellum, reticular activating system, basal ganglia, and other regions have been implicated in tinnitus.

Peripheral theories: Peripheral theories of tinnitus suggest that tinnitus is localized to the peripheral auditory system, here defined as the cochlea and auditory nerve. Significant research has sought to correlate tinnitus with spontaneous otoacoustic emissions; however, these efforts have been mostly unfounded and the prevalence of tinnitus directly related to spontaneous otoacoustic emissions is likely rare.[48,49] It is also worth noting that most spontaneous otoacoustic emissions occur in the range of 900 to 4,000 Hz and more common in normal hearing young people, whereas tinnitus is associated with perception at higher frequencies, hearing loss, and older age.

Another example of a peripheral theory is the discordant damage theory proposed by Jastreboff et al.[39] At that time, the primary pathological effects of noise and ototoxic drugs were believed to compromise outer hair cell (OHC) integrity in the basal turn, and subsequent or secondary impact on inner hair cells (IHC) and neural fibers. The discordant damage theory suggested that loss of OHCs and the decoupling from the tectorial membrane would result in the tectorial membrane then directly impinging on the stereocilia of the IHC, causing a constant depolarization. Another variation of the discordant theory suggests loss of OHC function decreases activity in type II afferent fibers resulting in loss of inhibition at the level of the cochlear nucleus.

More recently, the integrity of the afferent synapse has been implicated in tinnitus, particularly related to noise exposure. Animal models have demonstrated that noise does not necessarily cause primary damage to OHC, but rather the synapse may be the site of primary pathology. In these studies, rodents exposed to a moderate level of noise inducing a robust temporary threshold shift, show complete recovery of thresholds and OHC function as measured by DPOAEs. Anatomical studies show that both OHCs and IHCs remain intact. However, there is an immediate loss of afferent neural fibers, with preferential loss of high threshold low spontaneous rate fibers or activity. It has been suggested this loss in low spontaneous fiber activity then results in a net increase in excitation and tinnitus.[50] Tan et al[51] performed psychophysical tuning curves in tinnitus patients matched on hearing thresholds to controls. The findings, based on shape of psychophysical tuning curves, suggested that tinnitus was not strongly associated with OHC impairment, rather IHC or afferent function. In other words, patients with hearing loss and no tinnitus demonstrated broad tuning curves suggestive of OHC dysfunction, however those with hearing loss + tinnitus maintained sharp tuning curves suggesting intact OHC and loss of afferent output. The opposite was suggested in subjects with tinnitus, but normal hearing sensitivity.[52]

The major limitation of peripheral source of tinnitus is that ablation or destruction of the auditory nerve and cutting off of the peripheral portion of the system rarely results in eliminating tinnitus. Further information on ablation can be found in the Treatment section of this chapter.

Central theories: Currently, the evidence points to a centralization of neurophysiological changes that underlie tinnitus. In other words, peripheral changes to cochlear or auditory neural integrity results in maladaptive plasticity at more rostral segments of the pathway. For example, animals with behavioral evidence of tinnitus exhibit increased spontaneous firing rate in neurons of the cochlear nucleus (particularly of fusiform cells of the dorsal cochlear nucleus). Increases in net neural excitations are also demonstrated by changes in neurotransmitters (NT) with decrease in inhibitory NT (e.g., glycine and γ-aminobutyric acid [GABA]) and increase in excitatory NT (e.g., glutamate). Similar hyperactivity effects have been demonstrated in the inferior colliculus, medial geniculate body of the thalamus, and auditory cortex. Further, changes in peripheral auditory function can result in auditory frequency representation (mapping) where regions of the auditory cortex that correspond to the hearing loss shift their preferred tuning to frequencies near the audiometric edge creating an overrepresentation in the cortical tonotopic mapping. See a recent review by Henry et al[53] for more detailed summary.

These changes to auditory functionality are implicated in setting the conditions for the establishment of tinnitus. However, some of these changes may also be due to hearing loss or hyperacusis. This leads to the question: "Why do some people with hearing loss have tinnitus while others do not?" The answer may lie with the role of nonauditory regions in tinnitus.

Numerous nonauditory structures have been implicated in tinnitus. The somatosensory system is a complex system of neurons called sensory receptors that respond to changes to the surface or internal state of the body. The somatosensory system is integrated with the auditory system even at caudal levels as low as the cochlear nucleus. In animal studies, peripheral auditory damage can lead to increased activation in somatosensory neurons resulting in long-term potentiation of neurons affiliated with auditory regions and tinnitus. However, animals without long-term potentiation do not show evidence of tinnitus. This enhanced integration is also believed to underlie modulation of tinnitus with facial movement, sometimes referred to as somatic modulation or somatic tinnitus, as previously described.

Pearl ✔

Studies have shown that over 75% of individuals with tinnitus can modulate their tinnitus through stimulation or movement of the head or neck.[32]

In addition, to somatosensory effects, subcortical and cortical nonauditory structures have been implicated in the perception of tinnitus. The primary nonauditory regions of study are those that comprise the limbic system and its affiliated network, this includes but not limited to the thalamus, hypothalamus, amygdala, nucleus accumbens, hippocampus, parahippocampus, basal ganglia (caudate nucleus), anterior cingulate, insula, prefrontal cortex, and striatum. Theories incorporating nonauditory factors include thalamocortical dysrhythmia resulting in altered brain oscillatory activity, enhanced connectivity between auditory and frontoparietal attention networks, enhanced activity in limbic and basal ganglia structures, default mode network alterations, and striatal gating pathways. In general, these neural networks are involved in sound processing, detection, attention, salience, emotion, and stress. Brain changes recorded by electroencephalography (EEG) and its magnetic counterpart MEG show decreased oscillatory activity in the alpha band and increased slow-wave delta activity.[54] Increased gamma activity has also been reported.[55] These EEG/MEG findings further support the distributed brain network activity associated with tinnitus. Tinnitus and the experience of pain, in particular, chronic pain or pain with phantom limb syndrome have been suggested to have parallel mechanisms.[56] Similar to phantom limb pain, the patient often experiences the pain from the amputated site, as most individuals with tinnitus experience the percept from the ear.

Recently, two pathways have been suggested in mediating tinnitus perception (i.e., why do some people with hearing loss have tinnitus and others do not). Rauschecker and colleagues[56] have identified a primary role in the ventromedial prefrontal cortex and the nucleus accumbens[57] a gatekeeping system also involved in chronic pain. In brief, the model describes peripheral deafferentation (i.e., peripheral hearing damage) that creates a signal that travels rostral through the auditory pathway up to the auditory thalamus and auditory cortex. This signal is then assessed by the limbic frontostriatal network (which includes the ventromedial prefrontal cortex, nucleus accumbens, amygdala, and medial dorsal nucleus), which is part of the ventral striatum (a portion of the basal ganglia involved in decision making and reward). If the limbic frontostriatal network determines the signal is irrelevant, it is then suppressed. However, if suppression does not occur, chronic tinnitus results. Cheung and colleagues have also suggested the striatum, but the dorsal striatum rather than the ventral. They found enhanced activity in the LC area of caudate dorsal striatum (junction of the head and body of the caudate nucleus), caudate nucleus, other basal ganglia regions, and the auditory cortex in subjects with tinnitus.[58] These theoretical suggestions provide some explanation of why not all individuals with hearing loss develop tinnitus. Even if hyperactivity exists in more caudal portions of the pathway, these striatal networks determine salience, if the signal is determined to be noise or meaningless neural static, the brain suppresses or does not attend. The following papers provide excellent reviews of auditory and nonauditory regions implicated in tinnitus perception.[53,59,60,61]

17.3.1 Evaluation and Triage of the Tinnitus Patient

The evaluation and appropriate triage of the tinnitus patient is critical to success in treatment and management. Patients with tinnitus will often be evaluated by a variety of health care providers including audiologist, primary care physicians, specialty physicians, and mental health providers. A recent guideline was developed by the American Academy of Otolaryngology Head Neck Surgery to help clinicians involved in managing patients with tinnitus.[31] Despite or perhaps due to the high prevalence of tinnitus, the complaint is often dismissed or providers are uncertain about what to tell patients and when or whom to refer. As a consequence, patients are often told that "there is no cure or treatment and they will learn to live with it." Such negative messages from a trusted provider can lead to and reinforce negative reactions to the tinnitus and also delay appropriate evaluation and management.

A critical component of the tinnitus evaluation and triage of tinnitus patients is the case history. A comprehensive case history can help determine appropriate referral, further evaluation components, and management recommendations. Often management will involve a multidisciplinary team.

Red flags: In a case history we want to first consider clinical presentations or "red flags" that may be associated with serious and perhaps life-threatening medical pathology. Sudden onset of tinnitus with a sudden change in hearing can be a serious concern and should be considered an otologic emergency. Complaints of tinnitus accompanied by facial paralysis, severe vertigo, or head trauma should also receive emergent medical care. Somatic tinnitus of a pulsatile nature may also require immediate medical referral, particularly if acute in presentation. If a patient with tinnitus displays extreme anxiety or depression, he or she should be referred to a mental health professional on the day of presenting with symptoms. Suicidal ideation may require immediate referral to an emergency department. Nonemergency, but urgent care should be for any other somatic form of tinnitus or tinnitus accompanied by otalgia or otorrhea or nonsevere vertigo. Tinnitus that suggests a neurophysiological origin without the above symptoms should be considered nonurgent. ▶Table 17.1 provides a summary of tinnitus triage based on patient complaints and appropriate referral considerations.

Once the patient has been appropriately triaged, further case history is completed including hearing health, medical health, psychosocial health, and tinnitus. The sources of history can include electronic medical records (EMR), referring provider records, preassessment questionnaires, interview, and sub-

Table 17.1 Tinnitus triage

If the patient has tinnitus and	Refer to	Status
Sudden loss of hearing	Emergency department or otolaryngology ASAP within 48 hours	Emergency
Neural deficits, facial weakness, head trauma	Emergency department or otolaryngology ASAP	Emergency
Suicidal thoughts/behaviors	Emergency department or mental health	Emergency
Vertigo/dizziness, somatosound tinnitus, persistent ear pain, ear drainage	Otolaryngology and audiology	Urgent
Without above symptoms	Audiology and otolaryngology	Nonurgent

Abbreviation: ASAP, as soon as possible.
Source: Adapted with permission from Henry et al.[33]

jective assessments of tinnitus impact on function or quality of life (e.g., Tinnitus Functional Index [TFI]). Another important question is the referral source. Often the referring provider can be a key indicator to the questions you will ask and the testing you recommend. Another common question to all case histories is the purpose of the visit. Why is the patient there to see you and what are his or her expectations?

The hearing health history should include questions in regard to perception of hearing loss, onset and progression of hearing loss (gradual vs. sudden), symmetry of hearing loss, stability of hearing loss (fluctuating vs. constant), noise exposure, previous hearing test results, family history of hearing loss, history of ear infections, history of ear pain or drainage, and use of amplification. You may also include a measure of impact of hearing loss on function, such as the Hearing Handicap Inventory (HHI)[62] or the Self-Assessment of Communication.[63]

A second important element is a comprehensive medical history. This should include questions regarding acute event such as recent cold/infection or trauma and chronic conditions including those related to cardiovascular health, metabolic health, and neural health. Conditions specifically associated with tinnitus, hearing loss, and dizziness should be addressed including but not limited to hypertension, diabetes, autoimmune disorders, pregnancy, thyroid dysfunction, headaches/migraines, and use of ototoxic medications. A list of medications including over-the-counter products (e.g., salicylate-containing products) should be obtained. The patient should also be questioned on their psychosocial history including history of anxiety, depression, other psychological disorders, employment status, marriage status, and use of drugs, alcohol, and tobacco products. Other lifestyle questions in regard to quality of diet, physical activity, and quality of sleep should be discussed. Sexual history may also be important, specifically if a sexually transmitted disease (e.g., syphilis) or penile erectile dysfunction (PED) is indicated. Several medications used to treat PED may have a potential side effect of tinnitus.

Comparable questions should be directed specifically toward the patient's tinnitus complaints. When did the patient first perceive tinnitus, onset and progression of tinnitus (gradual vs. sudden), correlation of tinnitus with any temporal event, symmetry and localization of tinnitus, sound quality of the tinnitus, sensitivity to sounds, somatic quality to tinnitus, duration of time actively perceive tinnitus, activities that make tinnitus less noticeable, activities that make tinnitus worse, other auditory-vestibular complaints (e.g., aural fullness, vertigo, etc.), and specific concerns regarding the tinnitus and quality of life.

17.3.2 Establishing Tinnitus Severity

A number of tinnitus outcome measures exist to determine subjective nature of tinnitus and scaling the severity, reaction, and impact on quality of life. These include the TFI,[64] Tinnitus Handicap Inventory (THI),[65] Tinnitus Reaction Questionnaire,[66] Tinnitus Handicap Questionnaire,[67] Tinnitus Questionnaire,[68] and others. It has been well demonstrated that severity scales do not correlate with psychophysical measures.[69]

The most recent of these, the TFI, represents a collaborative effort of the majority of the authors of the outcome measures listed. The TFI was developed for assessing responsiveness to change and validity for establishing severity of multiple domains. The TFI consists of 25 questions and 8 subscales (intrusive, control, cognitive, sleep, auditory, relaxation, quality, and emotional). The patient responds by selecting items on a 10-point scale (percentage items are scored as equivalent point, 100% = 10 points) for each question. The maximum overall score is 250; the sum is then divided by the number of questions scored and multiplied by 10 to give a 0 to 100 range. Functional impact is interpreted: 0 to 17 not a problem, 18 to 31 small problem, 32 to 53 moderate problem, 54 to 72 big problem, 73 to 100 very big problem. A TFI score change of at least 13 is considered significant. Subscales can also be calculated.

The THI is one of the best known and widely used tinnitus instruments, with well-established reliability and construct validity. The THI consists of 25 questions pertaining to the patient's subjective experience of tinnitus. The subjects respond yes, sometimes, or no; scored 0, 2, and 4, respectively for a possible score of 0 to 100. There are three subscales: functional, emotional, and catastrophic. Handicap is graded based on the overall score, 0 to 16 slight or no handicap, 18 to 36 mild handicap, 38 to 56 moderate handicap, 58 to 76 severe handicap, 78 to 100 catastrophic handicap. A 20-point change is considered significant (Newman et al[70]). Subscale items can also be scored.

It is also important to discriminate between patients with primary complaints of hearing loss versus primary complaints of tinnitus. Often patients will report significant tinnitus, but after further inquiry, it is clear they attribute decreased hearing and reduced speech understanding to the tinnitus and really have a primary complaint of hearing loss. The Tinnitus and Hearing Survey[71] is useful to differentiate these two commonly confused complaints.

Pearl ✔
Scales of severity do not correlate with psychophysical measure of tinnitus (pitch match, loudness match, minimum masking level).

Other outcome measures: In addition to tinnitus specific surveys, it is common to use measures of psychological status. These include the Becks Depression Inventory (Beck and Beck[72]), Visual Analog Scales, State Trait Anxiety Inventory (Spielberger et al[73]), Yale-Brown Obsessive Compulsive Scale,[74] Hamilton Anxiety Scale,[75] and many more. Patients with anxiety and depression are likely to have greater difficulty with their tinnitus and may benefit from psychological or psychiatric evaluation for additional intervention options. Rarely has tinnitus been identified as the direct cause of suicide. In most cases, there are coinciding psychopathological issues.[76] However, patients reporting significant depression, anxiety, or thoughts of suicide should be appropriately referred for psychological/psychiatric evaluation and managements.

17.3.3 Physical Examination and Testing

Comprehensive case history will usually lead to appropriate triage of the patient. Patients reporting red flag symptoms or with significant complaint of tinnitus on their life should undergo a medical evaluation, preferably by an otolaryngologist and specifically an otologist or neuro-otologist.

Medical examination: The medical evaluation will include a review of systems, history, and an otoscopic examination to detect infection or occluding/impacted cerumen. A cranial nerve examination is performed as well as auscultation over the neck, periauricular area, orbits, and mastoid.[77] An otolaryngologist (ENT) will commonly perform tuning fork tests including the Weber and Rinne to determine asymmetry and clue into type of hearing loss. The physician may order specific laboratory examinations and imaging based on the outcomes of the physical examination. Laboratory tests may include complete blood count, lipid profile, serum glucose, fluorescent treponema antibodies, thyroid studies, and an autoimmune panel (antinuclear antibodies, sedimentation rate, and rheumatoid factor). Radiological evaluation may include magnetic resonance imaging (MRI) of the internal auditory canals, computerized topography (CT), or magnetic resonance angiography (MRA). In almost all cases, the patient will be referred for audiologic testing.

Audiological examination: The audiological examination is dependent on the presenting history and symptoms reported by the patient. The testing commonly includes otoscopy, a comprehensive audiometric evaluation (air-conduction thresholds, bone-conduction thresholds, and speech testing), immittance testing including middle ear muscle reflexes/reflex decay, and loudness discomfort level testing. Other testing can include otoacoustic emissions, eustachian tube dysfunction testing, and auditory-evoked potentials. The audiologist should exercise caution when using middle ear muscle reflexes and decay at higher levels in individuals with sound sensitivity. An alternative is to use broadband stimuli at which lower levels can be used to elicit the reflex.

Tinnitus examination: The tinnitus evaluation (CPT code 92599) involves a series of psychophysical assessment procedures to obtain information regarding the patient's tinnitus including pitch, loudness, and maskability. Edmund Fowler first introduced many of these assessment techniques in the 1930s and standardized recommendations were presenting in the 1980s.[78] Though the information obtained may be limited for modern intervention purposes, many patients get a certain comfort knowing their tinnitus has been quantified and objectified. There are numerous approaches to completing a tinnitus evaluation, outlined here are methods consistent with.[79] The tinnitus evaluation can be completed with a standard clinical audiometer. A first place to start is to establish the patient's thresholds for pure tone stimuli, white noise, and possibly narrowbands of noise (NBN). Second, you will want to counsel the patient on the difference between the terms "pitch"

and "loudness." Third, you will want to determine where the patient localizes the tinnitus and types of sounds perceived. If a patient reports a unilateral tinnitus, it is often easier to play the matching stimuli in the contralateral ear. If the tinnitus is localized to both ears or the head, then independent ear measures may be necessary if the patient reports asymmetry in loudness or pitch. In some cases, the tinnitus may be described as multiple sounds and the provider should be prepared to match multiple sounds. Although contralateral presentation is preferred, ipsilateral presentation may be more appropriate in some situations, such as a distorted perception (e.g., diplacusis).

Pitch matching (PM) involves playing sounds to the patient to match the pitch (i.e., perceived frequency) of their tinnitus. It is important to try to maintain comparable levels as you present different frequency stimuli to the patient. Levels presented at 10 to 20 dB sensation level (SL) are a good starting point. A second item to address is the type of sound stimulus. If the patient reports a tonal tinnitus, pure tone stimuli are recommended; if the patient reports a noise-like tinnitus, use NBN. By using narrowband noise, you will want to get thresholds at the test frequencies.

To perform PM, a forced choice procedure is recommended where two different frequencies are played and the patient is requested to select which frequency was closer in proximity to the match of their tinnitus pitch. Start with 1,000 Hz played at 10 to 20 dB SL (either pure tone or NBN). Play the stimulus for 2 to 3 seconds and then play the second sound (e.g., 4,000 Hz). Repeat this process using higher- and lower-frequency stimuli until confirming a closest match. Recognize, most audiometers have limited frequency resolution, so an exact match is not likely, nor necessary for most applications of this information. Often patients will match the pitch of their tinnitus to the region of hearing loss in their audiogram or at the edge frequency.[80] This presents an excellent counseling tool on the relationship between tinnitus and the individual's hearing loss. A limiting factor in PM is high variability (poor test-retest reliability) and possible fluctuating nature of tinnitus.

Loudness matching (LM) involves playing sounds to the patients to match the "loudness" of their tinnitus. Tinnitus LM is performed with the pitch match and/or at 1,000 Hz. The loudness match is often performed in the smallest step size available on the audiometer, usually 1 to 2 dB. The loudness match can be reported in dB SL or dB HL. To present in dB SL, it is recommended to determine threshold at the test frequency with the same 1 to 2 dB resolution.

The determination of loudness can be achieved in several ways. You can play the stimulus at a level just at audibility for 2 to 3 seconds and ask if the tinnitus is louder or softer. Then repeat at each level until the patient reports a loudness match. Another option is to start below the threshold of hearing and gradually increase the level and have the patient indicate when the sound you are playing matches the level of the tinnitus. The additional match at 1,000 Hz is to address issues of confusion between test stimuli and the tinnitus and influence of hearing loss on loudness match. The reliability of LM is usually within a few decibels of each other for most patients with chronic tinnitus. Despite the decent reliability, LM is not without its limitations. The most significant criticism of LM is that it is not a measure of the subjective magnitude of sound, rather a measure of physical magnitude and the lack of relationship to reported loudness. Numerous investigators have attempted to address these limitations with adjustments for recruitment, conversion to sones or phons, and alterations in subjective loudness scales (e.g., Likert's scale 0–7, 0 = silence and 7 = loudest sound ever heard). However, whether using dB HL, dB SL, sones, or some variation, only mild-to-moderate correlations have been found between loudness match and loudness scales. In other words, though two patients may have similar hearing loss, pitch match, and match their tinnitus at 10 dB SL; the perceived loudness may be of significant difference.

Minimum masking/suppression levels (MML) refers to the lowest level of a broadband noise (BBN) that renders a patient's tinnitus unperceivable. The use of the term masking in this instance has been debated and suppression is possibly a more appropriate term. Nonetheless, the aim of the MML test is to determine the maskability/suppressability of the patient's tinnitus and can indicate potential success with sound therapy. In some cases, complete masking or suppression cannot be achieved and only a partial masking/suppression is possible. Further, in a subpopulation of patients' presentation of external sounds result in exacerbation of the patient's tinnitus, sometimes referred to as reactive tinnitus. To complicate the test more, contralateral masking may be more effective than ipsilateral and monaural masking may be more effective than binaural.

To perform MML, first obtain a threshold for white noise in 1 to 2 dB steps for each ear. Often it can be confusing to attempt to establish ipsilateral and contralateral MMLs. Therefore, if a patient has bilateral tinnitus, bilateral MML testing is recommended. If they have unilateral tinnitus, monaural testing (both ipsi- and contra-) are recommended. Instruct the patient that you are going to play a noise and try to find the softest level required to cover up their perception of their tinnitus. The BBN is then raised in 1 to 2 dB steps until the patient raises their hand or presses the button indicating masking. The patients can raise their right hand when the tinnitus is masked in the right ear, left hand when masked in the left ear, and both hands when both ears masked. For unilateral tinnitus, the same procedure is performed, but with sound presented only to the ipsilateral ear or only to the contralateral ear. If during this testing in the unilateral case, the patient perceives tinnitus in the contralateral ear, noise is then introduced to that ear for binaural presentation. I mention in the case of unilateral tinnitus use of masking in the contralateral ear. In some cases, a patient may have a severe-to-profound hearing loss in the ear with the tinnitus, perhaps due to an idiopathic sudden sensorineural hearing loss. It is useful to be able to demonstrate that sound can still be used to provide relief from the tinnitus, even if the ear itself with the tinnitus cannot hear.

Residual inhibition (RI) is a phenomenon where tinnitus perception is reduced in intensity following auditory stimulation. Following establishment of MML, patients will sometimes report sustained reduction of their tinnitus, despite distinguishing of the BBN. The effect has been contributed neural adaptation. A minority of patients may experience exacerbated tinnitus, which may be consistent with a reactive tinnitus.

To perform RI, a BBN is presented at 10 dB above the MML. The patient is instructed that there will be a noise presented for 1 minute and sometimes this noise can alter the perception of the tinnitus. They should focus on the noise, but otherwise no response is necessary. The noise will then be discontinued and the patient should report when the tinnitus returns to its current sound quality. Allow the patient to focus on the sound of their tinnitus for a moment, then play the noise. You can use a stopwatch or timer to determine the length of time until the tinnitus returns to prenoise level (you can stop measurement at 1 minute). Be sure to ask the patient if the tinnitus got softer or louder after the exposure. Patients can experience partial or complete suppression.

Other testing: Other testing may be recommended based on the patient's complaints. Loudness discomfort level testing is common for patients experiencing sound sensitivity in addition to tinnitus. Further description of low-density lipoprotein (LDL) testing will be provided in the Sound Sensitivity section of this chapter. In addition, other testing elements may include measures to exclude middle ear dysfunction, cochlear dysfunction, and retrocochlear pathology.

Pearl	

Plot the tinnitus pitch and loudness on the patient's audiogram as a counseling tool.

17.3.4 Differential Diagnosis in the Tinnitus Patient

Somatosound Tinnitus

There are numerous types of somatosound tinnitus; we will discuss some of common causes for each. This type of tinnitus refers to a sound that originates within the body, often vascular or muscular in source. This form of tinnitus can be of serious consequence and usually warrants a medical referral.

Pulsatile tinnitus: Pulsatile tinnitus commonly originates from vascular structures within the cranial cavity, head and neck region, and thoracic cavity. Pulsatile tinnitus can be of a venous or arterial source. See Sismanis[81] for review. The history is the most important part of the pulsatile tinnitus evaluation. Typically, the patients will describe their symptoms as hearing their own heartbeat or a thumping noise.

Venous causes are thought to be more common due to the more torturous nature of the venous system. Venous causes include idiopathic intracranial hypertension (IHH; aka pseudotumor cerebri syndrome) and venous hum (aka essential pulsatile tinnitus). IHH is characterized by increased intracranial pressure without usual focal signs of neurologic dysfunction. It is more common in obese females of childbearing age. Patients report posture-dependent headaches and visual changes (e.g., blurred vision), often accompanied by hearing loss, dizziness, and aural fullness. The exact pathophysiology is not known, but believed to involve resistance to cerebrospinal fluid (CSF) absorption resulting in interstitial brain edema.[82] Venous hum also has a marked female preponderance. The pathophysiology is believed to be due to turbulent blood flow in the internal jugular vein. Other venous causes to consider include jugular bulb abnormalities, abnormal emissary veins, Arnold–Chiari syndrome, etc.

Arterial causes include atherosclerotic carotid artery disease (ACAD) and intracranial vascular abnormalities (e.g., dural arteriovenous fistulae). Pulsatile tinnitus related to ACAD is often secondary to carotid bruits (audible vascular sound usually heard with stethoscope) produced by turbulent blood flow at stenotic segments of the carotid artery. Dural arteriovenous fistulae and other arteriovenous malformations can also create pulsatile tinnitus, usually involving the transverse and sigmoid sinuses near the ear. As these venous channels are compromised, narrowed regions can be created resulting in bruits. Other arterial causes to consider include aneurysms, glomus tumors of the jugular foramen and middle ear, fibromuscular dysplasia, tortuous internal carotid artery, semicircular canal dehiscence, otosclerosis, vascular compression of the eighth nerve, hypertension, hyperthyroidism, etc.[81]

The diagnosis of somatosound tinnitus is dependent on a good case history and examination. If described as pulsatile, the next step is to determine synchrony with cardiac cycle. This can be accomplished by comparing patients' count of "tinnitus pulses" to patients' cardiac pulse over a short time. Otoscopy can reveal possible movement of the tympanic membrane or observation of a mass or other signs of pathology (e.g., crescent mass: glomus jugulare tumor; Schwartze's sign: otosclerosis); ophthalmoscopy may also be performed to look at vasculature of the eye. A physician may also compress the ipsilateral jugular or carotid to determine source. Changes in intensity with head turning often suggest a venous source. Otherwise ultrasound studies and imaging are a common next step (MRI, MRA, and CT). Lumbar puncture may be performed to measure CSF pressure.

Nonpulsatile somatosound tinnitus: Nonvascular sources of somatosound tinnitus are relatively rare. The primary nonvascular sources to consider are foreign bodies, myoclonus, and eustachian tube related. Myoclonic tinnitus refers to contraction in muscles creating fluttering sensations or clicking. Palatal myoclonus refers to a rhythmic involuntary movement of the muscles of the soft palate or throat. It is commonly associated with neurodegenerative disorders like multiple sclerosis. Palatal myoclonus often presents with a bilateral clicking. Other sources of myoclonic tinnitus include contractions of the tensor tympani, stapedius muscle or muscles of the eustachian tube, and nasopharyngeal muscles (dilator tubae, salpingopharyngeus, tensor veli, levator veli palatini, and superior constrictors). Inspection of the nasopharynx can show muscle contractions coincident with the clicking (with exception of tensor tympani and stapedius source). Stapedial muscle contractions can produce clicking, and also fluttering or crackling sound and can be exacerbated by outside sounds. Most commonly seen with recovery from Bell's palsy. Tensor tympani syndrome involves contraction of the tensor tympani muscle that can produce clicking and fluttering sensations, may be associated with noise exposure, hyperacusis, and anxiety. Patients with tensor tympani syndrome can report aural fullness, pain, and mild vertigo.

Other somatosounds include sounds coincident with jaw and head movements, which can be related to temporomandibular joint issues or foreign object in ear canal (e.g., water). Autophony or blowing tinnitus is related to a blowing-like sound with respiration or echoing of one's own voice. This can be caused by a patulous (chronically open) eustachian tube. Semicircular canal dehiscence can lead to perception of pulsatile tinnitus, also distortions in sound of own voice and even perception of sound of own eye movement.[83] Tinnitus of a typewriter/popcorn nature has been associated with vascular compression of the eighth nerve.

Audiological work-up is an important component to somatosound tinnitus including audiometry, immittance, electrophysiology, and balance assessment. It may be possible to acquire an objective measure using common immittance equipment. Tympanometry may show perturbations in the response related to myoclonic, vascular, or patulous eustachian tube changes in middle ear admittance. Another option is to perform low-level reflex decay to visualize changes in admittance. The procedure involves selecting reflex decay and lowering the stimulus level to the lowest possible (e.g., 35 dB HL). Frequency is not critical, but the author commonly uses 1,000-Hz stimulus. The pressure is introduced and the stimulus is presented. At this level, no middle ear muscle reflex is expected, nor a change in admittance. If the patient has a pronounced somatosound tinnitus, this may result in immittance changes that can be recorded. If the source is the stapedius muscle, you will not likely see tympanic membrane movement.

Neurophysiological Tinnitus

Tinnitus is significantly associated with hearing loss, however, not all individuals with hearing loss have tinnitus and not all individuals with tinnitus have hearing loss. The reason some people with hearing loss do not perceive tinnitus is not clear. Numerous theories exist including differences in peripheral damage and differences in central plasticity as a result of peripheral damage (see Neuroscience of Tinnitus section of this chapter).

Noise-induced tinnitus: Noise exposure represents a common variable in hearing loss and tinnitus. Noise is also a cause of hearing loss and tinnitus that is potentially 100% preventable. The common first complaint of an individual with noise exposure is tinnitus. Hearing loss may be a delayed complaint due to the initial limited effects of a mild noise-induced hearing loss on perception. Noise exposure can cause primary damage to sensory receptors of the inner ear (OHCs and IHCs) and to neural populations. Noise can cause both temporary and/or permanent changes in hearing referred to as temporary threshold shift (TTS) and permanent threshold shift (PTS). See the chapter on noise for further details (Chapter 16). In brief, a noise resulting in TTS creates a shift in threshold that recovers

to within baseline data within days. PTS refers to a noise exposure that does not completely recover to within 5 dB of the baseline test (or the normative of test–retest reliability). The pathological effects of noise can be both mechanical and metabolic in nature. TTS has been associated with effects on hair cell stereocilia, reticular lamina, and separation of OHCs from the tectorial membrane.[84] Recently, the temporary nature of TTS has been questioned with demonstration of loss of afferent neural synapses despite no loss of hair cells and recovery of thresholds. This primary afferent neural damage (primary in that the damage is not secondary to hair cell loss) is created by an excitotoxic event (excessive release of glutamate) that can be rapid and permanent (see Neuroscience section). PTS is associated with damage to cochlear hair cells, with initial damage to regions more basal than noise band, consistent with the resonance characteristics of the external, middle, and inner ear and half-octave shift. The half-octave shift refers to a basal shift in basilar membrane motion related to intense sound stimulation. These resonance characteristics are correlated with the "noise-notch" usually between 3 to 6 kHz. The damage can be due to mechanical disruption of hair cell integrity (e.g., broken stereocilia) or subsequent metabolic processes that activate stress signaling pathways that ultimately determine the fate of the cell. However, intense sounds such as blast can damage the conductive components of the auditory system (e.g., perforation of eardrum).

It is also possible that noise exposure can cause further exacerbation of existing tinnitus. At-risk individuals should be counseled on appropriate hearing conservation strategies to prevent noise-induced tinnitus and secondary prevention strategies to reduce risk for worsening of tinnitus.

Drugs: Ototoxic drugs can induce tinnitus as well as hearing loss. Well-known ototoxic agents include platinum-based neoplastic drugs (cisplatin and carboplatin), aminoglycoside antibiotics, loop diuretics, quinine, and nonsteroidal anti-inflammatory drugs (e.g., aspirin). However, even drugs not considered to be ototoxic have been reported to have a side effect of tinnitus, though the number of people who report tinnitus for many is very low and not necessarily confirmed by any mechanism. These include drugs for treating high blood pressure, cholesterol, penile erection dysfunction, and even drugs for anxiety and depression. A search of the Physicians' Desk Reference will list several hundred agents with tinnitus as a reported side effect, though most in less than 3% of patients. Some of these drugs may only have a temporary effect on hearing or cause transient tinnitus due to pharmacological site of action, dose, schedule, and duration of use.

Sodium salicylate (aspirin) in high doses reliability induces tinnitus, however, often transient. Recent work has suggested the mechanism is related to long-term potentiation of N-methyl-D-aspartate (NMDA) receptors. NMDA is a metabotropic glutamate receptor located on primary auditory afferent fibers and reported to orchestrate repair of the synapse after an excitotoxic event. However, NMDA is not believed to be a primary player in hearing, rather the fast excitatory neurotransmissions required for hearing are mediated by ionotropic receptors called AMPA and kainate. Guitton et al[85] suggested tinnitus was created by altered arachidonic acid metabolism that increases channel opening probability of NMDA receptors. Salicylate's effects on hearing are mediated through impact on chloride channels implicated in prestin and OHC motility.

Appropriate clinical correlation for drug-induced tinnitus is dependent on temporal elements. This is primarily obtained through a comprehensive history. The patient should be questioned as to what medications (prescribed and over the counter) and supplements they are taking and if onset or change in tinnitus was associated. This includes starting, stopping, or changing dose of a medication or supplement. Medications and/or interactions of medications can also induce musical hallucinations.

Pearl ✔

The synergistic effects of drugs and noise should also be a concern. Ototoxic medications in particular may increase the risk for noise-induced hearing loss and tinnitus.

Auditory pathology: Any pathology affecting the auditory pathway can result in perception of tinnitus, from as benign as cerumen to as serious as a retrocochlear mass. Auditory pathologies requiring exclusion for tinnitus include excessive cerumen, external ear infections (otitis externa), middle ear pathology (e.g., otitis media, otosclerosis, cholesteatoma, ossicular chain pathology, glomus tumor, etc.), inner ear–related disorders (Meniere's disease, other endolymphatic hydrops, autoimmune inner ear disease, labyrinthitis, perilymph fistulae, semicircular canal dehiscence, otosyphilis, idiopathic sudden sensorineural hearing loss, trauma, etc.), and disorders of the nerve or brain (e.g., vestibular schwannoma, multiple sclerosis, viral infection). However, other comorbidities can also contribute to hearing loss and therefore the development of tinnitus (e.g., diabetes mellitus, hypertension, thyroid dysfunction, trigeminal neuralgia, etc.).

Nonhearing loss: Tinnitus is often associated with peripheral hearing loss, but is not dependent on changes to peripheral auditory function to manifest. Tinnitus can manifest as a result of traumatic brain injury and whiplash/neck trauma despite no overt evidence of effect on hearing. The mechanism of trauma-induced tinnitus may involve ephaptic neural transmission. In other words, damage results in plasticity that now creates a pathway where neural stimulation is now being channeled to the auditory pathway and resulting in perception of a sound.[86] In addition to trauma, pathology of neurovascular systems may also be implicated in tinnitus presentation without evidence of hearing loss. Disorders such as stroke, trigeminal neuralgia, multiple sclerosis, thyroid dysfunction, fibromyalgia, Lyme disease can all present with tinnitus despite "normal" hearing sensitivity. There is also evidence of a stroke resulting in resolution of tinnitus perception without effect on hearing.[87]

17.3.5 Tinnitus Management Approaches

There are numerous approaches to the management of the tinnitus patient. For historical perspective, the interested reader is referred to Stephens.[88] Medical management is limited. There is no drug or surgery that is approved by the FDA for the treatment of tinnitus. However, numerous pharmacological and surgical approaches to tinnitus management are in variable developmental phases. A brief overview of these approaches is provided in the latter half of this section. In addition to contemporary medical reliance on drugs and surgery, there are a number of nonmedical tinnitus management approaches that involve some combination of counseling and sound therapy. The recent AAO-HNSF clinical guidelines[31] for tinnitus provide statements based on strength of evidence for management of tinnitus.

A principle to consider when considering treatment options for tinnitus and strength of evidence is the significant placebo effect seen with tinnitus, reported as high as 40%.[89] An effect of this magnitude has the potential to confound any clinical trial, particularly those focused on the subjective evaluation of tinnitus. An almost universal problem with clinical research in tinnitus is lack of well-designed, randomized, placebo-controlled studies in sizeable populations and universal outcome measures. There are no objective measures for tinnitus. Outcomes are based on reported tinnitus severity and psychophysical measures of loudness and pitch. Often studies will report objective measures were used, for example, pitch match and loudness. This is inaccurate;

all of these are dependent on the patient's report and are therefore subjective. Finally, greater emphasis needs to be placed on characteristics of the tinnitus population and understanding of factors' mediating effects. This is critically important to understand why one person may obtain benefit with an intervention while another does not.

17.3.6 Counseling-Based Approaches

Nonmedical approaches to tinnitus management commonly involve counseling and/or sound-based therapy. Counseling approaches include tinnitus retraining therapy (TRT), tinnitus activities treatment (TAT), progressive tinnitus management (PTM), integrative tinnitus patient management, cognitive behavioral therapy (CBT), mindfulness-based stress reduction (MBSR) therapy, acceptance and commitment therapy (ACT), and/or modified versions of the above (e.g., dialectical behavior therapy). All of these approaches can be successful in helping patients manage their tinnitus and there is limited data to support the superiority of one over the other. What studies do support is the significant clinician effect on success with therapy approaches. In other words, a clinician with cursory knowledge and experience with tinnitus will likely have less success than more seasoned clinicians. Henry et al[90] found no difference in the effectiveness of tinnitus therapies (masking, TRT, basic education) when performed by clinicians with limited training and experience. However, management by a seasoned clinician demonstrated significant differences,[91,92] indicative of a clinician effect, that is, the training and experience of the clinician directly influence the effectiveness and benefit perceived by the patient.

There are many commonalities among these approaches, but there are also some perceived fundamental philosophical differences. All of these approaches are based on the idea of counteracting the negative reaction to tinnitus. The difference is belief in how the negative reaction was learned which in turn influences the approach to altering the reaction. Classical and operant conditioning are forms of learning. Classical conditioning was first described by Ivan Pavlov in 1927 and involves pairing a previously neutral stimulus with an unconditioned stimulus and unconditioned response. After associating the neutral stimulus and the unconditioned stimulus, the neutral stimulus becomes a conditioned stimulus resulting in a conditioned response. Operant conditioning, first described by Skinner in the 1930s, focuses on using either reinforcement (positive or negative) or punishment (positive or negative) to increase or decrease behavior. The traditional difference between classical and operant conditioning is focus on whether the behavior is involuntary or voluntary, where classical conditioning leans toward passive association and reflexive behavior; operant conditioning leans toward voluntary behavior that is manipulated via reinforcement/punishment. Of course, learning is not this simple and there is often overlap. For example, an involuntary behavior such as heart rate can be modified though operant conditioning techniques.

Classical and operant conditioning principles underlie some differences in theoretical frameworks that underlie approaches to tinnitus management. TRT is based in and leans toward classical conditioning theory with tinnitus response viewed as being mediated by the subconscious. On the other hand, TAT, based in aspects of cognitive behavioral theory leans more toward operant theory with reinforcement of the negative response mediated by cognitive distortions and maladaptive thoughts/behaviors. However, as mentioned previously, there is room for both principles at play. Below you will find discussion of some common therapeutic/counseling approaches to tinnitus.

Cognitive behavioral therapy: Behavioral therapy emerged in the 1960s and cognitive therapy in the 1970s. Behavioral therapy placed emphasis on the stimulus or behavior and cognitive therapy on thoughts or perceptions of the stimulus or behavior. The inherent overlap of these approaches led to use of the term cognitive behavioral therapy (CBT). By the 1980s, CBT was applied to a wide range of psychological issues including tinnitus.[93,94,95,96,97] The aim of CBT as with other tinnitus management approaches is to alter the distress experienced rather than the tinnitus sound itself. This is accomplished by helping people identify and modify maladaptive thoughts and behaviors that accompany their tinnitus distress. Identification of these automatic thoughts (or images), which reflect the persons' appraisal of a situation rather than the objective reality, can help to alter the emotional or behavioral response. These automatic thoughts or cognitive distortions with tinnitus are usually negative and involve generalization, all or none thinking, disqualifying the positive, etc. CBT challenges these maladaptive thoughts and behaviors, teaches the patient to recognize them, and to reinterpret. CBT can also include relaxation training, including imagery and breathing exercises. Numerous randomized controlled trials (RCT) with CBT have suggested significant improvement in affective elements of tinnitus.[98] CBT typically involves eight or more weekly sessions, lasting 1 to 2 hours. CBT can be administered one-on-one (in person or remotely) or in group settings. CBT typically progresses through sessions covering principles of CBT to identifying thoughts/emotions, identifying distortions, establishing alternatives, discussing relaxation, increasing positive activities, and skill reviews. Homework is often assigned through the process, which may involve keeping a diary to performing a specific behavior.

Sweetow[96] stressed that the patient may reject a purely psychological approach. Instead, the patient should be informed that tinnitus has a physiological origin, but the reaction is ultimately a psychological interpretation. Therefore, a CBT-based approach is appropriate and does not imply mental illness. CBT reached the level of recommendation by the AAO-HNS.[31] The possibility of psychological intervention such as CBT should be discussed early in the tinnitus management process to diffuse the idea of need due to the patient being "crazy." Rather the benefit is to help mitigate stress and improve overall well-being, so the brain can more effectively habituate to the tinnitus.

Tinnitus retraining therapy (TRT) was developed by Pawel Jastreboff and Jonathan Hazell over 25 years ago.[45] The approach was significantly influenced by Jastreboff's own animal work,[40] expanding knowledge of peripheral auditory system changes with pathology,[99,100,101] and an evolving critical mass of literature suggesting nonauditory brain regions implicated in tinnitus response[102,103,104,105]; though no experimental evidence existed at the time. The idea being that tinnitus perception alone is not pathological, but activation of nonauditory regions and negative association lead to a pathological state. This activation depends on the strength of the negative association and not on the perceptual characteristics (psychoacoustic measures: pitch, loudness) of the tinnitus itself. TRT involves a combination of counseling and sound-based therapy. The counseling is primarily directive or educational in nature with focus and stress on the neurophysiological model of tinnitus. The neurophysiological model proposed by Jastreboff and colleagues suggests peripheral pathology that leads to parallel processing involving subconscious detection and conscious perception of the tinnitus. At this same time, the limbic system, involved in emotional association of sensory signals, is activated. This in turn facilitates enhancement of the tinnitus and induces activation of the autonomic nervous system. The reaction of the autonomic nervous system is conditioned to the tinnitus signal as a conditioned reflex (subcortical/subconscious). This negative reaction is further reinforced (operant conditioning) by conscious perception of the tinnitus and association with fear and/or negative feelings (cortical/conscious). The outcome is a vivious cycle, where the presence of tinnitus and accompany limbic response results in increased attention and perception of the tinnitus.[106] The neurophysiological model postulates that many regions of the brain are involved in tinnitus and the auditory system plays a secondary role. The main goal TRT counseling is to reclassify the tinnitus into the category of a neutral stimulus and the main goal of the sound therapy is to decrease the strength of tinnitus-related neuronal activity; this leads to habituation of reactions and/or perception of the tinnitus.

Habituation takes place when a new stimulus becomes "well known" and loses relevance. An example often cited is a ring on the finger. Habituation often fails if the stimulus is associated with a negative evaluation. Habituation of tinnitus was first suggested by Hallam et al,[103] in his approach tinnitus was equated with any other sound a person may or may not attend, and the natural process of the brain is to habituate.

In TRT, emphasis is placed on the conditioned reflex pathway as dominating the reaction with the primary goal to habituate the reaction and secondary goal to habituate the perception. The overarching goal is to reach a point where the tinnitus is having a minimal impact on the patient's life. TRT implementation can vary depending on the patient's complaints. Categories were developed based on impact of tinnitus, subjective perception of hearing loss, hyperacusis, reactivity to sound, and response to specific sounds (e.g., misophonia). The sound therapy component involves use of sound (should not be a sound perceived as negative) set at a mixing point to diminish perception of the tinnitus; masking of the tinnitus is considered counterproductive; too low of sound is suggested to lead to increased perception of tinnitus related to stochastic resonance (phenomenon where a signal that is normally too weak to detect can be boosted by adding a white noise). The sound therapy process is aimed at facilitating the process of habituation of both tinnitus-induced reaction and perception by decreasing the difference between tinnitus-related neural activity and background neural activity. Over the years, TRT has undergone slight modification to incorporate new advances in the neuroscience of tinnitus, greater stress on hearing rehabilitation, and misophonia strategies.[107]

Tinnitus activities treatment (TAT) was developed by Richard Tyler. TAT is based in principles of cognitive behavioral therapy and was influenced by work of Hallam and colleagues.[68,97,102,108,109,110] TAT involves a series of interactive counseling sessions that cover topics including thoughts and emotions (emotional well-being), hearing and communication, sleep, and concentration. The three main components are counseling, activities engagement, and sound therapy (when needed).[111] Picture-based material is used to reinforce concepts. Not all patients require all four activities, the Tinnitus Activities Questionnaire can be used to assist in this decision.

Thoughts and emotions in TAT include listening to the patient, providing information on hearing, hearing loss, tinnitus, attention, and alternative thoughts. The activities with this topic including altering attention to and away from tinnitus, identifying activities to reduce attention, trying different low-level sounds, and keeping a short-term tinnitus diary (2 weeks). All counseling material can be located at the University of Iowa Tinnitus Clinic website http://www.medicine.uiowa.edu/oto/research/tinnitus/.

Sleep category of TAT focuses on understanding normal sleep patterns, factors that affect sleep, and sleep hygiene activities. This can include identifying variables that facilitate sleep, use of relaxation techniques, use of sound therapy, and possible sleep diary.

Hearing and communication in TAT involves discussion of tinnitus and impact on hearing and communication and communication strategies. Part of this involves counseling on the minimal impact tinnitus has on hearing, in other words, tinnitus is not the cause of hearing loss and removal of tinnitus would not resolve hearing difficulties, with acknowledgement that tinnitus can cause distraction and affect listening. If hearing loss is present, treatment options are discussed (e.g., hearing aids, assistive listening devices). In addition, communication strategies are highlighted (e.g., repair strategies, positioning, lighting, etc.). Activities in this section include apply communication strategies and keeping a diary of their impact.

Concentration is the final problem category in TAT. Here discussion focuses on distractions in the visual and auditory domain. Patients attempt to identify situations and elements that contribute to the distracting nature of their tinnitus. Strategies discussed include working in shorter time spans, eliminating other distractors, escalating task complexity, and sound therapy. The patient performs activities including switching attention from one stimulus to another. They may start by focusing on a physical sensation like shoes on their feet and switch attention to another stimulus. This helps to demonstrate some level of self-control. This is eventually performed with the tinnitus itself.

Sound-based therapy is commonly used (as mentioned above), but not required and at times not recommended. The sound therapy approach in TAT uses "partial masking," that is, the lowest-level sound that provides adequate relief. Caution is placed on frequent changes to sound as to not draw attention to tinnitus. A slower approach with sound may be necessary for those with sound reactive tinnitus, or tinnitus that is exacerbated in the presence of other sound.

Progressive audiologic tinnitus management (PATM/PTM) was developed by James Henry and colleagues; PTM is a hierarchical approach to tinnitus management used primarily in the VA setting. There are five levels to PTM. Level 1 is the triage for appropriate referral of patients based on complaints and needs; these are guidelines for nonaudiologist to determine appropriate referral needs. Level 2 is an audiological evaluation. A standardized audiological assessment is performed. Patient with hearing loss and complaints of hearing problems are fit with hearing aids. A patient take-home workbook, "How to Manage Your Tinnitus: A Step-by Step Workbook" is provided. The workbook includes many of the topics discussed above in CBT, TRT, and TAT. If no resolve in issues, the patient moves to level 3, group education. The group sessions consist of two sessions separated by 2 weeks. The sessions involve counseling on tinnitus and use of concepts in the workbook. Level 4 is a formal tinnitus evaluation, trial use of tinnitus management devices (e.g., ear-level sound generators), and possible referral to mental health. Level 5 is individualized management, which involves further counseling and possible formal CBT and/or TRT. A recent review on PTM is available to the interested reader.[112]

17.3.7 Applications of Sound Therapy

Sound therapy in tinnitus management has been long recognized. Hippocrates, Aristotle, or Pseudo-Aristotle are often credited with the quote "Why is it that buzzing in the ears ceases if one makes a sound? Is it because a greater sound drives out the less?". One of the earliest recording of sound therapy for tinnitus comes from Jean-Marie Itard, who in 1821 noted in his medical textbook that running water or wood crackling on the fire can help those with tinnitus. Over the last two centuries, many techniques have been proposed to deliver sound for relief of tinnitus; see Stephens[88] for review. Modern approaches of sound therapy for therapeutic purposes for tinnitus can be traced to the work of Jack Vernon in the 1970s.[113,114] Please see Henry[91] for a recent review of sound therapy approaches.

Sound therapy here is defined as any use of sound intended to alter tinnitus perception or reaction. Sound therapy approaches include masking and partial masking by use of background noise, environmental sound generators, ear-level sound generators, personal listening devices, hearing aids, proprietary devices, or combination of the above. Another novel application of sound is for engaging neuroplasticity to alter the strength of the tinnitus signal. The term masking here does not refer to conventional sound on sound masking that is dependent on critical band as in psychoacoustic procedures. Such rules do not apply to the "maskability" of tinnitus.

Total masking involves application of sound to reduce the perception of the tinnitus using a sound more acceptable to the patient. Total masking can provide immediate relief from the bothersome nature of the tinnitus. However, it does have its criticisms including need for intense sound for some patients to achieve masking and concern for counterproductivity to habituation.[115] Tyler et al[116] demonstrated no significant effect of total masking on habituation outcomes.

Partial masking refers to use of sound at levels that does not completely mask the tinnitus. There are numerous descriptors for partial masking and specific guidelines depending on the tinnitus management approach. TRT uses a "mixing point,"[115] the mixing point is defined as the level above stochastic resonance and below masking or annoyance, usually in the range of 6 to 20 dB SL. To set the mixing point, the sound therapy is raised until tinnitus and therapy sound are of equal audibility; the therapy sound is then lowered to just below this mixing level and/or level of annoyance. The therapy sound should not alter the tinnitus percept, rather to increase background neural activity to diminish contrast to tinnitus-related neural activity. On the other hand, TAT recommends the lowest level that provides adequate relief.

Partial or total masking can be achieved with environmental, ear-level, or personal listening devices (e.g., MP3 player, smartphone, etc.). Fukuda et al[117] compared hearing aids, sound generator, and personal listening devices for provision of TRT. All methods were effective in reducing tinnitus distress, however, there was no difference in efficacy.

The type of sound used is another consideration. Everything from BBN to simple amplification of environmental sounds (hearing aids) has demonstrated benefit. Other sound-based approaches have been developed and incorporated into proprietary treatment approaches. Applications of music have seen a particular increase for tinnitus management. Music relates to many human brain functions, such as perception, action, cognition, emotion, learning, and memory; neural structures underlying these brain functions have also been identified in tinnitus perception. Currently, there is no overwhelming evidence to suggest one form of sound therapy is most effective for tinnitus. However, unless they are part of a hearing aid they will not be beneficial for hearing loss.

Pearl	✔

Not all patients will report benefit from sound therapy (reactive tinnitus) and counseling and CBT-based approaches without sound therapy may be preferred initial approaches for treatment.

Hearing aids: One of the earliest suggestions of hearing aids for tinnitus relief dates to Saltzman and Ersner.[118] Hearing aids by themselves have been reported to provide tinnitus relief.[119] The benefits of hearing aids include an enriched soundscape, reduced salience of tinnitus, partial masking, altered attention to real sound, and of course improved hearing and reduced listening fatigue. Often patient with tinnitus will mistakenly attribute hearing difficulties to tinnitus and therefore intervention that improves hearing results in resolving some of these misplaced beliefs. Linear octave frequency transposition has also been suggested for tinnitus relief.[120] Perhaps of importance is also the change of treatment focus. Often patients with tinnitus have hearing loss and hearing loss complaints. A direct approach to treating tinnitus may actually increase focus on the tinnitus. For example, if a patient is putting on a sound generator every day to treat his/her tinnitus, is that not a daily reminder of tinnitus? Hearing aids can help alter this perception by using amplification to not only help with the tinnitus, but to help improve hearing and communication, a focus on treating the auditory system and not the tinnitus.

Combination devices and use of wireless technology: Combination devices refer to a hearing aid with a built-in sound generator. Most of the major hearing aid manufacturers have combination devices available. Although there are limited data, there are some to suggest enhanced benefit of a combination device to hearing aid alone.[121] The author prefers use of combination devices for tinnitus therapy for patients with hearing loss. The advantages include ability to provide a constant sound therapy-based sound and benefit of improved access to sound through amplification at minimal additional cost. In addition, wireless capabilities of hearing aids are continuing to improve with "made for smartphone" devices that do not require an intermediary device for communication. Many apps already exist for and are being developed for sound therapy approaches for tinnitus (on multiple platforms) and can be leveraged through wireless capable devices. Wireless technology expands sound options to almost limitless bounds. The con for this approach is drain on battery life for hearing aid and smartphone.

Neuromonics: Neuromonics Tinnitus Treatment utilizes sound therapy with a structured program of counseling. The sound therapy component involves listening to music that is spectrally modified to the individual's hearing thresholds. In phase I (preconditioning), the patient listens to relaxing music embedded with a BBN at least 2 hours or more per day, particularly when tinnitus is disturbing. The level of the music and noise is set to essentially mask the patient's tinnitus with a comfortable relaxing sound. Phase I lasts approximately

8 weeks. Phase II (active) eliminates the embedded noise. During this phase, the tinnitus is no longer masked and tinnitus perception occurs in an intermittent fashion facilitated by dynamic of the music. In other words, the music provides some level of masking in the peaks of the music and momentary perception in the troughs. Phase II lasts approximately 4 months or more.

Neuromonics was previously only performed with a proprietary device with Bang & Olafsen nonoccluding high-fidelity earphones. However, recently an app-based platform was released in 2016 that uses a subscription-based payment approach. Several trials have been completed showing significant success of Neuromonics for tinnitus relief,[122,123,124] however, the quality of these studies and appropriate randomization and controls was questionable.[125] Newman and Sandridge[126] compared the benefit and economic value between Neuromonics and ear-level sound generators. They found both treatments provided significant reduction of tinnitus; however, there was no difference between the two treatments. The sound generators were reported as the more cost-effective alternative.

Sound cure: Sound Cure is a sound-based intervention delivered as part of a broader tinnitus treatment program packaged in a proprietary device, at the time of writing called the Serenade. The sounds, called "S tones" are modulated sounds customized to the individual's tinnitus. The premise is based on protocols used to deliver electrical stimulation to cochlear implant patients,[127] which have been shown to suppress tinnitus in cochlear implant users (low rate pulse at 100 Hz). Based on this idea Reavis et al[128] examined different modulation rates with carrier frequencies near the tinnitus pitch and found greatest "suppression" with 40-Hz amplitude-modulated tones. The researchers claim that the effect is not masking, rather suppression of the tinnitus through interruption of the tinnitus generation. Whether the S tones are no different than masking is unclear, but reduction in perception of tinnitus can be achieved with lower stimulus levels compared to white noise. Despite the name, the developers do not claim the device as a cure for tinnitus.

Music notch therapy: Notched music was introduced by Okamoto et al.[129] The approach involves listening to music notched in the frequency band of one octave width centered at the individual tinnitus frequency. This was based on work by Pantev et al[130] that demonstrated listening to spectrally "notched" music can reduce cortical activity corresponding to the notch center frequency, possibly through lateral inhibition. Okamoto et al[129] showed positive effects in reduction of tinnitus loudness and distress compared to placebo-notched and wait list controls. However, the effect was neither seen for tinnitus with pitch matched above 8,000 Hz, nor were the effects persistent.[131] Other variations of notched

therapy have used noise instead of music.[132] Several app/computer-based platforms exist; ProMedical Audio and AudioNotch are two examples.

Acoustic coordinated reset neuromodulation therapy: This approach was based on electrical stimulation used to treat Parkinson's disease to disrupt (reset) pathological neural synchrony. However, instead of electrical stimulation, sound is used. The sound stimulation is tailored to each individual's tinnitus with tones presented around the pitch of the perceived tinnitus. The treatment has been shown to be effective in diminishing tinnitus perception,[133,134] however, no appropriately controlled trials have been performed, thus there is currently no evidence that the treatment is greater than a placebo.

Otoharmonics Levo System: The Levo System is specifically designed for use during sleep. No peer-published research could be found on the system. However, the approach appears to be based out of a group in Uruguay. The system uses sounds to mimic the individual's tinnitus, the sound is played during sleep to attempt to "reinstall the normal balance in the central-level processing of information." Studies have demonstrated significant improvement in tinnitus loudness and distress, but have lacked placebo-controlled designs.[135]

Fractal tones (Widex Zen): The Widex Zen product uses fractal tones, melodic sound that have a recursive algorithm to limit prediction. The fractal tones sound similar to music and have a wind chime quality without sudden change in tonality or tempo. It is suggested that the musical quality and relaxing nature of the fractal tones can improve tinnitus outcomes.[136,137]

Ultrasonic treatment: The inhibitor is an ultrasonic tinnitus treatment device marketed by MelMedtronics. The device is held against the patient's mastoid and delivers a high-frequency stimulation. A similar device the Aurex-3 also did not survive the marketplace. A handful of studies have shown some support to ultrasonic treatment,[138] but all have lacked appropriate placebo-controlled design.

Phase inversion: Phase inversion therapy is based on the principle of noise cancellation, such as in feedback with hearing aids. Several methods have been attempted with variable success, but no greater than placebo control. The major limitation of this approach is that tinnitus is not an acoustic signal and therefore does not have an acoustic phase to cancel. Any benefit from phase inversion is likely due to general sound therapy effects.

17.3.8 Medical Management of Tinnitus

Currently there are no FDA-approved medical (pharmacological and surgical) treatments for tinnitus. Numerous attempts at medical resolution of tinnitus exist within the literature. However, intervention is limited by the highly heterogeneous nature of tinnitus. Medical management is also dependent on the type of tinnitus. In many cases, somatosound forms of tinnitus (pulsatile and nonpulsatile) may be alleviated through medical intervention. In addition, medical management for tinnitus must be divided into interventions directed at the elimination of tinnitus versus those directed at an independent primary otopathology whose symptoms include tinnitus, where altered tinnitus may be a secondary event. For example, an individual with chronic otitis media may experience tinnitus due to the conductive nature of the hearing loss, however, after myringotomy or placement of tympanostomy tube, the tinnitus is no longer perceivable. Here we will focus our conversation on medical management directed at resolution specifically of tinnitus.

Surgery: Surgical interventions for somatosound forms of tinnitus are dependent on the source of the somatosound. Benign intracranial hypertension may require placement of a shunt. ACAD may necessitate carotid endarterectomy or carotid angioplasty with stenting. Surgical repair of sinus aneurysms, removal of masses, ligation procedures, or microvascular decompression may also be performed. Myoclonic tinnitus can be resolved with sectioning of muscles contributing to the somatosound.[81]

Surgical intervention for neurophysiological tinnitus is less straightforward. Attempts to resolve tinnitus surgically have been made at various levels of the auditory system, with varying degrees of success. Surgical sectioning or ablation of the vestibulocochlear nerve (eighth nerve) was hypothesized as a potential treatment for tinnitus, under the premise that tinnitus has a peripheral source. There are reports of surgical sectioning of the eighth nerve resulting in the relief of tinnitus, however, in these cases relief was secondary in nature due to treatment of the primary pathology (e.g., vestibular schwannoma). House and Brackmann[139] described outcomes of several surgeries and the effect on tinnitus (nerve sectioning, stapedectomies, etc.) and found improvement in approximately 40% of patients and unchanged nature or worsening in 60%. Pulec[140] reported much greater success using a translabyrinthine section of the eighth nerve. Out of 93 cases, 62 reported complete relief, 26 showed improvement, and 5 showed no improvement. The majority of the patients had Meniere's disease. Interesting fact: the first eighth nerve section was performed in 1898 by Krause for intractable tinnitus, the attempt was unsuccessful and the operation eventually fatal.

Several forms of neuromodulation treatments for tinnitus are in development. Some of these neuromodulation approaches involve surgery while others do not. Deep brain stimulation (DBS) has been used to clinically treat several neurologic diseases, such as Parkinson's disease and essential tremor. A handful of studies have examined applications of DBS to tinnitus. The first study stimulated the ventral intermediate nucleus of the thalamus in patients with tinnitus and concomitant movement disorders. Three of the seven patients experienced a decrease in tinnitus without perceptual change in hearing.[141] A second study was performed in patients with Parkinson's disease or essential tremor patients. DBS was intraoperatively activated to stimulate the caudate nucleus. The patient was blinded to the stimulation. In five of six patients there was acute suppression of tinnitus during stimulation.[142] The exact mechanism by which DBS exerts therapeutic effect is not yet fully understood; hypotheses include silencing of neurons (inhibition of surrounding neurons) and modification of pathological activity.[143]

Vagus nerve stimulation via an implanted neurostimulator has been used to treat epilepsy for decades, the first human study was published in 1990.[144] However, vagus nerve stimulation alone does not seem to alter tinnitus. De Ridder et al[145] implanted 10 patients with neurostimulators and paired the stimulation with tones and saw reduction in tinnitus in four of the patients. The lack of effect in the remaining patients was attributed to concomitant medications.

Noninvasive neuromodulation alternatives to DBS and vagus stimulation include repetitive transcranial magnetic stimulation (TMS), transcranial direct current stimulation (tDCS), and transcutaneous electric nerve stimulation (TENS). TMS involves applying an impulse magnetic field that induces an electrical current and can alter neural activity, when repeated in trains of stimulation, it is referred to as repetitive TMS. In tDCS, a relatively weak constant current (between 0.5 and 2 mA) is passed to the cerebral cortex via scalp electrodes. Depending on the polarity, tDCS can increase or decrease cortical excitability. TENS is another method of applying electrical current, but to other regions such as the median nerve, temporomandibular joint, and upper cervical nerve region (C2). Randomized studies show some small improvements with these techniques, no effect at all, and even elicitation of tinnitus.[146]

Cochlear implants (CI) have shown success in alleviating tinnitus in patients with severe-to-profound hearing loss. Van de Heyning et al[147] demonstrated significant reduction in tinnitus loudness and distress with CI stimulation. Kim et al[148] showed elimination in 10 of 40 patients with tinnitus and improvement in 16 of 40. Some patients with CIs report sleep difficulties related to tinnitus. Pierzycki et al[149] suggested this was related to suppression of tinnitus while active electrical stimulation and return of tinnitus upon removal of external component during sleep. An alternative is to simply keep the CI on.

Pharmacological: Many drugs have been examined for treatment of tinnitus; unfortunately, there is not consistent therapeutic benefit, again reflective of the heterogeneous nature of tinnitus. Currently, there are no FDA- or EMEA-approved drugs for the treatment of tinnitus. Here we will review some of the more common drugs that have been studied.

Lidocaine was first found to suppress tinnitus in 1935. Lidocaine is generally used as a local anesthetic and for treatment of cardiac arrhythmias. The mode of action is complex, but involves modulation of voltage-gated sodium channels. Several clinical studies have demonstrated transient tinnitus suppression by intravenous administration. However, the effects are short-lived and risk of potentially life-threatening side effects limits application as a tinnitus treatment option. Tocainide is an oral analogue of lidocaine. Clinical studies have found no significant benefit for tinnitus.

Antidepressants have also been examined for application to tinnitus. Tricyclic antidepressants include nortriptyline (Sensoval, Aventyl, Norpress, Allegron, etc.), amitriptyline (Elavil), and trimipramine (Surmontil, Rhotrimine, Stangyl). In general, these drugs have roles in reuptake of serotonin and other NT (norepinephrine, dopamine, and noradrenaline), but differ in mode of action. Besides treatment for depression, tricyclic antidepressants have been shown to be effective for treatment of chronic pain. Effects on tinnitus have been inconsistent. Amitriptyline was shown to significantly reduce tinnitus complaints and loudness compared to a placebo group.[150] However, tricyclic antidepressants have also been shown to induce tinnitus.[151] Selective serotonin reuptake inhibitors (SSRIs) have also been examined. SSRIs are a class of antidepressants that function in part by increasing extracellular levels of the NT serotonin by blocking or limiting uptake increasing duration of serotonin available in the synaptic cleft to bind to postsynaptic receptors. Paroxetine (Paxil) was not found to be more effective than placebo; sertraline (Zoloft) was found to be more effective than placebo in reducing tinnitus severity, but not annoyance.[152] The general consensus is that tinnitus patients with depression and anxiety may benefit from antidepressants, but is related to benefit on the comorbid state of depression/anxiety. Use of antidepressants for tinnitus without comorbid depression or anxiety is not recommended.[153] Cyclobenzaprine a tricyclic

antidepressant analog and muscle relaxer at a high dose (30 mg) was able to significantly reduce THI scores, however, the findings were not placebo-controlled.[154,155]

Benzodiazepines enhance the effects of the NT gamma-aminobutyric acid (GABA) resulting in decreased excitability. They are commonly used as sedatives, antianxiety (anxiolytics), anticonvulsants, and muscle relaxants. Alprazolam (Xanax) has been shown to reduce tinnitus loudness compared to a control group, however, the findings have not been replicated.[156,157] Diazepam (Valium) has also been evaluated with no reported benefit for tinnitus.[158] Clonazepam (Klonopin) showed benefit for tinnitus in a small study.[159] The limitation of benzodiazepines is the high risk for drug dependency and protracted tinnitus upon discontinuation of drug.[152]

Antiseizure medications (anticonvulsants) have also been examined for treatment of tinnitus. Anticonvulsants work through numerous mechanisms, but in general involve stabilizing receptor states and reducing neural activity. Gabapentin is commonly used for treatment of neuropathic pain and migraines. Placebo-controlled study has found no benefit for tinnitus.[160] However, there has been some report of gabapentin supplemented with clonazepam for tinnitus relief.[161] Vigabatrin has shown promise in animal studies, but can cause visual field deficits in humans and application is restricted. Carbamazepine may provide relief for tinnitus in patients that respond to intravenous lidocaine.[162] A specific application of carbamazepine has been with "typewriter tinnitus" associated with vascular compression of the auditory nerve.[163]

Antiglutamatergic drugs function as glutamate antagonist, the primary excitatory NT of the auditory system. Caroverine, an antagonist of glutamate receptors, has shown some promise in reducing tinnitus loudness, but results have not been replicated. Acamprosate enhances GABAergic transmission and blocks NMDA receptors and is approved for the treatment of alcoholism. In a double-blind placebo-controlled study, acamprosate resulted in significant reduction in tinnitus loudness.[164] AM-101 or Keyzilen (Auris Medical) is an NMDA antagonist, applied to the middle ear space via transtympanic injection. The drug is the S-enantiomer of ketamine. Double-blind placebo-controlled randomized study found improvement in loudness and annoyance of tinnitus.[165]

Numerous other pharmacological agents are currently being explored for tinnitus including potassium ion channel modulators (e.g., Maxipost), antioxidants (e.g., ebselen), EGb-761 (concentrated version of Ginkgo biloba), and many more.

An excellent recent review is available to the interested reader—Langguth et al.[152]

17.4 Lifestyle Management of Tinnitus

A healthy lifestyle is important to our general health, mood, and well-being. Eating healthy, exercise and physical activity, sleep and stress reduction are all on the table when it comes to tinnitus.

Diet: There is limited study of the influence of diet on tinnitus. Most of the work on diet and tinnitus is challenged by lack of RCT. A handful of studies have suggested specific dietary deficiencies underlying risk for tinnitus, most commonly B-complex and zinc. However, the application of supplements to treat tinnitus is inconclusive at best. Despite lack of support to supplements, there is some support to healthy diet influencing susceptibility to hearing loss and tinnitus. Spankovich and colleagues demonstrated a significant relationship between dietary quality and both hearing and tinnitus. The findings suggested that a healthy diet that meets USDA recommendations is associated with better high-frequency hearing and decreased report of persistent tinnitus.[166,167,168] Other work has shown lower odds of tinnitus report with higher intake of fish, lower intake of eggs, and higher intake of caffeinated coffee. Increased odds were reported with greater bread intake and greater vegetable/fruit intake. However, the strengths of these relationships though statistically significant were small in effect size.[169] There are no conclusive data suggesting dietary changes that will cure existing tinnitus.

Patients commonly report effects of specific foods or drinks on their tinnitus, both positive and negative. These effects are most often transient in nature. The patient should be counseled on eating a healthy diet as to improve overall health, but not to cure the tinnitus. In addition, the patient needs to determine the cost–benefit of making specific changes. For example, a patient may experience transient spikes in their tinnitus with his or her morning coffee. It is not likely this will lead to permanent changes in the tinnitus perception. It is now the patient's decision to discontinue coffee intake, which may lead to headache or mood changes or is the morning coffee worth the transient tinnitus spike. Changes should be of a positive nature to improve general health and de-emphasis on tinnitus as the central reason for change. In some cases, such as Meniere's disease–specific dietary recommendations may be made, such as reduced sodium intake.

General recommendations include lowering overall caloric intake, lowering intake of high glycemic index foods (e.g., sugar sweetened foods), lowering intake of saturated fats, lowering intake of processed foods (often high sodium), and increasing intake of fruits, vegetables, seeds, nuts, and fish. Alcohol intake should be in moderation. The patient should discuss any dietary change with their primary care physician or dietician/nutritionist. An excellent diet to consider is the Dietary Approach to Stop Hypertension (DASH) diet.

Physical activity: Tinnitus can have significant impact on quality of life. However, individuals with higher levels of physical activity report lower tinnitus severity and reduced effects on life.[170] In addition, there is some suggestion to decreased odds of reporting tinnitus with greater physical activity.[171] Patients should be counseled on being active and exercise not only to improve general health, but also to help in distraction/attention to tinnitus, and improve sleep.

Sleep hygiene: Sleep issues remain a common complaint of individuals with tinnitus. Tinnitus can interfere with sleep and lack of sleep can lead to increased difficulty with tinnitus.[172] Often patients will report minimal difficulty during the day with their tinnitus (due to distraction or elevated sound) and issues only with sleep. Patients with CI that achieve suppression of tinnitus while wearing the implant will often complain of difficulty sleeping due to perceivable tinnitus once CI is deactivated. The CI problem is easy; wear the CI to sleep. Other patients can benefit from basic sleep hygiene recommendations. See the box on Sleep Hygiene Tips from the American Sleep Association. Sound therapy can also beneficial for sleep. The patient should use a relaxing and soothing sound, not a sound that incurs active listening. The sound can be played through tabletop speakers, earphones, or a sound pillow. A sound pillow is a pillow with a speaker inside and headphone jack attached. It can often be a good option for patients with spouses that do not wish to hear the sound therapy sound.

Smoking: Several studies have suggested greater odds of reporting tinnitus in smokers. This does indicate smoking causes tinnitus, but lifestyle and general health can influence tinnitus.

Social media and internet: The Internet, social media, online support groups are often negative influences on tinnitus. The patient should be instructed to avoid excessive searching and researching cures, as it will only bring greater attention to their tinnitus. The audiologist should serve as their resource.

Sleep Hygiene Tips from the American Sleep Association

- Go to sleep at same time (have a routine).
- Avoid naps.
- Don't just stay in bed with mind racing; get out of bed and sit in a chair with soothing sound and go back to bed when tired.
- Do not watch TV or read in bed, reserve for sleep and hanky-panky.
- Do not drink caffeine prior to bed, limit use to before noon.
- Cigarettes, alcohol, and medications can alter sleep, avoid if possible.
- Exercise regularly, but not right before bed.
- Do not drink or eat a large meal right before bed that may necessitate a trip to the bathroom in middle or night.
- Set your thermostat to a comfortable temperature, generally a little cooler. Keep pets where less likely to awaken you.
- Keep bedroom dark.
- Have a comfortable bed and pillow.
- Use a soft soothing sound to help diminish perception of tinnitus, the sound should engage passive not active listening; a sound pillow (pillow with speaker inside) is an excellent option.

17.4.1 Alternative Treatments for Tinnitus

Neurofeedback or biofeedback training: Neurofeedback or neurobiofeedback is a type of therapy that uses real-time displays of brain activity, most commonly with EEG, to teach self-regulation of brain function. Other forms of biofeedback also exist that use other functional measures to teach control and relaxation. Research has been inconclusive and often lacks appropriate placebo controls, but several reports suggest benefit. The effect is believed to be related to correcting abnormal oscillatory brain activity, that is, altered brain waves with enhancement in alpha activity and enhancement of tau activity and reduction in delta activity. It is believed the alpha activity has an inhibitory role.[54,173,174,175]

Hypnosis: Hypnotherapy for tinnitus has a long history. However, no large-scale, randomized control studies have been performed. Hypnotherapy can promote relaxation and reduce anxiety and therefore may have benefit for tinnitus patients. Self-hypnosis has also been shown to be beneficial.[176]

Laser treatment: Laser treatment involves use of a soft or low-powered laser focused into the patient's ear canal and directed toward the cochlea through the tympanic membrane. Studies including a placebo group have demonstrated no significant effects.[177,178]

Wearable magnets: Magnets have been purported as treatment for a variety of conditions. Devices are commonly worn as bracelets or necklaces. Takeda[179] found a magnet embedded in cotton and placed in the ear of tinnitus patients resulted in reduction in symptoms in 66% of cases. No control was employed. A placebo-controlled design found no effect of magnet in the ear canal.[180]

Hyperbaric oxygen therapy: Hyperbaric oxygen (HBO2) therapy involves breathing 100% oxygen at elevated ambient pressure. The therapy can reduce hematocrit and improve hemorheology. Application of HBO2 has been shown to have some effect on acute hearing loss and possibly acute tinnitus. However, improvement in chronic tinnitus is not supported[181] and has been shown to be influenced by psychological status and expectations of patients.[182]

Acupuncture/acupressure: There have been many reports on benefit of acupuncture for the treatment of tinnitus. The majority of the studies showing positive benefit are in Chinese, the majority showing no benefit are in English. Liu et al[183] performed a recent meta-analysis and found five blinded RCT examining acupuncture for tinnitus. Four out of the five found no significant effect. The authors suggest limited benefit of acupuncture for tinnitus and describe numerous methodological flaws that limit a definitive conclusion.

Supplements: Numerous supplements have been explored for tinnitus management. The biggest limitation to supplements is the lack of regulation in contents and quality of the agent. Recent random quality test has found that many popular supplements from places including GNC, Walgreens, CVS, and Target contained zero amounts of the purported agent (O'Connor[184]). One of the most popular herbal supplements proposed for tinnitus is Ginkgo biloba, a bioactive flavonoid with terpenes and both vasoactive and antioxidant properties. Some studies have suggested benefit of Ginkgo (in form of EGb-761) in comparison to control,[185] while others have not.[186,187] Currently, the evidence for Ginkgo biloba for tinnitus is inconclusive. Proponents and opponents to Ginkgo point to study design issues on either side, regardless no studies have shown that Ginkgo is a cure for tinnitus. In addition, Ginkgo can alter platelet-activating factor and lead to interactions in conjunction with other antiplatelet agents (e.g., aspirin, warfarin) and can potentially interact with other medications.

Melatonin is a naturally occurring hormone that plays a role in regulating circadian rhythms. Melatonin has shown some benefit for reduced subjective rating in tinnitus and improvement in sleep quality, whereas other studies have shown no benefit compared to placebo. The benefit associated with tinnitus seems to be limited to improvement in sleep disturbances.[188]

Bojungikgitang and banhabaekchulchonmatang are two herbal medicines used in Korea and are approved by the Korea Food and Drug Administration for the treatment of tinnitus. Kim et al[189] reported a study protocol for a randomized double-blind placebo-controlled study, however, no results were presented nor have been published to date. Anecdotal reports of other Oriental Medicine herbal treatments including Er Ming Fang and Yoku-kan-san for tinnitus relief have been reported, but lack any formal study.[190]

Currently, there are dozens of over-the-counter supplements with a variety of lipoflavanoids, vitamins, minerals, herbs, and spices. The audiologist is cautioned in recommending any of these supplements for treatment of tinnitus. Rationale for caution includes (1) lack of well-designed placebo-controlled studies, even compounds that have received significant study show questionable benefit (Ginkgo biloba) and (2) Lack of quality control and regulation of these products. Robert DiSogra, AuD has a text available on over-the-counter products for tinnitus that includes a breakdown of ingredients and review of the literature on effectiveness for tinnitus (Over-the-Counter Tinnitus Relief Products by DiSogra). A recent review of alternative treatments for tinnitus is recommended to the interested reader.[191]

17.4.2 Tips and Strategies for Working with Tinnitus Patients

Working with tinnitus patients can be a challenge, however, it is a challenge worth pursuing. Many of these patients simply need someone to acknowledge tinnitus as a real phenomenon and provide some simple explanations and tips and strategies for dealing with their tinnitus. There is a significant clinician effect. The more experienced and knowledgeable the clinician in a specific approach to tinnitus, often the better the outcomes.[90] Here we will review five take-home messages for tinnitus patients and useful analogies to incorporate into your dialogue.

> **Pearl** ✔
>
> The provider's experience, knowledge, and counseling skills can significantly influence outcomes.

1. *Understanding the source:* It is critical that the patient understand what tinnitus represents. A primary function of the audiologist and corresponding medical colleague (e.g., otolaryngologist) is to rule

out serious medical pathology related to the tinnitus percept. An appropriate audiological and medical evaluation can help alleviate concerns that the tinnitus is a symptom of something more significant. To help the patient understand tinnitus it is recommended to provide an overview of normal hearing. The objective is to enable the patient to understand that we hear with our brains and that the peripheral auditory system (external ear—auditory nerve) functions to take sound and convert to a signal the brain can interpret. After reviewing normal hearing, you can then talk about the patient's hearing and the type of hearing loss they may be experiencing. Next, it is helpful to discuss tinnitus as a nonpathological phenomenon. A great example is to review the work of Heller and Bergman and similar studies. Finally, you can move to discussion of tinnitus and provide a basic overview of the neuroscience of tinnitus as described earlier in the chapter.

A simple explanation is as follows (for someone with hearing loss) "we have ruled out significant medical disease underlying your tinnitus. The tinnitus you are experiencing is related to your hearing loss. When there is damage to the peripheral auditory system, central portions of the system change to try to adapt and/or compensate for the loss of input, this is called neural plasticity. These changes can include changes in neural mapping and increase in neural activity to try to essentially fill in the gap. The net effect is neural activity sending a signal to regions of the brain involved in sound processing; these brain regions interpret the signal as the tinnitus you perceive. I say regions of the brain because the perception of tinnitus involves a broad network of brain regions that are involved in sound perception, memory, attention, vigilance, and emotional response and changes to these different regions can alter perception of tinnitus. The difficulty for the brain is resolving the meaning of the tinnitus, which influences the attention and stress-based response the patient experiences. It makes sense for the brain to view tinnitus as something negative. Here is a sound that you were not perceiving previously or has worsened to a point where it is impacting your life. When you hear tinnitus, your first reaction is not this must mean I am healthier and my hearing has improved." I often incorporate visuals and discussion of specific parts of the brain involved in tinnitus perception and reaction.

Myth busting is also important. First, tinnitus will not cover up your ability to hear, nor is why the patient has difficulty understanding speech in noise, that is the patient's hearing loss. Second, tinnitus is not likely coming from the ear; rather the brain perceives this because a sound's usual pathway is from the external ear. Third, tinnitus is not commonly a sign of life-threatening disease; rather it is a common side effect of hearing loss and most people will experience tinnitus when in very quiet laboratory settings (subaudible tinnitus). Fourth, it makes sense for the brain to view as negative due to the novel and unexplained nature.

2. *Understanding habituation and cognitive restructuring:* Habituation is a psychophysiological process wherein there is a decrease in response to a stimulus after repeated exposure. The brain has a natural ability to habituate, in other words to filter out irrelevant stimuli and focus selectively on important stimuli. The brain is fairly effective at this process and the patient must understand this process. A simple explanation is as follows "your brain is constantly sent a stream of neural input all day, much of this information is determined to be noncritical and put to the background. Good examples are the shoes on your feet, the watch on your wrist, or ring on your finger. All day you have been wearing shoes (or watch, ring, etc.), but you were not actively feeling them until I just mentioned them. However, those shoes have been stimulating touch receptors on your feet all day and sending the message to your brain, but it has been going to the 'junk mail.' Now I mention the shoes and force your brain to read that message. Now, no matter how hard you try you will not be feeling the shoes on your feet by the end of this appointment. That is because your brain will have more important stimuli to attend too, that is habituation. Your brain does this not only with tactile input, but also sounds. You may hear the air conditioner turn on in your house. You notice it turn on because it is novel to the soundscape. However, you then go about what you are doing and no longer are actively listening to that sound even though it is there."

Cognitive restructuring represents an interactive identification of maladaptive thoughts and behaviors regarding the patient's tinnitus. The audiologist helps to identify these maladaptive patterns and provides alternative thoughts and behaviors with a more positive and logical view. For example, the patient may have a negative thought "my life used to be perfect before I had tinnitus, now it is terrible." This is an example of all or none thinking. An alternative thought is "life was never perfect, you likely had some problems before, and still have good things in your life."

3. *Sound and sound therapy:* Specific recommendations for sound therapy may be based on the management approach and hearing status. However, almost all approaches recommended keeping some soft soothing sound in the background and avoiding silence. This necessitates the discussion of "what is silence." The world is simply not devoid of sound. As I sit my "silent" office, I hear the air conditioning in the hallway, light conversation of colleagues, the fan in my computer, the clicking of my keystrokes, and even my own breathing. In truth, tinnitus or not, there is no such thing as silence, just what we subjectively perceive as silence. The purpose of sound therapy is to stimulate the brain with real sound and to train the brain to recognize that constant sound does not need to be annoying or bothersome, rather it can be soothing and relaxing. If your brain can find one sound to be meaningless and habituate, it can do the same thing with the tinnitus. In truth, they are both sounds, just one has an external source and one does not. The bothersome or annoyance of the tinnitus is subjective and can be altered. If you are going to be around high-level sounds (concerts, amplified music, power tools, etc.), use hearing protection devices. However, do not use hearing protection when in quiet or moderate-level environments. If the patient has hearing loss, hearing aids with a combination sound therapy option or wireless capability are the author's recommendation (see Sound Therapy section).

4. *Distraction:* Attention has significant role in tinnitus perception. Often patients will report they can hear their tinnitus 24/7. However, in most cases, tinnitus patients do not actively perceive their tinnitus 24/7. Very rarely do patient report also experiencing tinnitus even in their dreams. The 24/7 report is commonly based on the ability to listen for and hear tinnitus at any time. Rather, most people with tinnitus, if distracted, can go some duration of time without active perception of their tinnitus. Recommendations to distract from the tinnitus include not empowering tinnitus, try not to make it a central factor in your life, avoid doing research or online chat groups. Engage in activities that are positive and stimulating when bothered by the tinnitus.

If you are bothered by your tinnitus, don't just sit there and listen to it, get up and do something else to alter the brain's attention. Patients can consider practicing distraction with their tinnitus. Here the patient focuses on their tinnitus with minimal environmental stimuli (e.g., turn off other sounds, turn off TV, etc.) for 10 to 20 seconds and notes the loudness, sound quality, and annoyance. By focusing on the tinnitus, the patient may be able to change the loudness or notice modulations in the quality. Then the patient should engage in some positive enjoyable activity in a sound-enriched environment. The goal is try not to attend to the tinnitus during this exercise. With the practice, the patient will begin to improve his or her ability to disengage from the tinnitus. However, this is not an easy task. It is common for individuals to notice their tinnitus more after initiating a tinnitus management approach. Why? Well, how do you know if the treatment is working unless you monitor the effect on your tinnitus? The patient needs to push past this common reaction.

5. *Diet, exercise, and lifestyle:* Lifestyle is a critical element in diminishing tinnitus issues. Tinnitus should not be a central component of the patient's life. Keeping active and busy and exercise can help distract the brain from the tinnitus and aid in improved health in general, including improved sleep. Eating healthy is important to our general health and well-being. Eating healthy will not cure tinnitus, but can help and basic recommendations are provided above. If there are activities, the patient is longer participating in because of the tinnitus, they can feel free to do those things again and enjoy life again. They can still go to concerts, play music, etc., but just use hearing protection (only around loud sounds). Also, application of relaxation training and alternative therapies to reduce stress can be discussed. This can include progressive muscle relaxation, deep breathing, imagery, meditation, Tai Chi, yoga, etc, or extend to recommendation for formal CBT or other psychological therapy.

17.4.3 Analogies

Ear Lid's and Brain's Response to absence of sound: We were not born with ear lids, in other words we cannot voluntarily stop hearing. Even if you put your fingers in your ears or use hearing protection, you can still hear. We don't really ever stop hearing. Our auditory system is our built-in warning system. It is not the visual of a crying baby that wakes you up at night, but rather the sound. Therefore, when we are placed in an artificial environment with low sound levels, such as a sound-treated room, our brain increases sensitivity. Essentially, the brain is trying to hear something. This increase in sensitivity can lead to perception of tinnitus, or detection of underlying neural input without an external source. With hearing loss, now the brain changes to try to compensate (called neural plasticity) to fill in the gap, the result can also be tinnitus.

Tinnitus perception and car engine noise: Cars make sound, engine noise, road noise, stereo/radio, etc. Of these sounds, we don't often focus on the engine sound. However, if you were driving your car down the road and began to perceive a knocking noise from the engine, it would grab your attention. Your first reaction to hearing a knocking noise in your engine is not likely positive. You don't likely think to yourself, "Yes! This is a good sign" or "My engine must be working even better and I am going to get more miles per gallon and another 20 years out of this car." No, your first reaction is more likely "what is this sound and how much is this going to cost me." Now, the car engine was already making sound, but it was a sound that you perceived as "normal," the new unexpected sound was perceived as "abnormal." What if the sound was not an obvious "knocking" but rather a slight rougher engine sound. We all expect some wear and tear to our car engine and a car you purchased 10 years ago does not sound the exact same as when you drove off the lot. Yet, we don't pay more attention to that sound. What creates the difference is how we interpret the meaning of each sound, but both are sounds.

Same sound different meaning example (the Cat): Say you have family visiting for the weekend. It is late in the evening and you are lying in bed, about to drift off to sleep and you hear a creek in the floor and someone rummaging through the kitchen. Your reaction is likely fairly minor. You notice the sound and think to yourself that must be my visiting family member getting a glass of water. Now, say you are lying in bed, about to drift off to sleep and you hear a creek in the floor and someone rummaging through the kitchen, but no one is visiting. Your reaction is likely different. In both cases, the sound was the exact same, creek in floor and rummaging in kitchen. However, the response was very different. The difference is in part of the source, you know source of the first sound, in the second example, you don't know the source. In addition to the source is knowing the consequences. In the first case, this was perceived as benign and in the second as a sign of danger. It could be someone breaking in, someone there to hurt you, or it could be the cat.

Habituation: Classic examples include things you wear (e.g., watch, shoes), things you smell, and even sounds (HVAC system to refrigerator). See habituation example above.

Reduce tinnitus perception with sound, light example: If you turn all the lights on in a room and shine a flashlight on the wall, you will have limited ability to see the light from the flashlight. If you turn off the room lights, the flashlight is then very noticeable. Tinnitus will in most cases be less noticeable with a sound-enriched environment and perception will often increase without sound or with hearing loss that reduces sound to the system.

Ephaptic neural transmission/cross-talk: Ephaptic transmission refers to cross-talk between neural elements. If there is damage to a neural region due to a head–neck injury or disease, this can result in damage to the myelin sheathing and can lead to a neural leakage that can stimulate surrounding neural elements. This is similar to taking to electrical wires plugged into the wall and cutting off the insulation. If you bring those wires close to each other, you can see arching of the electricity across the wires. A similar event can happen with neural pathways. This may now result in a signal that normally only stimulated a motor or touch-associated region of the brain to now arch over and stimulate the auditory region. The auditory region does not know this signal is not coming from the ear, all it knows is that it is being stimulated, that means sound, in this case tinnitus.

Broken arm pain and hearing aids for tinnitus: If I was a primary care physician and you came to me with a broken arm complaining of pain, I could just give you aspirin and send you home. However, that is not the likely treatment. Rather, I would give you aspirin for the pain, and also set the broken bone and put you in a cast. Let's apply to tinnitus. In this case, tinnitus is like the pain, indeed there are many similarities between brain regions involved in pain perception and tinnitus, as well as the subjective nature. The hearing loss is the broken arm. Sound therapy and counseling is the aspirin. To appropriately address the pain (tinnitus), we must treat the break (hearing loss). Hearing aids are the tools we use to treat broken hearing and can be effective for tinnitus.

17.4.4 Tinnitus and Sound Sensitivity

Tinnitus can often present with a comorbidity of sound sensitivity. Sound sensitivity (SS) or decreased sound tolerance (DST) can manifest with a spectrum of complaints. Sound sensitivity can be classified based on presence of loudness intolerance or lack of loudness intolerance (▶**Fig. 17.1**). Loudness intolerance refers to an abnormal growth or perception of sound level, in other words, sound that others commonly find soft or moderate in loudness is perceived at a much greater subjective level. Hyperacusis and recruitment represent two forms of loudness intolerance. Nonloudness intolerance forms of sound sensitivity can include misophonia and phonophobia. In this, the patient does not necessarily report loudness complaints, rather an abnormally strong stress-based reaction to sounds. However, patients can present with both loudness intolerance and stress-based reaction. Sensory processing disorder (SPD) is recognized here as a separate phenomenon. Often SPD is associated with other sensory processing issues or disorders associated with sensory issues (e.g., autism spectrum disorder) and sound sensitivity related to louder unexpected sounds or sources with a conditioned fear or emotional response. It should be noted that there are other classification systems for sound sensitivity.

Hyperacusis: Hyperacusis is defined as an unusual tolerance to ordinary environmental sounds. The prevalence estimates of hyperacusis are primarily derived from smaller studies and vary between 3.2 and 17.6% depending on the study design and study population. No standard criteria exist to determine presence of hyperacusis.[27] However, these estimates are fairly comparable to tinnitus. Indeed, it has been reported that approximately 60% of tinnitus patients also report sound sensitivity, of these, approximately 30% have hyperacusis. On the other hand, it has been reported that 86% of patient with hyperacusis also report tinnitus.

The mechanism underlying hyperacusis has been attributed to changes in central gain. Determining the origin of central gain is complicated by the complex nature of the auditory system. Salvi et al's[192] noise exposed chinchillas and recorded potentials from the auditory nerve, cochlear nucleus, and inferior colliculus. Responses from the nerve and cochlear nucleus were reduced post noise, but responses from the inferior colliculus were enhanced with increased stimulus level. Nonauditory regions can also show enhancement including the amygdala, striatum, and hippocampus, and these regions can modulate enhancement in auditory regions. See Auerbach et al[193] for an excellent review of central gain mechanisms.

Individuals with hyperacusis can also experience pain with sound, sometimes called pain hyperacusis.[194] The pain is often described as a neural pain, sometimes reported as a stabbing pain or chronic burning sensation. Indeed, pain-transmitting neuropeptides and receptors are present in the cochlear

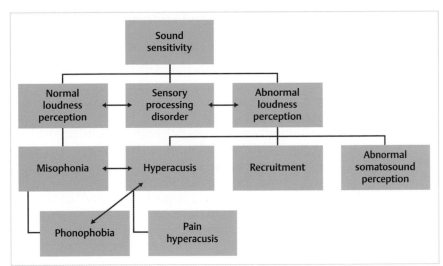

Fig. 17.1 Types of sound sensitivity. Sound sensitivity can be categorized as involving normal or abnormal perception of sound loudness. Overlap of subcategories is common. Sensory processing disorder is recognized here as a separate category with auditory sensitivity commonly associated with other sensory issues and emotional reactions. However, it may be just as prudent to place sound sensitivity as a variant of SPD.

nucleus and the auditory nerve. It has been suggested that damage to auditory nerve fibers results in spontaneous activity at the level of the cochlear nucleus leading to activation of these pain receptors. Type II afferents have recently been implicated in this noxacusis or painful form of hyperacusis.[195] It is also plausible that more central regions mediate pain response similar to phantom limb pain.

Recruitment: Recruitment refers to a form of sound sensitivity related to hearing loss and refers to an abnormal growth of loudness due to elevated hearing thresholds that compress the normal growth of loudness.[196] The normal auditory system has a large dynamic range detecting pressure variations of approximately 0.00002 Pa and reaching pressures 1,000,000 times greater before the sensation becomes painful. The dynamic range is largely established by mechanoelectrical transduction that takes place in the cochlea that provides amplification and nonlinearity. Damage to this normal mechanism results in an elevated threshold and loss of nonlinearity and a narrowed dynamic range. For example, a person has thresholds at 10 dB HL across the audiogram and their uncomfortable loudness level is 110 dB HL. This corresponds to a 100 dB dynamic range. If this same person acquires hearing loss, his or her threshold may now be 60 dB HL across the audiogram (moderate hearing loss). However, sounds may still become uncomfortably loud at 110 dB HL. The dynamic range is now 50 dB or half the normal range of loudness growth.

Misophonia: Misophonia refers to an abnormally strong reaction (anger, rage, crying) to specific sounds or specific types of sounds, commonly referred to as trigger sounds (Jastreboff and Jastreboff[197]). Selective sound sensitivity syndrome is a variant of misophonia characterized by sensitivity to soft sounds often related to chewing and breathing sounds. Another term is annoyance hyperacusis.[194] Misophonia can be

an independent symptom or related to other existing disorders. It is unclear what role the auditory pathway plays in misophonia; no comprehensive study of auditory physiology has been performed. Schröder et al[198] reported abnormalities in the N1 component of the auditory late-evoked response. However, the sample size was small, some subjects were on psychotropic medications, and the response can be influenced by general hyperarousal. In general, individuals first develop misophonia symptoms during childhood and usually have normal peripheral hearing sensitivity.

A potential correlate to misophonia is tinnitus. Indeed, similar areas of the brain are activated by sounds judged aversive as are activated by tinnitus (Mirz et al[199]), suggesting misophonia is like an external tinnitus. Currently, there are two main views on misophonia. The first view is that misophonia is a subvariant of obsessive-compulsive disorder or other psychological disorders. The second is that misophonia is an altered auditory-limbic response, where a negative conditioned reflex is established for the trigger sound, suggesting a physiological and psychological role in trigger establishment and response. Some individuals with misophonia can also present with other sensory sensitivities including visual, tactile, and olfactory triggers. Some can experience a trigger with anticipation of a sound. These triggers are not usually self-evoked. For a review, see Spankovich and Hall.[200]

Phonophobia: Phonophobia indicates actual fear of a sound. Another term used is fear hyperacusis.[194] Fear of sound can lead to self-withdrawal and avoidance of sound. True phonophobia, sometimes called ligyrophobia has no or minimal abnormality in the peripheral or central auditory pathway. It is believed the negative effect is conditioned leading to development of specific reactions and avoidance patterns. Like all fear phobias, phonophobia is created by the unconscious mind as a protective mechanism.[201]

Diplacusis and polyacusis: Diplacusis or polyacusis is characterized by the perception of two or more sounds when subject is exposed to a single pure tone. There are numerous variations depending if both ears are impacted and nature of the perception. It is believed that the experience is rare. For review see Jastreboff.[107]

Abnormal somatosound perception: Patients may present with unusual sound awareness/perception. For example, their breathing may sound loud, voice echoing, perceive loud footsteps, or even hear their eyes moving. These experiences are often related to pathologies such as superior canal dehiscence or fistula (perilymph fistula) of the oval or round window. Patients with a dehiscence or fistula may present with dizziness with loud sound (Tullio's phenomenon) or changes in pressure (Hennebert's sign).

17.4.5 Evaluation of Sound Sensitivity

The evaluation is similar to that described for tinnitus, including comprehensive evaluation to rule out pathology. There is general agreement to include measurement of loudness discomfort levels (LDLs). Not all forms of sound sensitivity will present with decreased LDLs (e.g., misophonia). Several studies indicate that normal LDLs fall in the range of 90 to 100 dB HL. When sound sensitivity is present that alters loudness tolerance, LDLs are typically in the 60 to 85 dB HL range. This range is consistent with hyperacusis. In the case of pure misophonia, LDLs can range from 30 to 120 dB HL depending on the sound.

A common method to determine LDLs is the contour test of loudness.[202] Warble tones are presented at frequency of interest using an ascending-level method. The starting level is commonly 20 dB HL and level is incremented in 5 dB steps with three to four pulses of tone presented at each level. The patient then responds to the subjective loudness on a 7-point scales from very soft to uncomfortably loud. This is performed for each ear, additional frequencies and speech can be incorporated. Other variations exist.

To establish sound sensitivity severity, several scales or questionnaires exist. The Khalfa Hyperacusis Questionnaire,[203] The Multipe-Activity Scale for Hyperacusis,[204] the Misophonia Assessment Questionnaire, and the Amsterdam Misophonia Scale.[205] Other scales exist, but limited research has been performed on validity and reliability. In addition, other scales for depression, anxiety, anger, obsessive-compulsive behavior are applicable.

17.4.6 Differential Diagnosis of Sound Sensitivity

Differential diagnosis begins with a comprehensive case history. Medical evaluation, preferably by an otologist or neurotologist, is recommended, particularly with complaints of otalgia (ear pain). Numerous medical conditions can present with sound sensitivity including migraine, dysfunction of the facial nerve (e.g., Bell's palsy), Lyme disease, Williams' syndrome, head injury, medications (e.g., benzodiazepines withdrawal), perilymph fistula, stapedectomy, semicircular canal dehiscence, Meniere's disease, otosyphilis, fibromyalgia, trigeminal neuralgia, chronic pain, autism spectrum disorder, acoustic trauma, and sensory processing disorder. In addition, psychophysiological condition should be considered including presence of obsessive-compulsive behavior, Tourette's syndrome, anxiety, depression, posttraumatic stress disorder, etc.

Differentiating sound sensitivity forms is important. Recruitment is associated with hearing loss and sensitivity usually to louder sounds only (e.g., clatter of dishes). Hyperacusis does not require hearing loss, but is often related to an acoustic trauma. Individuals with hyperacusis often present with sensitivity to all sounds, not just loud. The patients may even present to the office wearing hearing protection devices and complaint of pain. Individuals with misophonia commonly report sensitivity to specific sounds independent of level. The most common sounds are mouth-related sounds (e.g., chewing, breathing, throat clearing, scratching) and repetitive sounds (e.g., tapping, clicking). Patients with phonophobia are commonly extreme cases of hyperacusis or misophonia where the patient has now developed a fear of specific or all sounds. Another variant of sound sensitivity is related to sensory processing issues commonly seen in persons with autism spectrum disorder. The sounds found to be aversive in the population tend to be louder and of sudden onset (e.g., fireworks, toilet flush, and vacuum).

Patients may also report abnormally loud somatosounds, such as autophony, where one's own voice sounds loud or the ability to hear one's own eye movement or perception of louder footsteps. These experiences may be consistent with superior semicircular canal dehiscence, fistula, patulous eustachian tube, or stapedial reflex dysfunction.

17.4.7 Management of Sound Sensitivity

The management of sound sensitivity often follows the approaches used in tinnitus. There are specific recommendations in TRT and TAT for loudness intolerance and nonloudness intolerance variations of sound sensitivity. Often it is recommended to treat the sound sensitivity prior to tinnitus or hearing loss, if present as comorbidities. In addition, for most forms of sound sensitivity use of hearing protection devices is not recommended. Constant use of hearing protection can actually increase sound sensitivity.[206] Patients presenting with hearing protection or report use in moderate-level environments should be counseled on tapering off their use.

Pearl ✔

In most cases when a patient presents with both tinnitus and sound sensitivity, sound sensitivity should be addressed first.

The approach for treating sound sensitivity is a combination of counseling on the central gain theory or theoretical mechanism underlying misophonia/phonophobia and sound therapy. In this case, the sound is applied to help desensitize the system. Slightly different approaches are recommended for hyperacusis versus misophonia/phonophobia.[107,207] For hyperacusis, patients are counseled to avoid silence and begin continual exposure to sound. The sound level should never induce discomfort or annoyance; ear level devices can help keep a constant sound. The recommended level is from 9 to 20 dB SL. The level can be slightly increased over time or remain at same level depending on approach. The goal of constant sound stimulation is to recalibrate the system and reduce the central gain by increasing the level of the background sound. This approach is not recommended for misophonia, which needs to address the conditioned reflex. For misophonia, the patient is instructed to use highly pleasant sounds (e.g., favorite music). Eventually, the patient uses these highly pleasant sounds while in the presence of their trigger sound. Over time, the ratio of the positive to negative sound is decreased. This should be performed in a safe environment and with plenty of positive reinforcement. This may also involve relinquishing control over the pleasant sound to a trusted individual. CBT has also shown benefit for individuals with sound sensitivity and is a component of the TAT approach to hyperacusis (Juris et al[208]) that follows a similar format to the TAT tinnitus program (Pienkowski et al[207]).

17.5 Summary

Tinnitus and sound sensitivity are significant issues that can alter a patient's quality of life, in some cases to extreme levels. Our understanding of the mechanisms underlying tinnitus and sound sensitivity are growing exponentially. Tinnitus and sound sensitivity expand beyond the ear. Tinnitus and sound sensitivity are not simply auditory manifestations, rather involve numerous brain regions involved in attention, awareness, and emotional response. For most cases, there are no surgical or pharmacological treatments. Tinnitus and sound sensitivity patients are often dismissed by the medical community, not necessarily due to lack of compassion, rather due to lack of effective medical treatments. The audiologist is uniquely positioned with expertise in auditory physiology and use of sound-based treatments to evaluate and manage tinnitus and sound sensitivity patients. The audiologist must have in-depth knowledge of tinnitus and sound sensitivity neuroscience, differential diagnosis of medical pathologies contributing to tinnitus and sound sensitivity, adjustment-based counseling, lifestyle factors, and sound therapeutic options.

Numerous options exist for management of tinnitus and sound sensitivity. Counseling and sound-based therapy represent two approaches to tinnitus management often used in parallel by audiologists. Effective counseling involves an interactive discussion including (1) source theory and demystification of tinnitus, (2) the habituation process and cognitive restructuring (physiological and psychological elements, i.e., maladaptive thoughts and behaviors regarding the tinnitus and alternative thoughts/behaviors), (3) recommendations on sound therapy options, (4) role of distraction, and (5) education on lifestyle changes. Sound therapy options can include basic sound enrichment, amplification, and proprietary systems. Formal structured approaches exist and the reader is encouraged to expand his or her knowledge through coursework, professional lectures, and workshops.

References

[1] Bhatt JM, Lin HW, Bhattacharyya N. Prevalence, severity, exposures, and treatment patterns of tinnitus in the United States. JAMA Otolaryngol Head Neck Surg. 2016; 142(10):959–965

[2] Mahboubi H, Oliaei S, Kiumehr S, Dwabe S, Djalilian HR. The prevalence and characteristics of tinnitus in the youth population of the United States. Laryngoscope. 2013; 123(8):2001–2008

[3] Nondahl DM, Cruickshanks KJ, Huang GH, et al. Generational differences in the reporting of tinnitus. Ear Hear. 2012; 33(5):640–644

[4] Nondahl DM, Cruickshanks KJ, Wiley TL, et al. The ten-year incidence of tinnitus among older adults. Int J Audiol. 2010; 49(8):580–585

[5] Shargorodsky J, Curhan GC, Farwell WR. Prevalence and characteristics of tinnitus among US adults. Am J Med. 2010; 123(8):711–718

[6] Gallus S, Lugo A, Garavello W, et al. Prevalence and determinants of tinnitus in the Italian adult population. Neuroepidemiology. 2015; 45(1):12–19

[7] Gopinath B, McMahon CM, Rochtchina E, Karpa MJ, Mitchell P. Incidence, persistence, and progression of tinnitus symptoms in older adults: the Blue Mountains Hearing Study. Ear Hear. 2010a; 31(3):407–412

[8] Izuhara K, Wada K, Nakamura K, et al. Association between tinnitus and sleep disorders in the general Japanese population. Ann Otol Rhinol Laryngol. 2013; 122(11):701–706

[9] Jalessi M, Farhadi M, Asghari A, et al. Tinnitus: an epidemiologic study in Iranian population. Acta Med Iran. 2013; 51(12):886–891

[10] Kim HJ, Lee HJ, An SY, et al. Analysis of the prevalence and associated risk factors of tinnitus in adults. PLoS One. 2015; 10(5):e0127578

[11] McCormack A, Edmondson-Jones M, Fortnum H, et al. The prevalence of tinnitus and the relationship with neuroticism in a middle-aged UK population. J Psychosom Res. 2014; 76(1):56–60

[12] Oiticica J, Bittar RS. Tinnitus prevalence in the city of São Paulo. Rev Bras Otorrinolaringol (Engl Ed). 2015; 81(2):167–176

[13] Park KH, Lee SH, Koo JW, et al. Prevalence and associated factors of tinnitus: data from the Korean National Health and Nutrition Examination Survey 2009–2011. J Epidemiol. 2014; 24(5):417–426

[14] Xu X, Bu X, Zhou L, Xing G, Liu C, Wang D. An epidemiologic study of tinnitus in a population in Jiangsu Province, China. J Am Acad Audiol. 2011; 22(9):578–585

[15] Seidman MD, Jacobson GP. Update on tinnitus. Otolaryngol Clin North Am. 1996; 29(3):455–465

[16] Bauch CD, Lynn SG, Williams DE, Mellon MW, Weaver AL. Tinnitus impact: three different measurement tools. J Am Acad Audiol. 2003; 14(4):181–187

[17] Cima RF, Crombez G, Vlaeyen JW. Catastrophizing and fear of tinnitus predict quality of life in patients with chronic tinnitus. Ear Hear. 2011; 32(5):634–641

[18] Erlandsson SI, Hallberg LR. Prediction of quality of life in patients with tinnitus. Br J Audiol. 2000; 34(1):11–20

[19] Nondahl DM, Cruickshanks KJ, Dalton DS, et al. The impact of tinnitus on quality of life in older adults. J Am Acad Audiol. 2007; 18(3):257–266

[20] Gopinath B, McMahon CM, Rochtchina E, Karpa MJ, Mitchell P. Risk factors and impacts of incident tinnitus in older adults. Ann Epidemiol. 2010b; 20(2):129–135

[21] Nondahl DM, Cruickshanks KJ, Huang GH, et al. Tinnitus and its risk factors in the Beaver Dam offspring study. Int J Audiol. 2011; 50(5):313–320

[22] Nondahl DM, Cruickshanks KJ, Wiley TL, Klein R, Klein BE, Tweed TS. Prevalence and 5-year incidence of tinnitus among older adults: the epidemiology of hearing loss study. J Am Acad Audiol. 2002; 13(6):323–331

[23] Sindhusake D, Golding M, Newall P, Rubin G, Jakobsen K, Mitchell P. Risk factors for tinnitus in a population of older adults: the blue mountains hearing study. Ear Hear. 2003; 24(6):501–507

[24] US Department of Veterans Affairs. The Fiscal Year 2014 Annual Benefits Report. 2014. Available at: https://www.benefits.va.gov/REPORTS/abr/ABR-Combined-FY14-11052015.pdf . Accessed April 1, 2017

[25] Theodoroff SM, Lewis MS, Folmer RL, Henry JA, Carlson KF. Hearing impairment and tinnitus: prevalence, risk factors, and outcomes in US service members and veterans deployed to the Iraq and Afghanistan wars. Epidemiol Rev. 2015; 37:71–85

[26] Park B, Choi HG, Lee HJ, et al. Analysis of the prevalence of and risk factors for tinnitus in a young population. Otol Neurotol. 2014; 35(7):1218–1222

[27] Rosing SN, Schmidt JH, Wedderkopp N, Baguley DM. Prevalence of tinnitus and hyperacusis in children and adolescents: a systematic review. BMJ Open. 2016; 6(6):e010596

[28] Aarhus L, Engdahl B, Tambs K, Kvestad E, Hoffman HJ. Association between childhood hearing disorders and tinnitus in adulthood. JAMA Otolaryngol Head Neck Surg. 2015; 141(11):983–989

[29] Cianfrone G, Mazzei F, Salviati M, et al. Tinnitus Holistic Simplified Classification (THoSC): a new assessment for subjective tinnitus, with diagnostic and therapeutic implications. Ann Otol Rhinol Laryngol. 2015; 124(7):550–560

[30] Heller AJ. Classification and epidemiology of tinnitus. Otolaryngol Clin North Am. 2003; 36(2):239–248

[31] Tunkel DE, Bauer CA, Sun GH, et al. Clinical practice guideline: tinnitus. Otolaryngol Head Neck Surg. 2014; 151(suppl 2):S1–S40

[32] Simmons R, Dambra C, Lobarinas E, Stocking C, Salvi R. Head, neck, and eye movements that modulate tinnitus. Semin Hear. 2008; 29(4):361–370

[33] Henry JA, Zaugg TL, Myers PJ, Kendall CJ, Michaelides EM. A triage guide for tinnitus. J Fam Pract. 2010; 59(7):389–393

[34] Heller MF, Bergman M. Tinnitus aurium in normally hearing persons. Ann Otol Rhinol Laryngol. 1953; 62(1):73–83

[35] Knobel KA, Sanchez TG. Influence of silence and attention on tinnitus perception. Otolaryngol Head Neck Surg. 2008; 138(1):18–22

[36] Tucker DA, Phillips SL, Ruth RA, Clayton WA, Royster E, Todd AD. The effect of silence on tinnitus perception. Otolaryngol Head Neck Surg. 2005; 132(1):20–24

[37] Del Bo L, Forti S, Ambrosetti U, et al. Tinnitus aurium in persons with normal hearing: 55 years later. Otolaryngol Head Neck Surg. 2008; 139(3):391–394

[38] Schaette R, Turtle C, Munro KJ. Reversible induction of phantom auditory sensations through simulated unilateral hearing loss. PLoS One. 2012; 7(6):e35238

[39] Blom JD, Sommer IE. Auditory hallucinations: nomenclature and classification. Cogn Behav Neurol. 2010; 23(1):55–62

[40] Jastreboff PJ, Brennan JF, Sasaki CT. An animal model for tinnitus. Laryngoscope. 1988; 98(3):280–286

[41] Bauer CA, Brozoski TJ. Assessing tinnitus and prospective tinnitus therapeutics using a psychophysical animal model. J Assoc Res Otolaryngol. 2001; 2(1):54–64

[42] Lobarinas E, Hayes SH, Allman BL. The gap-startle paradigm for tinnitus screening in animal models: limitations and optimization. Hear Res. 2013; 295:150–160

[43] Lobarinas E, Sun W, Cushing R, Salvi R. A novel behavioral paradigm for assessing tinnitus using schedule-induced polydipsia avoidance conditioning (SIP-AC). Hear Res. 2004; 190(1–2):109–114

[44] Turner JG, Brozoski TJ, Bauer CA, et al. Gap detection deficits in rats with tinnitus: a potential novel screening tool. Behav Neurosci. 2006; 120(1):188–195

[45] Hazell JW, Jastreboff PJ. Tinnitus. I: auditory mechanisms: a model for tinnitus and hearing impairment. J Otolaryngol. 1990; 19(1):1–5

[46] Lockwood AH, Salvi RJ, Coad ML, Towsley ML, Wack DS, Murphy BW. The functional neuroanatomy of tinnitus: evidence for limbic system links and neural plasticity. Neurology. 1998; 50(1):114–120

[47] Melcher JR, Sigalovsky IS, Guinan JJ, Jr, Levine RA. Lateralized tinnitus studied with functional magnetic resonance imaging: abnormal inferior colliculus activation. J Neurophysiol. 2000; 83(2):1058–1072

[48] Norton SJ, Schmidt AR, Stover LJ. Tinnitus and otoacoustic emissions: is there a link? Ear Hear. 1990; 11(2):159–166

[49] Penner MJ. An estimate of the prevalence of tinnitus caused by spontaneous otoacoustic emissions. Arch Otolaryngol Head Neck Surg. 1990; 116(4):418–423

[50] Liberman MC. Noise-induced hearing loss: permanent versus temporary threshold shifts and the effects of hair cell versus neuronal degeneration. Adv Exp Med Biol. 2016; 875:1–7

[51] Tan CM, Lecluyse W, McFerran D, Meddis R. Tinnitus and patterns of hearing loss. J Assoc Res Otolaryngol. 2013; 14(2):275–282

[52] Mitchell CR, Creedon TA. Psychophysical tuning curves in subjects with tinnitus suggest outer hair cell lesions. Otolaryngol Head Neck Surg. 1995; 113(3):223–233

[53] Henry JA, Roberts LE, Caspary DM, Theodoroff SM, Salvi RJ. Underlying mechanisms of tinnitus: review and clinical implications. J Am Acad Audiol. 2014; 25(1):5–22, quiz 126

[54] Weisz N, Dohrmann K, Elbert T. The relevance of spontaneous activity for the coding of the tinnitus sensation. Prog Brain Res. 2007; 166:61–70

[55] Lorenz I, Müller N, Schlee W, Hartmann T, Weisz N. Loss of alpha power is related to increased gamma synchronization—a marker of reduced inhibition in tinnitus? Neurosci Lett. 2009; 453(3):225–228

[56] Rauschecker JP, May ES, Maudoux A, Ploner M. Frontostriatal Gating of Tinnitus and Chronic Pain. Trends Cogn Sci. 2015; 19(10):567–578

[57] Leaver AM, Turesky TK, Seydell-Greenwald A, Morgan S, Kim HJ, Rauschecker JP. Intrinsic network activity in tinnitus investigated using functional MRI. Hum Brain Mapp. 2016; 37(8):2717–2735

[58] Hinkley LB, Mizuiri D, Hong O, Nagarajan SS, Cheung SW. Increased striatal functional connectivity with auditory cortex in tinnitus. Front Hum Neurosci. 2015; 9:568

[59] Eggermont JJ, Roberts LE. Tinnitus: animal models and findings in humans. Cell Tissue Res. 2015; 361(1):311–336

[60] Husain FT. Neural networks of tinnitus in humans: elucidating severity and habituation. Hear Res. 2016; 334:37–48

[61] Leaver AM, Seydell-Greenwald A, Rauschecker JP. Auditory-limbic interactions in chronic tinnitus: challenges for neuroimaging research. Hear Res. 2016; 334:49–57

[62] Newman CW, Weinstein BE, Jacobson GP, Hug GA. The Hearing Handicap Inventory for Adults: psychometric adequacy and audiometric correlates. Ear Hear. 1990; 11(6):430–433

[63] Schow RL, Nerbonne MA. Communication screening profile: use with elderly clients. Ear Hear. 1982; 3(3):135–147

[64] Meikle MB, Henry JA, Griest SE, et al. The tinnitus functional index: development of a new clinical measure for chronic, intrusive tinnitus. Ear Hear. 2012; 33(2):153–176

[65] Newman CW, Jacobson GP, Spitzer JB. Development of the Tinnitus Handicap Inventory. Arch Otolaryngol Head Neck Surg. 1996; 122(2):143–148

[66] Wilson PH, Henry J, Bowen M, Haralambous G. Tinnitus reaction questionnaire: psychometric properties of a measure of distress associated with tinnitus. J Speech Hear Res. 1991; 34(1):197–201

[67] Kuk FK, Tyler RS, Russell D, Jordan H. The psychometric properties of a tinnitus handicap questionnaire. Ear Hear. 1990; 11(6):434–445

[68] Hallam RS, Jakes SC, Hinchcliffe R. Cognitive variables in tinnitus annoyance. Br J Clin Psychol. 1988; 27(pt 3):213–222

[69] Meikle MB, Sandridge SA, Johnson RM. The perceived severity of tinnitus. Some observations concerning a large population of tinnitus clinic patients. Otolaryngol Head Neck Surg. 1984; 92(6):689–696

[70] Newman CW, Sandridge SA, Jacobson GP. Psychometric adequacy of the Tinnitus Handicap Inventory (THI) for evaluating treatment outcome. J Am Acad Audiol 1998; 9(2):153–160

[71] Henry JA, Griest S, Zaugg TL, et al. Tinnitus and hearing survey: a screening tool to differentiate bothersome tinnitus from hearing difficulties. Am J Audiol. 2015; 24(1):66–77

[72] Beck AT, Beck RW. Screening depressed patients in family practice: A rapid technique. Postgrad Med. 1972; 52(6):81–85

[73] Spielberger CD, Gorsuch RL, Lushene R, Vagg PR, Jacobs GA. Manual for the State-Trait Anxiety Inventory. Palo Alto, CA: Consulting Psychologists Press. 1983

[74] Goodman WK, Price LH, Rasmussen SA, et al. The Yale-Brown Obsessive Compulsive Scale. I. Development, use, and reliability. Arch Gen Psychiatry. 1989; 46(11):1006–1011

[75] Maier W, Buller R, Philipp M, Heuser I. The Hamilton Anxiety Scale: reliability, validity and sensitivity to change in anxiety and depressive disorders. J Affect Disord. 1988; 14(1):61–68

[76] Pridmore S, Walter G, Friedland P. Tinnitus and suicide: recent cases on the public record give cause for reconsideration. Otolaryngol Head Neck Surg. 2012; 147(2):193–195

[77] Crummer RW, Hassan GA. Diagnostic approach to tinnitus. Am Fam Physician. 2004; 69(1):120–126

[78] Vernon JA, Meikle MB. Tinnitus masking: unresolved problems. Ciba Found Symp. 1981; 85:239–262

[79] Henry JA, Zaugg TL, Schechter MA. Clinical guide for audiologic tinnitus management I: assessment. Am J Audiol. 2005; 14(1):21–48

[80] Moore BC, Vinay, Sandhya. The relationship between tinnitus pitch and the edge frequency of the audiogram in individuals with hearing impairment and tonal tinnitus. Hear Res. 2010; 261(1–2):51–56

[81] Sismanis A. Pulsatile tinnitus: contemporary assessment and management. Curr Opin Otolaryngol Head Neck Surg. 2011; 19(5):348–357

[82] Sismanis A. Pulsatile tinnitus. Otolaryngol Clin North Am. 2003; 36(2):389–402, viii

[83] Adams ME, Levine SC. The first new otologic disorder in a century: superior canal dehiscence syndrome. Minn Med. 2011; 94(11):29–32

[84] Nordmann AS, Bohne BA, Harding GW. Histopathological differences between temporary and permanent threshold shift. Hear Res. 2000; 139(1–2):13–30

[85] Guitton MJ, Caston J, Ruel J, Johnson RM, Pujol R, Puel JL. Salicylate induces tinnitus through activation of cochlear NMDA receptors. J Neurosci. 2003; 23(9):3944–3952

[86] Kreuzer PM, Landgrebe M, Vielsmeier V, Kleinjung T, De Ridder D, Langguth B. Trauma-associated tinnitus. J Head Trauma Rehabil. 2014; 29(5):432–442

[87] Lowry LD, Eisenman LM, Saunders JC. An absence of tinnitus. Otol Neurotol. 2004; 25(4):474–478

[88] Stephens SD. The treatment of tinnitus – a historical perspective. J Laryngol Otol. 1984; 98(10):963–972

[89] Duckert LG, Rees TS. Placebo effect in tinnitus management. Otolaryngol Head Neck Surg. 1984; 92(6):697–699

[90] Henry JA, Stewart BJ, Griest S, Kaelin C, Zaugg TL, Carlson K. Multisite randomized controlled trial to compare two methods of tinnitus intervention to two control conditions. Ear Hear. 2016; 37(6):e346–e359

[91] Henry JA. Tinnitus management: state of the art and looking ahead. J Am Acad Audiol. 2014; 25(1):4

[92] Theodoroff SM, Schuette A, Griest S, Henry JA. Individual patient factors associated with effective tinnitus treatment. J Am Acad Audiol. 2014; 25(7):631–643

[93] Henry JL, Wilson PH. The Psychological Management of Tinnitus: Comparison of a Combined Cognitive Educational Program, Education Alone and a Waiting-List Control. Int Tinnitus J. 1996; 2:9–20

[94] Lindberg P, Scott B, Melin L, Lyttkens L. The psychological treatment of tinnitus: an experimental evaluation. Behav Res Ther. 1989; 27(6):593–603

[95] Sweetow R. Counseling the patient with tinnitus. Arch Otolaryngol. 1985; 111(5):283–284

[96] Sweetow RW. Cognitive aspects of tinnitus patient management. Ear Hear. 1986; 7(6):390–396

[97] Wilson PH, Henry JL, Andersson G, Hallam RS, Lindberg P. A critical analysis of directive counselling as a component of tinnitus retraining therapy. Br J Audiol. 1998; 32(5):273–286

[98] Cima RF, Andersson G, Schmidt CJ, Henry JA. Cognitive-behavioral treatments for tinnitus: a review of the literature. J Am Acad Audiol. 2014; 25(1):29–61

[99] Kiang NY, Moxon EC, Levine RA. Auditory-nerve activity in cats with normal and abnormal cochleas. In: Sensorineural hearing loss. Ciba Found Symp 1970:241–273

[100] Salvi RJ, Ahroon WA. Tinnitus and neural activity. J Speech Hear Res. 1983; 26(4):629–632

[101] Tonndorf J. Tinnitus and physiological correlates of the cochleo-vestibular system: peripheral; central. J Laryngol Otol Suppl. 1981(4):18–20

[102] Hallam RS, Jakes SC. Tinnitus: differential effects of therapy in a single case. Behav Res Ther. 1985; 23(6):691–694

[103] Hallam RS, Jakes SC, Chambers C, Hinchcliffe R. A comparison of different methods for assessing the 'intensity' of tinnitus. Acta Otolaryngol. 1985; 99(5–6):501–508

[104] Hazell JW. Management of tinnitus: discussion paper. J R Soc Med. 1985; 78(1):56–60

[105] Slater R. On helping people with tinnitus to help themselves. Br J Audiol. 1987; 21(2):87–90

[106] Jastreboff PJ, Gray WC, Gold SL. Neurophysiological approach to tinnitus patients. Am J Otol. 1996; 17(2):236–240

[107] Jastreboff PJ. 25 years of tinnitus retraining therapy. HNO. 2015; 63(4):307–311

[108] Coles RR, Hallam RS. Tinnitus and its management. Br Med Bull. 1987; 43(4):983–998

[109] Stephens SD, Hallam RS, Jakes SC. Tinnitus: a management model. Clin Otolaryngol Allied Sci. 1986; 11(4):227–238

[110] Sweetow RW. The evolution of cognitive-behavioral therapy as an approach to tinnitus patient management. Int Tinnitus J. 1995; 1(1):61–65

[111] Tyler RS, Gogel SA, Gehringer AK. Tinnitus activities treatment. Prog Brain Res. 2007; 166:425–434

[112] Myers PJ, Griest S, Kaelin C, et al. Development of a progressive audiologic tinnitus management program for Veterans with tinnitus. J Rehabil Res Dev. 2014; 51(4):609–622

[113] Vernon J. Attemps to relieve tinnitus. J Am Audiol Soc. 1977; 2(4):124–131

[114] Vernon J, Schleuning A. Tinnitus: a new management. Laryngoscope. 1978; 88(3):413–419

[115] Jastreboff PJ, Jastreboff MM. Tinnitus Retraining Therapy (TRT) as a method for treatment of tinnitus and hyperacusis patients. J Am Acad Audiol. 2000; 11(3):162–177

[116] Tyler RS, Noble W, Coelho CB, Ji H. Tinnitus retraining therapy: mixing point and total masking are equally effective. Ear Hear. 2012; 33(5):588–594

[117] Fukuda S, Miyashita T, Inamoto R, Mori N. Tinnitus retraining therapy using portable music players. Auris Nasus Larynx. 2011; 38(6):692–696

[118] Saltzman M, Ersner MS. A hearing aid for the relief of tinnitus aurium. Laryngoscope. 1947; 57(5): 358–366

[119] Searchfield GD, Kaur M, Martin WH. Hearing aids as an adjunct to counseling: tinnitus patients who choose amplification do better than those that don't. Int J Audiol. 2010; 49(8):574–579

[120] Peltier E, Peltier C, Tahar S, Alliot-Lugaz E, Cazals Y. Long-term tinnitus suppression with linear octave frequency transposition hearing AIDS. PLoS One. 2012; 7(12):e51915

[121] Henry JA, Frederick M, Sell S, Griest S, Abrams H. Validation of a novel combination hearing aid and tinnitus therapy device. Ear Hear. 2015; 36(1):42–52

[122] Davis PB, Paki B, Hanley PJ. Neuromonics Tinnitus Treatment: third clinical trial. Ear Hear. 2007; 28(2):242–259

[123] Hanley PJ, Davis PB, Paki B, Quinn SA, Bellekom SR. Treatment of tinnitus with a customized, dynamic acoustic neural stimulus: clinical outcomes in general private practice. Ann Otol Rhinol Laryngol. 2008; 117(11):791–799

[124] Vieira D, Eikelboom R, Ivey G, Miller S. A multi-centre study on the long-term benefits of tinnitus management using Neuromonics Tinnitus Treatment. Int Tinnitus J. 2011; 16(2):111–117

[125] Hoare DJ, Kowalkowski VL, Kang S, Hall DA. Systematic review and meta-analyses of randomized controlled trials examining tinnitus management. Laryngoscope. 2011; 121(7):1555–1564

[126] Newman CW, Sandridge SA. A comparison of benefit and economic value between two sound therapy tinnitus management options. J Am Acad Audiol. 2012; 23(2):126–138

[127] Zeng FG, Tang Q, Dimitrijevic A, Starr A, Larky J, Blevins NH. Tinnitus suppression by low-rate electric stimulation and its electrophysiological mechanisms. Hear Res. 2011; 277(1–2):61–66

[128] Reavis KM, Rothholtz VS, Tang Q, Carroll JA, Djalilian H, Zeng FG. Temporary suppression of tinnitus by modulated sounds. J Assoc Res Otolaryngol. 2012; 13(4):561–571

[129] Okamoto H, Stracke H, Stoll W, Pantev C. Listening to tailor-made notched music reduces tinnitus loudness and tinnitus-related auditory cortex activity. Proc Natl Acad Sci U S A. 2010; 107(3):1207–1210

[130] Pantev C, Wollbrink A, Roberts LE, Engelien A, Lütkenhöner B. Short-term plasticity of the human auditory cortex. Brain Res. 1999; 842(1):192–199

[131] Teismann H, Okamoto H, Pantev C. Short and intense tailor-made notched music training against tinnitus: the tinnitus frequency matters. PLoS One. 2011; 6(9):e24685

[132] Lugli M, Romani R, Ponzi S, Bacciu S, Parmigiani S. The windowed sound therapy: a new empirical approach for an effective personalized treatment of tinnitus. Int Tinnitus J. 2009; 15(1):51–61

[133] Hauptmann C, Ströbel A, Williams M, et al. Acoustic coordinated reset neuromodulation in a real life patient population with chronic tonal tinnitus. BioMed Res Int. 2015; 2015:569052

[134] Williams M, Hauptmann C, Patel N. Acoustic CR neuromodulation therapy for subjective tonal tinnitus: a review of clinical outcomes in an independent audiology practice setting. Front Neurol. 2015; 6:54

[135] Drexler D, López-Paullier M, Rodio S, González M, Geisinger D, Pedemonte M. Impact of reduction of tinnitus intensity on patients' quality of life. Int J Audiol. 2016; 55(1):11–19

[136] Sweetow RW. The use of fractal tones in tinnitus patient management. Noise Health. 2013; 15(63): 96–100

[137] Sweetow RW, Sabes JH. Effects of acoustical stimuli delivered through hearing aids on tinnitus. J Am Acad Audiol. 2010; 21(7):461–473

[138] Carrick DG, Davies WM, Fielder CP, Bihari J. Low-powered ultrasound in the treatment of tinnitus: a pilot study. Br J Audiol. 1986; 20(2):153–155

[139] House JW, Brackmann DE. Tinnitus: surgical treatment. Ciba Found Symp. 1981; 85:204–216

[140] Pulec JL. Tinnitus: surgical therapy. Am J Otol. 1984; 5(6):479–480

[141] Shi Y, Burchiel KJ, Anderson VC, Martin WH. Deep brain stimulation effects in patients with tinnitus. Otolaryngol Head Neck Surg. 2009; 141(2):285–287

[142] Cheung SW, Larson PS. Tinnitus modulation by deep brain stimulation in locus of caudate neurons (area LC). Neuroscience. 2010; 169(4):1768–1778

[143] Smit JV, Janssen ML, Schulze H, et al. Deep brain stimulation in tinnitus: current and future perspectives. Brain Res. 2015; 1608:51–65

[144] Penry JK, Dean JC. Prevention of intractable partial seizures by intermittent vagal stimulation in humans: preliminary results. Epilepsia. 1990; 31(suppl 2):S40–S43

[145] De Ridder D, Vanneste S, Engineer ND, Kilgard MP. Safety and efficacy of vagus nerve stimulation paired with tones for the treatment of tinnitus: a case series. Neuromodulation. 2014; 17(2):170–179

[146] Vanneste S, De Ridder D. Noninvasive and invasive neuromodulation for the treatment of tinnitus: an overview. Neuromodulation. 2012; 15(4):350–360

[147] Van de Heyning P, Vermeire K, Diebl M, Nopp P, Anderson I, De Ridder D. Incapacitating unilateral tinnitus in single-sided deafness treated by cochlear implantation. Ann Otol Rhinol Laryngol. 2008; 117(9):645–652

[148] Kim DK, Moon IS, Lim HJ, et al. Prospective, multicenter study on tinnitus changes after cochlear implantation. Audiol Neurootol. 2016; 21(3): 165–171

[149] Pierzycki RH, Edmondson-Jones M, Dawes P, Munro KJ, Moore DR, Kitterick PT. Tinnitus and sleep difficulties after cochlear implantation. Ear Hear. 2016; 37(6):e402–e408

[150] Bayar N, Böke B, Turan E, Belgin E. Efficacy of amitriptyline in the treatment of subjective tinnitus. J Otolaryngol. 2001; 30(5):300–303

[151] Feder R. Tinnitus associated with amitriptyline. J Clin Psychiatry. 1990; 51(2):85–86

[152] Langguth B, Salvi R, Elgoyhen AB. Emerging pharmacotherapy of tinnitus. Expert Opin Emerg Drugs. 2009; 14(4):687–702

[153] Salvi R, Lobarinas E, Sun W. Pharmacological treatments for tinnitus: new and old. Drugs Future. 2009; 34(5):381–400

[154] Coelho C, Figueiredo R, Frank E, et al. Reduction of tinnitus severity by the centrally acting muscle relaxant cyclobenzaprine: an open-label pilot study. Audiol Neurootol. 2012; 17(3):179–188

[155] Vanneste S, Figueiredo R, De Ridder D. Treatment of tinnitus with cyclobenzaprine: an open-label study. Int J Clin Pharmacol Ther. 2012; 50(5):338–344

[156] Jalali MM, Kousha A, Naghavi SE, Soleimani R, Banan R. The effects of alprazolam on tinnitus: a crossover randomized clinical trial. Med Sci Monit. 2009; 15(11):PI55–PI60

[157] Johnson RM, Brummett R, Schleuning A. Use of alprazolam for relief of tinnitus. A double-blind study. Arch Otolaryngol Head Neck Surg. 1993; 119(8):842–845

[158] Kay NJ. Oral chemotherapy in tinnitus. Br J Audiol. 1981; 15(2):123–124

[159] Han SS, Nam EC, Won JY, et al. Clonazepam quiets tinnitus: a randomised crossover study with Ginkgo biloba. J Neurol Neurosurg Psychiatry. 2012; 83(8):821–827

[160] Aazh H, El Refaie A, Humphriss R. Gabapentin for tinnitus: a systematic review. Am J Audiol. 2011; 20(2):151–158

[161] Shulman A. Gabapentin and tinnitus relief. Int Tinnitus J. 2008; 14(1):1–5

[162] Sanchez TG, Balbani AP, Bittar RS, Bento RF, Câmara J. Lidocaine test in patients with tinnitus: rationale of accomplishment and relation to the treatment with carbamazepine. Auris Nasus Larynx. 1999; 26(4):411–417

[163] Nam EC, Handzel O, Levine RA. Carbamazepine responsive typewriter tinnitus from basilar invagination. J Neurol Neurosurg Psychiatry. 2010; 81(4):456–458

[164] Azevedo AA, Figueiredo RR. Treatment of tinnitus with acamprosate. Prog Brain Res. 2007; 166: 273–277

[165] van de Heyning P, Muehlmeier G, Cox T, et al. Efficacy and safety of AM-101 in the treatment of acute inner ear tinnitus—a double-blind, randomized, placebo-controlled phase II study. Otol Neurotol. 2014; 35(4):589–597

[166] Spankovich C. The Role of Nutrition in Healthy Hearing. SIG 6 Perspectives on Hearing and Hearing Disorders Research and Diagnositcs. 2014; 18(2):27–34

[167] Spankovich C, Le Prell CG. Healthy diets, healthy hearing: National Health and Nutrition Examination Survey, 1999–2002. Int J Audiol. 2013; 52(6): 369–376

[168] Spankovich C, Le Prell CG. Associations between dietary quality, noise, and hearing: data from the National Health and Nutrition Examination Survey, 1999–2002. Int J Audiol. 2014; 53(11):796–809

[169] McCormack A, Edmondson-Jones M, Mellor D, et al. Association of dietary factors with presence and severity of tinnitus in a middle-aged UK population. PLoS One. 2014; 9(12):e114711

[170] Carpenter-Thompson JR, McAuley E, Husain FT. Physical activity, tinnitus severity, and improved quality of life. Ear Hear. 2015; 36(5):574–581

[171] Loprinzi PD, Lee H, Gilham B, Cardinal BJ. Association between accelerometer-assessed physical activity and tinnitus, NHANES 2005–2006. Res Q Exerc Sport. 2013; 84(2):177–185

[172] Pan T, Tyler RS, Ji H, Coelho C, Gogel SA. Differences among patients that make their tinnitus worse or better. Am J Audiol. 2015; 24(4):469–476

[173] Crocetti A, Forti S, Del Bo L. Neurofeedback for subjective tinnitus patients. Auris Nasus Larynx. 2011; 38(6):735–738

[174] Dohrmann K, Elbert T, Schlee W, Weisz N. Tuning the tinnitus percept by modification of synchronous brain activity. Restor Neurol Neurosci. 2007; 25(3–4):371–378

[175] Dohrmann K, Weisz N, Schlee W, Hartmann T, Elbert T. Neurofeedback for treating tinnitus. Prog Brain Res. 2007; 166:473–485

[176] Maudoux A, Bonnet S, Lhonneux-Ledoux F, Lefebvre P. Ericksonian hypnosis in tinnitus therapy. B-ENT. 2007; 3(suppl 7):75–77

[177] Nakashima T, Ueda H, Misawa H, et al. Transmeatal low-power laser irradiation for tinnitus. Otol Neurotol. 2002; 23(3):296–300

[178] Teggi R, Bellini C, Piccioni LO, Palonta F, Bussi M. Transmeatal low-level laser therapy for chronic tinnitus with cochlear dysfunction. Audiol Neurootol. 2009; 14(2):115–120

[179] Takeda G. Magnetic therapy for tinnitus. jibi to rinsho. 1987; 33(4):700–706

[180] Coles R, Bradley P, Donaldson I, Dingle A. A trial of tinnitus therapy with ear-canal magnets. Clin Otolaryngol Allied Sci. 1991; 16(4):371–372

[181] Desloovere C. Hyperbaric oxygen therapy for tinnitus. B-ENT. 2007; 3(suppl 7):71–74

[182] Porubsky C, Stiegler P, Matzi V, et al. Hyperbaric oxygen in tinnitus: influence of psychological factors on treatment results? ORL J Otorhinolaryngol Relat Spec. 2007; 69(2):107–112

[183] Liu F, Han X, Li Y, Yu S. Acupuncture in the treatment of tinnitus: a systematic review and meta-analysis. Eur Arch Otorhinolaryngol. 2016; 273(2):285–294

184] O'Connor A. What's in those supplements? New York Times. February 3, 2015

[185] Holstein N. [Ginkgo special extract EGb 761 in tinnitus therapy. An overview of results of completed clinical trials] Fortschr Med Orig. 2001; 118(4):157–164

[186] Drew S, Davies E. Effectiveness of Ginkgo biloba in treating tinnitus: double blind, placebo controlled trial. BMJ. 2001; 322(7278):73

[187] Rejali D, Sivakumar A, Balaji N. Ginkgo biloba does not benefit patients with tinnitus: a randomized placebo-controlled double-blind trial and meta-analysis of randomized trials. Clin Otolaryngol Allied Sci. 2004; 29(3):226–231

[188] Miroddi M, Bruno R, Galletti F, et al. Clinical pharmacology of melatonin in the treatment of tinnitus: a review. Eur J Clin Pharmacol. 2015; 71(3):263–270

[189] Kim NK, Lee DH, Lee JH, et al. Bojungikgitang and ban-habaekchulchonmatang in adult patients with tinnitus, a randomized, double-blind, three-arm, placebo-controlled trial—study protocol. Trials. 2010; 11:34

[190] Smith GS, Romanelli-Gobbi M, Gray-Karagrigoriou E, Artz GJ. Complementary and integrative treatments: tinnitus. Otolaryngol Clin North Am. 2013; 46(3):389–408

[191] Folmer RL, Theodoroff SM, Martin WH, Shi Y. Experimental, controversial, and futuristic treatments for chronic tinnitus. J Am Acad Audiol. 2014; 25 (1):106–125

[192] Salvi RJ, Saunders SS, Gratton MA, Arehole S, Powers N. Enhanced evoked response amplitudes in the inferior colliculus of the chinchilla following acoustic trauma. Hear Res. 1990; 50(1–2):245–257

[193] Auerbach BD, Rodrigues PV, Salvi RJ. Central gain control in tinnitus and hyperacusis. Front Neurol. 2014; 5:206

[194] Tyler RS, Pienkowski M, Roncancio ER, et al. A review of hyperacusis and future directions: part I. Definitions and manifestations. Am J Audiol. 2014; 23(4):402–419

[195] Liu C, Glowatzki E, Fuchs PA. Unmyelinated type II afferent neurons report cochlear damage. Proc Natl Acad Sci U S A. 2015; 112(47):14723–14727

[196] Moore BC, Glasberg BR, Vickers DA. Simulation of the effects of loudness recruitment on the intelligibility of speech in noise. Br J Audiol. 1995; 29(3):131–143

[197] Jastreboff MM, Jastreboff PJ. Hyperacusis. Audiology Online. 2001. Available at: HYPERLINK "http://www.audiologyonline.com/articles/hyperacusis-1223" www.audiologyonline.com/articles/hyperacusis-1223. Accessed March 27, 2018

[198] Schröder A, van Diepen R, Mazaheri A, et al. Diminished n1 auditory evoked potentials to oddball stimuli in misophonia patients. Front Behav Neurosci. 2014; 8:123

[199] Mirz F, Gjedde A, Södkilde-Jrgensen H, Pedersen CB. Functional brain imaging of tinnitus-like perception induced by aversive auditory stimuli. Neuroreport 2000; 11(3):633–637

[200] Spankovich C, Hall JW. The misunderstood misophonia. Audiology Today. 2014; 26(4):15–23

[201] Asha'ari ZA, Mat Zain N, Razali A. Phonophobia and hyperacusis: practical points from a case report. Malays J Med Sci. 2010; 17(1):49–51

[202] Cox RM, Alexander GC, Taylor IM, Gray GA. The contour test of loudness perception. Ear Hear. 1997; 18(5):388–400

[203] Khalfa S, Dubal S, Veuillet E, Perez-Diaz F, Jouvent R, Collet L. Psychometric normalization of a hyperacusis questionnaire. ORL J Otorhinolaryngol Relat Spec. 2002; 64(6):436–442

[204] Dauman R, Bouscau-Faure F. Assessment and amelioration of hyperacusis in tinnitus patients. Acta Otolaryngol. 2005; 125(5):503–509

[205] Schröder A, Vulink N, Denys D. Misophonia: diagnostic criteria for a new psychiatric disorder. PLoS One. 2013; 8(1):e54706

[206] Formby C, Sherlock LP, Gold SL. Adaptive plasticity of loudness induced by chronic attenuation and enhancement of the acoustic background. J Acoust Soc Am. 2003; 114(1):55–58

[207] Pienkowski M, Tyler RS, Roncancio ER, et al. A review of hyperacusis and future directions: part II. Measurement, mechanisms, and treatment. Am J Audiol 2014; 23(4):420–436

[208] Jüris L, Andersson G, Larsen HC, Ekselius L. Cognitive behaviour therapy for hyperacusis: a randomized controlled trial. Behav Res Ther 2014; 54:30–37

Note: Page numbers set **bold** or *italic* indicate headings or figures, respectively.